An Invitation to Wellness works chapter-by-chapter with HealthNow™ to help students take control of their personal wellness. *See page six for details.*

From the best-selling author of *An Invitation to Health . . .*

Focused on behavior modification and full of healthy strategies students can use *now*!

This dynamic new book from Dianne Hales helps your students take full charge of their wellness

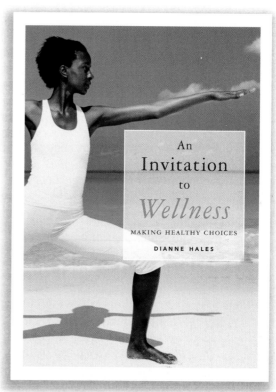

At last, the perfect book for your wellness course . . . researched and written by Dianne Hales, the respected author whose work you'll recognize from *Parade®* Magazine, as well as the best-selling text, **An Invitation to Health**.

Truly unmatched in her ability to inform, inspire change, and convey how attainable a lifestyle of wellness can be, Dianne Hales presents the latest information and recommendations related to wellness using stimulating visuals and an engaging writing style. She clearly presents extensive research that addresses those wellness-related issues that will affect your students—now and in the future. With a consistent theme of personalized health and behavior management, **An Invitation to Wellness** presents all course concepts within 15 captivating chapters. This interesting new book is a tool that will help your students take full charge of their own well-being and understand that wellness is not a subject to be memorized and mastered, but one to be both learned and lived.

From the engaging writing to the practical pedagogy, this new book gives students the tools they need to understand the relevance of good health to their own lives and education. Hales helps students make better decisions, assume responsibility for their own choices, and create and follow a healthy lifestyle. From the text, to the classroom, to the household, **An Invitation to Wellness** can support your course objectives and encourages your students to live a healthy lifestyle.

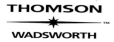

THOMSON

WADSWORTH

Your quick tour of this outstanding book starts here!

TURN THE PAGE...

Effective features, current topics, and the latest research get students engaged, motivated, and set to modify their own behavior!

Dianne Hales is known for the way she speaks *with* students—not at them. **An Invitation to Wellness**—with its emphasis on student awareness and behavior change—is the perfect tool to help students acquire the skills they need to ensure their well being and prevent serious health problems.

The book's strong emphasis on behavior change is reinforced with such pedagogy as:

■ The **Wellness Coach** sections
personalized features designed to engage students and inspire them to change behavior and make healthier choices

■ **Making Healthy Choices** features
positive summaries of practical behavior changes

■ **Action Plan** sections
practical guidelines to help students select a plan of action

■ The **Wellness Journal**
a powerful behavior modification tool to help students remain focused and motivated

With features like these, it's easy to see how Hales gets students involved and applying what they're learning to their own wellness.

WELLNESS COACH

Creating Your Wellness Toolbox

Wellness is your personal responsibility. Although products, programs, and people may offer quick and easy steps to feeling better, they almost always fail to live up to their promises. (See Savvy Consumer: "Too Good to Be True?") You have more control over how you feel now and in the future than anyone else.

The key to becoming your own wellness coach is self-responsibility. As Dr. John Travis defines this term in the context of wellness, this includes:

■ Developing awareness of your physical, mental, emotional, and spiritual processes and patterns.
■ Discovering your real needs and finding ways to meet them.
■ Making choices and living courageously in the midst of uncertainty.
■ Respecting your body through nutrition, exercise,
...cting
... tools

MAKING HEALTHY CHOICES

Lifelong Wellness

"Every man desires to live long," writes Jonathan Swift, "but no man would be old." We all wish for long lives, yet we want to avoid the disease and disability that can tarnish our golden years. Here are the best ways to ensure a lifetime of wellness.

■ **Exercise regularly.** By improving blood flow, staving off depression, warding off heart disease, and enhancing well-being, regular workouts help keep mind and body in top form.
■ **Don't smoke.** Every cigarette you puff can snuff out seven minutes of your life, according to the Centers for Disease Control and Prevention.
■ **Watch your weight and blood pressure.** Increases in these vital statistics can increase your risk of hypertension, cardiovascular disease, and other health problems.
■ **Eat more fruits and vegetables.** These foods, rich

your risk of cancer and damage from destructive free radicals.
■ **Cut down on fat.** Fatty foods can clog the arteries and contribute to various cancers.
■ **Limit drinking.** Alcohol can undermine physical health and sabotage mental acuity.
■ **Cultivate stimulating interests.** Elderly individuals with complex and interesting lifestyles are most likely to retain sharp minds and memories beyond age 70.
■ **Don't worry; be happy.** At any age, emotional turmoil can undermine well-being. Relaxation techniques, such as meditation, help by reducing stress.
■ **Reach out.** Try to keep in contact with other people of all ages and experiences. Make the effort to invite them to your home or go out with them. On a regular basis, do something to help another person.
■ **Make the most of your time.** Greet each day with a specific goal—to take a walk, write letters, visit a friend.

ACTION PLAN

Your Action Plan for Healthy Change

Now that you have a sense of your stage of readiness for change, use the following stage-specific ideas to get you going in the right direction.

Precontemplation (Not Active and Not Thinking about Becoming Active)

■ Commit yourself to attending class, reading the textbook, and completing assignments and labs.
■ List what you see as the disadvantages (or cons) of behavioral change. For example, do you fear making a change will be too difficult or will take up too much time? Write down a healthy change that you could make tomorrow that would take less than 15 minutes of your time.

Contemplation (Not Active but Thinking about Becoming Active)

■ Think back to activities and experiences you found enjoyable in the past. Did they include playing a sport, taking hikes, singing in a group? Ask friends and coworkers if they can put you in touch with others with the same interest.
■ Take a realistic look at your daily schedule and life circumstances. How much time could you carve out for a new healthy behavior? How much money could you invest in it?

WELLNESS JOURNAL

Countering the "Cons" of Change

One way to motivate yourself to initiate or maintain a health behavior change is to identify what you see as disadvantages, or "cons," and list ways to work over, around, or through them. Here are some examples of the cons of exercising. Read through them, then come up with your own list of cons and counters for your behavioral change goal:

Cons	Countercons
Too busy	■ Wake up half an hour earlier to get your workout done for the day. ■ Settle for half workouts if you can't do a full one. ■ Set aside exercise "appointments" on your schedule.
Boring	■ Mix it up. Walk one day; bike or jog the next. ■ Try something new, like tai chi.

ACTION PLAN

Your Action Plan for Healthy Change

Now that you have a sense of your stage of readiness for change, use the following stage-specific ideas to get you going in the right direction.

Precontemplation (Not Active and Not Thinking about Becoming Active)

- Commit yourself to attending class, reading the textbook, and completing assignments and labs.
- List what you see as the disadvantages (or cons) of behavioral change. For example, do you fear making a change will be too difficult or will take up too much time? Write down a healthy change that you could make tomorrow that would take less than 15 minutes of your time.

Contemplation (Not Active but Thinking about Becoming Active)

- Think back to activities and experiences you found enjoyable in the past. Did they include playing a sport, taking hikes, singing in a group? Ask friends and coworkers if they can put you in touch with others with the same interest.
- Take a realistic look at your daily schedule and life circumstances. How much time could you carve out for a new healthy behavior? How much money could you invest in it?

Self-Surveys allow students to assess their healthiness and relate chapter material to their own behaviors. The **Action Plan** and **Wellness Journal** features (described at left) as well as **Goal Setting** features follow each survey, providing specific guidelines on how to implement change.

HealthNow™ icons appear throughout the text and introduce a list of resources at http://healthnow.brookscole.com/itw that correspond with chapter concepts. Once at the **HealthNow** site, students can utilize the program to create and track a behavior change plan, as well as evaluate their knowledge of the material, take an exam-prep quiz, and receive a *Personalized Behavior Plan. See the inside front cover for more information on **HealthNow**.*

 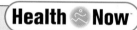

Health Now™

Don't forget to check out the wealth of resources on the HealthNow website at **http://healthnow.brookscole.com/itw** that will:
- Help you evaluate your knowledge of the material
- Allow you to take an exam-prep quiz
- Provide a Personalized Learning Plan targeting resources that address areas you should study
- Coach you through identifying target goals for behavior change and creating and monitoring your personal change plan throughout the semester.

The **Student Snapshot** sections present recent data on health, fitness, weight control, and other concerns of today's college students. These features reveal a compelling view of campus behaviors—representing all types of students in an eye-catching, thought-provoking format. Topics explored in the **Student Snapshot** feature include, "How Do Undergraduates Rate Themselves" and "Working Up a Sweat," (time spent on weight training.)

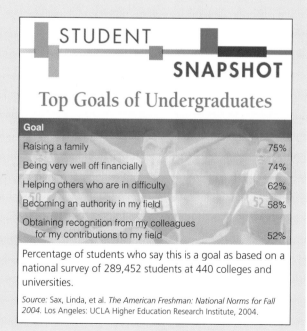

STUDENT SNAPSHOT

Top Goals of Undergraduates

Goal	
Raising a family	75%
Being very well off financially	74%
Helping others who are in difficulty	62%
Becoming an authority in my field	58%
Obtaining recognition from my colleagues for my contributions to my field	52%

Percentage of students who say this is a goal as based on a national survey of 289,452 students at 440 colleges and universities.

Source: Sax, Linda, et al. The American Freshman: National Norms for Fall 2004. Los Angeles: UCLA Higher Education Research Institute, 2004.

As students acquire new skills, Hales helps them…

Dianne Hales is masterful at helping students develop the skills they need to make better decisions, to assume responsibility for their own choices, to create and follow a healthy lifestyle, and most of all, to live what they learn.

▶ **Strategies for Change** boxes appear throughout the book and provide practical, checklist-style behavioral change strategies to help students achieve better health. **Strategies for Prevention** boxes provide effective, practical checklists for preventing health problems and reducing health risks.

▼ **Diversity coverage** is integrated throughout the text, including topics related to **dietary diversity** (Chapter 8, "Making Healthy Food Choices,") and **cancer risks for minority men and women** (Chapter 11, "Preventing Cancer and Other Illnesses.") An **icon** highlights where issues related to race, class, and gender are covered.

STRATEGIES for CHANGE

Use the Language of Change

Pay attention both to what you say when you talk or think about a health behavior change and how you say it. Then consciously edit the words in your mind and as you say them.

- **Watch out for weasel words.**
  Are you "planning" to quit smoking? "Hoping" to lose weight? When you use linguistic loopholes like "trying" or "hoping," you give yourself permission to settle for whatever happens. When you speak of goals, use definitive, unequivocal language.

- **Trade tenses.**
  When thinking or talking about bad health habits, switch to the past tense. Instead of saying, "I'm too lazy to exercise," tell yourself, "I used to be too lazy to exercise." This reminds you that you have changed, are changing, or at the least are capable of change.

- **Not "if" but "when."**
  Instead of saying, "If I could exercise more," say to yourself, "When I start exercising more." This simple switch sets the stage for believing that you will be able to change your lifestyle.

- **Just "because."**
  According to social psychology research, using the word "because" when making a request or seeking agreement can boost your compliance as high as 80 to 90 percent. For instance, you might tell yourself: "I won't buy dough-nuts *because* I don't want to be tempted."

- **Guard against demeaning words and phrases.**
  When a derogatory statement about yourself forms in your brain, say firmly, "Stop!" or "Delete!" If this is a hard habit to break, wear a rubber band on your wrist and snap it to alert yourself that you are thinking nega-tive, debilitating thoughts.

- **Don't focus on what you can't do.**
  Remind yourself of your strengths every day. Say to your-self, "I can go another five minutes on the treadmill," or "I can stand another half hour without a cigarette."

STRATEGIES for PREVENTION

Smart Steps to Take Now

- To lower your risk of heart disease, get your blood pres-sure and cholesterol checked. Don't smoke. Stay at a healthy weight. Exercise most days of the week. (See Chapter 9.)

- To lower your risk of major diseases, get regular check-ups. Make sure you are immunized against infec-tious illnesses. Know your family's health history. (See Chapter 11.)

- To lower your risk of substance abuse and related ill-nesses and injuries, don't drink, or limit how much you drink. Avoid illegal drugs. (See Chapter 13.)

- To lower your risk of sexually transmitted infections (STIs) or unwanted pregnancy, abstain from sex. If you decide to engage in potentially risky sexual activities, protect yourself with condoms and spermicides. (See Chapter 14.)

- To prevent car accidents, don't drive when road condi-tions are hazardous. When you drive, wear a seat belt and use defensive driving techniques. (See Chapter 15.)

goal is to eliminate health disparities among different seg-ments of the population.

Among the specific goals of Healthy People 2010 are:

- **Reduce the prevalence of cigarette smok-ing** among adults to 12 percent from the current 23.4 percent.
- **Reduce the number of new cancer cases** as well as the illnesses, disability, and death caused by cancer.
- **Promote the health of people with disabilities,** prevent secondary conditions, and eliminate disparities between people with and without disabilities in the U.S. population.
- **Reduce foodborne illnesses.**

Rates of obesity are about the same for men and women. Men are slightly more likely than women to smoke. They also are more physically active in their leisure time. Younger individuals are more physi-cally active than middle-aged adults; older Americans are less likely to be obese than middle-aged ones.

Asian adults are less likely to have unhealthy behaviors in terms of alcohol use, smoking, and body weight than other groups studied. Rates of leisure-time physical inactivity and obesity are higher among black adults than white adults. Black men are more likely than white men to be smokers, but among women the reverse is true. Hispanic women have low rates of smoking compared to non-Hispanic white women but higher rates of obesity.

As research on college students has shown, attitudes and feelings are related to stages of change. Smokers who believe that continuing to smoke would have only a minor or no impact on their health remain in the precontemplation stage; those with respiratory symptoms move on to contemplation and preparation.[5] In a study at Ohio State University, re-searchers classified student heavy drinkers according to the stages of change: Nearly two-thirds of the "precon-templators" continued to drink heavily and had no in-tention of changing their behavior. In the maintenance stage, students drank an average of one alcoholic drink a month even though they felt that heavy drinking was the norm on their campus.[6]

The Processes of Change

Anything you do to modify your thinking, feeling, or behavior can be called a change process. The nine in-cluded in the transtheoretical model are:

Consciousness-Raising The most widely used change process involves increasing knowledge about yourself or

Emotional Arousal This process, also known as dra-matic relief, works on a deeper level than consciousness-raising and is equally important in the early stages of change. Emotional arousal means experiencing and ex-pressing feelings about a problem behavior and its poten-tial solutions.
Example: Resolving never to drink and drive after the death of a friend in a car accident.

Self-Reevaluation This process requires a thoughtful reappraisal of your problem, including an assessment of the person you might be once you have changed the behavior.
Example: Recognizing that you have a gambling prob-lem and imagining yourself as a nongambler.

Commitment This process acknowledges—first pri-vately and then publicly—that you are responsible for your behavior and the only one who can change it.
Example: Joining a self-help or support group.

Countering Countering, or counterconditioning, sub-stitutes healthy behaviors for unhealthy ones.
Example: Chewing gum rather than smoking.

▲ **College icons** indicate where you'll find research on undergraduates that is especially relevant to students.

...aim for a happier, healthier, fuller life!

▼ **Making This Chapter Work for You** boxes review important chapter material by asking ten multiple-choice questions per chapter, with answers appearing at the end of the text. These questions are also within the **HealthNow™** online tutorial, and the results can be emailed to the instructor for credit. *See inside front cover for description of HealthNow™.*

Predisposing factors

Predisposing factors include knowledge, attitudes, beliefs, values, and perceptions. Unfortunately, knowledge isn't enough to cause most people to change their behavior; for example, people fully aware of the grim conse-

Young people, especially young men, are the greatest risk takers, a fact reflected in their high rates of auto accidents, binge drinking, drug use, and pathological gambling. The death rates for injuries related to swimming, boating, driving, cycling, and even crossing the street are higher in college-age men than women.

CHAPTER

2 Making This Chapter Work for You

1. The development of health behaviors is influenced by all of the following *except:*
   a. Reinforcing factors, which involve external recognition for achieving a goal.
   b. Preexisting health factors, which take into account the individual's current position on the wellness continuum.
   c. Predisposing factors, which include knowledge, attitudes, and beliefs.
   d. Enabling factors, which are related to an individual's skills and capabilities to make behavior changes.

2. Change processes, cognitive and behavior activities that facilitate change, include all of these *except:*
   a. Consciousness raising.
   b. Countering.
   c. Health awareness.
   d. Helping relationships.

3. Dylan decided to learn how to meditate to enhance his spiritual wellness and signed up for a workshop starting in two weeks. Dylan is in which stage of change?
   a. Precontemplation
   b. Contemplation
   c. Preparation
   d. Action

4. Bianca almost caused an accident last week when she was weaving between cars on the freeway. The incident scared her so much that she decided to change her driving habits and has stayed at the speed limit all this week. Which stage of change is Bianca in?
   a. Contemplation
   b. Preparation

5. According to the stages of change in the transtheoretical model of change, which statement is *incorrect?*
   a. In the maintenance stage, individuals have avoided relapse for six months.
   b. In the contemplation stage, individuals are considering changing a problem behavior in the next six months.
   c. In the action stage, individuals are actually modifying their behavior according to their plan.
   d. In the preparation stage, individuals intend to change a problem behavior in the next six months.

6. Michelle has a strong internal locus of control. According to research, she is more likely to
   a. Enjoy better health.
   b. Get a better job.
   c. Become a health-care professional.
   d. Be worried about the future.

7. If you want to change unhealthy behavior, which of the following strategies is least likely to promote success?
   a. Believe that you can make the change.
   b. Reward yourself regularly.
   c. During self-talks, remind yourself about all your faults.
   d. Accept that you are in control of your health.

8. Some effective strategies for achieving your wellness goals are:
   a. Set "step and stretch" goals.
   b. Use affirmations with the present tense.
   c. Visualize possible obstacles.
   d. All of the above.

9. Cameron feels good because he has made the decision to get fit. What does Cameron have to do next?
   a. Get more specific about his goal.
   b. Start working out.

▲ **Male and female icons** have been added throughout that indicate where specific gender health issues are covered. These highlight how men and women are alike—and different—with respect to a variety of health issues, such as nutritional needs, handling stress, and effects of exercise.

SAVVY CONSUMER

ASSESSING RISKS

At any age, the greatest health threats stem from high-risk behaviors—smoking, excessive drinking, not getting enough exercise, eating too many high-fat foods, driving recklessly, and not getting regular medical checkups, to name just a few. That's why changing unhealthy habits is the best way to reduce risks and prevent health problems.

Environmental health risks are the subject of newspaper headlines. Every year brings calls of alarm about a new hazard to health: electromagnetic radiation, fluoride in drinking water, hair dyes, silicone implants, radon, lead. Often the public response is panic. Consumers picket and protest. Individuals arrange for elaborate testing. Yet how do we

know whether or not alleged health risks are acceptable? Some key factors to consider are:

■ **Are there possible benefits?** Advantages—such as the high salary paid for working with toxic chemicals or radioactive materials—may make some risks seem worth taking.

■ **Is the risk voluntary?** All of us tend to accept risks that we freely choose to take, such as playing a sport that could lead to injuries, as opposed to risks imposed on us, such as threats of terrorism.

■ **Is the risk fair?** The risk of skin cancer affects us all. We may worry about it and take action to protect ourselves

and our planet, but we don't resent it the way we resent living with the risk of violence because the only housing we can afford is in a high-crime area.

■ **Are there alternatives?** As consumers, we may become upset about cancer-causing pesticides or food additives when we learn about safer chemicals or methods of preservation.

■ **Are lives saved or lost?** Our thinking about risks often depends on how they're presented. For instance, if we're told that a new drug may kill 1 out of every 100 people, we react differently than if we're told that it may save the lives of 99 percent of those who use it.

◄ The **Savvy Consumer** feature offers specific advice on getting the best possible health care services and information, whether students are interested in spotting nutrition misinformation or evaluating the risks of different types of contraceptives. Some examples include "Too Good To Be True?" (regarding advertising claims), "Selecting a Personal Trainer," and "The Perils of Performance-Boosting Drugs."

Unparalleled learning resources help students incorporate new behaviors and aim for fitness

Health Now™

Class-tested and student-praised, **HealthNow** offers a variety of features that support course objectives and interactive learning. This online tutorial for students, packaged with each new text, offers a **Personalized Change Plan**, pre- and post-tests, a wellness journal, and a variety of activities, all designed to get students involved in their learning progress and to be better prepared for class participation and class quizzes and tests. Students log on to **HealthNow** by using the access code available with the text.

See the inside front cover of the text for more information.

Visit http://www.thomsonedu.com/thomsonnow for more information on packaging **HealthNow** with Hales' new text.

Lab Booklet for An Invitation to Wellness: Making Healthy Choices... *packaged with all new student copies of the text!*

0-495-10857-X

The **Lab Booklet** includes activities that can be completed in or outside of class. Each activity is printed on perforated pages so they can easily be turned in for credit.

PLUS: Two outstanding resources that you can order with the text!

New from Thomson and in alliance with Walk4Life®
Walk4Life® Elite Model Pedometer
0-495-01315-3 • packaged with the text 0-495-21991-6

A $29.00 value! This pedometer tracks steps, elapsed time, distance, includes a calorie counter, and a clock... all at a significantly reduced price when you order it packaged with the text. Whether to be used as an activity in class or as a tool to encourage students to simply track their steps and walk towards better fitness awareness, this is a valuable item for everyone.

Dianne Hales' *Readings in Healthy Living*
0-759-35944-X

As a frequent author of health-related articles produced by *Parade®* Magazine, Dianne Hales has published numerous articles that students will find useful and interesting. This 12-article reader is a collection of some of Hales' key articles, and you can order it packaged with the text at great value. Articles include *Take Your Meds—The Right Way* and *You Can Think Yourself Thin.*

Contact your Thomson sales representative for ordering information.

Behavior Change Workbook

0-495-01145-2 • packaged with the text: 0-495-22299-2

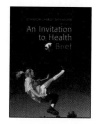

The **Behavior Change Workbook** includes a brief discussion of the current theories behind making positive lifestyle changes, along with exercises to help students effect those changes in their everyday lives.

TestWell

Access packaged with the text: 0-495-21990-8

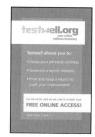

This online assessment tool allows students to complete a 100-question wellness inventory related to the dimensions of wellness. Students complete the personal assessment in order to evaluate their personal health status related to nutrition, emotional health, spirituality, sexuality, physical health, self-care, safety, environmental health, occupational health, and intellectual health. *Not sold separately.*

InfoTrac® College Edition with InfoMarks™

Access available with new copies of the text

When you adopt this text, you and your students can gain anytime, anywhere access to reliable resources with **InfoTrac College Edition**, the online library! This fully searchable database offers more than 20 years' worth of full-text articles (not abstracts) from almost 5,000 diverse sources. Certain restrictions may apply. *For additional information, please consult your local Thomson representative. Not sold separately.*

Careers in Health, Physical Education, and Sport

0-534-60785-3 • packaged with the text 0-495-21992-4

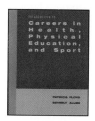

Unique to Thomson Wadsworth! This booklet takes students through the complicated process of picking the type of careers they want to pursue, how to prepare for the transition into the working world, and insight to different types of career paths, education requirements, and reasonable salary expectations. Included is also a designated chapter that discusses some of the legal issues that surround the workplace, including discrimination and harassment. This supplement is complete with personal development activities designed to encourage the students to focus and develop better insight into their future.

Health and Wellness Resource Center

http://www.gale.com/health

Gale's **Health and Wellness Resource Center** is a new comprehensive website that provides easy-to-find answers to health questions. For more information, contact your Thomson Wadsworth representative.

Instructor's Manual & Test Bank

0-495-01464-8

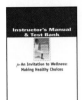

The **Instructor's Manual** provides learning objectives, detailed chapter outlines, a list of chapter-specific labs, a list of websites, classroom activities and teaching strategies. The **Test Bank** provides true/false, multiple choice, critical thinking/short answer questions, and essay questions.

Multimedia Manager: A Microsoft® PowerPoint® Tool

0-495-01468-0

This dual-platform presentation CD-ROM includes hundreds of Microsoft® PowerPoint® slides, an electronic version of the **Instructor's Manual** and **Test Bank**, and digital video from our ABC® Video Series.

JoinIn®

0-495-12678-0

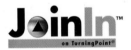

Thomson Wadsworth is now pleased to offer you book-specific **JoinIn**™ content for Response Systems tailored to Hales' text, allowing you to transform your classroom and assess your students' progress with instant in-class quizzes and polls. Our exclusive agreement to offer **TurningPoint**® software lets you pose book-specific questions and display students' answers seamlessly within the Microsoft® PowerPoint® slides of your own lecture, in conjunction with the "clicker" hardware of your choice. Enhance how your students interact with you, your lecture, and each other. *For college and university adopters only. Contact your local Thomson representative to learn more.* For more information, visit http://www.thomsonlearningconnections.com.

ExamView® Computerized Testing . . .

including online testing!

0-495-01467-2

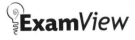

Create, deliver, and customize tests and study guides (both print and online) in minutes with this easy-to-use assessment and tutorial system. ExamView offers both a quick test wizard and an online test wizard that guide you step-by-step through the process of creating tests. The test appears on screen exactly as it will print or display online. Using ExamView's complete word processing capabilities, you can enter an unlimited number of new questions or edit existing questions.

Turnitin™ Online Originality Checker

This online "originality checker" is a simple solution for professors who want to put a strong deterrent against plagiarism into place, and make sure their students are employing proper research techniques. Students upload their papers to their professor's personalized website and within seconds, the paper is checked against three databases—a constantly updated archive of over 4.5 billion web pages; a collection of millions of published works, including a number of Thomson Higher Education texts; and the millions of student papers already submitted to **Turnitin**. At a glance, the professor can see if the student has used proper research and citation skills. Our exclusive agreement gives instructors the ability to package **Turnitin**™ with Hales' text. Please consult with your Thomson sales representative to find out more!

Transparency Acetates

0-495-10855-3

Approximately 80 full-color transparencies are correlated to the text to enhance your lectures.

ABC® Video Series . . .

0-495-11206-2

ABC Videos feature short, high-interest clips from current news events as well as historic raw footage going back 40 years. Perfect for discussion starters or to enrich your lectures and spark interest in the material in the text, these brief videos provide students with a new lens through which to view the past and present, one that will greatly enhance their knowledge and understanding of significant events and open up to them new dimensions in learning.

Wadsworth Health, Fitness, and Wellness Video Library

A comprehensive library of videos is available for adopters of this textbook. Topics include weight control and fitness, AIDS, sexual communication, peer pressure, compulsive and addictive behaviors and the relationship between alcohol and violence. *Restrictions apply.*

Trigger Video Series

Fitness 0-534-36233-8

Exclusive to Thomson Wadsworth! This video is designed to promote or "trigger" classroom discussion on a variety of important topics related to physical fitness.

Relaxation Video: A Personal Guide to Stress Management

0-534-58928-6

Covering the causes, symptoms, and effects of stress, this video helps students develop lifelong strategies for stress management.

www.wadsworth.com

www.wadsworth.com is the World Wide Web site for Thomson Wadsworth and is your direct source to dozens of online resources.

At *www.wadsworth.com* you can find out about supplements, demonstration software, and student resources. You can also send e-mail to many of our authors and preview new publications and exciting new technologies.

www.wadsworth.com
Changing the way the world learns®

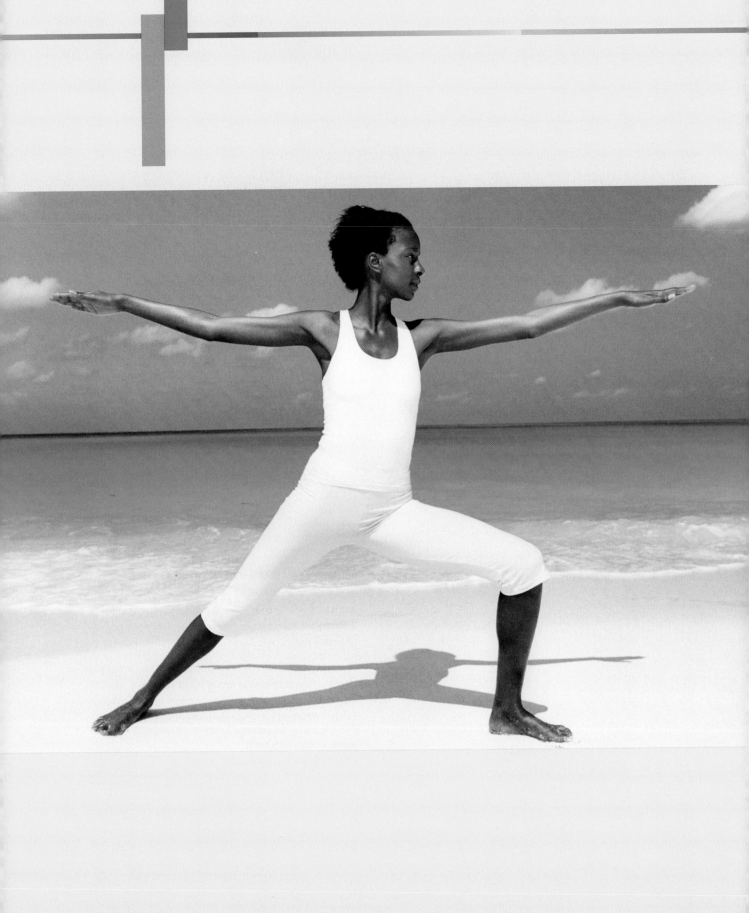

An Invitation to Wellness

MAKING HEALTHY CHOICES

Dianne Hales

THOMSON

WADSWORTH

Australia • Brazil • Canada • Mexico • Singapore
Spain • United Kingdom • United States

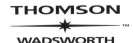

THOMSON
™
WADSWORTH

An Invitation to Wellness
Dianne Hales

Editor: *Nedah Rose*
Development Editor: *Pat Brewer*
Assistant Editor: *Kari Hopperstead*
Editorial Assistant: *Colin Blake*
Technology Project Manager: *Donna Kelley*
Marketing Manager: *Jennifer Somerville*
Marketing Assistant: *Michele Colella*
Marketing Communications Manager: *Bryan Vann*
Project Manager, Editorial Production: *Andy Marinkovich*
Creative Director: *Rob Hugel*
Art Director: *Lee Friedman*
Print Buyer: *Doreen Suruki*

Permissions Editor: *Kiely Sisk*
Production Service: *Dusty Friedman, The Book Company*
Text Designer: *Tani Hasegawa*
Photo Researcher: *Myrna Engler*
Copy Editor: *Yonie Overton*
Illustrator: *Hespenheide Design*
Cover Designer: *Gia Giasullo*
Cover Image: *Photo by John Hicks, for Getty Images*
Cover Printer: *Quebecor World / Dubuque*
Compositor: *G & S Typesetters, Inc.*
Printer: *Quebecor World / Dubuque*

Library of Congress Control Number: 2005934427

ISBN 0-495-01463X

Thomson Higher Education
10 Davis Drive
Belmont, CA 94002-3098
USA

For more information about our products, contact us at:
Thomson Learning Academic Resource Center
1-800-423-0563
For permission to use material from this text or product, submit a request online at **http://www.thomsonrights.com.**
Any additional questions about permissions can be submitted by e-mail to **thomsonrights@thomson.com.**

In memoriam

We dedicate this edition to our colleague and friend, Myrna Engler, whose photo selections brought our recent Invitations to life.

Brief Contents

Contents

CHAPTER
8

Making Healthy Food Choices 150

CHAPTER 11

Preventing Cancer and Other Illnesses 234

CHAPTER 12

Taking Care of Yourself 266

CHAPTER

15 Protecting Your Safety and Your Environment   352

Key Features

STRATEGIES for CHANGE

STUDENT SNAPSHOT

STRATEGIES for PREVENTION

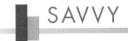

SAVVY CONSUMER

Preface

To the Student

This book invites you to begin a journey to a healthier, happier, fuller life. As you'll discover, wellness is not simply a state of body, mind, and spirit. It is a choice, a conscious decision that you make in order to move toward your maximum potential. This book will guide you as you learn about taking charge of your life. Of all the skills that you acquire in college, none may be more important than knowing how to make healthy choices. In the final analysis you choose what to eat, how much to exercise, whether to smoke or drink, how to cope with stress, whether to practice safer sex. The bottom line is that your choices and health behaviors can determine how long and how well you live. By reading and using *An Invitation to Wellness,* you can make healthy choices that will affect how you look, feel, and function—not just now but for decades to come.

To achieve your highest level of wellness, you may have to change some of your behaviors or habits. Change may seem scary or difficult. However, *An Invitation to Wellness* will help you through every step and stage.

Based on the latest research, *An Invitation to Wellness* is packed with information, advice, recommendations, and activities that serve as tools for building the best possible you. However, knowledge alone can't assure you a lifetime of wellness. That depends on you. The skills you acquire, the habits you form, the choices you make, the ways you live day by day will all shape your health and your future. You cannot simply read this book and study wellness the way you study chemistry or history. You must decide to make it part of your daily life.

This is our invitation to you. We hope you choose to accept it.

To the Instructor

In my career as a health writer, I have watched—and reported on—a revolution in health care. A few decades ago medicine began moving away from the disease model, with its focus on treating serious illnesses after they occur. This approach led to the conquest of infectious diseases, such as tuberculosis, malaria, polio, whooping cough, and diphtheria, that had claimed millions of lives. However, it wasn't enough for the major killers of the twentieth century.

Problems such as high blood pressure, cardiovascular illness, and diabetes progress steadily through life, first eroding well-being, then causing symptoms, and leading, in many cases, to disability and death. Even the best treatments often provide too little, too late. Prevention has proved to be our best hope against them.

The emphasis on prevention shifted responsibility for health from physicians to patients. The ability to make healthy choices has become the ultimate self-care tool. We've seen dramatic payoffs. Death rates from cardiovascular disease, the nation's number-one killer, have dropped by 60 percent since 1950, one of the major health achievements of the twentieth century.

We've now entered a new era. Today consumers can aim to do more than stave off illness. They can take steps to achieve the state of optimal functioning of mind, body, and spirit that we call wellness.

An Invitation to Wellness defines wellness in the broadest possible sense—as a journey of discovery and development of one's maximum potential. Covering all dimensions of life—physical, psychological, spiritual, social, occupational, and environmental—*An Invitation to Wellness* provides the most recent, state-of-the-science information on health as well as the insight and strategies students need to apply these findings in their quest for wellness.

This book views wellness through the lens of personal responsiblity, healthy lifestyle choices, and positive behavioral change. Our premise is that individuals have more control over their lives and well-being than anyone or anything else has. We believe that the choices your students make and the habits they develop will influence how long and how well they live. We have created this book to help.

Chapter 2 introduces students to the latest insights into behavioral change, including how people change, the stages of change, and change processes. Every chapter provides practical application of these theories in features such as the Wellness Coach, Strategies for Change, and Strategies for Prevention.

The Making Healthy Choices sections at the end of each chapter present Self-Survey personal assessments, Setting Goals exercises, Action Plans, and Wellness Journal activities. A separate Lab Booklet bundled with the text, offers more activities for students to assess where they are now and to determine goals.

Although your students may not be aware of it, this textbook works to promote change in indirect as well as direct ways. Simply reading the text and taking a health or wellness course can have a significant impact. One reason is what psychologists call the *exposure effect*. The more that individuals see, hear, or read about a topic, the more positively they view it. Because of the sheer quantity of information your students receive in the classroom and in their readings, they will want to heed at least some of the suggestions for change.

Once they do, another law of influence kicks in: the consistency principle. Students begin to see themselves as individuals who have control over their actions and who can change the way they think and behave. Without any conscious effort, their commitment to change grows, and the process of change takes on a momentum of its own.

By using this book and taking your course, students also acquire a special type of power—the power to make good decisions, to assume responsibility, and to create and follow a healthy lifestyle. This textbook is our invitation to them to live what they learn and make the most of their bodies and minds and of their lives.

This textbook also is an invitation to you as an instructor. We share your passion for education and would like to enter into a partnership with you. The editorial team at Thomson-Wadsworth welcomes your feedback and suggestions. Please let us hear from you at http://www.thomsonedu.com/health. I personally look forward to working with you toward our shared goal of preparing a new generation for a lifetime of wellness.

✚ Student Resources

Lab Booklet   The Lab Booklet, prepared by Dr. Roy Wohl of Washburn University, is available bundled with new copies of the text. This essential ancillary contains exploratory lab activities that can be completed in or outside of class. Labs include self-assessments, exercise programs, and research activities—all designed to help students evaluate and improve their personal wellness. The Lab Booklet pages are perforated, so individual activities can easily be turned in for credit.

HealthNow™   Class-tested and student-praised, HealthNow™ offers a variety of features that support course objectives and interactive learning. This online

tutorial available with new texts offers a Personalized Behavior Change Plan that guides students through a behavior change process tailored specifically to their needs and personal motivation. Fun and interesting to use, the Personalized Change Plan includes a Wellness Assessment, a Readiness Planner, tools for creating SMART goals and a Behavior Change Contract, a Change Tracker, and a Change Journal. Additional study help is available on HealthNow in the form of chapter-specific pre- and post-tests. These diagnostic tests are correlated to online tutorials and study tools, all aimed at helping students assess their own understanding and target their studying. HealthNow is also valuable for instructors, as the Personalized Behavior Change Plan, the pre-tests, and the post-tests are all easy to assign, track, and grade—even for large sections.

Walk4Life® Elite Model Pedometer   This pedometer tracks steps, elapsed time, and distance, and includes a calorie counter. Whether to be used as an activity in class or as a tool to encourage students to simply track their steps and walk towards better fitness awareness, this is a valuable item for everyone.

Readings in Healthy Living   As a frequent author of health-related articles produced by Parade® Magazine, Dianne Hales has published numerous articles that students will find useful and interesting. This 12-article reader is a collection of key articles, including *Take Your Meds—The Right Way* and *You Can Think Yourself Thin*.

Behavior Change Workbook   The Behavior Change Workbook includes a brief discussion of the current theories behind making positive lifestyle changes, along with exercises to help students effect those changes in their everyday lives.

TestWell   This online assessment tool allows students to complete a 100-question wellness inventory related to the dimensions of wellness. Students complete the personal assessment in order to evaluate their personal health status related to nutrition, emotional health, spirituality, sexuality, physical health, self care, safety, environmental health, occupational health, and intellectual health.

InfoTrac®College Edition with InfoMarks™   This fully searchable online database offers more than 20 years' worth of full-text articles (not abstracts) from almost 5,000 diverse sources. Access to InfoTrac is available with new texts.

InfoTrac College Edition Student Guide for Health   This 24-page booklet offers detailed guidance for students on how to use the *InfoTrac® College Edition* database. It includes log-in help, a complete search tips "cheat sheet," and a topic list of key word search terms for health, fitness, and wellness.

Health, Fitness, and Wellness Internet Explorer   A handy full-color trifold brochure contains dozens of useful health, fitness, and wellness Internet links.

Health and Wellness Resource Center at http://www .gale.com/health Gale's Health and Wellness Resource Center is a new comprehensive website that provides easy-to-find answers to health questions.

Careers in Health, Physical Education, and Sport
This is the essential manual for majors who are interested in pursuing a position in their chosen field. It guides them through the complicated process of picking the type of career they want to pursue, suggests how to prepare for the transition into the working world, and offers information about different career paths, education requirements, and reasonable salary expectations. The supplement also describes the differences in credentials found in the field and testing requirements for certain professions.

∎ Instructor Resources

http://www.thomsonedu.com/health When you adopt *An Invitation to Wellness: Making Healthy Choices,* you and your students will gain access to a rich array of teaching and learning resources that you won't find anywhere else. This outstanding site features access to both student resources for the text, including quizzes, web links, suggested online readings, and discussion forums, and instructor resources, including downloadable supplementary resources and multimedia presentation slides. You will also find an online catalog of Wadsworth's health, fitness, wellness, and physical education books and supplements.

Instructor's Manual and Test Bank These two essential ancillaries are bound together for your convenience. The Instructor's Manual provides chapter outlines, learning objectives, classroom handouts, discussion questions, a media resource list, and more. The test bank contains a variety of questions to test students' understanding, comprehension, and application of the text.

ExamView® Computerized Testing Create, deliver, and customize the thorough Test Bank in minutes with this easy-to-use assessment and tutorial system. *Exam View* offers both a *Quick Test Wizard* and an *Online Test Wizard* that guide you step-by-step through the process of creating tests, while it allows you to see the test you are creating on the screen exactly as it will print or display online. You can build tests of up to 250 questions using up to 12 question types. Using *Exam View's* complete word-processing capabilities, you can enter an unlimited number of new questions or edit existing questions.

Multimedia Manager for An Invitation to Wellness: A Microsoft® PowerPoint® Link Tool This dual-platform presentation CD-ROM includes Microsoft® PowerPoint® slides featuring text art, an electronic version of the Instructor's Manual and Test Bank, and digital video from our ABC Video Series.

JoinIn®on TurningPoint™ Enhance how your students interact with you, your lecture, and each other using JoinIn™ content for Response Systems tailored to this text. Thomson's exclusive agreement to offer TuringPoint® software lets you pose book-specific questions and display students' answers seamlessly within the Microsoft® PowerPoint® slides of your own lecture, in conjunction with the "clicker" hardware of your choice.

Transparency Acetates This set of approximately 80 transparency acetates of art taken from the text can be used to enhance lectures and provide visual support in the classroom.

ABC Videos for Health and Wellness These videos allow you to integrate the newsgathering and programming power of the ABC News networks into the classroom to show students the relevance of course topics to their everyday lives. The videos include news clips correlated directly with the text and can help you launch a lecture, spark a discussion, or demonstrate an application. Students can see firsthand how the principles they learn in the course apply to the stories they hear in the news.

Relaxation: A Guide to Personal Stress Management
This 30-minute video shows students how to manage their stress and what is a healthy stress level in their life. Experts explain relaxation techniques and guide the student through progressive relaxation, guided imagery, breathing, and physical activity.

Trigger Video Series: Fitness This 60-minute video focuses on changing concepts of fitness, contains five 8–10 minute clips followed by questions for answer or discussion, and material appropriate to the fitness chapters in the text.

Trigger Video Series: Stress This 60-minute video focuses on stress, contains five 8–10 minute clips followed by questions for answer or discussion, and material appropriate to the text chapters concerning stress and its positive and negative effects on health.

∎ Acknowledgments

Creating a new book always demands a team effort. Fortunately, I got to work once again with the team I consider the very best of the best in textbook publishing. They have my unending admiration and appreciation.

This book would not have taken life without Nedah Rose and her support, enthusiasm, creativity, and good humor. My deepest thanks go to Pat Brewer, the developmental editor, whose contributions always extend far beyond the demands of duty. I consider her a partner, co-conspirator, and friend. Once again I have come to think of Dusty Friedman of The Book Company as a worker of miracles and other marvels. Andy Marinkovich, Production Project Manager, has guided us all with wisdom and unfailing professionalism.

My thanks extend to Jennifer Somerville, Senior Marketing Manager, for her energy and commitment, to Jessica Perry for her work on the promotional materials, and to Kari Hopperstead, the creative force behind the ancillaries. Editorial assistant Colin Blake, ever-efficient and helpful, made all of our lives easier and contributed to this project in countless ways. Thanks also to Tani Hasegawa for our new design and cover, and to Hespenheide Design for art. Myrna Engler, to whom we dedicate this book, brought her usual flair and highest standard of excellence to the photo selections.

I especially thank Dr. Roy Wohl of Washburn University for his substantial contributions to the Lab Booklet and to the Making Healthy Choices feature in each chapter. Finally, I would like to thank the reviewers and focus group participants whose input has been so valuable:

Suzanne Zelnik-Geldys, Eastern Michigan University
Trey Cone, University of Central Oklahoma
Tanya R. Littrell, Oregon State University
Elaine Bryan, Georgia Perimeter College
James Padfield, Truman State University
Roy Wohl, Washburn U
Brady Redus, U. of Central Oklahoma
Stephen Sowulewski, J.S. Reynolds Community College
Jessica Poole, North Georgia College & State University
Carolyn Clancy, Phillips Community College
William J. Duey, Concordia University
Lance Lamport, St. Petersburg College
Joanna Hayden, William Paterson University
Marshall Meyer, Portland CC
Derek Suranie, North Georgia College
Vincent Mumford, University of Central Florida

Bonnie Young, Georgia Perimeter College—Dunwoody
Jeffrey Hoffman, Central Connecticut State U.

Dianne Hales

✚ About the Author

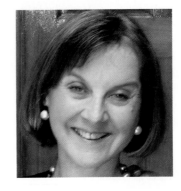

Dianne Hales, a contributing editor for *Parade,* has written more than 2,000 articles for national publications. Her trade books include *Think Thin, Be Thin; Just Like a Woman: How Gender Science Is Redefining What Makes Us Female* and the award-winning compendium of mental health information, *Caring for the Mind: The Comprehensive Guide to Mental Health.* Dianne Hales is one of the few journalists to be honored with national awards for excellence in magazine writing by both the American Psychiatric Association and the American Psychological Association. She also has won the EMMA (Exceptional Media Merit Award) for health reporting from the National Women's Political Caucus and Radcliffe College and numerous writing awards from various organizations, including the Arthritis Foundation, California Psychiatric Society, CHAAD (Children and Adults with Attention-Deficit Disorders), Council for the Advancement of Scientific Education, National Easter Seal Society, and the New York City Public Library.

An Invitation to Wellness

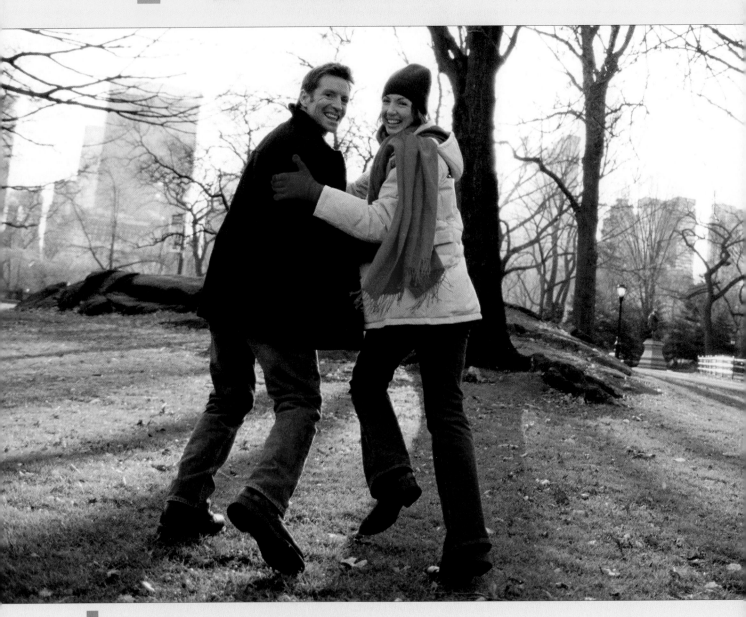

This is a book about you: your body and your mind, your habits and your hopes, your potential and your past. It is also a book that could change your life—by changing the way you live.

Every day you make choices, some small and trivial, some bigger and more important. You decide whether to skip breakfast and what to eat for lunch, whether to walk to class or hop on a bus, whether to spend a free hour in a gym or at a mall, whether to smoke, drink, or get a checkup. Over the course of a lifetime, these seemingly insignificant choices can make the difference between health and disease. But every single day, starting now, they also can make the difference between health and the state of optimal physical, mental, and spiritual well-being that we call wellness.

This chapter explores the meaning and interrelationship of health and wellness, discusses the six dimensions of wellness, reports on health and wellness in the 21st century, and provides guidance on how to make healthful choices so you can live long and well.

Rolf Bruderer

After studying the material in this chapter, you should be able to:

❚ **Identify** and **describe** the components of wellness.

❚ **Describe** Healthy People 2010 and some of its goals.

❚ **Explain** how gender, race, and ethnicity can influence wellness.

❚ **Name** at least three ways to help become your own wellness coach responsible for your own well-being.

Health Now™

Don't forget to check out the wealth of resources on the HealthNow website at **http://healthnow.brookscole.com/itw** that will:
• Help you evaluate your knowledge of the material
• Allow you to take an exam-prep quiz
• Provide a Personalized Learning Plan targeting resources that address areas you should study
• Coach you through identifying target goals for behavior change and creating and monitoring your personal change plan throughout the semester.

✚ What Is Wellness?

Wellness has been defined as purposeful, enjoyable living or, more specifically, a deliberate lifestyle choice characterized by personal responsibility and optimal enhancement of physical, mental, and spiritual health. Wellness means more than not being sick; it means taking steps to prevent illness and to lead a richer, more balanced, and more satisfying life.

Wellness also can be defined in other ways, for example:

■ as a choice, a decision you make to move toward optimal health

■ as a way of life you design to achieve your highest potential

■ as a process of developing awareness that health and happiness are possible in the present moment

■ as the integration of body, mind, and spirit

■ as the belief that everything you do, think, and feel has an impact on your state of health and the health of the world.[1]

"The 'well' person is not necessarily the strong, the brave, the successful, the young, the whole, or even the illness-free being," notes John Travis, M.D., author of *The Wellness Workbook*. "No matter what your current state of health, you can begin to appreciate yourself as a growing, changing person and allow yourself to move toward a happier life and positive health."

Wellness and health are related, but are not the same. By the simplest definition, health means being sound in body, mind, and spirit. The World Health Organization defines health as "not merely the absence of disease or infirmity," but "a state of complete physical, mental, and social well-being."[2]

Although physical well-being is essential to health, the term *wellness,* as used by health professionals, has a broader meaning. To understand how the concepts of wellness and health fit together, think of an automobile transmission: Having a disease (illness) is like being in reverse; absence of disease (health) puts you in neutral; but positive health changes (wellness) push you into drive—forward motion. When your entire lifestyle is based on health-enhancing behaviors, you're in high gear and going at top speed—and you've achieved total wellness.

✚ The Dimensions of Wellness

The various states of wellness and illness can be viewed as points on a continuum (**Figure 1-1**). At one end is early and needless death; at the other is optimal wellness, in which you feel and perform at your very best. In the middle, individuals are neither sick enough to need medical attention nor well enough to live each day with zest and vigor.

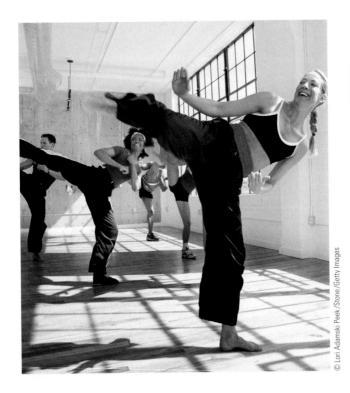

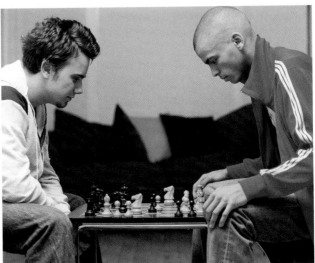

Wellness refers to creating a way of life that enables you to reach your highest potential.

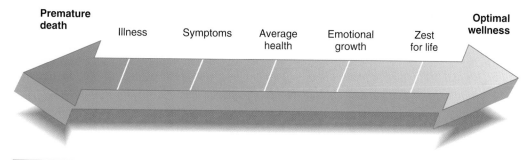

Premature death ← Illness — Symptoms — Average health — Emotional growth — Zest for life → **Optimal wellness**

FIGURE 1-1 ▍ The Wellness–Illness Continuum

Dr. Travis, who created the Wellness Inventory (see Self-Survey on page 11), uses another analogy to describe wellness. He compares the various dimensions of wellness to an iceberg (**Figure 1-2**). Only about one-tenth of the mass of an iceberg is visible; the rest is submerged. Your current state of health is like the tip of the iceberg—the part that shows.

"To understand all that creates and supports your current state of health," says Dr. Travis, "you have to look 'underwater.'" The first hidden level—the "lifestyle/behavioral" level—consists of what you eat, how active you are, how you manage stress, and how you protect yourself from hazards. Below this dimension is the

"cultural/psychological/motivational" level, the often-invisible influences that lead us to choose a certain lifestyle. The foundation of the iceberg is the "spiritual/being/meaning" realm, which encompasses issues such as your reason for being, the meaning of your life, and your place in the universe. "Ultimately," says Dr. Travis, "this realm determines whether the tip of the iceberg, representing your state of health, is one of disease or wellness." [3]

Physical Wellness

For the sake of optimal physical wellness, we must take positive steps away from illness and toward well-being. We must feed our bodies nutritiously, exercise them regularly, avoid harmful behaviors and substances, watch out for early signs of sickness, and protect ourselves from accidents.

Psychological Wellness

Like physical well-being, psychological wellness is more than the absence of problems or illness. Psychological wellness refers to both our emotional and our mental states—that is, to our feelings and our thoughts. It involves awareness and acceptance of a wide range of feelings in oneself and others, the ability to express emotions, to function independently, and to cope with the challenges of daily stressors.

Spiritual Wellness

Being *spiritual* doesn't mean belonging to a formal religion. Its essential component is a belief in some meaning or order in the universe, a higher power that gives greater significance to individual life. Spiritually healthy individuals identify their own basic purpose in life; learn how to experience love, joy, peace, and fulfillment; and help themselves and others achieve their full potential. They concern themselves with "giving, forgiving, and attending to others' needs before one's own," says Dr. Roger Smith of Michigan State University. Smith notes that

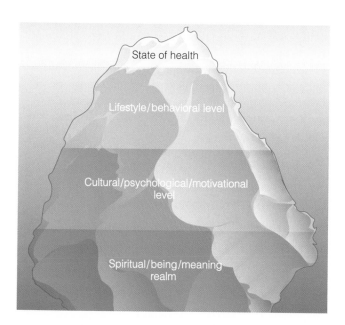

FIGURE 1-2 ▍ Iceberg Model of Wellness

Like an iceberg, only a small part of your total wellness is visible: your current state of health. Just as important are hidden dimensions, including lifestyle habits, cultural and psychological factors, and the realm of spiritual meaning and being.

spiritual development "produces a new meaning in one's life through a connectedness to something greater and mysterious."[4]

Americans tend to be both spiritual and religious. According to the most recent in a series of national Gallup polls conducted over the last 60-plus years, 90 percent of Americans believe in God—an all-time high. Most Americans also say that prayer is an important part of their lives, that they believe that miracles are performed by a divine power, and that they are sometimes conscious of the presence of God. Faced with physical or psychological difficulties, most Americans turn to prayer, reading the Bible, or meditation as a way of coping.

"Deeply religious people of all faiths appear to benefit in five major areas," reports Dr. Dale Matthews of Georgetown School of Medicine, who reviewed more than 300 studies on healing and religion.[5] These areas are less substance abuse; lower rates of depression and anxiety, especially among women; enhanced quality of life; quicker recovery from injury or illness; and longer life expectancy.

Social Wellness

Social wellness refers to the ability to interact effectively with other people and the social environment, to develop satisfying interpersonal relationships, and to fulfill social roles. It involves participating in and contributing to your community, living in harmony with fellow human beings, developing positive interdependent relationships with others, and practicing healthy sexual behaviors.

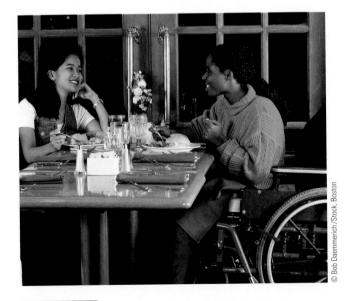

▮ As humans, we are social beings, and social interactions enhance our health and wellness.

In times of crisis, social connections provide comfort and support. Even in tranquil times, social isolation increases the risk of sickness and mortality. In a landmark study in Alameda County, California, death rates were twice as high for loners as for those with strong social ties. In other studies, social isolation greatly increased the risk of dying of a heart attack. Heart attack patients have a better chance of long-term survival if they believe they have adequate help in performing daily tasks from family and friends. People with spouses, friends, and a rich social network may outlive isolated loners by as much as 30 years.

Health educators are placing greater emphasis on social wellness in its broadest sense as they expand the traditional individualistic concept of health to include the complex interrelationships between one person's health and the health of the community and environment.

Intellectual Wellness

Your brain is the only one of your organs capable of self-awareness. Every day you use your mind to gather, process, and act on information; to think through your values; to make decisions, set goals, and figure out how to handle a problem or challenge. Intellectual wellness refers to your ability to think and learn from life experience, your openness to new ideas, and your capacity to question and evaluate information. Throughout your life, you'll use your critical thinking skills, including your ability to evaluate health information to safeguard your well-being.

Another important component of intellectual well-being is "emotional intelligence," which consists of self-awareness, altruism, personal motivation, empathy, and the ability to love and be loved by friends, partners, and family. People with high emotional intelligence succeed at home and at work by building fulfilling relationships and careers.

Environmental Wellness

You live in a physical and social setting that can affect every aspect of your health. Environmental wellness refers to the impact that your world has on your well-being. It means protecting yourself from dangers in the air, water, and soil, and in products you use—and also working to preserve the environment itself. (See Chapter 15 for a discussion of environmental health issues.)

✚ How Well Are We?

Americans are living longer and healthier lives than ever before in history. Life expectancy has reached a new high of 77.4 years, increasing for both men and women and blacks and whites. The gender gap between male and female life expectancies has narrowed to 5.2 years. The age-adjusted death rate has hit an all-time low of 847 deaths per 100,000 people, with declines in mortality from stroke, heart disease, cancer, and accidents.[6]

Yet we could be doing much better. Lifestyle factors remain the primary causes of disease and premature death in our country. Two out of every three deaths and one in three hospitalizations could be prevented by changes in six main risk factors: tobacco use, alcohol abuse, accidents, high blood pressure, obesity, and gaps in screening and primary health care.

Many college students think they are too young to worry about serious health conditions. Yet many chronic problems begin early in life. Two percent of college-age women already have osteoporosis, a bone-weakening disease; another 15 percent have osteopenia, that is, low bone densities that put them at risk of osteoporosis.[7] Many college students have several risk factors for heart disease, including high blood pressure and high cholesterol. Others increase their risk by eating a high-fat diet and not exercising regularly.

The greatest threat to American wellness may be the obesity epidemic. (See Chapter 9.) Current life expectancy at birth would be one-third to three-quarters of a year higher if all overweight adults were at their ideal weight.[8] In the next 50 years, the rapid rise in obesity among children and teenagers could have such a drastic impact on life expectancy—from two to five years—that it may eventually exceed the current impact of cancer or heart disease.[9]

Healthy People 2010

Healthy People 2010 is the prevention agenda for the nation. Every decade the federal government identifies the most significant preventable threats to health and creates leading indicators that assess the health of Americans. Its first goal is to help individuals of all ages increase life expectancy *and* improve their quality of life. Its second goal is to eliminate health disparities among different segments of the population.

Among the specific goals of Healthy People 2010 are:

▊ **Reduce the prevalence of cigarette smoking** among adults to 12 percent from the current 23.4 percent.

▊ **Reduce the number of new cancer cases** as well as the illnesses, disability, and death caused by cancer.

▊ **Promote the health of people with disabilities,** prevent secondary conditions, and eliminate disparities between people with and without disabilities in the U.S. population.

▊ **Reduce foodborne illnesses.**

▊ **Reduce the proportion of obese children and adolescents** from 11 percent to 5 percent.

▊ **Reduce the number of adolescents and adults** using illegal substances.

▊ **Reduce the number of adults** engaging in binge drinking.[10]

Health and Wellness Behaviors

In a national survey by the Centers for Disease Control (CDC), 79 percent of American adults described themselves as in excellent or very good health.[11] However, far fewer report excellent health habits. Another analysis by the CDC focused on four important health behaviors:[12]

▊ **Alcohol Use.** Six in ten adults are current drinkers; about 1 in 4 are lifetime abstainers. Nearly one-third of adults are light drinkers (3 or fewer drinks per week); and about 5 percent are heavier drinkers (7 or more drinks per week for women; 14 or more for men). About 20 percent of adults had 5 or more drinks per day at least once in the past year.

▊ **Smoking.** About 23 percent smoke every day or some days; another 23 percent are former smokers. More than half of adults in the United States have never smoked. About 40 percent of smokers attempted to quit in the past year.

▊ **Leisure-time Physical Activity.** Sixty-one percent of adults report at least some leisure-time activity. About one in four engage in light to moderate physical activity; about one in ten opt for vigorous activity at least five times per week.

▊ **Body Weight.** According to this survey, about 22 percent of adults are obese (defined as a body mass index of 30 or higher; see Chapter 9); 35 percent are overweight (defined as a body mass index of 25 but less than 30) but not obese; 40 percent are in a healthy weight range; and approximately 2 percent are underweight.

Rates of obesity are about the same for men and women. Men are slightly more likely than women to smoke. They also are more physically active in their leisure time. Younger individuals are more physically active than middle-aged adults; older Americans are less likely to be obese than middle-aged ones.

Asian adults are less likely to have unhealthy behaviors in terms of alcohol use, smoking, and body weight than other groups studied. Rates of leisure-time physical inactivity and obesity are higher among black adults than white adults. Black men are more likely than white men to be smokers, but among women the reverse is true. Hispanic women have low rates of smoking compared to non-Hispanic white women but higher rates of obesity.

STRATEGIES

for PREVENTION

Smart Steps to Take Now

▪ To lower your risk of heart disease, get your blood pressure and cholesterol checked. Don't smoke. Stay at a healthy weight. Exercise most days of the week. (See Chapter 9.)

▪ To lower your risk of major diseases, get regular checkups. Make sure you are immunized against infectious illnesses. Know your family's health history. (See Chapter 11.)

▪ To lower your risk of substance abuse and related illnesses and injuries, don't drink, or limit how much you drink. Avoid illegal drugs. (See Chapter 13.)

▪ To lower your risk of sexually transmitted infections (STIs) or unwanted pregnancy, abstain from sex. If you decide to engage in potentially risky sexual activities, protect yourself with condoms and spermicides. (See Chapter 14.)

▪ To prevent car accidents, don't drive when road conditions are hazardous. When you drive, wear a seat belt and use defensive driving techniques. (See Chapter 15.)

Diversity and Wellness

We live in the most diverse nation on Earth, one that is becoming increasingly diverse. For society, this variety can be both enriching and divisive. Tolerance and acceptance of others have always been part of the American creed. By working together, Americans have created a country that remains, to those outside our borders, a symbol of opportunity. Yet members of different ethnic groups still have to struggle against discrimination.

Despite improvements in economic and educational opportunities, discrepancies in health care for African Americans persist. Poverty remains a major barrier to quality health care for minorities. Without adequate insurance or the ability to pay, many cannot afford the tests and treatments that could prevent illness or overcome it at the earliest possible stages.

Black patients and white patients, to a large extent, receive care from different doctors. Those treating African-American patients may be less well trained and may have less access to health resources than those who treat white patients.

In some cultures, physicians are seen as less effective than other healers, who are believed to cure illness

caused by bad karma or evil spirits. American physicians, trained to believe that high-tech medicine is best, may not understand or appreciate traditional healing practices. In many communities, innovative programs have begun to educate patients from other cultures about the American health-care system, as well as to educate American health-care providers about the beliefs and health practices of their diverse patients.

Why Gender Matters

"Sex does matter. It matters in ways that we did not expect. Undoubtedly, it also matters in ways that we have not begun to imagine." This was the conclusion of the Institute of Medicine Committee on Understanding the Biology of Sex and Gender Differences in the first significant review of the status of sex and gender differences in biomedical research.

Sex, the committee stated, is "a classification, generally as male or female, according to the reproductive organs and functions that derive from the chromosomal complement." *Gender* refers to "a person's self-representation as male or female or how that person is responded to by social institutions on the basis of the individual's gender presentation." Rooted in biology, gender is shaped by environment and experience.

The experience of being male or female in a particular culture and society can and does have an effect on physical and psychological well-being. In fact, sex and gender may have a greater impact than any other variable on how our bodies function, how long we live, and the symptoms, course, and treatment of the diseases that strike us.

This realization is both new and revolutionary. For centuries, scientists based biological theories solely on a male model and viewed women as shorter, smaller, and rounder versions of men. Even modern medicine is based on the assumption that, except for their reproductive organs, both sexes are biologically interchangeable. We now know that this simply isn't so (**Figure 1-3**). Sex begins in the womb, but sex and gender differences affect behavior, perception, and health throughout life.

Recognition of these gender differences is transforming medical research and practice. *Gender-specific medicine* is replacing one-size-fits-all health care with new definitions of what is normal in both men and women, more complex concepts of disease, more precise diagnostic tests, and more effective treatments.

Does Race Affect Wellness?

Different racial and ethnic groups often face different wellness challenges. Consider the following statistics:

▪ The infant mortality rate for African-American babies remains higher than for white babies.

- Life expectancy for African Americans, though increasing, is five years lower than for whites.
- African Americans have higher rates of high blood pressure (hypertension), develop this problem earlier in life, suffer more severe hypertension, and have higher rates of stroke.
- African Americans have higher rates of glaucoma, systemic lupus erythematosus, liver disease, and kidney failure than whites.
- Overall, black Americans are more likely to develop cancer than persons of any other racial or ethnic group. Black Americans have higher than average colon and rectal cancer incidence and death rates than other racial and ethnic groups. Black Americans also have twice the average death rates from prostate cancer.[13]
- Latinos living in the United States have high rates of eye disease and visual impairment, particularly of diabetic retinopathy, an eye complication of diabetes; and open-angle glaucoma, a disease that damages the optic nerve.[14]
- Women of Filipino, Hawaiian, Indian, Pakistani, Mexican, South and Central American, and Puerto Rican descent are 20 to 260 percent more likely to be diagnosed with late-stage breast cancer than white women.[15]
- Caucasians are prone to osteoporosis (progressive weakening of bone tissue); cystic fibrosis; skin cancer; and phenylketonuria (PKU), a metabolic disorder that can lead to mental retardation.
- Native Americans have the highest rate of diabetes in the world. Among the Pima Indians, half of all adults have diabetes.

Are these increased susceptibilities the result of genetics, an unhealthy lifestyle, lack of access to health services, poverty, or the stress of living with discrimination? It is hard to say precisely. Certainly, poverty presents a major barrier to seeking preventive care and getting timely and effective treatment.

In some cases, both genetic and environmental factors may play a role. Take, for example, the high rates of diabetes among the Pima Indians. Until 50 years ago, these Native Americans were not notably obese or prone to diabetes. After World War II, the tribe started trading handmade baskets for lard and flour. Their lifestyle became more sedentary and their diet higher in fats. In addition, researchers have discovered that many Pima Indians have an inherited resistance to insulin that increases

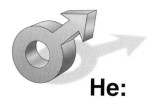
He:

- averages 12 breaths a minute
- has lower core body temperature
- has a slower heart rate
- has more oxygen-rich hemoglobin in his blood
- is more sensitive to sound
- produces twice as much saliva
- has a 10 percent larger brain
- is 10 times more likely to have attention deficit disorder
- as a teen, has an attention span of 5 minutes
- is more likely to be physically active
- is more prone to lethal diseases, including heart attacks, cancer, and liver failure

- is five times more likely to become an alcoholic
- has a life expectancy of 74.7 years

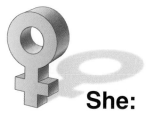
She:

- averages 9 breaths a minute
- has higher core body temperature
- has a faster heart rate
- has higher levels of protective immunoglobulin in her blood
- is more sensitive to light
- takes twice as long to process food
- has more neurons in certain brain regions
- is twice as likely to have an eating disorder
- as a teen, has an attention span of 20 minutes
- is more likely to be overweight
- is more vulnerable to chronic diseases, like arthritis and autoimmune disorders, and age-related conditions like osteoporosis
- is twice as likely to develop depression

- has a life expectancy of 79.9 years

FIGURE 1-3 ▮ Men and Women *Are* Different

their susceptibility to diabetes. The combination of a hereditary predisposition and environmental factors may explain why the Pimas now have epidemic levels of diabetes.

Ending Health Disparities

In the words of a National Institutes of Health report, minorities have carried "an unequal burden with respect to disease and disability, resulting in a lower life expectancy." Each year minorities in the United States—African Americans, Hispanics, Asian Americans, Pacific Islanders, Native Americans, and other groups—experience as many as 75,000 more deaths than they would if they lived under the same health conditions as the white population.

But race itself isn't the primary reason for the health problems faced by minorities in the United States. Poverty is. One in three Hispanics under age 65 has no health insurance. According to public health experts, low income may account for one-third of the racial differences in death rates for middle-aged African-American adults. High blood pressure, high cholesterol, obesity, diabetes, and smoking are responsible for another third. The final third has been blamed on "unexplained factors," which may well include poor access to health care and the stress of living in a society in which skin color remains a major barrier to equality.

When African Americans receive the same cancer treatments as whites, they are equally likely to survive. In

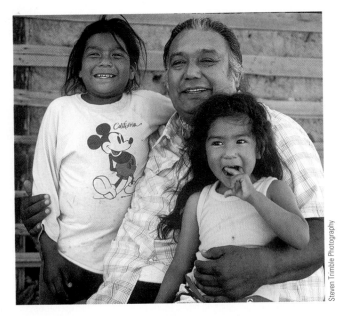

Steven Trimble Photography

▌ Both genetic and environmental factors have contributed to the increase in obesity and diabetes among the Pima tribe.

a study of nearly 3,400 colon cancer patients, white and black patients treated with surgery and chemotherapy had virtually the same five-year survival rates. Yet in past studies, African Americans were less likely to survive for five years than whites. When blacks and whites have equal access to quality health care, perhaps some of the racial-based differences in overall health will also be reduced.

✚ Staying Well on Campus

As one of the nation's 16.3 million undergraduate or graduate students, you belong to one of the most diverse groups in the United States. More than half—57 percent—are female; 63 percent are white; 11 percent, black; 9 percent, Hispanic. Among the 13.7 million undergraduates, about two-thirds are between the ages of 18 and 24, while a third are older than 25.[16] More than 3 million are enrolled in community colleges.[17]

The majority of college students are in the physical prime of life. As young, healthy adults, they are statistically less likely to develop life-threatening illnesses than older men and women. But contrary to what they may believe, they are not invincible. College students can and do develop a wide range of illnesses, from allergies (which afflict more than half of undergraduates) to potentially deadly cancers and heart conditions.

The number of college students with disabilities has tripled in the last two decades. According to the National Center for Educational Statistics, about 9 percent of full-time undergraduates report disabilities. The most common involve learning or health.[18]

College itself can seem hazardous to well-being. Dormitories have proved to be breeding grounds for serious infectious diseases, such as meningitis and Group B streptococcus (discussed in Chapter 11). Secondhand smoke can present a long-term threat to smokers' roommates. Binge drinking imperils not only the drinkers but those in their immediate environment, including anyone on the road if an intoxicated student gets behind the wheel of a car. However, most potential threats on campus stem from unhealthy habits or risky behaviors.

How Do College Students Rate Themselves?

College students, who have a greater tendency to worry in general, worry less about health than older adults. In fact, researchers describe them as having "an optimism bias," tending to underestimate their health risks and overestimate their level of wellness. About two-thirds of those surveyed at a large state university rated their risk of heart disease as lower or much lower than their peers—regardless of their family history or lifestyles.[19]

When asked to rate their physical and emotional health, about half of incoming freshmen say they're "above average" or "in the top 10 percent" compared with others their age. Men are much more likely to give themselves high health grades than women.[20] (See "Student Snapshot: How Do Undergraduates Rate Themselves?")

STUDENT SNAPSHOT
How Do Undergraduates Rate Themselves?

	All	Men	Women
Physical health	52%	64%	43%
Emotional health	51%	57%	46%
Self-confidence (intellectual)	58%	66%	50%
Self-confidence (social)	49%	54%	46%
Self-understanding	51%	56%	48%
Spirituality	37%	35%	38%

Based on a national survey of 289,452 students at 440 colleges and universities.
Source: Sax, Linda et al. *The American Freshman: National Norms for Fall 2004.* Los Angeles: UCLA Higher Education Research Institute, 2004.

© Jeff Greenberg/Alamy

Creating Your Wellness Toolbox

Wellness is your personal responsibility. Although products, programs, and people may offer quick and easy steps to feeling better, they almost always fail to live up to their promises. (See Savvy Consumer: "Too Good to Be True?") You have more control over how you feel now and in the future than anyone else.

The key to becoming your own wellness coach is self-responsibility. As Dr. John Travis defines this term in the context of wellness, this includes:

■ Developing awareness of your physical, mental, emotional, and spiritual processes and patterns.

■ Discovering your real needs and finding ways to meet them.

■ Making choices and living courageously in the midst of uncertainty.

■ Respecting your body through nutrition, exercise, and personal safety.

■ Creating the life you want rather than just reacting to whatever comes along.[21]

Throughout this book you will find practical tools that can help you reach a higher level of wellness.

Those tied to specific topics and dimensions of wellness can be found in the Lab Booklet that follows each chapter and those in your Lab Booklet.

Investigate Your Family Health History

Mapping your family medical history can help identify health risks you may face in the future. One way of charting your health history is to draw a medical family "tree" that includes your parents and siblings (who share half your genes), as well as grandparents, uncles, aunts, and cousins. Depending on how much information you're able to obtain for each relative, your medical family tree can include health issues each family member has faced, including illnesses with a hereditary component, such as high blood pressure, diabetes, some cancers, and certain psychiatric disorders. Although having a relative with a certain disease may increase your risk, your likelihood of ending up with the same condition also depends on your health habits, such as diet and exercise. Knowing now that you're at risk can motivate you to change any unhealthy behaviors.

"Family history is the single greatest risk factor for disease," says Dr. Paula Yoon of the CDC's Family Health Initiative, which is encouraging consumers to complete a family history and discuss it with their doctors. Physicians spend less than 2.5 minutes discussing family history and rarely include a family tree in a pa-

TOO GOOD TO BE TRUE?

Almost every week you're likely to come across a commercial or an ad for a new health product that promises better sleep, more energy, clearer skin, firmer muscles, lower weight, brighter moods, longer life—or all of these combined. As the Savvy Consumer throughout this book points out, you can't believe every promise you read or hear. Keep these general guidelines in mind the next time you come across a health claim:

■ **If it sounds too good to be true, it probably is.** If a magic pill could really trim off excess pounds or banish wrinkles, the world would be filled with thin people with unlined

skin. Look around, and you'll realize that's not the case.

■ **Look for objective evaluations.** If you're watching an infomercial for a treatment or technique, you can be sure that the enthusiastic endorsements have been skillfully scripted and rehearsed. Even ads that claim to be presenting the science behind a new breakthrough are really sales pitches in disguise.

■ **Consider the sources.** Research findings from carefully controlled scientific studies are reviewed by leading experts in the field and published in scholarly journals. Just because

someone has conducted a study doesn't mean it was a valid scientific investigation.

■ **Check credentials.** Anyone can claim to be a scientist or a health expert. Find out if advocates of any type of therapy have legitimate degrees from recognized institutions and are fully licensed in their fields.

■ **Do your own research.** Check with your doctor or with the student health center. Go to the library or do some online research to gather as much information as you can.

tient's file. Yet realizing that you have a relative with, say, colon cancer could mean that you should start screening tests ten years before others because you're at risk of developing a tumor at an earlier age. Says Yoon, "Knowing your family history could save your life."[22] (See your Lab booklet for instructions on taking a family health history.)

Discover the Joys of Journaling

Putting feelings into words and words onto paper is a powerful tool for behavior change. The process of expressive writing, or "journaling," provides an opportunity to reflect, evaluate past, present, and future behavior, and gain insight into your feelings. More than a decade of research has shown that writing about your inner life has a positive effect on both mental and physical health.

Think of your Wellness Journal as a chronicle of your journey to a higher level of well-being. Focus not just on events but on your underlying emotions, thoughts, dreams, and wishes. You can use the Wellness Journal pages included in every chapter's Labs, a separate notebook or a computer file.

Set aside a time and place to write. You don't have to write every day, but aim to do so at least three or four days a week. Try to write continuously for at least 15 minutes. Don't worry about spelling or grammar or how much or how little you write. Remember that your words are for your eyes only. Don't censor yourself. (See the Wellness Journal at the end of the chapter for ideas for getting started.)

Monitor Your Progress

Take stock of how you're doing on a regular basis. At the end of each day, you might jot down the most pos-

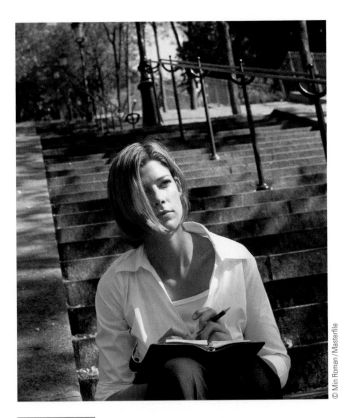

You don't need to be a journalist. Just write about *you*. Remember that your words are for your eyes only.

itive things you did for your well-being—and the most negative. At the end of each week, look back on the highs and lows. Use the "Wellness Report Card" (in your Lab booklet) to provide another snapshot of where you are on your wellness journey.

╬ MAKING HEALTHY CHOICES

To Live Long and Well

Change always begins with a single step. Use this course as an opportunity to zero in on at least one less-than-healthful behavior and improve it. Here are some suggestions:

▌ **Use seat belts.** In the last decade, seat belts have saved more than 40,000 lives and prevented millions of injuries.

▌ **Eat an extra fruit or vegetable every day.** Adding more fruit and vegetables to your diet can improve your digestion and lower your risk of several cancers.

▌ **Get enough sleep.** A good night's rest provides the energy you need to make it through the following day.

▌ **Take regular stress breaks.** A few quiet minutes spent stretching, looking out the window, or simply letting yourself unwind are good for body and soul.

▌ **Lose a pound.** If you're overweight, you may not think a pound will make a difference, but it's a step in the right direction.

▌ **If you're a woman, examine your breasts regularly.** Get in the habit of performing a breast self-examination every month after your period (when breasts are least swollen or tender).

- **If you're a man, examine your testicles regularly.** These simple self-exams can spot the early signs of cancer when they're most likely to be cured.
- **Get physical.** Just a little exercise will do some good. A regular workout schedule will be good for your heart, lungs, muscles, bones—even your mood.
- **Drink more water.** Eight glasses a day are what you need to replenish lost fluids, prevent constipation, and keep your digestive system working efficiently.
- **Do a good deed.** Caring for others is a wonderful way to care for your own soul and connect with others.

SELF-SURVEY

Wellness Inventory

What is Wellness?*

by John W. Travis M.D.

Go to Health Now™ for more activities.

Most of us think in terms of illness and assume that the absence of illness indicates wellness. There are actually many degrees of wellness, just as there are many degrees of illness. The Wellness Inventory is designed to stir up your thinking about many areas of wellness.

While people often lack physical symptoms, they may still be bored, depressed, tense, anxious, or generally unhappy with their lives. Such emotional states often set the stage for physical and mental disease. Even cancer may be brought on through the lowering of the body's resistance from excessive stress. These same emotional states can also lead to abuse of the body through smoking, overdrinking, and overeating. Such behaviors are usually substitutes for other, more basic human needs such as recognition from others, a more stimulating environment, caring and affection from friends, and greater self-acceptance.

Wellness is not a static state. High-level wellness involves giving good care to your physical self, using your mind constructively, expressing your emotions effectively, being creatively involved with those around you, and being concerned about your physical, psychological, and spiritual environments.

Instructions

Set aside a half hour for yourself in a quiet place where you will not be disturbed while taking the Inventory. Record your responses to each statement in the columns to the right where:

2 = Yes, usually
1 = Sometimes, maybe
0 = No, rarely

Select the answer that best indicates how true the statement is for you presently.

After you have responded to all the appropriate statements in each section, compute your average score for that section and transfer it to the corresponding box provided around the Wellness Inventory Wheel on page 12. Your completed Wheel will give you a clear presentation of the balance you have given to the many dimensions of your life.

You will find some of the statements are really two in one. We do this to show an important relationship between the two parts—usually an awareness of an issue, combined with an action based on that awareness. Mentally average your score for the two parts of the question.

Each statement describes what we believe to be a wellness attribute. Because much wellness information is subjective and "unprovable" by current scientific methods, you (and possibly other authorities as well) may not agree with our conclusions. Many of the statements have further explanation in a footnote. We ask only that you keep an open mind until you have studied available information, then decide.

This questionnaire was designed to educate more than to test. All statements are worded so that you can easily tell what we think are wellness attributes (which also makes it easy to "cheat" on your score). This means there can be no trick questions to test your honesty or consistency—the higher your score, the greater you believe your wellness to be. Full responsibility is placed on you to answer each statement as honestly as possible. It's not your score but what you learn about yourself that is most important.

If you decide that a statement does not apply to you, or you don't want to answer it, you can skip it and not be penalized in your score.

Transfer your average score from each section to the corresponding box around the Wheel. Then graph your score by drawing a curved line between the "spokes" that define each segment. (Use the scale provided—beginning at the center with 0.0 and reaching 2.0 at the circumference.) Last, fill in the corresponding amount of each wedge-shaped segment, using different colors if possible.

*Abridged from the Wellness Index in *The Wellness Workbook*, Travis & Ryan, Ten Speed Press, 1988. Used with the permission of John W. Travis, M.D. www.thewellspring.com.

Sample Questions

	Yes, usually	Sometimes, maybe	No, rarely
	2	**1**	**0**
1. I am an adventurous thinker.	✔		
2. I have no expectations, yet look to the future optimistically.		✔	
3. I am a nonsmoker.	✔		
4. I love long, hot baths.			✔

Total points for this section = **5**   4   +   1   +   0

Divided by   4   (number of statements answered) = 1.3 Average score for this section.

Your completed Inventory Wheel may look something like this:

2 Breathing — .4

3 Sensing — 1.1

4 Eating

12 Transcending
11 Finding Meaning
10 Sex
9 Communicating
8 Playing/Working
7 Thinking

1 Self-Responsibility and Love
2 Breathing
3 Sensing
4 Eating
5 Moving
6 Feeling

Section 1   WELLNESS, SELF-RESPONSIBILITY, AND LOVE

	Yes, usually	Sometimes, maybe	No, rarely
	2	1	0

1. I believe how I live my life is an important factor in determining my state of health, and I live it in a manner consistent with that belief.
2. I vote regularly.[1]
3. I feel financially secure.
4. I conserve materials/energy at home and at work.[2]
5. I protect my living area from fire and safety hazards.
6. I use dental floss and a soft toothbrush daily.
7. I am a nonsmoker.
8. I am always sober when driving or operating dangerous machinery.
9. I wear a safety belt when I ride in a vehicle.
10. I understand the difference between blaming myself for a problem and simply taking responsibility (ability to respond) for that problem.

Total points for this section = ☐ _____ + _____ + _____

Divided by ____ **(number of statements answered)** = ____ **Average score for this section.**
(Transfer to the Wellness Inventory Wheel on **p. 12**)

Section 2   WELLNESS AND BREATHING

	Yes, usually	Sometimes, maybe	No, rarely
	2	1	0

1. I stop during the day to become aware of the way I am breathing.
2. I meditate or relax myself for at least 15 to 20 minutes each day.
3. I can easily touch my hands to my toes when standing with knees straight.[3]
4. In temperatures over 70°F (21°C), my fingers feel warm when I touch my lips.[4]
5. My nails are healthy and I do not bite or pick at them.
6. I enjoy my work and do not find it overly stressful.
7. My personal relationships are satisfying.
8. I take time out for deep breathing several times a day.
9. I have plenty of energy.
10. I am at peace with myself.

Total points for this section = ☐ _____ + _____ + _____

Divided by _____ **(number of statements answered)** = ____ **Average score for this section.**
(Transfer to the Wellness Inventory Wheel on **p. 12**)

---

[1] Voting is a simple measure of your willingness to participate in the social system, which ultimately impacts your state of health.

[2] Besides recycling glass, paper, aluminum, and other recyclables, if you purchase products that are reusable rather than disposable, and are packaged with a minimum of material, you will reduce the drain of resources and the toxic load on the environment caused by the disposal of wastes.

[3] A lack of spinal flexibility is usually a symptom of chronic muscle tension as well as indicative of a poor balance of physical activities.

[4] If your hand temperature is below 85°F (30°C) in a warm room, you're cutting off circulation to your hands via an overactive sympathetic nervous system. You can learn to warm your hands with biofeedback and to thereby better relax.

Section 3 WELLNESS AND SENSING

	Yes, usually	Sometimes, maybe	No, rarely
	2	1	0
1. My place of work has mostly natural lighting or full-spectrum fluorescent lighting.[5]	___	___	___
2. I avoid extremely noisy areas or wear protective ear covers.[6]	___	___	___
3. I take long walks, hikes, or other outings to actively explore my surroundings.	___	___	___
4. I give myself presents, treats, or nurture myself in other ways.	___	___	___
5. I enjoy getting, and can acknowledge, compliments and recognition from others.	___	___	___
6. It is easy for me to give sincere compliments and recognition to other people.	___	___	___
7. At times I like to be alone.	___	___	___
8. I enjoy touching or hugging other people.[7]	___	___	___
9. I enjoy being touched or hugged by others.[8]	___	___	___
10. I get and enjoy backrubs or massages.	___	___	___

Total points for this section = ☐ ___ + ___ + ___

Divided by ___ **(number of statements answered)** = ___ **Average score for this section.**
(Transfer to the Wellness Inventory Wheel on **p. 12**)

Section 4 WELLNESS AND EATING

	Yes, usually	Sometimes, maybe	No, rarely
	2	1	0
1. I am aware of the difference between refined carbohydrates and complex carbohydrates and eat a majority of the latter.[9]	___	___	___
2. I think my diet is well balanced and wholesome.	___	___	___
3. I drink fewer than five alcoholic drinks per week.	___	___	___
4. I drink fewer than two cups of coffee or black (nonherbal) tea per day.[10]	___	___	___
5. I drink fewer than five soft drinks per week.[11]	___	___	___
6. I add little or no salt to my food.[12]	___	___	
7. I read the labels for the ingredients of all processed foods I buy and I inquire as to the level of toxic chemicals used in production of fresh foods—choosing the purest available to me.	___	___	___
8. I eat at least two raw fruits or vegetables each day.	___	___	___
9. I have a good appetite and am within 15% of my ideal weight.	___	___	___
10. I can tell the difference between "stomach hunger" and "mouth hunger," and I don't stuff myself when I am experiencing only "mouth hunger."[13]	___	___	___

Total points for this section = ☐ ___ + ___ + ___

Divided by ___ **(number of statements answered)** = ___ **Average score for this section.**
(Transfer to the Wellness Inventory Wheel on **p. 12**)

[5] Full-spectrum light, like sunlight, contains many different wavelengths. Most eyeglasses, and the glass windows in your home or car, block the "near" ultraviolet light needed by your body. Special bulbs and lenses are available.

[6] Loud noises that leave your ears ringing cause irreversible and cumulative nerve damage over time. Ear plugs/muffs, obtained in sporting goods stores, should be worn around power saws, heavy equipment, and rock concerts!

[7,8] Long recognized by hospitals as therapeutic, touch can be a powerful preventative as well.

[9] Refined carbohydrates (white flour, sugar, white rice, alcohol, and others) are burned up by the body very quickly and contain no minerals or vitamins. Complex carbohydrates (fruits and vegetables) burn evenly and provide the bulk of dietary nutrients.

[10] Coffee and nonherbal teas contain stimulants that, when overused, abuse your body's adrenal glands.

[11] Besides caffeine, the empty calories in these chemical brews may cause a sugar "crash" shortly after drinking. Artificially sweetened ones may be worse. Consider the other nutrients you won't be getting, and the prices!

[12] In addition to having a presumed connection with high blood pressure, the salting of foods during cooking draws out minerals, which are lost when the water is poured off.

[13] Stomach hunger is a signal that your body needs food. Mouth hunger is a signal that it needs something else (attention/acknowledgment), which you are not getting, so it asks for food, a readily available "substitute."

Section 5 WELLNESS AND MOVING

	Yes, usually	Sometimes, maybe	No, rarely
	2	**1**	**0**
1. I climb stairs rather than ride elevators.[14]	____	____	____
2. My daily activities include moderate physical effort.[15]	____	____	____
3. My daily activities include vigorous physical effort.[16]	____	____	____
4. I run at least 1 mile three times a week (or equivalent aerobic exercise).[17]	____	____	____
5. I run at least 3 miles three times a week (or equivalent aerobic exercise).	____	____	____
6. I do some form of stretching/limbering exercise for 10 to 20 minutes at least three times per week.[18]	____	____	____
7. I do some form of stretching/limbering exercise for 10 to 20 minutes at least six times per week.	____	____	____
8. I enjoy exploring new and effective ways of caring for myself through the movement of my body.	____	____	____
9. I enjoy stretching, moving, and exerting my body.	____	____	____
10. I am aware of and respond to messages from my body about its needs for movement.	____	____	____

Total points for this section = ☐ ____ + ____ + ____

Divided by _____ **(number of statements answered)** = ____ **Average score for this section.**
(Transfer to the Wellness Inventory Wheel on **p. 12**)

Section 6 WELLNESS AND FEELING

	Yes, usually	Sometimes, maybe	No, rarely
	2	**1**	**0**
1. I am able to feel and express my anger in ways that solve problems, rather than swallow anger or store it up.[19]	____	____	____
2. I allow myself to experience a full range of emotions and find constructive ways to express them.	____	____	____
3. I am able to say "no" to people without feeling guilty.	____	____	____
4. I laugh often and easily.	____	____	____
5. I feel OK about crying and allow myself to do so when appropriate.[20]	____	____	____
6. I listen to and consider others' criticisms of me rather than react defensively.	____	____	____
7. I have at least five close friends.	____	____	____
8. I like myself and look forward to the rest of my life.	____	____	____
9. I easily express concern, love and warmth to those I care about.	____	____	____
10. I can ask for help when needed.	____	____	____

Total points for this section = ☐ ____ + ____ + ____

Divided by _____ **(number of statements answered)** = ____ **Average score for this section.**
(Transfer to the Wellness Inventory Wheel on **p. 12**)

[14] If a long elevator ride is necessary, try getting off five flights below your destination. Urge building managers to keep stair doors unlocked.

[15] Moderate = rearing young children, gardening, scrubbing floors, brisk walking, and so on.

[16] Vigorous = heavy construction work, farming, moving heavy objects by hand, and so on.

[17] An aerobic exercise (like running) should keep your heart rate at about 60% of its maximum (120–150 bpm) for 12–20 minutes. Brisk walking for 20 minutes every day can produce effects similar to aerobic exercise.

[18] The stretching of muscles is important for maintaining maximum flexibility of joints and ligaments. It feels good, too.

[19] Learning to take charge of your emotions and using them to solve problems can prevent disease, improve communications, and increase your self-awareness. Suppressing emotions or using them to manipulate others is destructive to all.

[20] Crying over a loss relieves the body of pent-up feelings. In our culture males often have a difficult time allowing themselves to cry, while females may have learned to cry when angry, using tears as a means of manipulation.

Section 7 WELLNESS AND THINKING

	Yes, usually	Sometimes, maybe	No, rarely
	2	**1**	**0**
1. I am in charge of the subject matter and the emotional content of my thoughts, and I am satisfied with what I choose to think about.[21]	_____	_____	_____
2. I am aware that I make judgments wherein I think I am "right" and others are "wrong."[22]	_____	_____	_____
3. It is easy for me to concentrate.	_____	_____	_____
4. I am conscious of changes (such as breathing pattern, muscle tension, skin moisture, and so on) in my body in response to certain thoughts.[23]	_____	_____	_____
5. I notice my perceptions of the world are colored by my thoughts at the time.[24]	_____	_____	_____
6. I am aware that my thoughts are influenced by my environment.	_____	_____	_____
7. I use my thoughts and attitudes to make my reality more life-affirming.[25]	_____	_____	_____
8. Rather than worry about a problem when I can do nothing about it, I temporarily shelve it and get on with the matters at hand.	_____	_____	_____
9. I approach life with the attitude that no problem is too big to confront, and some mysteries aren't meant to be solved.	_____	_____	_____
10. I use my creative powers in many aspects of my life.	_____	_____	_____

Total points for this section = ☐ _____ + _____ + _____

Divided by _____ **(number of statements answered)** = _____ **Average score for this section.**
(Transfer to the Wellness Inventory Wheel on **p. 12**)

Section 8 WELLNESS AND PLAYING/WORKING

	Yes, usually	Sometimes, maybe	No, rarely
	2	**1**	**0**
1. I enjoy expressing myself through art, dance, music, drama, sports, or other activities and make time to do so.	_____	_____	_____
2. I regularly exercise my creativity "muscles."	_____	_____	_____
3. I enjoy spending time without planned or structured activities and make the effort to do so.	_____	_____	_____
4. I can make much of my work into play.	_____	_____	_____
5. At times I allow myself to do nothing.[26]	_____	_____	_____
6. At times I can sleep late without feeling guilty.	_____	_____	_____
7. The work I do is rewarding to me.	_____	_____	_____
8. I am proud of my accomplishments.	_____	_____	_____
9. I am playful and the people around me support my playfulness.	_____	_____	_____
10. I have at least one activity, hobby, or sport that I enjoy regularly but do not feel compelled to do.	_____	_____	_____

Total points for this section = ☐ _____ + _____ + _____

Divided by _____ **(number of statements answered)** = _____ **Average score for this section.**
(Transfer to the Wellness Inventory Wheel on **p. 12**)

---

[21] When you are unconscious of the content of your thoughts, they are more likely to control you. Observing them objectively develops self-awareness and strengthens your ability to take charge.

[22] Rather than trying to completely stop yourself from judging, you can observe your judgments as efforts by your ego to avoid getting on with life and hiding behind "right/wrong" game playing.

[23] Both biofeedback and the field of psycho-neuro-immunology have shown the connections between the mind, nervous system and body. The more you become consciously aware of that connection, the greater responsibility you can take for your health.

[24] Being aware of your internal distortion of perceptions can allow you to step back and reassess a situation more objectively.

[25] Honesty, tempered with care and concern, clears out many negative thoughts that can clutter up your mind, thus making your reality more fun. "Positive thinking" without honesty and truthfulness can backfire by suppressing valid concerns that must be addressed.

[26] Doing "nothing" can give us access to the more creative and nonverbal aspects of our being, so from another perspective, doing nothing becomes doing much more.

Section 9   WELLNESS AND COMMUNICATING

	Yes, usually	Sometimes, maybe	No, rarely
	2	**1**	**0**
1. In conversation I can introduce a difficult topic and stay with it until I've gotten a satisfactory response from the other person.	_____	_____	_____
2. I enjoy silence.	_____	_____	_____
3. I am truthful and caring in my communications with others.	_____	_____	_____
4. I assert myself (in a nonattacking manner) in an effort to be heard rather than be passively resentful of others with whom I don't agree.[27]	_____	_____	_____
5. I readily acknowledge my mistakes, apologizing for them if appropriate.	_____	_____	_____
6. I am aware of my negative judgments of others and accept them as simply judgments—not necessarily truth.[28]	_____	_____	_____
7. I am a good listener.	_____	_____	_____
8. I am able to listen to people without interrupting them or finishing their sentences for them.	_____	_____	_____
9. I can let go of my mental "labels" (for example, this is good, that is wrong) and judgmental attitudes about events in my life and see them in light of what they offer me.	_____	_____	_____
10. I am aware when I play psychological "games" with those around me and work to be truthful and direct in my communications.[29]	_____	_____	_____

Total points for this section = ☐ _____ + _____ + _____

Divided by _____ (number of statements answered) = _____ **Average score for this section.**
(Transfer to the Wellness Inventory Wheel on **p. 12**)

Section 10   WELLNESS AND SEX

	Yes, usually	Sometimes, maybe	No, rarely
	2	**1**	**0**
1. I feel comfortable touching and exploring my body.	_____	_____	_____
2. I think it's OK to masturbate if one chooses to do so.	_____	_____	_____
3. My sexual education is adequate.	_____	_____	_____
4. I feel good about the degree of closeness I have with men.	_____	_____	_____
5. I feel good about the degree of closeness I have with women.	_____	_____	_____
6. I am content with my level of sexual activity.[30]	_____	_____	_____
7. I fully experience the many stages of lovemaking rather than focus only on orgasm.[31]	_____	_____	_____
8. I desire to grow closer to some other people.	_____	_____	_____
9. I am aware of the difference between needing someone and loving someone.	_____	_____	_____
10. I am able to love others without dominating or being dominated by them.	_____	_____	_____

Total points for this section = ☐ _____ + _____ + _____

Divided by _____ (number of statements answered) = _____ **Average score for this section.**
(Transfer to the Wellness Inventory Wheel on **p. 12**)

[27] Attacking others rarely accomplishes your goals in the long run. Persisting in your convictions without using force is more effective and usually solves the problem without creating new ones.

[28] It is important to recognize that our internal judgments of others are based on personal biases that often have little objective basis.

[29] Psychological games, as defined by Eric Berne in *Games People Play,* are complex unconscious manipulations that result in the players getting negative attention and feeling bad about themselves.

[30] Including the choice to have no sexual activity.

[31] A common problem for many people is an overemphasis on performance and orgasm, rather than on enjoying a close sensual feeling with their partner whether or not they experience orgasm.

Section 11 WELLNESS AND FINDING MEANING

	Yes, usually	Sometimes, maybe	No, rarely
	2	**1**	**0**
1. I believe my life has direction and meaning.	_____	_____	_____
2. My life is exciting and challenging.	_____	_____	_____
3. I have goals in my life.	_____	_____	_____
4. I am achieving my goals.	_____	_____	_____
5. I look forward to the future as an opportunity for further growth.	_____	_____	_____
6. I am able to talk about the death of someone close to me.	_____	_____	_____
7. I am able to talk about my own death with family and friends.	_____	_____	_____
8. I am prepared for my death.	_____	_____	_____
9. I see my death as a step in my evolution.[32]	_____	_____	_____
10. My daily life is a source of pleasure to me.	_____	_____	_____

Total points for this section = [ ] _____ + _____ + _____

Divided by _____ **(number of statements answered)** = _____ **Average score for this section.**
(Transfer to the Wellness Inventory Wheel on **p. 12**)

This portion of the Inventory goes beyond the scope of most generally accepted "scientific" principles and expresses the values and beliefs of the authors. It is intended to stimulate interest in these areas. If you have strong beliefs to the contrary, you can skip the questions or make up your own.

Section 12 WELLNESS AND TRANSCENDING

	Yes, usually	Sometimes, maybe	No, rarely
	2	**1**	**0**
1. I perceive problems as opportunities for growth.	_____	_____	_____
2. I experience synchronistic events in my life (frequent "coincidences" seeming to have no cause–effect relationship).[33]	_____	_____	_____
3. I believe there are dimensions of reality beyond verbal description or human comprehension.	_____	_____	_____
4. At times I experience confusion and paradox in my search for understanding of the dimensions referred to above.	_____	_____	_____
5. The concept of God has personal definition and meaning to me.	_____	_____	_____
6. I experience a sense of wonder when I contemplate the universe.	_____	_____	_____
7. I have abundant expectancy rather than specific expectations.	_____	_____	_____
8. I allow others their beliefs without pressuring them to accept mine.	_____	_____	_____
9. I use the messages interpreted from my dreams.	_____	_____	_____
10. I enjoy practicing a spiritual discipline or allowing time to sense the presence of a greater force in guiding my passage through life.	_____	_____	_____

Total points for this section = [ ] _____ + _____ + _____

Divided by _____ **(number of statements answered)** = _____ **Average score for this section.**
(Transfer to the Wellness Inventory Wheel on **p. 12**)

[32] Seeing your death as a stage of growth and preparing yourself consciously is an important part of finding meaning in your life.

[33] Modern physics reveals that the idea of cause and effect may be as limited as Newton's theory of a mechanical universe. It suggests that we must expand our view to see that everything in the universe is connected to everything else. (Synchronicity describes that experience.)

ACTION PLAN

Your Action Plan for Maximum Wellness

When you have completed the Wellness Inventory, study your wheel's shape and balance. How smoothly would it roll? What does it tell you? Are there any surprises in it? How does it feel to you? What don't you like about it? What do you like about it?

We recommend that you use colored pens to go back over the questions, noting the ones on which your scores were low and choosing some areas on which you are interested in working. It is easy to overwhelm yourself by taking on too many areas at once. Ignore, for now, those of lower priority to you. Remember, if you don't enjoy at least some aspects of the changes you are making, they probably won't last.

Here are some guidelines to help you:

▪ Read the following chapter on "Making Healthy Changes." It will provide you with detailed guidance on formulating and achieving goals.

▪ Get support from friends, but don't expect them to supply all the reinforcement you need. You may join a group of overweight individuals and rely on their encouragement to stick to your diet. That's a great way to get going. In the long run, your own commitment to losing weight has got to be strong enough to help you keep eating right and light.

▪ Focus on the immediate rewards of your new behavior. You may stop smoking so that you'll live longer, but take note of every other benefit it brings you—more stamina, less coughing, more spending money, no more stale tobacco taste in your mouth.

▪ Remind yourself of past successes you've had in making changes. Give yourself pep talks, commending yourself on how well you've done so far and how well you'll continue to do. This will boost your self-confidence.

▪ Reward yourself regularly. Plan a pleasant reward as an incentive for every week you stick to your new behavior—sleeping in on a Saturday morning, going out with some friends, or spending a sunny afternoon outdoors. Small, regular rewards are more effective in keeping up motivation than one big reward that won't come for many months.

▪ Expect and accept some relapses. The greatest rate of relapse occurs in the first few weeks after making a behavior change. During this critical time, get as much support as you can. In addition, work hard on self-motivation, reminding yourself daily of what you have to gain by sticking with your new health habit.

WELLNESS JOURNAL

Your Wellness Journey

Experiment with these styles of journaling to find which one works best for you.

"Stream-of-Consciousness" Journaling

You might begin with "stream-of-consciousness" journaling and simply record whatever thoughts come into your mind. Sit quietly and breathe deeply. Once relaxed and settled, begin to write. Don't be surprised at the number and intensity of thoughts and feelings that emerge. As they become part of your awareness, they may lead to insights that have eluded you in the past. Psychologists believe that this happens because you are taking the time to "hear" what you are thinking.

If you run into writer's block, complete one of the following sentences:

When I think about my current level of wellness, I wish I had _____.

Thinking about the way I treat my body, I feel _____.

Journaling for Specific Solutions

You also can use your journal to tackle specific issues and challenges.

▪ Write when you need to sort out complicated feelings about your body image.

▪ Write when you're struggling to stick with your action plan.

▪ At the end of the day, chronicle the good choices you made or note what you'll do differently the next day.

"Reflective" Journaling

Try "reflective" journaling and write about yourself and your life in the third person. For example, you might write: "This morning as she lay in bed she knew that she couldn't stand to live another day in her out-of-shape body. She decided at that very moment to. . . ."

"Dialogue" Journaling

You might experiment with "dialogue" journaling, in which you split yourself in two. In essence, you compose a script with two characters. One character might talk only of the benefits of a behavioral change. The other might complain about the drawbacks and difficulties. Write a back-and-forth conversation giving each character equal opportunity to make points and counterpoints.

Making This Chapter Work for You

1. Wellness is defined as
   a. purposeful, enjoyable living, characterized by personal responsibility and enhancement of physical, mental, and spiritual health.
   b. a state of complete physical, mental, and social well-being.
   c. attitudes and beliefs that contribute to a healthy state of mind.
   d. the absence of physical or mental illness.

2. The components of wellness include all of the following *except:*
   a. supportive friends and family.
   b. a well-paying job.
   c. energy and vitality.
   d. a clean environment.

3. Which of the following statements about the dimensions of health are true?
   a. Spirituality provides solace and comfort for those who are severely ill, but it has no health benefits.
   b. The people who reflect the highest levels of social health are usually among the most popular individuals in a group and are often thought of as the life of the party.
   c. Intellectual health refers to one's academic abilities.
   d. Optimal physical health requires a nutritious diet, regular exercise, avoidance of harmful behaviors and substances, and self-protection from accidents.

4. The most important dimension of wellness is
   a. physical wellness.
   b. spiritual wellness.
   c. psychological wellness.
   d. trick question—all of the dimensions of wellness are vital to leading a balanced and satisfying life.

5. What is probably the greatest current threat to American wellness?
   a. cancer.
   b. lowered life expectancies.
   c. smoking rate among adolescents.
   d. obesity epidemic.

6. The goals of the Healthy People 2010 initiative include all of the following *except:*
   a. reduce the proportion of obese adults and children in the population.
   b. decrease the number of teens using illegal substances.
   c. increase the number of adults engaging in daily vigorous physical activity for 30 minutes per occasion.
   d. reduce the percentage of teens and adults who report smoking cigarettes in the past month.

7. A group of students is discussing the differences between the sexes. Whose statement is incorrect?
   a. Matt: "Men breathe faster but have a slower heart rate—and have a larger brain."
   b. Elena: "But women have more neurons in certain brain regions."
   c. Kristin: "And women are less likely to get arthritis."
   d. Rick: "Got me there—men *are* more likely to have heart attacks and to get cancer."

8. Health risks faced by different ethnic and racial groups include all of the following *except:*
   a. Whites have higher rates of hypertension, lupus, liver disease, and kidney failure than African Americans.
   b. Native Americans have a higher rate of diabetes than other racial and ethnic groups.
   c. Infant mortality is higher for African-American babies than for white babies.
   d. Latinos living in the United States have high rates of eye disease.

9. The majority of college students are in the physical prime of their lives. To stay well, you should avoid:
   a. binge drinking.
   b. unprotected sex.
   c. smoking.
   d. all of the above.

10. Tools to help you reach a higher level of wellness include:
    a. investigation of your family history.
    b. writing a journal.
    c. noting the positive actions you take each day.
    d. all of the above.

Answers to these questions can be found on page 376.

Critical Thinking

1. What is the definition of wellness according to the text? Does your personal definition differ from this? If so, in what ways? How would you have defined wellness before reading this chapter?

2. Talk to classmates from different racial or ethnic backgrounds than yours about their culture's attitudes toward wellness. Are psychological and social wellness considered necessary for wellness in their cultures? Does spirituality play a role in their cultures?

3. Where are you on the wellness–illness continuum? What variables might affect your place on the scale? What do you consider your optimum state of health to be?

Media Menu

Health Now™

Don't forget to check out the wealth of resources on the HealthNow website at **http://healthnow.brookscole.com/itw** that will:

- Help you evaluate your knowledge of the material
- Allow you to take an exam-prep quiz
- Provide a Personalized Learning Plan targeting resources that address areas you should study
- Coach you through identifying target goals for behavior change and creating and monitoring your personal change plan throughout the semester.

INTERNET CONNECTIONS

Go Ask Alice

www.goaskalice.columbia.edu/index.html
Sponsored by Columbia University, this site offers questions and answers as well as an interactive service on a wide variety of health-related topics.

Lifescan Health Risk Appraisal

http://wellness.uwsp.edu/other/lifescan/lifescan.htm
This site, created by Bill Hettler, M.D. of the National Wellness Institute, helps you identify specific lifestyle factors that can impair your health and longevity. Take the health questionnaire to determine your personal lifestyle risks. Your results provide a score for general results, nutrition results, and height/weight results. Your ranking among the top ten causes of death is provided, as well as suggestions on how to improve.

Healthy People 2010

www.healthypeople.gov
Healthy People 2010 is a statement of national health objectives developed by the Office of Disease Prevention and Health Promotion, U.S. Department of Health and Human Services. This collection of national health objectives is designed to identify the most significant preventable causes of acute and chronic illnesses and accidents and to establish national goals to reduce these threats to health. The goals are aimed at improving the health of all Americans by the year 2010.

InfoTrac College Edition Activity Healthy doctors, healthy communities. (Healthy People 2010) by Donna Cameron; Ellen Katch; Patricia Anderson; Mary A. Furlong. *The Journal of Ambulatory Care Management,* Oct–Dec 2004 v27 i4 p328(11).

1. What health behaviors typically characterize medical students?

2. Why did the American Medical Student Association (AMSA) initiate the Train the Trainer program designed to promote student wellness in medical schools nationwide?

3. Describe three evaluation and assessment techniques presented by the authors.

4. What are the Multidimensional Model of Wellness and the Stages of Change Model as described in the medical students' course experiences?

You can find additional readings related to personal health with InfoTrac College Edition, an online library of more than 900 journals and publications. Follow the instructions for accessing InfoTrac College Edition that were packaged with your textbook; then search for articles using a keyword search.

For additional links, resources, and suggested readings on the InfoTrac College Edition, visit our Health and Wellness Resource Center at **http://health.wadsworth.com**.

Key Term

The term listed is used on the page indicated. Definition of the term is in the Glossary at the end of the book.

wellness 2

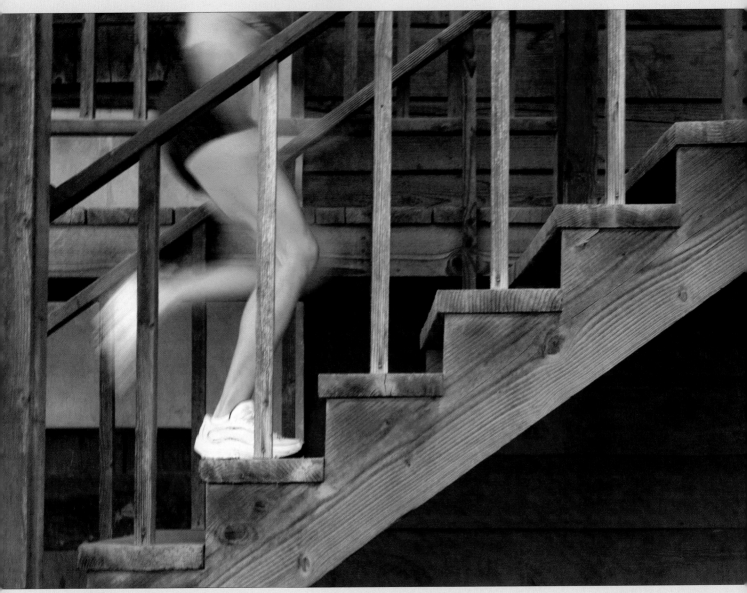

Jessica describes herself as an average college student in almost every way: grades, looks, athletic ability—and wellness. Yes, she could make better food choices. Yes, she should exercise more consistently. Yes, she gets stressed out and doesn't get enough sleep. Occasionally she drinks too much. She smokes with friends when they light up. She knows that heart disease "runs" in her family, but she doesn't understand exactly what that means. Ask Jessica if she'd like to be better than average, and she'll say "yes." But she doesn't know where to begin.

Do you want to be and feel and do as well as possible, to live and work at your maximum potential? This chapter can help you begin. Whatever physical shape and psychological state you're in, you can enhance your wellness and improve your fitness and health. But doing so requires more than reading this book or taking this course. You have to commit yourself to change.

Personal change always begins in the same place: the brain. As decades of research have shown, your thoughts determine how you feel and how you behave. Your thoughts determine every choice that you make. The discovery that thoughts create feelings and drive behavior—one of the most important psychological breakthroughs of the last 50 years—is the foundation of all cognitive and behavioral therapy approaches. These methods emphasize setting goals (defining what you intend to accomplish) and changing the way you think about or interpret a situation.

This chapter is a primer in behavioral change. It describes the factors that influence health behavior and the stages of readiness for change. As you read it, you can immediately apply the information and insights to your own health behaviors. As you do, you will develop goals and begin moving toward them—and toward the level of wellness that can lift your life well above average.

After studying the material in this chapter, you should be able to:

▌ Define the three factors that shape health behaviors.

▌ Name the three key components of the Transtheoretical Model of Change.

▌ Describe the stages of change and give an example of each.

▌ Name at least two mental attitudes that can help you successfully make a change.

Health ☁ Now™

Don't forget to check out the wealth of resources on the HealthNow website at **http://healthnow.brookscole.com/itw** that will:

• Help you evaluate your knowledge of the material
• Allow you to take an exam-prep quiz
• Provide a Personalized Learning Plan targeting resources that address areas you should study
• Coach you through identifying target goals for behavior change and creating and monitoring your personal change plan throughout the semester.

✚ Changing Health Behaviors

Nothing is certain in life except change. Every day ushers in changes large and small, but the changes that matter most are those we make ourselves. In recent decades behavioral scientists have dissected the process of how people change, mapping the stages of change and identifying the components of successful change. The following sections describe some of the steps that can help you make changes for the better.

Understanding Health Behavior

Your choices and behaviors affect how long and how well you live. Nearly half of all deaths in the United States are linked to behaviors such as tobacco use, improper diet, abuse of alcohol and other drugs, use of firearms, motor vehicle accidents, risky sexual practices, and lack of exercise.

If you would like to improve your health behavior, you have to realize that change isn't easy. Between 40 and 80 percent of those who try to kick bad health habits lapse back into their unhealthy ways within six weeks. To make lasting beneficial changes, you have to understand the three types of influences that shape behavior: predisposing, enabling, and reinforcing factors (**Figure 2-1**).

Predisposing factors

Predisposing factors include knowledge, attitudes, beliefs, values, and perceptions. Unfortunately, knowledge isn't enough to cause most people to change their behavior; for example, people fully aware of the grim conse-

quences of smoking often continue to puff away. Nor is attitude—one's likes and dislikes—sufficient; an individual may dislike the smell and taste of cigarettes but continue to smoke regardless.

Beliefs are more powerful than knowledge and attitudes, and researchers report that people are most likely to change health behavior if they hold three beliefs:

❚ **Susceptibility.** They acknowledge that they are at risk for the negative consequences of their behavior.
❚ **Severity.** They believe that they may pay a very high price if they don't make a change.
❚ **Benefits.** They believe that the proposed change will be advantageous to their health.

There can be a gap between stated and actual beliefs, however. Young adults may say they recognize the very real dangers of casual, careless sex in this day and age. Yet, rather than act in accordance with these statements, they may impulsively engage in unprotected sex with individuals whose health status and histories they do not know. The reason: Like young people everywhere and in every time, they feel invulnerable, that nothing bad can or will happen to them, that if there were a real danger, they would somehow know it. Often it's not until something happens—a former partner may admit to having a sexually transmitted infection—that their behaviors become consistent with their stated beliefs.

Young people, especially young men, are the greatest risk takers, a fact reflected in their high rates of auto accidents, binge drinking, drug use, and pathological gambling. The death rates for injuries related to swimming, boating, driving, cycling, and even crossing the street are higher in college-age men than women.

The value or importance we give to health also plays a major role in changing behavior. Many people aren't concerned about their health just for the sake of being healthy. Usually, they want to look or feel better, be more productive or competitive, or behave more independently. They're more likely to change, and to stick with a change, if they can see that the health benefits also enhance other important aspects of their lives.

Perceptions are the way we see things from our unique perspective; they vary greatly with age. As a student, you may not think that living a few hours longer is a significant gain; as you grow older, however, you may prize every additional second.

Enabling factors

Enabling factors include skills, resources, accessible facilities, and physical and mental capacities. Before you initiate a change, assess the means available to reach your goal. No matter how motivated you are, you'll become frustrated if you keep encountering obstacles. That's why breaking a task or goal down into step-by-step strategies is so important in behavioral change.

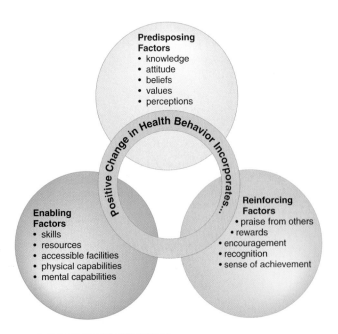

Predisposing Factors
• knowledge
• attitude
• beliefs
• values
• perceptions

Positive Change in Health Behavior Incorporates...

Enabling Factors
• skills
• resources
• accessible facilities
• physical capabilities
• mental capabilities

Reinforcing Factors
• praise from others
• rewards
• encouragement
• recognition
• sense of achievement

FIGURE 2-1 ❚ Factors that Shape Positive Behavior

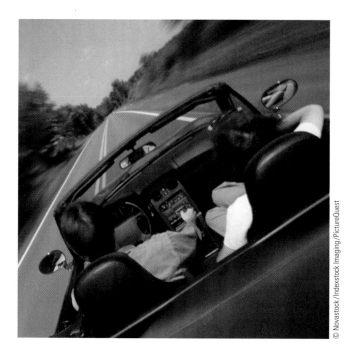

▌ Your *stated* belief and knowledge may be that unsafe driving can cause accidents, but your *actual* belief is that it won't happen to you. To learn how to change predisposing factors that influence your behavior, read this chapter carefully.

Reinforcing factors

Reinforcing factors may be praise from family and friends, rewards from teachers or parents, or encouragement and recognition for meeting a goal. Although these help a great deal in the short run, lasting change depends not on external rewards but on an internal commitment and sense of achievement. To make a difference, reinforcement must come from within.

A decision to change a health behavior should stem from a permanent, personal goal, not from a desire to please or impress someone else. If you lose weight for the homecoming dance, you're almost sure to regain pounds afterward. But if you shed extra pounds because you want to feel better about yourself or get into shape, you're far more likely to keep off the weight.

✚ The Transtheoretical Model of Change

This theoretical model of behavioral change, developed by psychologist James Prochaska and his colleagues, focuses on the individual's decision making rather than on social or biological influences on behavior.[1] It is the foundation of programs for smoking cessation, exercise, healthy food choices, alcohol abuse, weight control, condom use, drug abuse, mammography screening, and stress management. However, conclusive scientific evidence for its usefulness in lifestyle change remains limited.[2]

These key components of the **transtheoretical model of change** are described in the following sections:

▌ **Stages of Change**
▌ **Processes of Change**—cognitive and behavior activities that facilitate change
▌ **Self-efficacy**—the confidence people have in their ability to cope with challenge.

What are the Stages of Change?

According to the transtheoretical model of change, individuals progress through a sequence of stages as they make a change (**Figure 2-2**). No one stage is more important than another, and people often move back and forth between them. Most "spiral" from stage to stage, slipping from maintenance to contemplation or from action to precontemplation before moving forward again. People usually cycle and recycle through the stages several times. Smokers, for instance, report making three or four serious efforts to quit before they succeed.

The six stages of change are:

1. **Precontemplation.** Whether or not they're aware of a problem behavior, people in this stage have no intention of making a change in the next six months. Busy college students in good health, for instance, might never think about getting more exercise.
2. **Contemplation.** Individuals in this stage are aware they have a problem behavior and are considering changing it within the next six months. However, they may be torn between the positives of the new behavior and the amount of energy, time, and other resources required to change.[3] Students in a health course, for instance, may start thinking about exercising but struggle to balance potential benefits with the effort of getting up early to jog or go to the gym.
3. **Preparation.** People in this stage intend to change a problem behavior within the next month. Some focus on a master plan. For instance, they might look into fitness classes, gyms, or other options for working out. Others might start by making small changes, such as walking to classes rather than taking a campus shuttle bus.
4. **Action.** People in this stage are modifying their behavior according to their plan. For instance, they might be jogging or working out at the gym three times a week.
5. **Maintenance.** In this stage, individuals have continued to work at changing their behavior and have avoided relapse for at least six months. New exercisers are likely to stop during the first three to six months. One reason that researchers have identified: the temptation to not exercise. However, follow-up,

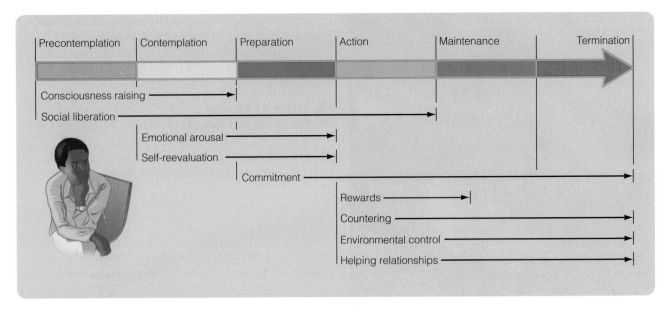

FIGURE 2-2 ▌ The Stages of Change and Some Change Processes

These change processes can help you progress through the stages of change. Each may be most useful at particular stages.

whether by mail, e-mail, or phone calls from supportive friends, family, or a counselor, can help maintain physical activity levels.[4]

6. **Termination.** While it may take two to five years, a behavior becomes so deeply ingrained that a person can't imagine abandoning it. More than eight in ten college seniors who exercised regularly for example, remain as active, or even more active, after graduation.

As research on college students has shown, attitudes and feelings are related to stages of change. Smokers who believe that continuing to smoke would have only a minor or no impact on their health remain in the precontemplation stage; those with respiratory symptoms move on to contemplation and preparation.[5] In a study at Ohio State University, researchers classified student heavy drinkers according to the stages of change: Nearly two-thirds of the "precontemplators" continued to drink heavily and had no intention of changing their behavior. In the maintenance stage, students drank an average of one alcoholic drink a month even though they felt that heavy drinking was the norm on their campus.[6]

The Processes of Change

Anything you do to modify your thinking, feeling, or behavior can be called a change process. The nine included in the transtheoretical model are:

Consciousness-Raising The most widely used change process involves increasing knowledge about yourself or the nature of your problem. As you learn more, you gain understanding and feedback about your behavior.
Example: Reading Chapter 8 on making healthy food choices.

Social Liberation This process takes advantage of alternatives in the external environment that can help you begin or continue your efforts to change.
Example: Spending as much time as possible in no-smoking areas.

Emotional Arousal This process, also known as dramatic relief, works on a deeper level than consciousness-raising and is equally important in the early stages of change. Emotional arousal means experiencing and expressing feelings about a problem behavior and its potential solutions.
Example: Resolving never to drink and drive after the death of a friend in a car accident.

Self-Reevaluation This process requires a thoughtful reappraisal of your problem, including an assessment of the person you might be once you have changed the behavior.
Example: Recognizing that you have a gambling problem and imagining yourself as a nongambler.

Commitment This process acknowledges—first privately and then publicly—that you are responsible for your behavior and the only one who can change it.
Example: Joining a self-help or support group.

Countering Countering, or counterconditioning, substitutes healthy behaviors for unhealthy ones.
Example: Chewing gum rather than smoking.

Environmental Control This action-oriented process restructures your environment so you are less likely to engage in a problem behavior.
Example: Getting rid of your stash of sweets.

Rewards This process reinforces positive behavioral changes with self-praise or small gifts.
Example: Getting a massage after a month of consistent exercise.

Helping Relationships This process recruits individuals —family, friends, therapist, coach—to provide support, caring, understanding, and acceptance.
Example: Finding an exercise buddy.

Self-Efficacy and Locus of Control

Do you see yourself as master of your fate, asserting control over your destiny? Or do so many things happen in your life that you just hang on and hope for the best? The answers to these questions reveal two important characteristics that affect your wellness: your sense of **self-efficacy** (the belief in your ability to change and to cope with challenge) and your **locus of control** (the sense of being in control of your life).

Your confidence in your ability to cope with challenge can determine whether you can and will succeed in making a change. In his research on self-efficacy, psychologist Albert Bandura of Stanford University found that the individuals most likely to reach a goal are those who believe that they can. The stronger their faith in themselves, the more energy and persistence they put into making a change. The opposite is also true, especially for health behaviors. Among people who begin an exercise program, those with lower self-efficacy are more likely to drop out.

If you believe that your actions will make a difference in your health, your locus of control is internal. If you believe that external forces or factors play a greater role, your locus of control is external. Hundreds of studies have compared people who have these different perceptions of control. "Internals," who believe that their actions largely determine what happens to them, act more independently, enjoy better health, and are more optimistic about their future. "Externals," who perceive that chance or outside forces determine their fate, find it harder to cope with stress and feel increasingly helpless over time. When it comes to weight, for instance, they see themselves as destined to be fat.

How You Change

Awareness of a negative behavior is always the first step toward changing it. Once you identify what you'd like to change, use your Wellness Journal as a behavioral diary for one or two weeks, noting what you do, when, where, and what you're feeling at the time. If you'd like, enlist the help of friends or family to call attention to your be-

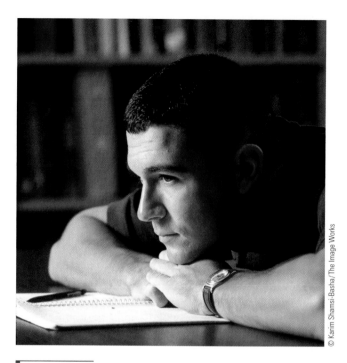

Do you picture yourself as master of your own destiny? You are more likely to achieve your wellness goals if you believe that you are in control of your life.

havior. Sometimes self-observation in itself proves therapeutic: Just the act of keeping a journal can be enough to help you lose weight or kick the smoking habit.

Decisional Balance

In making a change, you have to weigh its potential pluses and minuses. Decisional balance involves consideration of the consequences of change to yourself and others and the reactions of both yourself and others as a result of change. These can be both positive and negative.

For instance, if your target health behavior goal is to stop smoking, you will definitely benefit in many ways, such as breathing more easily and lowering your risk of heart disease and cancer. But you may gain a few pounds or miss the camaraderie of hanging out with fellow smokers. You are more likely to make —and maintain— a health change if you see the pros of the change outweighing the cons.

Self-Management

Once you've identified the situations, moods, thoughts, or people that act as cues for a behavior, identify the most powerful ones and develop a plan to avoid them. For instance, if you snack continuously when studying in your room, try working in the library, where food is forbidden.

Planning ahead is a crucial part of successful change. If you can't avoid certain situations, anticipate how you might cope with the temptation to return to your old behavior. Develop alternatives. Visualize yourself walking past the desserts in the cafeteria or chewing gum instead of lighting a cigarette.

Some people find it helpful to sign a "contract," a written agreement in which they make a commitment to change, with their partner, parent, or health educator. Spelling out what they intend to do, and why, underscores the seriousness of what they're trying to accomplish (see the example at the end of the chapter).

Norms

Social and cultural **norms**—behaviors that are expected, accepted, or supported by a group—can make change much harder if they're constantly working against a person's best intentions. You may resolve to eat less, for instance, yet your mother may keep offering you homemade fudge and brownies because your family's norm is to show love by making and offering delicious treats. Or you might decide to drink less, yet your friends' norm may be to equate drinking with having a good time.

If you're aware of the norms that influence your behavior, you can devise strategies either to change them (by encouraging your friends to dance more and drink less at parties, for example) or adapt to them (having just a bite of your mother's sweets). Another option is to develop relationships with people who share your goals and whose norms can reinforce your behavior.

Self-Talk

Your **self-talk**—the messages you send yourself—also can play a role. In recent decades, mental health professionals have recognized the conscious use of positive self-talk as a powerful force for changing the way individuals think, feel, and behave. "We have a choice about how we think," explains psychologist Martin Seligman, Ph.D., author of *Learned Optimism*. As he notes, by learning to challenge automatic negative thoughts that enter our brains and asserting our own statements of self-worth, we can transform ourselves into optimists who see what's right rather than pessimists forever focusing on what's wrong.[7]

Incentives

Get support from friends, but don't expect them to supply all the motivation you need. You may join a group of overweight individuals and rely on their encouragement to stick to your diet. That's a great way to get going; but in the long run, your own commitment to making a change has got to be strong enough to help you sustain your new behaviors.

Reinforcements—either positive (a reward) or negative (a punishment)—also can play a role. Plan a pleasant reward as an incentive for every week you stick to your new behavior—sleeping in on a Saturday morning, going out with some friends, or spending a sunny afternoon outdoors. Small, regular rewards are more effective in keeping up motivation than one big reward that won't come for many months.

STRATEGIES for CHANGE

Use the Language of Change

Pay attention both to what you say when you talk or think about a health behavior change and how you say it. Then consciously edit the words in your mind and as you say them.

▍ **Watch out for weasel words.**
Are you "planning" to quit smoking? "Hoping" to lose weight? When you use linguistic loopholes like "trying" or "hoping," you give yourself permission to settle for whatever happens. When you speak of goals, use definitive, unequivocal language.

▍ **Trade tenses.**
When thinking or talking about bad health habits, switch to the past tense. Instead of saying, "I'm too lazy to exercise," tell yourself, "I used to be too lazy to exercise." This reminds you that you have changed, are changing, or at the least are capable of change.

▍ **Not "if" but "when."**
Instead of saying, "If I could exercise more," say to yourself, "When I start exercising more." This simple switch sets the stage for believing that you will be able to change your lifestyle.

▍ **Just "because."**
According to social psychology research, using the word "because" when making a request or seeking agreement can boost your compliance as high as 80 to 90 percent. For instance, you might tell yourself: "I won't buy doughnuts *because* I don't want to be tempted."

▍ **Guard against demeaning words and phrases.**
When a derogatory statement about yourself forms in your brain, say firmly, "Stop!" or "Delete!" If this is a hard habit to break, wear a rubber band on your wrist and snap it to alert yourself that you are thinking negative, debilitating thoughts.

▍ **Don't focus on what you can't do.**
Remind yourself of your strengths every day. Say to yourself, "I can go another five minutes on the treadmill," or "I can stand another half hour without a cigarette."

WELLNESS COACH

✚ Going for Your Goals

Think of goals as road maps that give you both a destination and a planned itinerary for getting there. "To set goals means to set a course for your life," says psychologist James Fadiman, author of *Unlimit Your Life:*

Setting and Getting Goals, "Without goals, you remain what you were. With goals, you become what you wish."[8] As studies of performance in students, athletes, and employees have shown, the one single characteristic that separates high- and low-achievers is having a clear, specific goal.[9] (See Student Snapshot: "Top Goals of Undergraduates.") The following sections describe the most effective strategies for using goals to map your way to the life you want.

Set Your Sights on a Destination

You wouldn't board a bus without knowing where you want to go, but it's easy to drift through life with only a vague sense of where you're heading. Unfortunately, goals that don't lead somewhere—like wanting to be healthy—tend to go nowhere. A specific, focused, realistic goal—like developing your upper body strength or reaching a certain weight—can fast-forward you into the future.

The more vividly that you can see, feel, touch, and taste what you want, the more likely you are to achieve it. The reason, explains psychologist Kenneth W. Christian, author of *Your Own Worst Enemy,* is that a destination goal transforms your brain into a satellite dish picking up the signals that are most relevant to your quest. "You begin to see possibilities that pull you closer to your goal. You meet people who can help you. It can seem magical, but it's not. Your unconscious mind is working on your goal while you go on with your life."[10]

Take a Step and a Stretch

With your target goal in sight, set "step and stretch" goals. Think of them like stair steps that lift you out of your comfort zone and keep you moving forward. It doesn't matter how many there are. In some instances, it may be six; in others, sixty. Every goal should be a reach from where you are that will bring you to the next level.

Break down each step goal into projects, and every project into tasks. Ask yourself the following questions, and write down the answers.

- What skills do I need to achieve this?
- What information and knowledge must I acquire?
- What help, assistance, or resources do I need?
- What can block my progress? (For each potential barrier, list solutions.)
- Whom can I turn to for support?
- Who or what is likely to get in my way?
- How am I most likely to sabotage myself?

As you develop your game plan, make sure each goal is within your control. "Other people should not have to change in order for you to meet your goal," emphasizes Fadiman. Don't depend on your roommate to jump on your get-organized bandwagon, or your friends to sizzle with the same enthusiasm for

---

STRATEGIES *for* CHANGE

Is Your Goal S.M.A.R.T.?

Many professional coaches use the following questions to help clients set effective goals:

- **Specific?**
  Identifying exactly what you want to accomplish helps you plan the steps that lead to your goal.

- **Measurable?**
  Your goal should be concrete enough so that both you and others can see the progress you're making.

- **Achievable?**
  Set goals that are slightly out of your immediate grasp, but not so far that there is no hope of achieving them.

- **Rewarding?**
  You will be more motivated to reach your goals if you can clearly define the benefits of doing so.

- **Time Defined?**
  Set a timeframe for the goal. Putting an end point on your goal gives you a clear target to work towards.

---

shaping up for a marathon. Focus on the process not the outcome.

What is an Affirmation?

Once you've pictured your goal in detail, express it in an **affirmation,** a single positive sentence. As decades

---

STUDENT SNAPSHOT

Top Goals of Undergraduates

Goal	
Raising a family	75%
Being very well off financially	74%
Helping others who are in difficulty	62%
Becoming an authority in my field	58%
Obtaining recognition from my colleagues for my contributions to my field	52%

Percentage of students who say this is a goal as based on a national survey of 289,452 students at 440 colleges and universities.

Source: Sax, Linda, et al. *The American Freshman: National Norms for Fall 2004.* Los Angeles: UCLA Higher Education Research Institute, 2004.

of psychological research have shown, affirmations serve as powerful tools for behavioral change. One key to their success is the present tense. "In your mind's inner grammar, the present tense predicts the future while the words 'I will' delay it," says Fadiman. "The impact is subtle but critical when you're setting goals."

In Fadiman's work with smokers, those who repeated the phrase "I am not a smoker" daily—even though they were allowed to continue smoking—typically threw away their cigarettes within a few weeks. "If you are not a smoker, you don't need or want cigarettes," he explains. "If you hold any statement in your conscious mind, there is an effort to bring it into reality. That's why when you change your thoughts and attitudes, your behavior follows." You don't need to tag a deadline onto a destination goal. "If you tell yourself you're going to lose weight by the end of the year, that's how long it will take," says Fadiman. "Why wait?"

Once you've polished your affirmation, put it on paper. By putting it in writing, you become more committed to making your words come true. Some people post their affirmations on their computers and night stands or carry them in their wallets; others scrawl them in big letters across the bathroom mirror. Wherever you jot yours, look at your affirmation often—ideally at least once a day.

Visualize the Hurdles

During training, many athletes visualize crossing the finish line or scoring the winning point. Gold medal Olympian Edwin Moses used a different technique: He visualized every hurdle in a 400-meter race, calculating the distance between each and seeing himself clearing each one. Goal-getters do the same. If you think ahead to what might go wrong, you can come up with ways of going over, under, around, or through whatever obstacles you encounter. If you don't anticipate and problem-solve, obstacles turn into excuses.

Remember that you don't have to go it alone. A buddy or accountability partner can help—by checking in every week, joining you if you're going to the gym, or reminding you of why you set your goal in the first place.

Go All the Way

Despite good intentions and considerable progress, many people give up their goals just before the rainbow's end—and congratulate themselves for getting that far. "Would you ever board a plane for Chicago and say, 'Well, we got three-quarters of the way there!' as if that were good?" asks psychologist Christian, who urges goal-seekers to persist, persevere, and "not settle for almost-there." If you stall on the final stretch, do a quick reality check. Maybe you need to add some smaller step goals, seek more support, or simply allow yourself more time.

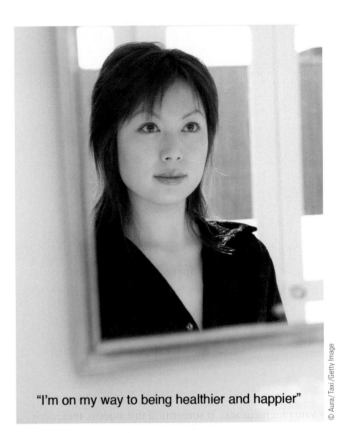

"I'm on my way to being healthier and happier"

▍ An affirmation, a single positive statement, is a powerful tool to help you make a change.

Set aside a page or section in your Wellness Journal to amend, modify, refine, expand, and extend your goals. Whenever you achieve one, check it off, acknowledge it, tell a friend, or just raise your hands above your head like a runner crossing the finish line. This is what builds your sense of "I can do it. I AM doing it. Look how far I've come!"

✚ Making Good Wellness Decisions

Every day you make decisions that have immediate and long-term effects on your health. You decide what to eat, whether to drink or smoke, when to exercise, and how to cope with a sudden crisis. Beyond these daily matters, you decide when to see a doctor, what kind of doctor, and with what sense of urgency. You decide what to tell your doctor and whether to follow the advice given, whether to keep up your immunizations, whether to have a prescription filled and comply with the medication instructions, and whether to seek further help or a second opinion. The entire process of maintaining or restoring health depends on your decisions; it cannot start or continue without them.

The small decisions of everyday life—what to eat, where to go, when to study—are straightforward choices. Larger decisions—which major to choose, what to do about a dead-end relationship, how to handle an awkward work situation—are more challenging. However, if you think of decision making as a process, you can break down even the most difficult choices into manageable steps:

▌ **Set priorities.** Rather than getting bogged down in details, step back and look at the big picture. What matters most to you? What would you like to accomplish in the next week, month, year? Look at the decision you're about to make in the context of your values and goals.

▌ **Inform yourself.** The more you know—about a person, a position, a place, a project—the better you'll be able to evaluate it. Gathering information may involve formal research, such as an online or library search for relevant data, or informal conversations with teachers, counselors, family members, or friends.

▌ **Consider all your options.** Most complex decisions don't involve simple either-or alternatives. List as many options as you can think of, along with the advantages and disadvantages of each.

▌ **Tune in to your gut feelings.** After you've gotten the facts and analyzed them, listen to your intuition. While it's not infallible, your sixth sense can provide valuable feedback. If something just doesn't feel right, try to figure out why. Are there any fears you haven't dealt with? Do you have doubts about taking a certain path?

▌ **Consider a worst-case scenario.** When you've come close to a final decision, imagine what will happen if everything goes wrong—the workload becomes overwhelming, your partner betrays your trust, your expectations turn out to be unrealistic. If you can live with the worst consequences of a decision, you're probably making the right choice.

Unhealthy Habits on Campus

Often on their own for the first time, college students leave behind their family's ways of eating, sleeping, and relaxing and develop new habits and routines—usually not healthier ones. Many simply don't get enough sleep or keep irregular schedules that throw their sleep patterns off. Often it seems that there aren't enough hours in the day for all the things undergraduates need or want to do—study, socialize, pursue extracurricular activities, surf the Internet, work at part-time jobs, participate in community service. Sleeping less, juggling more, students can quickly end up exhausted—and at greater risk for colds, flus, digestive problems, and other maladies.

Poor sleep can be both a symptom and a cause of stress, which, as discussed in Chapter 7, is especially common among freshmen. More undergraduates are seeking psychological counseling to deal with the strain they feel as well as mental disorders such as anxiety and depression.

Students who endure harassment or abuse of any sort are more likely to report health-related symptoms. Those most at risk include minority students as well as gay, lesbian, and bisexual undergraduates.

SAVVY CONSUMER

ASSESSING RISKS

At any age, the greatest health threats stem from high-risk behaviors—smoking, excessive drinking, not getting enough exercise, eating too many high-fat foods, driving recklessly, and not getting regular medical checkups, to name just a few. That's why changing unhealthy habits is the best way to reduce risks and prevent health problems.

Environmental health risks are the subject of newspaper headlines. Every year brings calls of alarm about a new hazard to health: electromagnetic radiation, fluoride in drinking water, hair dyes, silicone implants, radon, lead. Often the public response is panic. Consumers picket and protest. Individuals arrange for elaborate testing. Yet how do we know whether or not alleged health risks are acceptable? Some key factors to consider are:

▌ **Are there possible benefits?** Advantages—such as the high salary paid for working with toxic chemicals or radioactive materials—may make some risks seem worth taking.

▌ **Is the risk voluntary?** All of us tend to accept risks that we freely choose to take, such as playing a sport that could lead to injuries, as opposed to risks imposed on us, such as threats of terrorism.

▌ **Is the risk fair?** The risk of skin cancer affects us all. We may worry about it and take action to protect ourselves and our planet, but we don't resent it the way we resent living with the risk of violence because the only housing we can afford is in a high-crime area.

▌ **Are there alternatives?** As consumers, we may become upset about cancer-causing pesticides or food additives when we learn about safer chemicals or methods of preservation.

▌ **Are lives saved or lost?** Our thinking about risks often depends on how they're presented. For instance, if we're told that a new drug may kill 1 out of every 100 people, we react differently than if we're told that it may save the lives of 99 percent of those who use it.

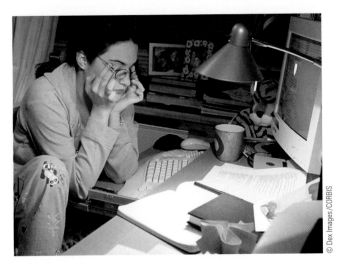

▌ Unhealthy habits often become routine for college students—and may make them more susceptible to health problems both in the short and long term.

Nutrition habits also change during college. As discussed in Chapter 8, the majority of freshmen say their diet has changed for the worse. During their first year, students often gain a few pounds (although less than the notorious "freshman 15").

Students also become more sedentary in college, as they log more hours in classes and in front of computers. The combination of a high-fat diet and a sedentary lifestyle in college can set the stage for the development of health problems that include obesity, diabetes, metabolic syndrome, heart disease, and certain cancers.

How Can I Change ▄▇ a Bad Health Habit?

Change is never easy—even if it's done for the best possible reasons. When you decide to change a behavior, you have to give up something familiar and easy for something new and challenging. Change always involves risk —and the prospect of rewards.

Researchers have identified approaches other than the transtheoretical model that people use to make beneficial changes. In the moral model, you take responsibility for a problem (such as smoking) and its solution; success depends on adequate motivation, while failure is seen as a sign of character weakness. In the enlightenment model, you submit to strict discipline to correct a problem; this is the approach used in Alcoholics Anonymous. The behavioral model involves rewarding yourself when you make positive changes. The medical model sees the behavior as caused by forces beyond your control (a genetic predisposition to being overweight, for example) and employs an expert to provide advice or treatment. For many people, the most effective approach is the compensatory model, which doesn't assign blame but puts responsibility on individuals to acquire whatever skills or power they need to overcome their problems.

Before they reach the stage where they can and do take action to change, most people go through a process comparable to religious conversion. First, they reach a level of accumulated unhappiness that makes them ready for change. Then they have a moment of truth that makes them want to change. One pregnant woman, for instance, felt her unborn baby quiver when she drank a beer and swore never to drink again. As people change their behavior, they change their lifestyles and identities as well. Ex-smokers, for instance, may start an aggressive exercise program, make new friends at the track or gym, and participate in new types of activities, like racquetball games or fun runs.

Think about the behavior you want to change. Now think about which of the six stages of change you are in with regard to that behavior. Table 2-1 lists some appropriate change goals for each stage. Set your goal and go for it!

TABLE 2-1 ▮ Stages of Lifestyle Change

Stage of Change	Appropriate Change Goal
1. Precontemplation: you are not truly convinced about the importance of the lifestyle goal.	Get more information about the value of the lifestyle change goal.
2. Contemplation: you have no definite plan for when to begin but would like to change.	Set a date for making the change.
3. Preparation: you have set a date to begin the new behavior and are planning the best strategy to carry out the change.	Develop a plan and tell others about the change.
4. Action: you are engaged in making changes.	Adjust to new lifestyle and manage unexpected emotional and physical reactions.
5. Maintenance: you are working to integrate the lifestyle change into normal day-to-day life.	Continue to pay attention to the behavior and work through any relapse. Help others achieve similar lifestyle goals.
6. Termination: you have maintained the change for six months to a year and are ready to move on to other lifestyle interests.	Set new health-enhancing goals. Move on from support systems that are focused exclusively on the prior lifestyle goal.

Source: Human Resources Institute. www.healthyculture.com/Articles/mentoarticle.html

Recovering from a Relapse

Once you are ready to change, getting started with an action plan is not the greatest challenge you'll face. That usually comes weeks or months later, when your progress hits a wall or you return to your old, unhealthy habits. Rather than looking for someone or something to help you get back on track, try the following:

▌ Gather data. Use your Wellness Journal to keep a detailed log of your behavior for a week, including a weekend. If you're trying to make healthier food choices, record everything you put in your mouth. If your goal is to get into better shape, keep track of how much time you spend on sedentary pursuits, on what derails your plans to exercise, of the types of activities you most enjoy, and so on.

▌ Reassess your goals. Are your expectations too high? Is your timetable unrealistic? Have you been derailed by finals, stress, the flu, a family crisis?

▌ Check with your doctor. Various medical conditions (such as infections, depression, diabetes) and certain medications (including corticosteroids and hormones) can undermine your energy and ability to pursue your wellness goals.

▌ Problem-solve your way around the wall. Ask yourself the following questions, and write your answers in your Wellness Journal.
1. What is your biggest wellness problem right now? Make it specific: For example, I stick to my diet during the week but blow it on weekends. Or I smoke when I play poker with my friends.
2. List every way you can think of to solve this problem. The more solutions you list, the greater your chance of finding the one that will work best for you. For instance, to avoid weekend overeating, you might volunteer at a hospice or library. Or you might change your poker site to a nonsmoking setting.
3. Read over your solution list, and put a check by those that make the most sense for your lifestyle. Pick one solution and implement it this week. If after a month, this solution has failed you or you have failed it, read over your list again, and pick the next one on the list.

▌ Autopsy setbacks. If you blow your diet or slide back into couch-potato habits, analyze what went wrong and why. Start with the following questions, which you can answer in your Wellness Journal.
1. What blindsided, distracted, demoralized, or otherwise derailed your plan?
2. What excuses did you use?
3. Who were the saboteurs who undermined your efforts?
4. How did they sidetrack you?

▌ Now focus on the future.
1. What potential pitfalls do you anticipate?
2. How will you overcome them?
3. What are your backup plans in case something or someone unexpectedly tries to sabotage your current efforts to change a health behavior?

MAKING HEALTHY CHOICES

Lifelong Wellness

"Every man desires to live long," writes Jonathan Swift, "but no man would be old." We all wish for long lives, yet we want to avoid the disease and disability that can tarnish our golden years. Here are the best ways to ensure a lifetime of wellness.

▌ **Exercise regularly.** By improving blood flow, staving off depression, warding off heart disease, and enhancing well-being, regular workouts help keep mind and body in top form.

▌ **Don't smoke.** Every cigarette you puff can snuff out seven minutes of your life, according to the Centers for Disease Control and Prevention.

▌ **Watch your weight and blood pressure.** Increases in these vital statistics can increase your risk of hypertension, cardiovascular disease, and other health problems.

▌ **Eat more fruits and vegetables.** These foods, rich in vitamins and protective antioxidants, can reduce your risk of cancer and damage from destructive free radicals.

▌ **Cut down on fat.** Fatty foods can clog the arteries and contribute to various cancers.

▌ **Limit drinking.** Alcohol can undermine physical health and sabotage mental acuity.

▌ **Cultivate stimulating interests.** Elderly individuals with complex and interesting lifestyles are most likely to retain sharp minds and memories beyond age 70.

▌ **Don't worry; be happy.** At any age, emotional turmoil can undermine well-being. Relaxation techniques, such as meditation, help by reducing stress.

▌ **Reach out.** Try to keep in contact with other people of all ages and experiences. Make the effort to invite them to your home or go out with them. On a regular basis, do something to help another person.

▌ **Make the most of your time.** Greet each day with a specific goal—to take a walk, write letters, visit a friend.

SELF-SURVEY

Where Are You? The Readiness for Change Ruler

1. On the ruler below, mark where you are now on this line that measures change in behavior. Are you not prepared to change, already changing, or someplace in the middle?

Not prepared
to change

Already
changing

2. Answer the questions that apply to you.

▮ If your mark is on the left side of the line:
How will you know when it's time to think about changing?
What signals will tell you to start thinking about changing?
What qualities in yourself are important to you?
What connection is there between those qualities and "not considering a change"?

▮ If your mark is somewhere in the middle:
Why did you put your mark there and not further to the left?
What might make you put your mark a little further to the right?
What are the good things about the way you're currently trying to change?
What are the not-so-good things?
What would be the good result of changing?
What are the barriers to changing?

▮ If your mark is on the right side of the line:
Pick one of the barriers to change and list some things that could help you overcome this barrier.
Pick one of those things that could help and decide to do it by _____ (write in a specific date).

▮ If you've taken a serious step in making a change:
What made you decide on that particular step?
What has worked in taking this step?
What helped it work?
What could help it work even better?
What else would help?
Can you break that helpful step down into smaller pieces?
Pick one of those pieces and decide to do it by _____ (write in a specific date).

▮ If you're changing and trying to maintain that change:
Congratulations! What's helping you?

What else would help?
What are your high-risk situations?

▮ If you've "fallen off the wagon":
What worked for a while?
Don't kick yourself—long-term change almost always takes a few cycles.
What did you learn from the experience that will help you when you give it another try?

3. The following are stages people go through in making important changes in their health behaviors. All the stages are important. We learn from each stage. We go **from** "not thinking about it" **to** "weighing the pros and cons" **to** "making little changes and figuring out how to deal with the really hard parts" **to** "doing it!" **to** "making it part of our lives." Many people "fall off the wagon" and go through all the stages several times before the change really lasts.

Source: Zimmerman, Gretchen, et al. "A 'Stages of Change' Approach to Helping Patients Change Behavior." American Academy of Family Physicians, March 1, 2000, www.aafp.org/afp/20000301/1409.html

ACTION PLAN

Your Action Plan for Healthy Change

Now that you have a sense of your stage of readiness for change, use the following stage-specific ideas to get you going in the right direction.

Precontemplation (Not Active and Not Thinking about Becoming Active)

▮ Commit yourself to attending class, reading the textbook, and completing assignments and labs.

▮ List what you see as the disadvantages (or cons) of behavioral change. For example, do you fear making a change will be too difficult or will take up too much time? Write down a healthy change that you could make tomorrow that would take less than 15 minutes of your time.

Contemplation (Not Active but Thinking about Becoming Active)

▮ Think back to activities and experiences you found enjoyable in the past. Did they include playing a sport, taking hikes, singing in a group? Ask friends and coworkers if they can put you in touch with others with the same interest.

▮ Take a realistic look at your daily schedule and life circumstances. How much time could you carve out for a new healthy behavior? How much money could you invest in it?

▌ Find an image of the life you'd like to have—from a magazine article or advertisement, for example—and post it where you can see it often.

Preparation (Active but Not at Recommended Levels)

▌ Identify specific barriers that limit your activity. If you live in a dorm, your food choices may be limited. If you have a part-time job, you may feel you're constantly on the run and can't take steps to de-stress your life.

▌ Set specific daily and weekly goals. Your daily goal might begin with 10 or 15 minutes of exercise or relaxation and increase by 5 minutes every week or two. If you're trying to overcome shyness, your weekly goal might be to strike up a conversation with five strangers or to attend one social event.

▌ Document your progress. Use your Wellness Journal to track what's going right and what's not. Take time to brainstorm every night about what you might do differently the next day.

Action and Maintenance (Active at Recommended Levels for Less than Six Months)

▌ Reach out for support. If you're dieting, log on to a diet blog. If you're shaping up, join a team that's training for a charity run or an intramural competition.

▌ Develop new interests and skills that reinforce your goal. If you are quitting smoking, spend more and more time in places where you can't smoke and with people who don't smoke.

▌ Become a mentor. As you incorporate your healthy new behavior into your identity, reach out to help others who want to do the same. Swap diet strategies with a friend who's just committed to losing weight. Demonstrate some of the more challenging postures and exercises to a newcomer to your Pilates or yoga class.

SETTING GOALS

Identifying Your Target Goal

1. Choose four health or fitness goals that you believe would change the quality of your life. Word them in a positive way. What do you want?
   1. _____
   2. _____
   3. _____
   4. _____

2. To focus your behavior and be successful, you must first decide which goal is the MOST important for you to take care of right away. Analyze your goals by answering these questions. Give each question a value based on a scale of 1–10: 10 = most valuable and/or easiest to attain; 1 = least valuable and/or hardest to attain.

Goal #1 _____
   How important is this goal to me? _____
   How attainable is the goal? _____
   Are resources available to help me attain this goal? _____
   Do I have the time needed to reach this goal? _____
   How will reaching this goal affect my overall happiness? _____
   Will the rewards be worth the time and effort? _____

Goal #2 _____
   How important is this goal to me? _____
   How attainable is the goal? _____
   Are resources available to help me attain this goal? _____
   Do I have the time needed to reach this goal? _____
   How will reaching this goal affect my overall happiness? _____
   Will the rewards be worth the time and effort? _____

Goal #3 _____
   How important is this goal to me? _____
   How attainable is the goal? _____
   Are resources available to help me attain this goal? _____
   Do I have the time needed to reach this goal? _____
   How will reaching this goal affect my overall happiness? _____
   Will the rewards be worth the time and effort? _____

Goal #4 _____
   How important is this goal to me? _____
   How attainable is the goal? _____
   Are resources available to help me attain this goal? _____
   Do I have the time needed to reach this goal? _____
   How will reaching this goal affect my overall happiness? _____
   Will the rewards be worth the time and effort? _____

3. The goal that has the highest priority value will be your first "target goal." You have given it the most value. Make achieving it your priority!

   Target goal: _____

4. Now turn to Chapter 2 of your Lab Booklet and use this new target goal when working through Lab 1: Setting a S.M.A.R.T. Goal and Lab 2: Behavior Change Contract.

*My Contract For Change**

Note: See your Lab Booklet for a goal-setting activity.

Date: _____

Wellness goal: _____

_____

_____

_____

Change(s) I promise to make to reach this goal:

_____

Plan for making this change: _____

_____

_____

Start date: _____

Short-term goals: _____

_____

_____

_____

If I need help: _____

_____

_____

Target date for reaching goal: _____

Reward for achieving goal: _____

Penalty for failing to achieve goal: _____

_____

Signed: _____

Witnessed by: _____

*Also available on HealthNow

WELLNESS JOURNAL

Countering the "Cons" of Change

One way to motivate yourself to initiate or maintain a health behavior change is to identify what you see as disadvantages, or "cons," and list ways to work over, around, or through them. Here are some examples of the cons of exercising. Read through them, then come up with your own list of cons and counters for your behavioral change goal:

Cons	Countercons
Too busy	▌ Wake up half an hour earlier to get your workout done for the day.
	▌ Settle for half workouts if you can't do a full one.
	▌ Set aside exercise "appointments" on your schedule.
Boring	▌ Mix it up. Walk one day; bike or jog the next.
	▌ Try something new, like tai chi.

CHAPTER

2 Making This Chapter Work for You

1. The development of health behaviors is influenced by all of the following *except:*
   a. Reinforcing factors, which involve external recognition for achieving a goal.
   b. Preexisting health factors, which take into account the individual's current position on the wellness continuum.
   c. Predisposing factors, which include knowledge, attitudes, and beliefs.
   d. Enabling factors, which are related to an individual's skills and capabilities to make behavior changes.

2. Change processes, cognitive and behavior activities that facilitate change, include all of these *except:*
   a. Consciousness raising.
   b. Countering.
   c. Health awareness.
   d. Helping relationships.

3. Dylan decided to learn how to meditate to enhance his spiritual wellness and signed up for a workshop starting in two weeks. Dylan is in which stage of change?
   a. Precontemplation
   b. Contemplation
   c. Preparation
   d. Action

4. Bianca almost caused an accident last week when she was weaving between cars on the freeway. The incident scared her so much that she decided to change her driving habits and has stayed at the speed limit all this week. Which stage of change is Bianca in?
   a. Contemplation
   b. Preparation
   c. Action
   d. Maintenance

5. According to the stages of change in the transtheoretical model of change, which statement is *incorrect?*
   a. In the maintenance stage, individuals have avoided relapse for six months.
   b. In the contemplation stage, individuals are considering changing a problem behavior in the next six months.
   c. In the action stage, individuals are actually modifying their behavior according to their plan.
   d. In the preparation stage, individuals intend to change a problem behavior in the next six months.

6. Michelle has a strong internal locus of control. According to research, she is more likely to
   a. Enjoy better health.
   b. Get a better job.
   c. Become a health-care professional.
   d. Be worried about the future.

7. If you want to change unhealthy behavior, which of the following strategies is least likely to promote success?
   a. Believe that you can make the change.
   b. Reward yourself regularly.
   c. During self-talks, remind yourself about all your faults.
   d. Accept that you are in control of your health.

8. Some effective strategies for achieving your wellness goals are:
   a. Set "step and stretch" goals.
   b. Use affirmations with the present tense.
   c. Visualize possible obstacles.
   d. All of the above.

9. Cameron feels good because he has made the decision to get fit. What does Cameron have to do next?
   a. Get more specific about his goal.
   b. Start working out.
   c. Find a friend to work out with.
   d. Jog regularly.

10. Relapses are common (you're human, aren't you?), but don't let them keep you from your goal. Which of these strategies might help you recover from a re-lapse?
    a. Have a hot fudge sundae.
    b. Decide to think about it after finals.
    c. Analyze what went wrong and why.
    d. Put yourself back into the contemplation stage.

Answers to these questions can be found on page 376.

Critical Thinking

1. Think about a behavioral change you have made in your life in the past three years in any of the dimensions of wellness (physical, psychological, spiritual, social, intellectual, environmental). Can you remember going through each of the six stages of the transtheoretical model of change?

2. Self-control is a basic human trait usually learned as a child. How might feelings of self-control differ between individuals with an internal locus of control and those with an external locus of control? How do you think "internals" and "externals" differ in their approach to personal change?

3. It is normal for people to require several trips through the stages of change to make a lasting change, and relapse is viewed as a normal part of the change process, just as in the learning process. What do we learn from our relapses? And how do they help us focus?

Media Menu

Health☺Now™

Don't forget to check out the wealth of resources on the HealthNow website at **http://healthnow.brookscole.com/itw** that will:
- Help you evaluate your knowledge of the material
- Allow you to take an exam-prep quiz
- Provide a Personalized Learning Plan targeting resources that address areas you should study
- Coach you through identifying target goals for behavior change and creating and monitoring your personal change plan throughout the semester.

INTERNET CONNECTIONS

The Transtheoretical Model

www.med.usf.edu/~kmbrown/Stages_of_Change_ Overview.htm
This site, from the University of South Florida Community and Family Health, describes the historical development of the Transtheoretical Model and features several useful print references.

Transtheoretical Model-Cancer Prevention Research Center

www.uri.edu/research/cprc/TTM/detailedoverview.htm
This site describes the Transtheoretical Model, including descriptions of effective interventions to promote health behavior change, focusing on the individual's decision-making strategies.

Theories of Behavioral Change

www.csupomona.edu/~jvgrizzell/best_practices/bctheory .html
This very comprehensive site, by the Department of Health Promotion at California Polytechnic University at Pomona, describes all of the theories of behavioral change, including Learning Theories, Transtheoretical Model, Health Belief Model, Relapse Prevention Model, Reasoned Action and Planned Behavior, Social Learning/Social Cognitive Theory, and Social Support.

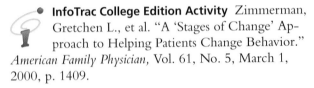 **InfoTrac College Edition Activity** Zimmerman, Gretchen L., et al. "A 'Stages of Change' Approach to Helping Patients Change Behavior." *American Family Physician,* Vol. 61, No. 5, March 1, 2000, p. 1409.

1. What does the Stages of Change Model reveal about behavior changes?

2. According to the Health Belief Model and the External Locus of Control Model, why don't people stop destructive behaviors during the precontemplation stage?

3. What are some successful approaches to help someone move beyond the contemplation phase?

4. How can a relapse prove helpful to future efforts at behavior modification?

"The Effects of a Transtheoretical Model Physical Activity Intervention Program on the Physical Activity Behavior of Female Adolescents." *Research Quarterly for Exercise and Sport,* Vol. 71, No. 1, March 2000, p. A–78.

1. What are the two objectives of this study?

2. What were the barriers to physical activity noted in this study?

3. What are the results of this study using the Transtheoretical Model for physical activity intervention?

You can find additional readings related to personal health with InfoTrac College Edition, an online library of more than 900 journals and publications. Follow the instructions for accessing InfoTrac College Edition that were packaged with your textbook; then search for articles using a keyword search.

For additional links, resources, and suggested readings on the InfoTrac College Edition, visit our Health and Wellness Resource Center at **http://health .wadsworth.com**.

Key Terms

The terms listed are used on the page indicated. Definitions of the terms are in the Glossary at the end of the book.

affirmation 29

enabling factors 24

locus of control 27

norms 28

predisposing factors 24

reinforcements 28

reinforcing factors 25

self-efficacy 27

self-talk 28

transtheoretical model of change 25

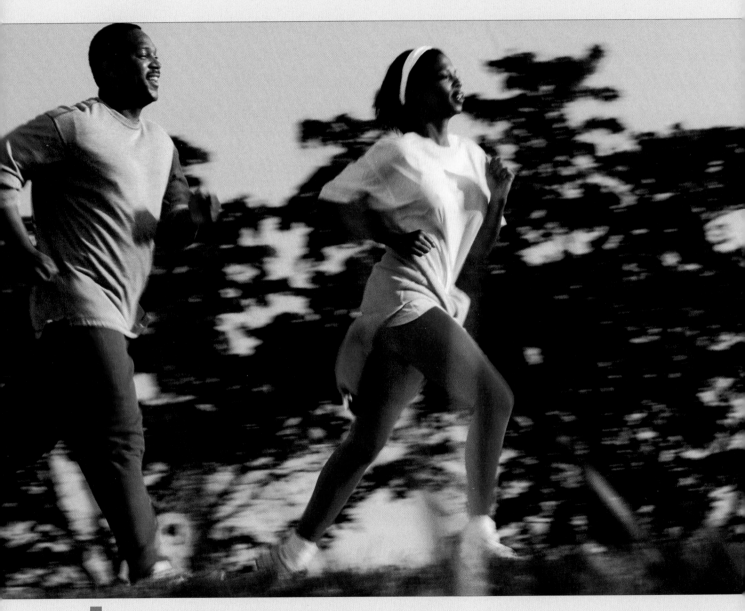

CHAPTER 3

The Joy of Fitness

FREQUENTLY ASKED QUESTIONS

FAQ: Can a person be fat and fit? 48

FAQ: How much exercise is enough? 51

FAQ: How can I prevent injuries? 54

FAQ: What causes cramps and sore muscles? 55

FAQ: How much water should I drink while exercising? 56

As a boy, Derek never thought about doing anything special to stay physically fit. He loved sports so much that he spent every free moment on a softball field or basketball court. He could sprint faster, jump higher, and hit a ball harder than any of his friends. In high school Derek's life revolved around practices and games. He was a varsity athlete and a regional all-star.

Early in his first year in college, an injury sidelined Derek. Frustrated that he had to sit out the season, he gave up his rigorous training routine. As he became immersed in academics and other activities, Derek stopped going to the gym or working out on his own. Yet he continued to think of himself as an athlete in excellent physical condition. When Derek went home for spring break, he joined his younger brothers on a neighborhood basketball court. While he wasn't surprised that his long shots were off, Derek was amazed by how quickly he got winded. In 15 minutes, he was panting for breath. "Getting old," one of his brothers joked. "Getting soft," the other teased.

Often the college years represent a turning point in physical fitness. Like Derek, many students, busy with classes and other commitments, devote less time to physical activity. About four in ten undergraduates do not participate in moderate or vigorous physical activity on a regular basis.[1]

The choices you make and the habits you develop now can affect how long and how well you'll live. As you'll see in this chapter, exercise yields immediate rewards: It boosts energy, improves mood, soothes stress, improves sleep, and makes you look and feel better. In the long term, physical activity slows many of the changes associated with chronological aging, such as loss of calcium and bone density, lowers the risk of serious chronic illnesses, and extends the lifespan.

This chapter can help you reap these rewards. It presents the latest activity recommendations, documents the benefits of exercise, describes types of exercise, and provides guidelines for getting into shape and exercising safely.

After studying the material in this chapter, you should be able to:

▌ **List** the five components of health-related fitness.

▌ **Describe** the health benefits of regular physical activity.

▌ **Explain** the overload principle.

▌ **Define** the four parts of the FITT principle.

▌ **Describe** the PRICE plan for handling an exercise injury.

Health ☾ Now™

Don't forget to check out the wealth of resources on the HealthNow website at **http://healthnow.brookscole.com/itw** that will:

• Help you evaluate your knowledge of the material
• Allow you to take an exam-prep quiz
• Provide a Personalized Learning Plan targeting resources that address areas you should study
• Coach you through identifying target goals for behavior change and creating and monitoring your personal change plan throughout the semester.

✚ What Is Physical Fitness?

The simplest, most practical definition of **physical fitness** is the ability to respond to routine physical demands, with enough reserve energy to cope with a sudden challenge. You can consider yourself fit if you meet your daily energy needs; can handle unexpected extra demands; and are protecting yourself against potential health problems, such as heart disease. Fitness is important both for health and for athletic performance.

Health-Related Fitness

The five health-related components of physical fitness include aerobic or cardiorespiratory endurance, muscular strength, muscular endurance, flexibility, and body composition (the ratio of fat to lean body tissue).

Cardiorespiratory fitness refers to the ability of the heart to pump blood through the body efficiently. It is achieved through **aerobic exercise**—any activity, such as brisk walking or swimming, in which sufficient or excess oxygen is continually supplied to the body. In other words, aerobic exercise involves working out strenuously without pushing to the point of breathlessness.

Muscular strength refers to the force within muscles; it is measured by the absolute maximum weight that you can lift, push, or press in one effort. Strong muscles help keep the skeleton in proper alignment, improve posture, prevent back and leg aches, help in everyday lifting, and enhance athletic performance. Muscle mass increases along with strength, which makes for a healthier body composition and a higher metabolic rate.

Muscular endurance is the ability to perform repeated muscular effort; it is measured by counting how many times you can lift, push, or press a given weight. Important for posture, muscular endurance helps in everyday work as well as in athletics and sports.

Flexibility is the range of motion around specific joints—for example, the stretching you do to touch your toes or twist your torso. Flexibility depends on many factors: your age, gender, and posture; how muscular you are, and how much body fat you have. As children develop, their flexibility increases until adolescence. Then a gradual loss of joint mobility begins and continues throughout adult life. Both muscles and connective tissue, such as tendons and ligaments, shorten and become tighter if not consistently used through their full range of motion.

Body composition refers to the relative amounts of fat and lean tissue (bone, muscle, organs, water) in the body. As discussed in detail in Chapter 9, a high proportion of body fat has serious health implications, including increased incidence of heart disease, high blood pressure, diabetes, stroke, gallbladder problems, back and joint problems, and some forms of cancer.

Physical **conditioning** (or training) refers to the gradual building up of the body to enhance cardiorespiratory or aerobic fitness, muscular strength, muscular endurance, flexibility, and a healthy body composition.

Athletic or Performance-Related Fitness

You may jog five miles, work out with weights, and start each day with a stretching routine. This doesn't qualify you for the soccer team. Most sports, including softball, tennis, and basketball, require additional skills, including:

- Agility, the ability to change direction rapidly.
- Balance, or equilibrium, the ability to maintain a certain body position.
- Coordination, the ability to integrate the movement of body parts to produce smooth, fluid movements.
- Power, the product of force and speed.
- Reaction time, the time required to respond to a stimulus.
- Speed, or velocity, the ability to move rapidly.

While many amateur and professional athletes are in superb overall condition, you do not need athletic skills to keep your body operating at maximum capacity throughout life.

Fitness and Wellness

The concept of fitness is evolving. Rather than focusing only on miles run or weight lifted, instructors, coaches, and consumers are pursuing a broader vision of total fitness that encompasses wellness and wholeness. A key trend in fitness is blending traditional forms of exercise with popular mind–body approaches such as yoga and Pilates (both discussed in Chapter 6). These methods, offered in gyms, fitness centers, and sports medicine facilities across the country, integrate breathing into movement, focus mental awareness, and help us connect with and draw on our internal strengths.

Total fitness enhances every dimension of wellness. Here are some of the ways:

- Physical. As described later in this chapter, becoming fit reduces your risk of major diseases, increases energy and stamina, and may prolong your life.
- Emotional. Fitness lowers tension and anxiety, lifts depression, relieves stress, improves mood, and promotes a positive self-image.
- Social. Physical activities provide opportunities to meet new people and to work out with friends or family.

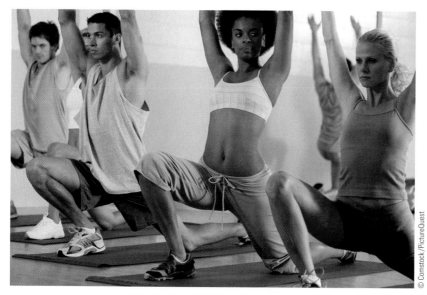

Through mind–body approaches, such as yoga or Pilates, you can develop dimensions of wellness that go beyond the physical.

	Female	Male
Percent fat	27%	15%
Lean body mass	107.8 pounds	134.2 pounds
Blood volume	4.5–5 liters	5–6 liters
Maximum oxygen consumption	3–3.5 liters per minute	5.5–5.9 liters per minute

FIGURE 3-1 ▌ Physiological Differences Between Men and Women

▌ Intellectual. Fit individuals report greater alertness, better concentration, more creativity, and improved personal health habits.

▌ Occupational. Fit employees miss fewer days of work, are more productive, and incur fewer medical costs.

▌ Spiritual. Fitness fosters appreciation for the relationship between body and mind and may lead to greater realization of your potential.

▌ Environmental. Fit individuals often become more aware of their need for healthy air and food and develop a deeper appreciation of the physical world.

Fitness, Gender, and Race

Men and women of all racial backgrounds benefit equally from fitness. However, there are some physiological differences between men and women, many of which are related to size.

On average, men are 10 to 15 percent bigger than women, with roughly twice the percentage of muscle mass and half the percentage of body fat. Overall, men are about 30 percent stronger, particularly above the waist. They have more sweat glands and a greater maximum oxygen uptake. A man's bigger heart pumps more blood with each beat. His larger lungs take in 10 to 20 percent more oxygen (**Figure 3-1**). His longer legs cover more distance with each stride. If a man jogs along at 50 percent of his capacity, a woman has to push to 73 percent of hers to keep up.

Women have a higher percentage of body fat than men, and more is distributed around the hips and thighs; men carry more body fat around the waist and stomach.

College-age men average 15 percent body fat; college-age women, 23 percent. On average, women have 11 percent more body fat and 8 percent less muscle mass than men.[2]

The average woman has a smaller heart and blood volume than a man. Because women have a lower concentration of red blood cells, their bodies are less effective at transporting oxygen to their working muscles during exercise.

Even though training produces the same relative increases for both genders, a woman's maximum oxygen intake remains about 25 to 30 percent lower than that of an equally well-conditioned man. In elite athletes, the gender difference is smaller: 8 to 12 percent. Because the angle of the upper leg bone (femur) to the pelvis is greater in a woman, she is less efficient at running.

In some endurance events, such as ultramarathon running and long-distance swimming, female anatomy and physiology may have some aerobic advantages. The longer a race—on land, water, or ice—the better women perform.

Racial and ethnic background also influences fitness. According to recent research, white men perform better than African-American men on exercise stress tests, which evaluate the heart's health. Among women, physical fitness levels are similar between whites and blacks, but obesity is more common among African Americans.[3] These findings suggest that if you are African American, you may need to place even greater emphasis on improving your overall fitness to reduce your risk of heart disease.[4]

© Comstock/PictureQuest

✚ The Inactivity Epidemic

One in four Americans reports no physical activity at all, according to the Centers for Disease Control and Prevention (CDC). About half exercise occasionally, but not at the levels recommended by the National Center for Chronic Disease Prevention and Health Promotion. Only one in four adults meets the levels of physical activity recommended by federal health officials.[5]

Many factors affect physical activity levels, including geographic location, gender, education, and income. According to the CDC, city-dwellers are more active than country folks, westerners more active than those in other regions. Men, people with higher education levels, and high-income earners work out more often.

How do Americans spend most of their leisure time? Watching television. According to a national survey, adult men spend about 29 hours a week watching television; women average 34 hours per week. The more time that individuals spend in front of the TV, the greater their risk of obesity and related chronic diseases. Compared with other sedentary activities, such as reading, writing, or driving, watching TV lowers metabolic rate so people burn fewer calories. TV viewers are likely to snack as they watch, so they also take in more calories.

The Toll of Sedentary Living

Sedentary living is as great a hazard to health as obesity.[6] Inactivity increases all causes of mortality, doubles the risk of cardiovascular diseases, diabetes, and obesity, and increases the risk of colon cancer, high blood pressure, osteoporosis, depression, and anxiety.[7] The combination of physical inactivity and being overweight is responsible for more than 300,000 deaths a year.[8] Epidemiologists predict that this deadly duo may soon overtake tobacco as the nation's number-one killer.[9]

The economic impact is equally staggering: an estimated $1 trillion in health-care bills a year. As a risk factor for heart disease, physical inactivity ranks as high as elevated cholesterol, high blood pressure, or cigarette smoking.[10]

The inactivity epidemic doesn't stop at the border. According to the College of Family Physicians of Canada, an estimated 21,000 Canadians die prematurely every year because of medical problems related to physical inactivity.[11] Two-thirds of Canadian children and young people are not active enough for optimal growth and development.[12]

The Campus Couch Potato Crisis

Although most are young and healthy, college students aren't necessarily more active or fit than the general population. In one national survey, 57 percent of male and 61 percent of female college

---

STRATEGIES for CHANGE

Couch Potatoes, Arise!

❚ Turn commercials into mini-workouts. Stand up; sit down (better yet, don't sit down all the way), then stand. Continue these squats through one commercial; gradually increase the time to two or three commercials.

❚ At the next break, march in place, moving both your arms and legs. Work up to doing jumping jacks as well.

❚ Using books, bottles of water, cans of soup, or hand weights, work your upper body with biceps curls, overhead shoulder presses, and side arm raises.

❚ Lying on the floor, do side-lying leg raises and crunches. Alternate with push-ups, either from your knees or toes.

---

students reported performing no vigorous or moderate exercise on at least three of the previous seven days. Another study of almost 500 undergraduates at a large midwestern university found that students spent almost 30 hours a week on sedentary behaviors, mainly studying. Although men reported more time in front of a television or computer, they were generally more physically active than women.[13] (See Student Snapshot: "How Physically Active Are Undergraduates?")

Mexican-American students, both male and female, and African-American women report the lowest rates of physical activity. The most physically active men are African American; the most active women, white.[14]

While 70 percent of 12-year-olds engage in vigorous physical activity on a regular basis, only 35 percent of 21-year-olds maintain this level.[15] A study of 145 first-year students found a significant drop in self-reported physical activity among both male and female freshmen —from 66 percent to 44 percent. The students who were active reported higher levels of energy and less anxiety than those who became or remained inactive.[16]

Patterns set in college influence lifelong activity levels. In a survey of 367 alumni who graduated two to ten years previously from a southern university, more than half of those who had exercised regularly in college were even more physically active. The irregular exercisers were more likely to remain at the same or a lower level of activity. The nonexercisers tended to become less active after graduation.[17]

Poor fitness in young adults increases the likelihood of later cardiovascular problems. In a study that followed men and women between ages 18 and 30 for 15 years,

STUDENT SNAPSHOT

How Physically Active Are Undergraduates?

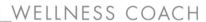

	Men	Women
Sedentary behaviors		
Studying	12.9 hours/week	13.5 hours/week
TV/Videos / DVDs	12.0	9.6
Computer	6.7	5.2
Physical activity		
Vigorous	3.3 hours/week	2.5 hours/week
Moderate	2.9	3.0

Based on a study of 439 undergraduates at a large midwestern university. *Source:* Buckworth, Janet, and Claudio Nigg. "Physical Activity, Exercise, and Sedentary Behavior in College Students." *Journal of American College Health,* July/August 2004, Vol. 53, No. 1, p. 28.

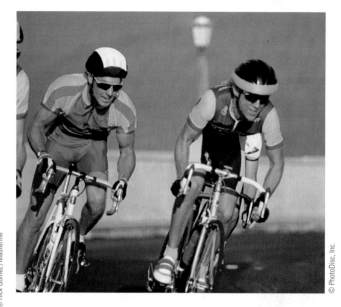

Find a group of friends who are as interested in physical fitness as you are to help keep your motivation high.

those with the lowest fitness levels were three to six times more likely to develop diabetes, hypertension, and metabolic syndrome (discussed in Chapter 10) than those with higher fitness levels.[18]

WELLNESS COACH

Motivating Yourself to Get Moving

Before you move a muscle, you need to be motivated. You may never even have thought about becoming more active. You may be thinking about getting into shape—someday. You may exercise, but not on a regular basis. Or you may have started working out in the last six months.

Each of these statements applies to a different stage of motivational readiness for change, discussed in Chapter 2. In studies on increasing activity in adults, researchers have found that strategies tailored to an individual's stage of readiness for change are effective in boosting motivation and getting people moving.[19]

Both cognitive and behavioral strategies are effective in motivating change. Cognitive strategies, such as learning about the risks of remaining sedentary, typically work best in the contemplation and preparation stages. Behavioral strategies, such as keeping athletic shoes in the car or in a locker at the gym, are most effective at the action stage.[20]

In a study of the stages and processes of change in college students, the most widely used behavioral processes were countering (going for a run instead of slumping in front of a television), environmental control (blocking out times for weight training), and self-liberation (enrolling in a cardio-kickboxing class).[21]

Your health or wellness course may help you get motivated and moving. In a study of 1,625 undergraduates enrolled in Personal Wellness classes, attitudes toward exercise and physical activity improved significantly over the course of a semester. Students who were not active or engaged only in light exercise registered positive changes in addition to the more active students. The women students, who had been less active than the males, showed the greatest boost in attitudes toward exercise and fitness.[22]

In another study at a Colorado university, students enrolled in a fitness and wellness course were more likely to participate in regular physical activity when tired, in a bad mood, in bad weather, time-pressured, or unsure of their ability to perform an activity.[23]

Physical Activity and Wellness

If exercise could be packed into a pill, it would be the single most widely prescribed and beneficial medicine in the nation. Why? Because nothing can do more to help

STRATEGIES

for CHANGE

Motivating Yourself to Move

Here are some of the best ways to get moving:

▮ **Sign up for a fitness class,** such as spinning or step-aerobics, so that exercise is built into your weekly schedule.

▮ **Go to the gym with friends.** "Even if it's rainy and cold, I know they're waiting for me so I go," one woman explained.

▮ **Find a fun workout.** "I love working out when it's something different—like water aerobics, ice skating, or swing dance," said one student.

▮ **Join a team—or root for one.** College sports, whether competitive or informal, can help maintain fitness levels. So can cheerleading, which has become so physically demanding that college cheerleaders have scored as high a fitness level as college athletes.[24]

▮ **Do double-duty.** Some students read class notes while on a Stairmaster or stationary bicycle. Others listen to required reading books as they work out.

your body function at its best (**Figure 3-2**). With regular activity, your heart muscles become stronger and pump blood more efficiently. Your heart rate and resting pulse slow down. Your blood pressure may drop slightly from its normal level.

Regular physical activity thickens the bones and can slow the loss of calcium that normally occurs with age. Exercise increases flexibility in the joints and improves digestion and elimination. It speeds up metabolism, so the body burns up more calories and body fat decreases. It heightens sensitivity to insulin (a great benefit for diabetics) and may lower the risk of developing diabetes. In addition, exercise enhances clot-dissolving substances in the blood, helping to prevent strokes, heart attacks, and pulmonary embolisms (clots in the lungs).[25] Regular, vigorous exercise can actually extend the lifespan.

The Benefits of Physical Activity

What can exercise do for you? It can boost your energy, lower stress, improve sleep, increase stamina and focus, brighten your mood—and that's just for starters. Here are some of its other proven benefits:

Longer Life

Capacity for exercise has proved a better predictor of whether a man would die in the next few years than other risk factors, such as high blood pressure, high total cholesterol, or smoking. Formerly sedentary people, even the elderly, who begin to exercise live longer, on average, than those who remain inactive. However, for active people light to moderate exercise won't do it—only vigorous exercise reduces the risk of dying of heart disease and of premature death from other causes.[26]

Healthier Heart and Lungs

Sedentary people are about twice as likely to die of a heart attack as people who are physically active. (See Chapter 10 for a discussion of heart disease.) Regular physical activity makes blood less likely to clot and cause a stroke or heart attack.

Exercise also lowers levels of one of the indicators of increased risk of heart disease and diabetes, (C-reactive protein, which is discussed in Chapter 10).[27] Exercise itself, even without weight loss, may reduce the risk of developing the prediabetic condition called metabolic syndrome, which if untreated can lead to type 2 diabetes and increase the risk of heart disease.[28]

In addition to its effects on the heart, exercise makes the lungs more efficient. The lungs take in more oxygen, and their vital capacity (the maximum amount of air volume the lungs can take in and expel) increases, providing more energy for you to use.

Even in young men, physical fitness is associated with improvements in blood pressure and the makeup of blood fats, including cholesterol and triglycerides.[29] Exercise, along with a healthy weight, keeps blood fats at healthy levels over time.[30] Prolonged, sustained endurance training prevents the stiffening of the heart muscle once thought to be an inevitable consequence of aging.[31]

Protection Against Cancer

As discussed in Chapter 9, fatness increases the risk of several cancers; fitness decreases it. The evidence for exercise's protective effects is strongest for colon and rectal cancer, possibly because it enhances digestion and elimination. Physical activity also lowers the risk of breast cancer in women.[32]

In a study that followed more than 5,000 men and women for more than 20 years, fitness was a strong predictor of cancer death rates for men, but not for women. The fittest men had the lowest cancer death rates. But for women, body weight, as measured by body mass index (BMI), discussed in Chapter 9, proved more significant.[33]

Less Risk of Disease

Moderate exercise correlates with a reduced number of sick days. Researchers speculate that exercise may en-

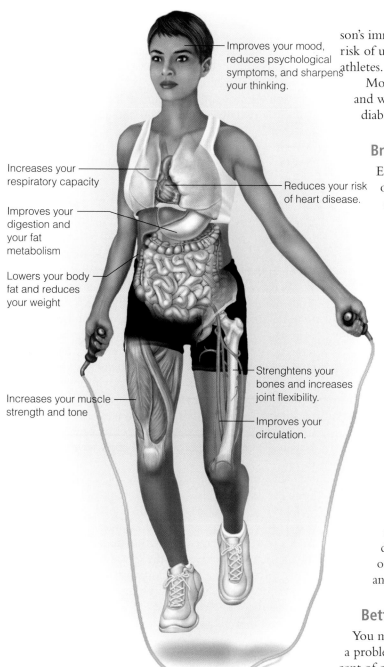

Improves your mood, reduces psychological symptoms, and sharpens your thinking.

Increases your respiratory capacity

Improves your digestion and your fat metabolism

Lowers your body fat and reduces your weight

Increases your muscle strength and tone

Reduces your risk of heart disease.

Strenghtens your bones and increases joint flexibility.

Improves your circulation.

FIGURE 3-2 ▌ The Benefits of Exercise

Regular physical activity enhances your overall health and helps prevent disease.

son's immune system, heavy training may increase the risk of upper respiratory tract infections for endurance athletes.

Moderate exercise, combined with a balanced diet and weight loss, can cut in half the risk of developing diabetes among those at high risk.[34]

Brighter Mood

Exercise makes people feel good from the inside out. Exercise boosts mood, increases energy, reduces anxiety, improves concentration and alertness, and enables people to handle stress better. During long workouts, some people experience what is called "runner's high," which may be the result of increased levels of mood-elevating brain chemicals called **endorphins.**

Better Mental Health and Functioning

Exercise is an effective—but underused—treatment for mild to moderate depression and may help in treating other mental disorders. Regular, moderate exercise, such as walking, running, or lifting weights, three times a week, has proved helpful for depression and anxiety disorders, including panic attacks. Exercise is as effective as medication in improving mood and also helps prevent relapse.

According to numerous long-term studies, physically fit adults perform better on cognitive tests than their less-fit peers.[35] Improving cardiorespiratory fitness reduces the harmful effects of aging on brain structures as well as on memory and other functions.[36]

Better Bones

You may think that weak, brittle bones are a problem only for the elderly. However, 2 percent of college-age women already have **osteoporosis,** a condition in which bones lose their mineral density and become susceptible to injury. According to a recent study, another 15 percent have already sustained significant losses in bone density and are at high risk of osteoporosis. Women who did not participate in high school sports were 7 times more likely to have low bone density than were those who had.[37]

In the study, the college women at greatest risk often were extremely skinny and maintained their low weights and slim looks by dieting and by avoiding exercise (which would increase their muscle mass). Some had eliminated dairy products, an important source of calcium, from their diets. Depo-Provera, a method of birth control that consists of hormone injections every three months, also was associated with low bone density, especially with long-term use.

hance immune function by reducing stress hormones like cortisol that can dampen resistance to disease.

Women who walk briskly for 35 to 45 minutes five days a week experience half the number of sick days with cold symptoms as inactive women. While moderate exercise seems to bolster a per-

Bone mass peaks at about age 30, and college is the ideal time to improve bone density. Regular weight-bearing exercise (jogging, walking, aerobics, resistance training) is the best means of strengthening your bones. Think of it as an investment in your bones' future.

Lower Weight

Aerobic exercise burns off calories during your workout because as your body responds to the increased demand from your muscles for nutrients, your metabolic rate rises. Moreover, this surge persists for as long as 12 hours after exercise, so you continue to use up more calories than usual, even after you've stopped sweating. Resistance training builds muscle tissue, which burns up more calories throughout the day.

For individuals on a diet, exercise provides extra benefits: A combination of dietary change and moderate to high-level intensity of exercise leads to greater weight loss than either alone. Dieters who work out lose more fat than lean muscle tissue, which improves their body composition.

In one study, college-age men who started exercising lost abdominal fat, which poses the greatest risk to health.[38] (See Chapter 9 for information on exercise and weight control.)

Sexuality

By improving physical endurance, muscle tone, blood flow, and body composition, exercise improves sexual functioning. Simply burning 200 extra calories a day can significantly lower the risk of erectile dysfunction in sedentary men. Exercise also may increase sexual drive, activity, and sexual satisfaction in people of all ages.

In a recent study of about 400 students at a southeastern university, college students who exercise frequently and see themselves as physically fit rate themselves higher with regard to sexual performance and sexual desirability than those who exercise less and don't describe themselves as fit. All the men who exercised six to seven days per week rated their sexual desirability as above or much above average.[39]

A More Active Old Age

Exercise slows the changes that are associated with advancing age: loss of lean muscle tissue, increase in body fat, and decrease in work capacity. In addition to lowering the risk of heart disease and stroke, exercise also helps older men and women retain the strength and mobility needed to live independently. Even in old age, exercise boosts strength and stamina, lessens time in wheelchairs, and improves outlook and sense of control.

Benefits for Students

Unlike middle-aged and older individuals, traditional-age college students cite fitness as the number-one advantage that exercise offers, followed by improved appearance and muscle tone. Undergraduates who recognize the benefits of exercise are more likely to be physically active than those who focus on barriers to working out.[40]

Will exercise improve your grades? Not necessarily. A study at two Texas universities found that the fittest students didn't necessarily have higher GPAs. However, increasing their level of physical fitness did have a positive impact on the GPAs of the female students.

Can a Person Be Fat and Fit?

Most people assume that fitness comes in only one size: small. That's not necessarily so. There is considerable controversy over how to define a healthy weight. But individuals of every size can improve their physical fitness.

In ten years of research on 25,000 men and 8,000 women, scientists at the Cooper Institute for Aerobics Research in Dallas have found that heavier individuals can be just as healthy and physically fit as their leaner counterparts. In their studies, obese people who exercised moderately (30 minutes of daily walking at three or four miles per hour) had half the death rate of those who were slimmer but more sedentary. Low cardiorespiratory fitness, regardless of an individual's weight, is as great a risk factor for dying of heart disease or other causes such as diabetes, high blood pressure, and other well-recognized threats.

Nonetheless, fitness doesn't completely reverse the increased risks associated with excess weight. If you're obese, even a high level of physical activity does not protect you from premature death. And if you're sedentary, being thin does not cancel out the dangers of inactivity. In the long-term Nurses Health Study, which has followed more than 100,000 women for decades, women who were both obese and inactive were most likely to die. Those who were fit but fat and those who were thin but sedentary also had higher death rates than others.[41]

Exercise Guidelines for Americans

Because inactivity is so hazardous to our well-being, public health officials have tried many approaches to get Americans moving. Rather than emphasizing vigorous cardiorespiratory or aerobic activity, a landmark report by the Surgeon General in 1996 recommended 30 minutes of moderate-intensity exercise—such as brisk walking, bicycling, or gardening—on all or most days of the week.

Exercise is a component of the Dietary Guidelines for Americans, released by the federal government in 2005. The most recent recommendations, which call for more physical activity for added health benefits, include the following:

▍ Engage in regular physical activity and reduce sedentary activities to promote health, psychological well-being, and a healthy body weight.

- To reduce the risk of chronic disease in adulthood, engage in at least 30 minutes of moderate-intensity physical activity, above usual activity, at work or home on most days of the week. For most people, greater health benefits can be obtained by engaging in physical activity of more vigorous intensity or longer duration.
- To help manage body weight and prevent gradual, unhealthy weight gain in adulthood, engage in approximately 60 minutes of moderate- to vigorous activity on most days of the week while not exceeding caloric intake requirements.
- To sustain weight loss in adulthood, participate in at least 60 to 90 minutes of daily moderate-intensity physical activity while not exceeding caloric intake requirements. Some people may need to consult with a health-care provider before participating in this level of activity.
- Achieve physical fitness by including cardiovascular conditioning, stretching exercises for flexibility, and resistance exercises or calisthenics for muscle strength and endurance.[42]

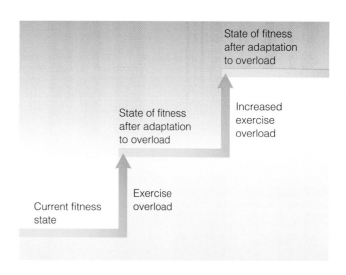

FIGURE 3-3 ▌The Overload Principle

By increasing frequency, intensity, or duration, you will improve your level of fitness. Once your body adapts (becomes comfortable) to the demands, you can again apply the overload principle to achieve a higher level of fitness.

✚ The Principles of Exercise

Your body is literally what you make of it. Superbly designed for multiple uses, it adjusts to meet physical demands. If you need to sprint for a bus, your heart will speed up and pump more blood. Beyond such immediate, short-term adaptations, physical training can produce long-term changes in heart rate, oxygen consumption, and muscle strength and endurance. Although there are limits on the maximum levels of physical fitness and performance that any individual can achieve, regular exercise can produce improvements in everyone's baseline wellness and fitness.

As you begin the process of working toward total fitness, it's important to keep in mind the principles of exercise, discussed next.

Overload Principle

The **overload principle** requires a person exercising to provide a greater stress or demand on the body than it's usually accustomed to handling. For any muscle, including the heart, to get stronger, it must work against a greater-than-normal resistance or challenge. To continue to improve, you need further increases in the demands—but not too much too quickly. **Progressive overloading**—gradually increasing physical challenges —provides the benefits of exercise without the risk of injuries (**Figure 3–3**).

Overloading is specific to each body part and to each component of fitness. Leg exercises develop only the lower limbs; arm exercises, only the upper limbs. This is why you need a comprehensive fitness plan that includes a variety of exercises to develop different parts of the body. If you play a particular sport, you also need training to develop sports-specific skills, such as a strong, efficient stroke in swimming.

FITT Principle

Although low-intensity activity can enhance basic health, you need to work harder—that is, at a greater intensity—to improve fitness. Whatever exercise you do, there is a level, or threshold, at which fitness begins to improve; a target zone, where you can achieve maximum benefits; and an upper level, at which potential risks outweigh any further benefits. The acronym **FITT** sums up the four dimensions of progressive overload: *frequency* (how often you exercise) *intensity* (how hard), *time* (how long), and *type* (specific activity). (See **Table 3–1**.)

Frequency

To attain and maintain physical fitness, you need to exercise regularly, but the recommended frequency varies with different types of exercise and with an individual's fitness goals. Health officials urge Americans to engage in moderate-intensity aerobic activity most days and in resistance and flexibility training two or three days a week.

Intensity

Exercise intensity varies with the type of exercise and with personal goals. To improve cardiorespiratory fitness, you need at a minimum to increase your heart rate to a target zone (the level that produces benefits). To develop muscular strength and endurance, you need to increase the amount of weight you lift or the resistance you work

TABLE 3-1 ▌ Guidelines for Physical Fitness: The FITT Principle

	Cardiorespiratory	Strength	Flexibility
	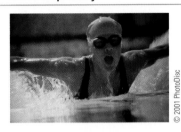	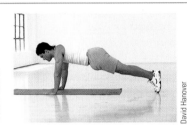	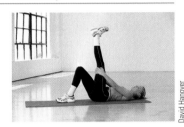

Frequency: Most days of the week. Start with three days and gradually increase frequency.

	Almost every day	A minimum of 2 to 3 days per week	A minimum of 2 to 3 days per week

Intensity: Start at low to moderate intensity and gradually increase to more vigorous efforts over several weeks.

	60 to 85% of maximum heart rate	Enough to enhance muscle strength and improve body composition	Enough to develop and maintain a full range of motion

Time: 30 to 60 minutes, using a gradual progression.

	20 to 60 minutes	8 to 12 repetitions of 8 to 10 different exercises (minimum)	4 repetitions of 10 to 30 seconds per muscle group (minimum)

Type of activity: Start with low-impact activities (walking, cycling, low-impact aerobics, water exercise); resistance or weight training; flexibility exercises.

	Aerobic activity that uses large-muscle groups and can be maintained continuously	Resistance activity that is performed at a controlled speed and through a full range of motion	Stretching activity that uses the major muscle groups

Source: Adapted from American College of Sports Medicine, "Position Stand: The Recommended Quantity and Quality of Exercise for Developing and Maintaining Cardiorespiratory and Muscular Fitness and Flexibility in Healthy Adults." *Medicine and Science in Sports and Exercise,* Vol. 30, 1998, pp. 975–991; and from McInnis, Kyle, et al., "Counseling for Physical Activity in Overweight and Obese Patients." *American Family Physician,* Vol. 67, No. 6, March 15, 2003, p. 1254.

against and/or the number of repetitions. For enhanced flexibility, you need to stretch muscles beyond their normal length.

"Moderate" intensity activities burn 3.5 to 7 calories per minute. They include brisk walking, dancing, bicycling, and mowing the lawn. "Vigorous" intensity activities—jogging, cycling uphill, swimming continuous laps, and heavy yard work—burn more than 7 calories per minute. The more vigorous an activity is, the less time needed to burn the same number of calories. As **Figure 3-4** shows, you can burn 150 calories in just 15 minutes on a stair machine, while you would have to shoot hoops for half an hour or play touch football for up to 45 minutes in order to burn the same amount.

Another way to determine how much physical activity a particular exercise provides is by its MET, or metabolic equivalent, a measurement of how much oxygen, or energy, it uses. One MET is the amount of energy you use when you are resting. Two METS is twice resting energy expenditure; three METS is three times, and so on. The harder a person exercises, the higher the MET level. A 10-MET activity, such as jogging, requires a tenfold increase in the body's resting energy requirements.

Time (Duration)

The amount of time, or duration, of your workouts is also important, particularly for cardiorespiratory exercise. As noted in Table 3-1, the American College of Sports Medicine recommends 30 to 45 minutes of aerobic exercise, preceded by 5 to 10 minutes of warm-up and followed by 5 to 10 minutes of stretching. However, experts have found similar health benefits from a single 30-minute session of moderate exercise or from several shorter sessions throughout the day. Duration and intensity are interlinked. If you're exercising at high intensity (biking or running at a brisk pace, for instance), you don't need to exercise as long as when you're working at lower intensity (walking or swimming at a moderate pace). For muscular strength and endurance and for flexibility, duration is defined by the number of sets or repetitions rather than total time.

Type (Specificity)

The **specificity principle** refers to the body's adaptation to a particular type of activity or amount of stress placed upon it. Jogging, for instance, trains the heart and lungs

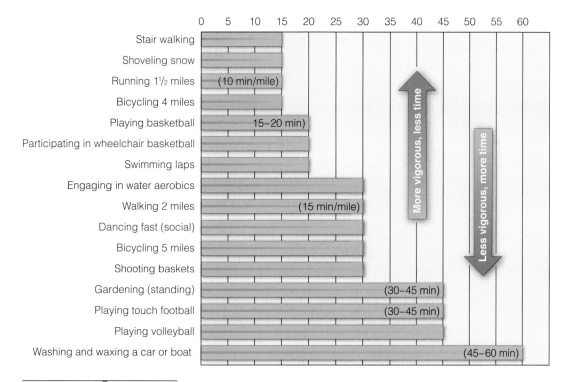

FIGURE 3-4 ▮ Minutes of Activity Required to Burn 150 kcalories

Source: www.cdc.gov/nccdphp/dnpa/physical/recommendations/adults.htm

to work more efficiently and strengthens certain leg muscles. However, it does not build upper body strength or enhance flexibility.

Reversibility Principle

The **principle of reversibility** is the opposite of the overload principle. Just as the body adapts to greater physical demands, it also adjusts to lower levels. If you stop exercising, you can lose as much as 50 percent of your fitness improvements within two months. If you have to curtail your usual exercise routine because of a busy schedule, you can best maintain your fitness by keeping the intensity constant and reducing frequency or duration. The principle of reversibility is aptly summed up by the phrase, "Use it or lose it."

Diminishing Returns Principle

If you haven't been exercising regularly, you can expect to see dramatic improvements in your fitness and health when you begin, even if you can't run very far or lift heavy weights. If you're already in fair shape and step up from a moderate workout program to a more rigorous one, you'll see further improvements, but they won't be as dramatic. This is the principle of **diminishing returns.**

Individuality

No two bodies are alike, and the same is true of fitness, athletic performance, and sports skills. There are individual limits on each person's adaptability and potential for improvement. Most people can improve their vital capacity—their maximum oxygen intake—by about 15 to 30 percent through training. This may not be enough to qualify for competitive sports, but it can produce lifelong health benefits.

How Much Exercise is Enough?

The answer depends on your reasons for working out. If you want to feel better, boost your energy, tone your muscles, condition your heart, strengthen your bones, protect your heart, and lower your risk of major diseases, leading medical authorities, including the American College of Sports Medicine, the U.S. Surgeon General, and Health Canada's Physical Activity Guide to Healthy Active Living, recommend a minimum of 30 to 60 minutes of moderate activity (such as walking at a speed of three to four miles per hour) most days of the week. According to the most recent research, a minimum of 150 minutes a week of moderate-intensity exercise lifts men and women out of the "low-fitness" category and lowers their risk of cardio-

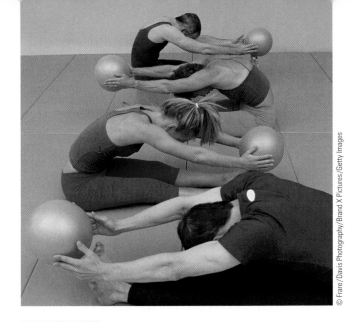

© Frare/Davis Photography/Brand X Pictures/Getty Images

STRATEGIES

for CHANGE

Mini-Workouts for Busy People

If you enjoy vigorous workouts but can't always find the time to do them regularly, you can increase the intensity to compensate for the reduced duration. Here are some examples:

▌ Run faster over a shorter distance or choose an uphill course to walk, bicycle, or skate.

▌ Split your exercise time in two. Do a strength or flexibility routine in the morning and a cardiovascular workout later. Or divide your cardiovascular exercise into three 10-minute sessions.

▌ For a more time-efficient strength workout, take an unloaded barbell and perform as many repetitions (reps) as possible of an exercise like curls in 30 seconds. Shoot for 30 reps, or 1 per second, and maintain strict form throughout. Rest only 30 seconds, then shift immediately to the next exercise, and perform as many reps as possible in 30 seconds. Continue this work/rest pace through eight or ten exercises that work the major muscle groups of the body. If you have little or no experience with weights, rest longer between sets.

▌ Do flexibility exercises wherever you are. Stretch the calf muscles by leaning forward against a wall with one leg extended back. While sitting at your desk, do side-to-side looks and ear-to-shoulder stretches for the neck, shoulder shrugs and rolls, and circles with arms extended out to the sides.

▌ The goal of exercise isn't to become a competitive athlete but to improve your well-being and achieve your maximum fitness potential.

vascular disease[43] and diabetes,[44] regardless of weight or body composition.

While half an hour of exercise five days a week is good, according to a recent review of current research, working out more often and more intensely can yield more health dividends, including improved muscular strength and endurance.[45] You may also need to exercise longer and harder to maintain a healthy weight and lose excess pounds. As discussed on page 48, the latest Dietary Guidelines for Americans concluded that individuals who've lost weight may need to exercise 60 to 90 minutes a day to keep off the pounds.[46] Vigorous physical activity (such as jogging or spinning) burns calories more rapidly per unit of time than moderate activities like walking. It doesn't matter if your goal is to improve fitness or avoid fatness. The same strategy—regular physical activity—is the key to both.[47]

✚ Evaluating Fitness Products and Programs

As fitness has become a major industry in the United States, consumers have been bombarded with pitches for products that promise to do everything from whittle a waistline to build up biceps. As always, you have to ask questions and do your own research—whether you're buying basic exercise aids or joining a health club. Beware of any promise that sounds too good to be true. And keep in mind that nothing matters more than your own commitment.

Exercise Equipment

Always try out equipment before buying it. If you decide to purchase a stationary bicycle, for instance, read all the product information. Ask someone in your physical education department or at a local gym for recommendations. Try out a bicycle at the gym. Make sure any equipment you purchase is safe and durable.

Not all fitness equipment comes with a big price tag. If you're considering strength-training equipment, remember that free weights are your least expensive option. You can purchase light weights to carry when walking and jogging to build and firm arm muscles. Training with heavier weights increases muscle strength and endurance, improves balance and body composition, and may reverse some bone loss.

Other options, discussed in Chapter 5, are resistance bands and tubes and fitness balls. Some trainers think these aids add fun and variety to a workout; others question their conditioning value.

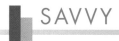

SAVVY
CONSUMER

HOW TO BUY ATHLETIC SHOES

Footwear has come a long way from the days of canvas sneakers. With so many new materials and high-tech options, choosing the right shoes for working out can be confusing. The best shoes aren't necessarily the most expensive but the ones that fit you best. Here are some basic guidelines:

■ **Choose the right shoes for your sport.** If you're a walker or runner, you want maximum overall shock absorption for the foot, with extra cushioning in the heel and under the ball of the foot (the metatarsal area) to prevent pain, burning, and tenderness. If you also participate in other types of exercise, consider "cross-trainers," shoes that are flexible enough in the front for running but provide the side-to-side, or lateral, control you need for aerobics or tennis.

■ **Check out the shoe.** A "slip-last" shoe, made by sewing together the upper like a moccasin and gluing it to the sole, is lightweight and flexible. A "board-last" shoe has a leather, nylon mesh, or canvas upper sewn to a cardboard-like material, which provides more support and control. A "combination-last" shoe offers the advantages of both other shoes and works well for a variety of foot types.

■ **Shop late.** Try on shoes at the end of the day or after a workout, when your foot size is at its maximum (sometimes half a shoe size larger than in the morning). Wear socks similar to those you'll wear for workouts.

■ **Give your toes room.** Allow a half inch, or the width of your index finger, between the end of your longest toe and the tip of the shoe. Try on both shoes. If one foot is larger than the other, buy the larger size.

■ **Check the width.** A shoe should be as wide as possible across the forefoot without allowing the heel to slip. Lace up the shoe completely and walk or jog a few steps to make sure the shoes are comfortable.

■ **Replace shoes when they lose their cushioning.** After about 300 to 500 miles of running or 300 hours of aerobic activity, your shoes are no longer absorbing the pounding and jarring of your sport. Don't put yourself at risk for knee and ankle injuries.

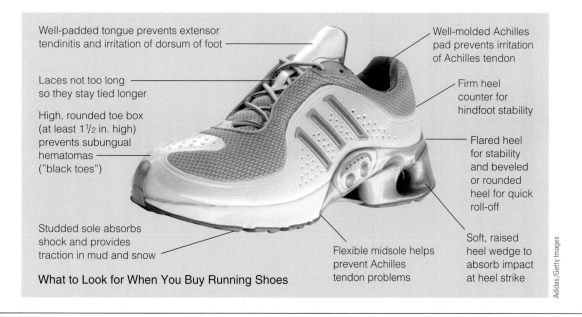

Well-padded tongue prevents extensor tendinitis and irritation of dorsum of foot

Well-molded Achilles pad prevents irritation of Achilles tendon

Laces not too long so they stay tied longer

Firm heel counter for hindfoot stability

High, rounded toe box (at least 1½ in. high) prevents subungual hematomas ("black toes")

Flared heel for stability and beveled or rounded heel for quick roll-off

Studded sole absorbs shock and provides traction in mud and snow

What to Look for When You Buy Running Shoes

Flexible midsole helps prevent Achilles tendon problems

Soft, raised heel wedge to absorb impact at heel strike

Adidas/Getty Images

✚ Safe and Healthy Workouts

Whenever you work out, you don't want to risk becoming sore or injured. Starting slowly when you begin any new fitness activity is the smartest strategy. Use your Wellness Journal to record the time and duration of each workout. Get accustomed to an activity first and then begin to work harder or longer. In this way, you strengthen your musculoskeletal system so that you're less likely to be injured; you lower the cardiovascular risk; and you build the exercise habit into your schedule.

Before You Start

Most people don't need to see a doctor before beginning a gradual, sensible exercise program. However, seek medical advice if you match any of the following descriptions:

▌ You've had a heart attack; your doctor has told you that you have heart trouble or a heart murmur; or your father, mother, brother, or sister had a heart attack before age 50.

▌ You often have pains or pressure in your left or mid-chest area or in your left neck, shoulder, or arm during or right after exercise; or you feel faint or have spells of dizziness; or you experience extreme breathlessness after mild exertion (such as a short walk at a moderate pace).

▌ Your doctor has told you that you have high blood pressure that is not under control or bone or joint problems, such as arthritis.

▌ You have a medical condition, such as diabetes, that might need special attention in an exercise program.

▌ You should also check with your doctor if you are over 40 and haven't been exercising two or three times a week.

The American College of Sports Medicine recommends that anyone with an unstable medical condition or with a previous injury seek medical evaluation before starting or returning to exercise. Individuals with heart, lung, or metabolic diseases should begin their exercise program "in a medically supervised environment."

How Can I Prevent Injuries?

According to the American Physical Therapy Association, the most common exercise-related injury sites are the knees, feet, back, and shoulders, followed by the ankles and hips. **Acute injuries**—sprains, bruises, and pulled muscles—are the result of sudden trauma, such as a fall or collision. **Overuse injuries,** on the other hand, are the result of overdoing a repetitive activity, such as running. When one particular joint is overstressed—such as a tennis player's elbow or a swimmer's shoulder—tendinitis, an inflammation at the point where the tendon meets the bone, can develop. Other overuse injuries include muscle strains and aches and stress fractures, which are hairline breaks in a bone, usually in the leg or foot.

Men and women may be vulnerable to different types of injuries. Studies of male and female college basketball and soccer players have shown that gender differences in the neuromuscular control of the knee places female athletes at higher risk for knee injuries.[48] Balance training may reduce the risk.[49]

To prevent exercise-related problems before they happen, use common sense and take appropriate precautions, including the following:

STRATEGIES for PREVENTION

Avoiding Injury

▌ Dress appropriately, and invest in good shoes (see Savvy Consumer: "How to Buy Athletic Shoes").

▌ Always warm up before and cool off after a workout.

▌ Don't push yourself; always build up frequency, intensity, and duration gradually.

▌ Keep high-impact exercises to a minimum.

▌ Rather than being sedentary all week and then training hard on weekends, try to stay active throughout the week and not overdo on weekends.

▌ Get proper instruction and, if necessary, advanced training from knowledgeable instructors.

▌ Make sure you have good equipment and keep it in good condition. Know how to check and do at least basic maintenance on the equipment yourself. Always check your equipment prior to each use (especially if you're renting it).

▌ Always make sure that stretching and exercises are preventing, not causing, injuries.

▌ Use reasonable protective measures, including wearing a helmet when cycling or skating.

▌ For some sports, such as boating, always go with a buddy.

▌ Take each outing seriously—even if you've dived into this river a hundred times before, even if you know this mountain like you know your own backyard. Avoid the unknown under adverse conditions (for example, hiking unfamiliar terrain during poor weather or kayaking a new river when water levels are unusually high or low) or when accompanied by a beginner whose skills may not be as strong as yours.

▌ Never combine alcohol or drugs with any sport.

Beyond the Gym

Many people are trying exhilarating sports that, by their very nature, entail some risk. If you choose these activities, you're responsible for learning how to stay safe as you push to the limit. Here are some sport-specific guidelines:

▌ **Inline skating.** The most common injuries are to the wrists. Skaters should always wear protective gear, including helmet, wrist guards, and knee pads, and should warm up before strapping on their skates.

Learn how to fall: Relax, go down to your knees, and roll to one side.

■ **Mountain biking.** Off-road biking requires knowing how to shift your weight to keep a bike stable on rough trails. Know the limits of your endurance and your equipment. Wear a helmet, bicycle gloves, and glasses or goggles to protect your eyes from dirt and overhanging branches. Carry a bike repair kit and a first aid kit if you head for a remote area.

■ **Rock climbing.** Rock climbing takes strength, balance, and hand-eye coordination. Training with a qualified instructor is essential to learn proper technique. The best place to learn is indoors, with supervised instruction and controlled conditions.

■ **Snowboarding.** Well-fitted snowboarding boots are essential, as is training in how to fall. The most common injuries are to the wrist or thumb, which can fracture if snowboarders put out their palms to break a fall. Sunburn and frostbite are both risks, and snow-boarders should wear sunscreen and monitor weather conditions closely.

Taking Care of Injuries

Sooner or later most active people suffer an injury. Although most are minor, they all require attention. Ignoring a problem or trying to push through the pain can lead to more serious complications. If you develop aches and pains beyond what you might expect from an activity, stop. Never push to the point of fatigue. If you do, you could end up with sprained or torn muscles. **Figure 3-5** gives the PRICE prescription for coping with an exercise injury.

What Causes Cramps and Sore Muscles?

You can develop abdominal cramps if you become dehydrated while exercising, particularly in warm weather. Pain felt during and immediately after exercise usually results from tissue **edema** (swelling) and a buildup of the chemical end products of exercise. This type of muscle soreness usually disappears within several hours after a workout. If your muscles feel sore a day or two after a workout, this could be a condition called **delayed-onset muscle soreness (DOMS).** Some researchers believe it is caused by damage to muscle fibers and supporting connective tissue.

When to Seek Medical Care

You should seek immediate medical attention anytime you suspect that an injury is serious, particularly if it's an injury to the eye or head, if a bone may be broken or a ligament may be torn, if heat exhaustion is a possibility, if symptoms such as chest pain develop, or if there was a loss of consciousness. You also should consult a health professional if a minor injury does not get better within a reasonable amount of time.

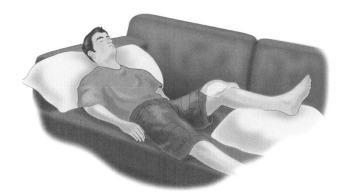

- **P**rotect the area with an elastic wrap, a sling, splint, cane, crutches or an air cast.
- **R**est to promote tissue healing. Avoid activities that cause pain, swelling or discomfort.
- **I**ce the area immediately, even if you're seeking medical help (don't put the ice pack directly on the skin). Repeat every two or three hours while you're awake for the first 48 to 72 hours. Cold reduces pain, swelling and inflammation in injured muscles, joints and connecting tissues and may slow bleeding if a tear has occurred.
- **C**ompress the area with an elastic bandage until the swelling stops. Begin wrapping at the end farthest from your heart. Loosen the wrap if the pain increases, the area becomes numb or swelling occurs below the wrapped area.
- **E**levate the area above your heart, especially at night. Gravity helps reduce swelling by draining excess fluid.

After 48 hours, if the swelling is gone, you may apply warmth or gentle heat, which improves the blood flow and speeds healing.

FIGURE 3-5 ▌ **PRICE: Coping with an Exercise Injury**

Overtraining

About half of all people who start an exercise program drop out within six months. One common reason is that they **overtrain,** pushing themselves to work too intensely too frequently. Signs of overdoing it include persistent muscle soreness, frequent injuries, unintended weight loss, nervousness, and an inability to relax. Overtraining for endurance sports like marathon running can damage the lungs and intensify asthma symptoms. You may find yourself unable to complete a normal workout or to recover after a normal workout.

If you develop any of the symptoms of overtraining, reduce or stop your workout sessions temporarily. Make gradual increases in the intensity of your workouts. Allow 24 to 48 hours for recovery between workouts. Make sure you get adequate rest. Check with a physical education instructor, coach, or trainer to make sure your exercise program fits your individual needs.

Excessive exercise can become a form of addiction, and "exercise dependence" is not uncommon among young men and women. Although most physically active college students work out at healthy levels, some exercise to an extent that could signal dependence. In one study of 257 students at an East

Coast university (none athletes in training or in season), about one in five exercised more than six hours a week and did so for reasons or in ways that appeared unhealthy. For example, they felt compelled to exercise even when ill or injured and felt guilty if they didn't work out.[50]

How Much Water Should I Drink While Exercising?

Water, which we need more than any other nutrient, is even more important during exercise and exertion. Thirst, the body's way of telling you to replace lost fluids, is not a good way for athletes to monitor their fluid needs. Rather than waiting until you're already somewhat dehydrated, you should be fully hydrated when you begin your activity or exercise and, depending on the duration and intensity of your workout, continue to replace fluids both during and afterward.

The American College of Sports Medicine recommends fluid intake before, during, and after exercise to regulate body temperature and replace body fluids lost through sweating. The failure to replace fluids during exercise can lead to dehydration, which can cause muscle fatigue, loss of coordination, heat exhaustion, and an elevation of body core temperature to dangerously high levels. To avoid this danger, the ACSM advises:

∎ Consume a nutritionally balanced diet and drink adequate fluids in the 24 hours before an exercise event.
∎ Drink about 17 ounces of fluid about two hours before.
∎ During exercise, start drinking early and at regular intervals to replace all the water lost through sweating (that is, body weight loss).
∎ Drink fluids with carbohydrates and/or electrolytes for exercise lasting more than an hour. For shorter periods, there is little evidence of differences between drinking a carbohydrate-electrolyte drink and plain water.

Too much water during prolonged bouts of exercise, such as a marathon, can lead to *hyponatremia*, or water intoxication. This condition occurs when the body's sodium level falls below normal as a result of salt loss from sweat and dilution of sodium in the bloodstream by overdrinking. Hyponatremia can cause nausea, vomiting, weakness, and, in severe cases, seizures, coma, and death.

✚ Special Health Concerns

Some form of physical activity is possible for almost everyone with a chronic health problem. However, certain adjustments must be made to ensure safety.

If You Have a Disability

Participation in sports and physical activity is one means by which individuals with physical and sensory disabilities can empower themselves. In a survey of disabled college students, the overwhelming

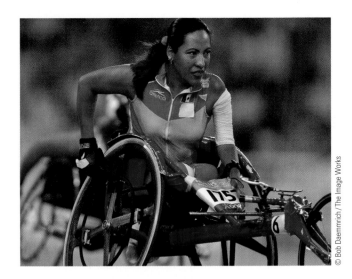

∎ Physical limitations are not a barrier to fitness but may require special training and adaptations.

STRATEGIES
for CHANGE

Are You Too Sick to Work Out?

∎ If your only symptoms are above the neck—a runny nose, sneezing, or a sore throat—moderate exercise is generally safe as long as you do not have a fever. Don't exercise more intensely until your symptoms disappear.

∎ If you have below-the-neck symptoms, such as extreme tiredness, muscle aches, vomiting, diarrhea, chills, swollen lymph glands, or a hacking cough, allow at least two weeks before returning to intense training.

∎ Don't exercise with a fever. Doing so increases the risk of dehydration, heat stroke, and even heart failure.

∎ Don't push yourself. More intense workouts may make your illness worse. Stop exercising if you feel dizzy or nauseous or experience any other exacerbated symptoms.

∎ Don't infect others or become infected. During cold and flu seasons, exercise during less crowded hours to avoid catching or transmitting viruses.

∎ Don't let a temporary illness stop you permanently. Focus on flexibility, stress management, and mind–body awareness during down times.

∎ Return to exercise slowly. Exercise for two days at a lower intensity for each day you were sick.

majority reported positive responses to exercise. Physical activity increased their perceptions of competence, facilitated goal attainment, and enhanced social integration.

Ask your physician or physical therapist for specific recommendations. Find out about special limitations you should be aware of, or ask for a referral to a fitness professional experienced in training clients with your condition. A qualified trainer can design a program tailored to your current abilities and fitness level. As you work, you should progress from an initial, easy effort to gradual increases in the intensity and duration of your workouts. In time your exercise program should prove to be an important, fulfilling part of coping with a chronic health challenge.

If You Have a Chronic Disease

Individuals with heart disease who participate in an exercise program have a 20 to 25 percent lower death rate than those who do not participate. Unfortunately, only 11 to 20 percent of cardiac patients participate in a supervised rehabilitation program, and many programs have dropout rates averaging 50 percent after three to six months. High-intensity activities such as sprinting can place undue stress on the heart and should be avoided. However, heart patients can begin a walking program and gradually increase the intensity of their workouts.

People with diabetes should consult their physicians if they are planning an intensive exercise program. Be-cause exercise can lead to hypoglycemia (a drop in blood sugar), diabetics should carry crackers or juice with them whenever they plan to increase their activity level. Those who take insulin should avoid giving themselves injections at a body site that typically is active during exercise. For example, a jogger might inject insulin in the abdomen instead of a leg, which undergoes more movement during running.

If You Are a Woman

Women often wonder about the impact of exercise on their menstrual cycles—and vice versa. Exercise physiologists have found no significant differences in aerobic capabilities throughout a woman's menstrual cycle. Indeed, many women report fewer menstrual cramps as they become more active, and women who engage in aerobic exercise are no more likely than others to suffer menstrual irregularities unless they are training extremely strenuously or their body fat drops very low.

Women who exercised before pregnancy generally can continue the same activities, possibly at a slightly lower intensity during pregnancy, provided they have no medical complications. Women who are physically active throughout their pregnancies may be better able to tolerate labor and more likely to have shorter labor and delivery times than their sedentary counterparts.

▮ MAKING HEALTHY CHOICES

To Improve Your Fitness

This chapter has given you the basic information you need to launch a fitness program. However, you're more likely to succeed if you create a plan and follow it. The labs at the end of this chapter can help you determine where you are now and how to get to where you want to be. Here are the basic steps:

- **Evaluate your readiness for change.** Use the Self-Survey on page 58 to determine your stage of behavioral change. Don't expect to progress directly from one stage to another just once. Most people "recycle" several times before a change becomes permanent.
- **Consider your fitness goals.** Use the goal-setting tool on page 59 to determine what you want from a fitness program. Do you have an overall conditioning goal, such as losing weight? Or do you have a training goal, such as preparing for a 5K race or the tryouts for the volleyball team? Break down your goal into smaller "step" goals that lead you toward it.
- **Think through your personal preferences.** What are your physical strengths and weaknesses? Do you have good upper body strength but easily get winded? Do you have a stiff back? Do your allergies flare up when you exercise outdoors? By paying attention to your needs, likes, and dislikes, you can choose activities you enjoy—and are more likely to continue.
- **Schedule exercise into your daily routine.** If you can, block out a half hour for working out at the beginning of the day, between classes, or in the evening. Write it into your schedule as if it were a class or doctor's appointment. If you can't find 30 minutes, look for two 15-minute or three 10-minute slots that you can use for "mini-workouts." Once you've worked out a schedule, write it down. A written plan encourages you to stay on track.
- **Assemble your gear.** Make sure you put your athletic shoes in your car or in the locker at the gym. Lay out the clothes you'll need to shoot hoops or play racquetball.
- **Start slowly.** If you are just beginning regular activity or exercise, begin at a low level. If you have an injury, disability, or chronic health problem, be sure you get medical clearance from a physician.
- **Progress gradually.** If you have not been physically active, begin by incorporating a few minutes of physical activity into each day, building up to 30 minutes or more of moderate-intensity activities. If you have been active but not as often or as intensely as recommended, become more consistent. Continue to increase the frequency, intensity, and duration of your workouts.

❚ After a few months of leading a more active life, take stock. Think of how much more energy you have at the end of the day. Ask yourself if you're feeling any less stressed, despite the push and pull of daily pressures. Focus on the unanticipated rewards of exercise. Savor the exhilaration of an autumn morning's walk; the thrill of feeling newly toughened muscles bend to your will; or the satisfaction of a long, smooth stretch after a stressful day. Enjoy the pure pleasure of living in the body you deserve.

SELF-SURVEY

Are You Ready to Become More Active?

For each of the following questions, please circle Yes or No. Please be sure to read the questions carefully.

Physical activity or exercise includes activities such as walking briskly, jogging, bicycling, swimming, or any other activity in which the exertion is at least as intense as these activities.

1. I am currently physically active.　　No　Yes

2. I intend to become more physically active in the next 6 months.　　No　Yes

For activity to be regular, it must add up to a total of 30 minutes or more per day and be done at least 5 days per week. For example, you could take one 30-minute walk or take three 10-minute walks for a daily total of 30 minutes.

3. I currently engage in regular physical activity.　　No　Yes

4. I have been regularly physically active for the past 6 months.　　No　Yes

Scoring Algorithm:

Precontemplation:　Question One = No
　　　　　　　　　Question Two = No
Contemplation:　　Question One = No
　　　　　　　　　Question Two = Yes
Preparation:　　　Question One = Yes and
　　　　　　　　　Question Three = No
Action:　　　　　Question One = Yes
　　　　　　　　　Question Three = Yes and
　　　　　　　　　Question Four = No
Maintenance:　　　Question One = Yes
　　　　　　　　　Question Three = Yes
　　　　　　　　　Question Four = Yes

Sources: Marcus, Bess, and Beth Lewis. "Physical Activity and the Stages of Motivational Readiness for Change Model." *President's Council on Physical Fitness and Sports Research Digest,* Series 4, No. 1, March 2003, p. 1. Marcus, H., and L. J. Forsyth. *Motivating People to Be Physically Active.* Champaign, Il.: Human Kinetics, 2003. Reprinted, by permission, from Marcus, B. H., and L. H. Forsyth, 2003, *Motivating People to be Physically Active,* Champaign, IL: Human Kinetics, p. 21.

ACTION PLAN

Your Action Plan for Physical Fitness

Once you know your stage of motivational readiness, you can employ the cognitive and behavioral strategies most likely to work for you now. As you progress through the stages of change, you can shift to other approaches. Here are some suggestions:

Precontemplation (not active and not thinking about becoming active)

❚ Use this course as an opportunity to learn about the benefits of physical activity, including better mood, lower stress, stronger bones, and a lower risk of cardiovascular disease.

❚ Set a small, reasonable goal that does not involve working up a sweat, such as looking up "exercise, benefits of" in the index of this book and reading the pages cited.

❚ List what you see as the cons of physical activity. For example, do you fear it would take time you need for your studies? Think of small changes that don't require time, for instance, standing rather than sitting when talking on the phone, doing stretches while watching television, or taking a quick walk down the hall or up the stairs while waiting for a friend or a class to begin.

❚ Identify barriers to physical activity, such as lack of money. Take advantage of your student status and check out facilities, such as the swimming pool at the athletic center, or opportunities, such as an intramural soccer team, available to you free (or almost).

Contemplation (not active but thinking about becoming active)

❚ Think back to activities you found enjoyable in the past. You might consider inline skating to class or around campus, or plan a hike for a weekend or school break.

❚ Determine the types of activity you can realistically fit into your daily schedule. You might join friends for softball every Saturday, or sign up for an evening body-sculpting class.

❚ Visualize success. Focus on the person you want to become: How would you look? What would you do differently? Find an image—from a magazine advertisement, for example—and post it where you can see it often.

❚ Plan your rewards. Use a technique called shaping, which reinforces progress on the way to a goal. For instance, initially you might reward yourself once you engage in physical activity for 15 minutes a day. After a week, you get the reward only after 20 minutes a day. Over time you increase the number of days you are physically active as well as the number of minutes of activity per day.

▌ Reach out for support. Find a friend, family member, or classmate who is willing or able to provide support for being active. Or join an organized martial arts class or an informal team.

Preparation (active but not at recommended levels)

▌ Identify specific barriers that limit your activity. If your daily jogs are rained or snowed out, develop a list of indoor alternatives, such as walking stairs or working out to an exercise video.

▌ Set specific daily and weekly goals. Your daily goal might begin with 10 or 15 minutes of activity. Your weekly goal might be to try a new activity, such as spinning or a dance class.

▌ Divide physical activity over the course of the day with a 10 or 15 minute walk in the morning, another at lunch, and a third at the end of the day.

▌ Document your progress. You could use a monthly calendar to keep track of the number of days you've exercised as well as the length of each workout. Or you can keep a more detailed record, noting the types of exercise you do every day, the intensity you work at, the duration of each workout, and so forth.

Action and Maintenance (active at recommended levels for less than six months)

▌ Identify risk factors that might lead to relapse. If vacations or holiday breaks disrupt your routine, make a plan for alternative ways to remain active before you leave campus.

▌ Stress proof your fitness program. In crunch times, you may feel you don't have time to spare for exercise. Multiple 10-minute walks during the day may be particularly useful both to keep up your fitness and to relieve stress buildup.

▌ Avoid boredom. Think through ways to vary your exercise routine. Take different routes on your walks. Invite different friends to join you. Alternate working with free weights and resistance machines at the gym.

▌ Set secondary goals. Once you've reached and maintained your goal for physical activity, set goals related to secondary benefits of exercise, for instance, losing weight or changing your body composition.

SETTING GOALS

Setting Personal Fitness Goals

Your Personal Total Fitness Goal:

Is it S.M.A.R.T.?
    Specific? _____

Measurable? _____
Achievable? _____
Rewarding? _____
Time Defined? _____

Strategies for Success:
    1. _____
    2. _____
    3. _____

Potential Obstacles:
    1. _____
    2. _____
    3. _____

Ways Around Them:
    1. _____
    2. _____
    3. _____

Daily Report

The Week That Was:
What went right?
What could I do better?

WELLNESS JOURNAL

Feelings About Physical Activity

The following statements will help you clarify your feelings toward physical activity. Complete each statement and write a few sentences that expand on these feelings.

1. When I think about physical activity, I . . .

2. When I am physically active, I enjoy/don't enjoy exercising because . . .

3. When I take part in physical activity, I usually, . . .

4. During physical activity, others see me as . . .

5. I like physical activities that are . . .

Are most of your responses positive regarding physical activity? If not, why do you feel this way? Identify barriers to increasing your activity and begin formulating strategies to overcome them. Review in your textbook the health benefits of being active and start with small goals to get you going. Ask your friends and family members if they want to become more active and then support each other's efforts. Also, check with the intramural sports department on campus and see what opportunities are there for you.

Adapted from "Finding Your Workout Personality". Pamela Peeke, MD, University of Maryland and Melanie Polk, RD, American Institute for Cancer Research.

Making This Chapter Work for You

1. Health-related fitness has five components: Three are cardiorespiratory endurance, muscular strength, and muscular endurance. Name the other two:
   a. Flexibility and physical conditioning.
   b. Balance and flexibility.
   c. Flexibility and body composition.
   d. Flexibility and coordination.

2. Which of the following statements is true?
   a. Inactivity does not affect health until middle age.
   b. Men and women have the same physiological capacities.
   c. Total wellness is one dimension of physical fitness.
   d. Physical fitness is one dimension of total wellness.

3. On average, undergraduates
   a. Spend more time studying than exercising.
   b. Spend more time exercising than studying.
   c. Spend more time exercising than 12-year-olds.
   d. Spend more time exercising than watching TV.

4. To motivate yourself to stick to an exercise program:
   a. Watch professional athletic competitions.
   b. Set a long-term goal, then break it down into short-term goals that can be achieved in a few months.
   c. Keep a detailed record of all the times that you avoided working out.
   d. Join an expensive health club so that you feel pressured to get your money's worth.

5. The benefits of regular physical activity include:
   a. Decreased bone mass.
   b. Lowered risk of shin splints.
   c. Enhanced immune response.
   d. Altered sleep patterns.

6. The new Exercise Guidelines for Americans recommend all of these except:
   a. Engage in at least 30 minutes of moderate-intensity physical activity on most days of the week.
   b. Engage in physical activity of more vigorous intensity or longer duration for greater health benefits.
   c. Engage in 60 minutes of moderate- to vigorous-intensity activity on most days of the week to prevent gradual weight gain.
   d. Engage in 120 minutes of vigorous-intensity activity to really get fit.

7. For any muscle to get stronger, it must work against a greater than-normal resistance. This is called the
   a. Reversibility principle.
   b. Overload principle.
   c. FITT principle.
   d. Principle of diminishing returns.

8. Which of the following precautions could help prevent a serious injury from occurring?
   a. Wear swimming goggles when doing laps to decrease the irritating effects of chlorine.
   b. Wear knee pads when cycling to prevent knee gashes if you fall off your bicycle.
   c. To eliminate persistent muscle soreness, increase the frequency and/or time period of your workout.
   d. Wear a helmet, wrist guards, and knee pads when inline skating to help prevent fractures and head injuries.

9. The PRICE prescription for coping with an exercise injury is
   a. Pamper, Rest, Insure, Compress, Elevate.
   b. Protect, Rest, Ice, Condition, Elevate.
   c. Protect, Rest, Ice, Compress, Elevate.
   d. Protect, Rest, Ice, Cold, Elevate.

10. Which of the following statements is true?
    a. People with heart disease should not exercise.
    b. People with diabetes should not exercise.
    c. People over 40 should not exercise.
    d. Almost all people can participate in some form of exercise.

Answers to these questions can be found on page 376.

Critical Thinking

1. Allison knows that exercise is good for her health, but she figures she can keep her weight down by dieting and worry about her heart and health when she gets older, "I look good, I feel okay. Why should I bother exercising?" she asks. What would you reply?

2. Your friend Tony is convinced that his asthma attacks have diminished since he joined the rowing team. Do you think this is possible? How might rowing and exercise be affecting Tony's respiratory system?

3. Your younger brother Andre is hoping to get a starting position on his high school football team, although he is not the biggest or the strongest. What advice would you give him to help prevent his getting injured during practice?

Media Menu

Health ⊗ Now™

Don't forget to check out the wealth of resources on the HealthNow website at **http://healthnow.brookscole.com/itw** that will:
- Help you evaluate your knowledge of the material
- Allow you to take an exam-prep quiz
- Provide a Personalized Learning Plan targeting resources that address areas you should study
- Coach you through identifying target goals for behavior change and

creating and monitoring your personal change plan throughout the semester.

INTERNET CONNECTIONS

American Council on Exercise

www.acefitness.org

This website features information for the general public as well as for certified fitness trainers. The comprehensive site includes health and fitness news headlines, Fit Facts information sheets, a question and answer site, whole body exercise workouts, daily fitness tips, discussion boards, newsletters, and information on ACE certification.

American Alliance for Health, Physical Education, Recreation, and Dance

www.aahperd.org

This organization provides legislative advocacy for healthy lifestyles through high-quality programs in health and physical education. The website features consumer news, career links, a listing of graduate programs, research, and a link for the *International Electronic Journal of Health Education.*

Shape Up America

www.shapeup.org/fitness.html

At this site, you can perform a battery of physical fitness assessments, including activity level, strength, flexibility, and aerobic fitness. You get started by entering your weight, height, age, and gender, and then take a quick screening test to assess your physical readiness for physical activity. Your final results in each area will be based on your personal data.

Just Move

www.justmove.org

At this website sponsored by the American Heart Association, after a free registration, you can access an interactive exercise diary, where you can keep track of your own exercise progress. In addition, an information resource called My Fitness provides recommendations for optimizing your exercise program to match your lifestyle, as well as a list of health and fitness resources.

InfoTrac College Edition Activities

Check "Health benefits of exercise," *JAAPA-Journal of the American Academy of Physicians Assistants,* Feb 2005 v18 i2 p30.

1. List five proven benefits of exercise.
2. What are some examples of moderate intensity activities?
3. Describe ways to get started exercising.

You can find additional readings related to personal health with InfoTrac College Edition, an online library of more than 900 journals and publications. Follow the instructions for accessing InfoTrac College Edition that were packaged with your textbook; then search for articles using a keyword search.

For additional links, resources, and suggested readings on the InfoTrac College Edition, visit our Health and Wellness Resource Center at **http://health .wadsworth.com.**

Key Terms

The terms listed are used on the page indicated. Definitions of the terms are in the Glossary at the end of the book.

acute injuries 54
aerobic exercise 42
body composition 42
cardiorespiratory fitness 42
conditioning 42
delayed-onset muscle soreness (DOMS) 55
diminishing returns principle 51
edema 55
endorphins 47
FITT 49

flexibility 42
muscular endurance 42
muscular strength 42
osteoporosis 47
overload principle 49
overtrain 55
overuse injuries 54
physical fitness 42
principle of reversibility 51
progressive overloading 49
specificity principle 50

Improving Cardio-respiratory Fitness

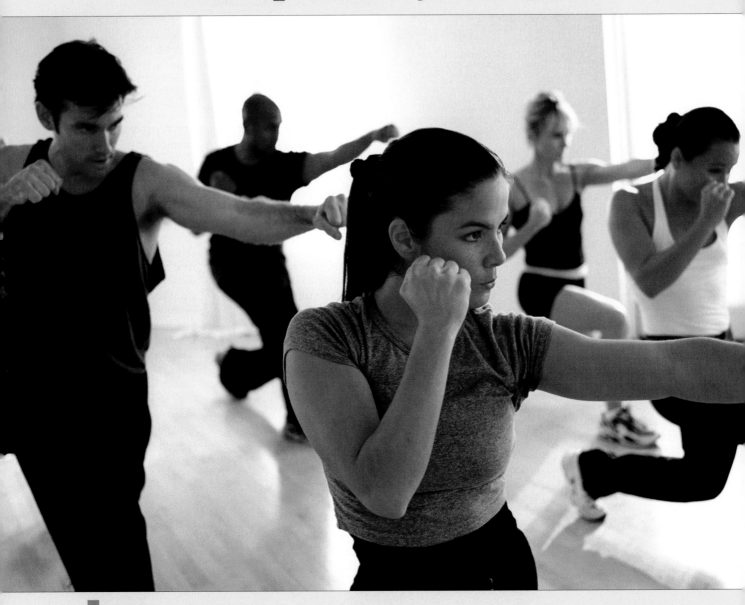

As a bicycle messenger in San Francisco, Manny would smile at the joggers huffing and puffing up the steep hills. "At least I get paid to work up a sweat," he'd think to himself. After Manny had saved enough money to study full-time at a community college, he spent more time on a bus than on a bike. Between classes and a new weekend job, he never thought about taking time to exercise.

Manny's mother was the one who insisted he get his blood pressure and cholesterol levels checked. "I'm too young to worry about heart attack," he told her. "Not with a family history like ours," she replied. Manny's father had his first heart attack when he was just 34; both of his grandfathers died of heart disease before age 55.

"I've got good news and bad news," the doctor told Manny after examining him and evaluating his blood tests. "The bad news is that you have several risk factors for heart disease. The good news is that you can do a lot to lower that risk." When she reached for her prescription pad, Manny thought he'd have to start taking medicine. Instead she wrote a prescription for 30 to 60 minutes of "cardio" a day.

Like other muscles, the heart becomes stronger and more efficient when challenged regularly by exercise—and weaker and less efficient when unexercised. Over years of sedentary living, an extremely inactive person has six times the risk of heart disease as someone who is active. It's never too late to reverse this situation, however. A three-month moderate-intensity cardiorespiratory fitness program can boost cardiorespiratory fitness by 15 to 20 percent.

This chapter describes the workings of the heart, blood vessels, and lungs; explains how exercise conditions the heart; reports on the benefits of heart-strengthening workouts; and provides guidelines on ways to keep your heart healthy throughout your life.

Marc Romanelli GETTY

After studying the material in this chapter, you should be able to:

▌ **Explain** the functions of the cardiovascular and respiratory systems.

▌ **Define** cardiorespiratory endurance and aerobic exercise.

▌ **Explain** how cardiorespiratory fitness is assessed and **list** tests commonly used to determine cardiovascular endurance.

▌ **Discuss** the stages of an aerobic workout and explain the benefits of each stage.

▌ **Compare** and **contrast** different forms of aerobic exercise and **determine** the most effective activity for your exercise program.

Health❀Now™

Don't forget to check out the wealth of resources on the HealthNow website at **http://healthnow.brookscole.com/itw** that will:
- Help you evaluate your knowledge of the material
- Allow you to take an exam-prep quiz
- Provide a Personalized Learning Plan targeting resources that address areas you should study
- Coach you through identifying target goals for behavior change and creating and monitoring your personal change plan throughout the semester.

✚ Inside the Cardiovascular and Respiratory Systems

The **cardiovascular system** consists of the heart and the blood vessels within the body. *Cardio* refers to the anatomical and functional aspects of the heart; *vascular,* to the vessels that carry blood to and from it. The cardiovascular system's fundamental job is to provide every cell with a continuous supply of nutrients and oxygen and to remove carbon dioxide and other waste materials from the body. The respiratory system works in tandem with the cardiovascular system to accomplish this mission.

The Heart

The heart is a hollow, muscular organ with four chambers that serve as two pumps (**Figure 4-1**). Each pump consists of a pair of chambers formed of muscles. The two upper chambers—each called an **atrium**—receive blood, which then flows through valves into the two lower chambers, the **ventricles,** which contract to pump blood

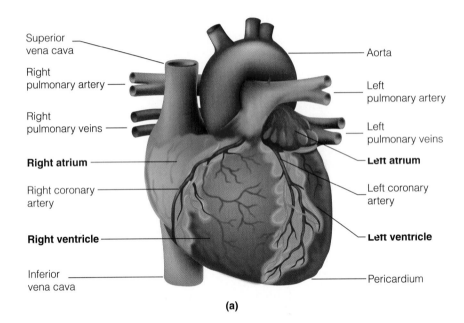

Superior vena cava
Right pulmonary artery
Right pulmonary veins
Right atrium
Right coronary artery
Right ventricle
Inferior vena cava

Aorta
Left pulmonary artery
Left pulmonary veins
Left atrium
Left coronary artery
Left ventricle
Pericardium

(a)

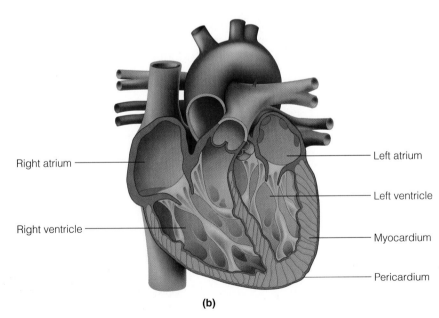

Right atrium
Right ventricle

Left atrium
Left ventricle
Myocardium
Pericardium

(b)

FIGURE 4-1 ▌ **The Healthy Heart**

(a) The heart muscle is nourished by blood from the coronary arteries, which arise from the aorta.
(b) The cross section shows the four chambers and the myocardium, the muscle that does the heart's work. The pericardium is the outer covering of the heart.

out into the arteries through a second set of valves. A thick wall called the septum divides the right side of the heart from the left, but even though the two halves are separated, they contract at almost the same time. The contraction of the ventricles is called **systole;** the period of relaxation between contractions is called **diastole.** The heart valves, located at the entrance to and exit from the ventricular chambers, have flaps that open and close to allow blood to flow through the chambers of the heart.

The heart muscle, or **myocardium,** consists of branching fibers that enable the heart to contract, or beat, about 100,000 times a day. With each beat, the heart pumps about 2 ounces of blood. Although this may not sound like much, it adds up to nearly 5 quarts of blood pumped by the heart in one minute and about 75 gallons in one hour. In a single year, the heart beats about 40 million times.

The Blood Vessels

The heart pumps oxygen-rich blood from the lungs to all parts of the body through a network of **arteries** and smaller branches called arterioles (**Figure 4-2**). The arterioles, in turn, are linked to smaller vessels called metarterioles and ultimately to **capillaries,** tiny blood vessels only slightly larger in diameter than a single red blood cell that serve as transfer stations. The network of tiny capillaries is where the exchange of oxygen and carbon dioxide between blood and body cells takes place. The blood within the capillaries supplies oxygen and nutrients and takes up various waste products.

From the capillaries, blood returns to the heart via another series of metarterioles, which are linked to small venules, which in turn lead to the larger **veins.** Veins, which are smaller and thinner than arteries, are intertwined with skeletal muscles. The blood from the upper body (except the lungs) drains into the heart through the *superior vena cava,* and blood from the lower body returns via the *inferior vena cava.*

The Respiratory System

The **respiratory system** is responsible for supplying oxygen to the blood and expelling waste gases. Ten to 20 times a minute, every day of your life, the lungs expand and contract. With every inhalation, air passes through the nasal passages, throat, larynx, trachea (windpipe), and bronchi into the lungs and travels through their many branching tubes to tiny air sacs called **alveoli.** There, in thousands of tiny chambers, oxygen is picked up by hemoglobin, a protein carried by red blood cells, and transferred through the membrane of the alveolar walls to the blood cells in the capillaries. At the same time, carbon dioxide passes from blood cells into the air in the alveoli and is exhaled.

Within cells oxygen converts nutrients into adenosine triphosphate (ATP), a compound that provides energy for maintaining internal equilibrium, body functions, and physical activity. Physical exertion requires more ATP, so the heart, lungs, and blood vessels have to deliver more oxygen.

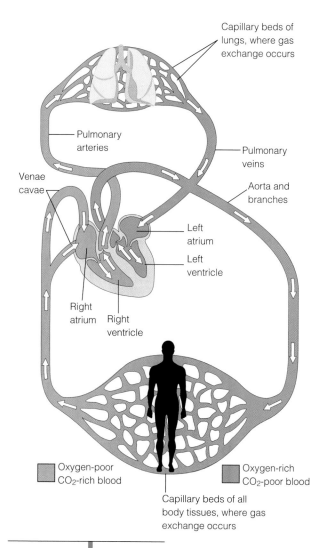

Capillary beds of lungs, where gas exchange occurs

Pulmonary arteries

Pulmonary veins

Venae cavae

Aorta and branches

Left atrium

Left ventricle

Right atrium

Right ventricle

☐ Oxygen-poor CO₂-rich blood

☐ Oxygen-rich CO₂-poor blood

Capillary beds of all body tissues, where gas exchange occurs

FIGURE 4-2 ▮ The Path of Blood Flow

Blood is pumped from the right ventricle into the pulmonary arteries, which lead to the lungs, where gas exchange (oxygen for carbon dioxide) occurs. Oxygenated blood returning from the lungs drains into the left atrium and is then pumped into the left ventricle, which sends the blood into the aorta and its branches. The oxygenated blood flows through the arteries, which extend to all parts of the body. Again, gas exchange occurs in the body tissues; this time oxygen is "dropped off" and carbon dioxide "picked up."

✚ Working Hearts

The hearts you hear about in poems and love songs get stolen or broken. We lose them or give them away. In real life, the heart does much more: it provides nourishment, protects against infection, maintains body temperature, and even hauls away garbage. The heart never rests, even when you do. Whenever you move, it responds immediately. The greater the demand, the harder it works to ensure that all of your bodily systems are functioning at their peak efficiency.

Aerobic training increases your **maximal oxygen uptake (VO$_2$ max),** the amount of oxygen you can use during physical activity. Depending on your initial level of fitness, you may be able to increase your maximal oxygen uptake by as much as 30 percent. As a result, you will be able to exercise longer and more intensely before becoming fatigued.

If your level of cardiorespiratory endurance is high, your heart and lungs can deliver the extra oxygen needed for prolonged exercise relatively easily. If your cardiorespiratory endurance is poor, your heart has to work at a higher rate, your tissues receive less oxygen, and you become fatigued more quickly. The greater your **oxygen uptake (VO$_2$),** the more efficiently your cardiorespiratory system is working.

As discussed in Chapter 5, muscles grow stronger and bigger when exercised. The same is true of the heart. As it becomes stronger, the heart muscle contracts more forcefully, which helps the heart eject more blood with

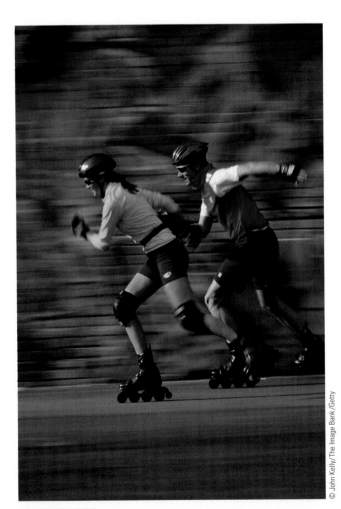

▌ With aerobic exercise, your heart will get stronger and your resting heart rate will decrease. This will save your heart millions of beats every year.

© John Kelly/The Image Bank /Getty

each beat. Because of this increase in **stroke volume,** the heart can rest longer between beats.

Heart rate—the number of beats per minute (bpm)—is higher in sedentary people and lower in those who exercise regularly. If you engage in no or very little physical activity, your resting heart rate, measured when you are doing nothing, is likely to be between 70 and 80 bpm. If you are active and fit, your resting heart rate might range from 45 to 55 bpm. A reduction of 20 bpm—which can occur with six to eight weeks of training—saves your heart about 10.5 million beats per year.

Aerobic training produces other beneficial changes in the cardiovascular system, including increases in red blood cells and the oxygen-carrying capacity of the blood, in the number and size of the mitochondria (the energy packets that provide fuel for work), and in the number of capillaries, which allow for the exchange of oxygen and carbon dioxide between the blood and the cells.

✚ Cardiorespiratory, or Aerobic, Fitness

Cardiorespiratory endurance refers to the ability of the heart, lungs, and circulatory system to deliver oxygen to muscles working rhythmically over an extended period of time. Unlike muscular endurance (discussed in Chapter 5), which is specific to individual muscles, cardiorespiratory endurance involves the entire body. **Aerobic exercise** improves cardiorespiratory endurance. Aerobic exercise can take many forms, as noted later in this chapter, but all involve working strenuously without pushing to the point of breathlessness. A person who builds up good aerobic capacity can maintain long periods of physical activity without great fatigue.

In **anaerobic exercise,** the amount of oxygen taken in by the body cannot meet the demands of the activity. This quickly creates an oxygen deficit that must be made up later. Anaerobic activities are high in intensity but short in duration, usually lasting only about ten seconds to two minutes. An example is sprinting the quarter-mile, which leaves even the best-trained athletes gasping for air. In *nonaerobic exercise,* such as bowling, softball, or doubles tennis, there is frequent rest between activities. Because the body can take in all the oxygen it needs, the heart and lungs really don't get much of a workout.

✚ The Benefits of Aerobic Exercise

Working the heart and lungs may indeed be the best prescription for optimal health and wellness. Among the benefits are the following:

▌ **Lower risk of cardiovascular disease and heart attack.** Sedentary men and women are about twice as

STUDENT SNAPSHOT

The Exercise I.Q.s of Undergraduates

Exercise Fact	Students Who Knew It*
Physical activity can prevent heart disease.	81%
Exercise can help prevent obesity.	89%
Exercise can help treat obesity.	83%
Exercise can help prevent diabetes.	36%
Exercise increases or maintains bone density.	45%

*Based on a study of 241 third-year students. Of these, 71 percent exercised regularly, and 58 percent met the minimum recommended guidelines for fitness.

Source: Hussey, J. M., et al. "Physical Activity Behavior and Knowledge of Effects of Physical Activity and Exercise Recommendations among University Students." *Journal of Sports Sciences,* March 2004, Vol. 22, No. 3, p. 282.

likely as active ones to suffer a heart attack and die as a result of coronary heart disease (CHD). The less active a person is, the greater the risk of a first heart attack and of fatal CHD. Yet not all college students know that exercise can prevent heart disease.[1] (See Student Snapshot "The Exercise I.Q.s of Undergraduates.")

- **Lower risk of dying prematurely.** When researchers have followed men from the time of one routine medical exam to the next, those who remained unfit had the highest all-cause mortality rates. Only exercise at a level that burns up 1,500 calories a week, however, has been shown to actually extend lifespan.
- **Improved blood flow and cholesterol levels.** Aerobic exercise decreases total cholesterol and low-density lipoproteins (LDL, the "bad" cholesterol) and slightly increases the good form of cholesterol, high-density lipoproteins (HDL).
- **Lower blood pressure.** Aerobic exercise has been shown to bring down blood pressure readings, perhaps by reducing body weight and fat stores.
- **Healthier blood vessels.** Aerobic exercise may reduce the risk of heart disease by improving the functioning of the **endothelium,** the specialized layer of tissue inside blood vessels, perhaps by improving its ability to produce nitric oxide, a substance that causes blood vessels to relax and contract more efficiently. (Abnormal endothelial function is believed to be the underlying cause of coronary artery disease.)
- **Lower levels of C-reactive protein.** Exercise is one of the best ways to reduce this indicator of increased

risk of heart disease and diabetes, discussed in depth in Chapter 10.[2]

- **Less risk of blood clots.** Aerobic exercise reduces the body's ability to produce dangerous blood clots that can obstruct blood vessels and cause heart attacks or strokes. Men who exercise have greater blood flow and less constriction in their coronary arteries than those who do not exercise.
- **Help in managing weight and preventing obesity.** Even relatively small amounts of excess fat—as little as 5 pounds—can add to the dangers in those already at risk for hypertension and diabetes. Other hazards of being overweight include higher rates of heart disease, gallbladder disease, osteoarthritis, and certain cancers.
- **Improved immune system.** Regular exercisers are less susceptible to minor viral illnesses, such as colds and the flu. The reason may be that aerobic exercise helps activate the immune system so that it can fight off infection.[3]
- **Increased bone mass and reduced risk of osteoporosis.** Aerobic exercise can help maintain bone health and lower vulnerability to bone injury and weakening.
- **Greater sense of well-being, increased energy, and more self-confidence.** These benefits may be due to increases in brain chemicals, including beta-endorphin and serotonin. Even a program of mild aerobic exercise can improve depression, particularly in people with chronic illnesses such as coronary heart disease.
- **Enhanced athletic performance.** Endurance training improves performance by increasing fat oxidation

STRATEGIES for CHANGE

How to Add Years to Your Life

The exercise-equivalent of 1,500 calories a week can affect the quantity as well as the quality of your life. Here are some aerobic options to meet this level. To exercise vigorously enough to burn up 1,500 calories a week, you could:

- Walk at a rate of three to four miles an hour for at least 30 minutes five times a week.
- Jog at a rate of six to seven miles an hour for three hours a week.
- Cycle for an hour four times a week.
- Swim laps for three hours a week.
- Play singles tennis for an hour three days a week.

and lowering the accumulation of **lactic acid,** a by-product of the breakdown of glucose that causes muscle fatigue.

❚ Assessing Your Cardiorespiratory Fitness

You probably have some idea of how hard your heart has to work to propel you as you go up a flight of stairs or sprint for a bus. If you're easily winded, chances are your cardiorespiratory fitness is less than ideal. There are more reliable and precise ways of assessing the state of your heart and lungs, however, including the following (see your Lab Booklet for the details):

❚ **One-mile walking test.** This test is based on the amount of time you take to complete a mile of brisk walking and your exercise heart rate at the end of your walk. A fast time and a low heart rate indicate good cardiorespiratory endurance. One advantage of this test is that individuals who haven't been exercising or who have suffered injuries can complete it safely.

❚ **Three-minute step test.** This test measures the rate at which the pulse returns to normal after exercise. A quick recovery is an indicator of physical fitness. To do the test, you step continuously at a steady rate for three minutes and then monitor your heart rate as it returns to normal. This test is not advised for those who are obese or who have joint problems in their hips, knees, or ankles.

❚ **1.5-mile run test.** This test is field measure of aerobic capacity. The greater your speed in traveling 1.5 miles, the higher your maximal oxygen consumption. This test works best for healthy individuals who have been moderately active. You should not perform this test in extremely hot or cold temperatures if you aren't accustomed to exercising in such weather.

❚ **Astrand-Rhyming cycle ergometer test.** The cycle ergometer measures the amount of resistance against a person's pedaling. The higher this power output, the harder or faster the cyclist is working. The test estimates maximal oxygen consumption from the exercise heart rate reached after pedaling for six minutes at a constant rate and resistance. A low exercise heart rate after pedaling at high intensity indicates high maximal oxygen consumption. This test is recommended for healthy people who have been at least moderately active and individuals with joint problems.

How Can I Tell If I'm Working Hard Enough?

To be sure you're working hard enough to condition your heart and lungs, but not overdoing it, use your pulse, or heart rate, as a guide. One of the easiest places to feel your pulse is in the carotid artery in your neck. Slightly

tilt your head back and to one side. Use your middle finger or fore-finger, or both, to feel for your pulse. (Do not use your thumb; it has a beat of its own.) To determine your heart rate, count the number of pulses you feel for 10 seconds and multiply that number by six, or count for 30 seconds and multiply that number by two. Learn to recognize the pulsing of your heart when you're sitting or lying down. This is your **resting heart rate.**

Start taking your pulse during, or immediately after, exercise, when it's much more pronounced than when you're at rest. Three minutes after heavy exercise, take your pulse again. The closer that reading is to your resting heart rate, the better your condition. If it takes a long time for your pulse to recover and return to its resting level, your body's ability to handle physical stress is poor. As you continue working out, however, your pulse will return to normal much more quickly.

You don't want to push yourself to your maximum heart rate, yet you must exercise at about 60 to 85 percent of that maximum to get cardiorespiratory benefits from your training. This range is called your **target heart rate.** If you don't exercise intensely enough to raise your heart rate at least this high, your heart and lungs won't reap the most benefit from the workout. If you push too hard and exercise at or near your absolute maximum heart rate, you run the risk of placing too great a burden on your heart. **Figure 4-3** shows the target heart rate for

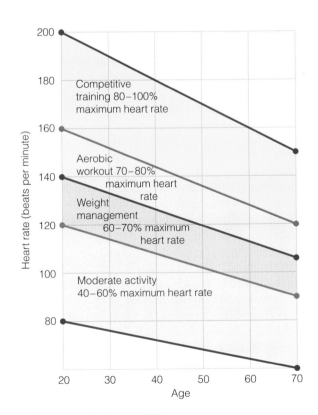

FIGURE 4-3 ❚ Target Heart Rates for Different Ages and Various Levels of Activity

Your maximum heart rate is 220 minus your age.

various ages and activities. Find your age at the bottom of the figure and move up the grid to find your target heart rate for "aerobic workout."

You can also use the following steps to determine your maximum heart rate and target heart rate (in beats per minute):

1. Maximum heart rate: Subtract your age from 220. So if you are 20, your maximum heart rate is $220 - 20 = 200$ beats per minute.
2. Lower-limit target heart rate: Multiply your maximum heart rate by 0.6. So if you are 20, your lower-limit target heart rate is $200 \times 0.6 = 120$ beats per minute.
3. Upper-limit target heart rate. Multiply your maximum heart rate by 0.85. If you are 20, your upper-limit target heart range is $200 \times 0.85 = 170$.

Your target heart rate range is between your lower and upper limits (Table 4-1).

According to the American College of Sports Medicine, for most people, exercising at the lower end of the target heart rate range for a long time is more beneficial than exercising at the higher end of the range for a short time. If your goal is losing weight, exercise at 60 to 70 percent of your maximum heart rate in order to burn fat calories. To improve aerobic endurance and strengthen your heart, work at 70 to 80 percent of your maximum heart rate. Competitive athletes may train at 80 to 100 percent of their maximum heart rate (See Figure 4-3).

Although many fitness experts still believe that maximum target heart rate, also known as the Karvonen formula, is the best measurement of exercise intensity, others have doubts because many factors (caffeine, stress, lack of sleep) can affect heart rate. According to research at the University of Colorado, Boulder, the Karvonen formula overestimates maximum heart rate in young

adults and underestimates it in older adults. One alternative formula, developed by Hirofumi Tanaka, is

208 minus 70% of age.

However, Tanaka notes that actual maximum heart rate may vary by as many as ten beats per minute.[4]

Rating of Perceived Exertion

Another option besides heart rate for monitoring your exercise intensity is the **Rating of Perceived Exertion (RPE),** a self-assessment scale that rates symptoms of breathlessness and fatigue. You can use the RPE scale to describe your sensation of effort when exercising and gauge how hard you are working. The American College of Sports Medicine revised the original RPE scale to a range of 0 to 10 (**Figure 4-4**). Most exercisers should aim for a perceived exertion of "Somewhat strong" or "strong," the equivalent of 4 or 5 on the RPE scale.

RPE is considered fairly reliable, but about 10 percent of the population tends to over- or underestimate their exertion. Your health or physical education instructor can help you learn to match what your body is feeling to the RPE scale. By paying attention to how you feel at different exercise intensities, you can learn how to challenge yourself without risking your safety.

TABLE 4-1 ▌ Target Heart Rate

Age	Average Maximum Heart Rate (100%)	Target Heart Rate (60–85%)	
20	200	120	170
25	195	117	166
30	190	114	162
35	185	111	157
40	180	108	153
45	175	105	149
50	170	102	145
55	165	99	140
60	160	96	136
65	155	93	132
70	150	90	128

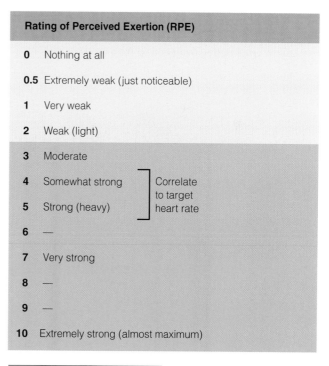

Rating of Perceived Exertion (RPE)

0	Nothing at all
0.5	Extremely weak (just noticeable)
1	Very weak
2	Weak (light)
3	Moderate
4	Somewhat strong
5	Strong (heavy)
6	—
7	Very strong
8	—
9	—
10	Extremely strong (almost maximum)

Correlate to target heart rate (bracketing 4 and 5)

FIGURE 4-4 ▌ Revised Scale for Rating of Perceived Exertion (RPE)
You can learn to rate your exertion based on this scale.

Source: Original scale from G. Borg. "Psychophysical Bases of Perceived Exertion." *Medicine and Science in Sports and Exercise,* Vol. 14, No. 5, 2003, pp. 377–381.

You can also experiment with other alternative ways for determining exercise intensity. One of the easiest follows.

The "Talk Test"

During "aerobic" exercise, you should be able to carry on a somewhat stilted conversation, if you are indeed "with oxygen"—which is what the word "aerobic" means.

If you are gasping for air and unable to talk, you are most likely working at or beyond the anaerobic "without oxygen" threshold—a very, very, very hard intensity level at or beyond the high end of the aerobic zone.

If you can sing the entire Star Spangled Banner, you are probably not exerting much effort. If you can sing "Row Row Row Your Boat," but have to take a breath after every other word, you are probably working pretty hard—and just where you should be.

✚ Designing an Aerobic Workout

Whatever activity you choose, your aerobic workout should consist of several stages: a warm-up, an aerobic activity, and a cool-down (**Figure 4-5**).

Warm-Up

Just as you don't get in your car and immediately gun your engine to 60 miles per hour, you shouldn't do the same with your body. You need to prepare your car-

diorespiratory system for a workout, speed up the blood flow to your lungs, and increase the temperature and elasticity of your muscles and connective tissue to avoid injury.

After reviewing more than 350 scientific studies, the American College of Sports Medicine (ACSM) concluded that preparing for sports or exercise should involve a variety of activities and not be limited to stretching alone. They found little to no relationship between stretching and injuries or postexercise pain. A better option, according to the ACSM, is a combination of warm-up, strength training, and balance exercises.[5]

Start by walking briskly for about 5 minutes. This helps your body make the transition from inactivity to exertion. Follow this general warm-up with about 5 minutes of simple stretches of the muscles you'll be exercising most. Before a jog, for instance, you can stretch the muscles in your ankle and the back of your leg by leaning against a wall, with one leg bent and tilted forward and the other straight. Lean forward until you feel the stretch and hold.

Aerobic Activity

The two key components of this part of your workout are intensity and duration. As described in the previous section, you can use your target heart rate range to make sure you are working at the proper intensity. The current recommendation is to keep moving for 20 to 60 minutes, either in one session or several briefer sessions, each lasting at least 10 minutes.

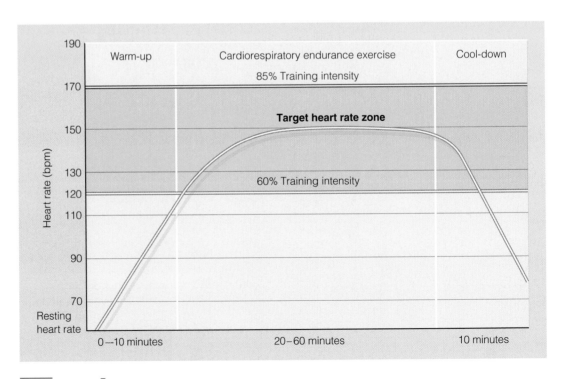

FIGURE 4-5 ▌ A Cardiorespiratory Endurance Workout

Why Do I Have to Cool Down?

After you've pushed your heart rate up to its target level and kept it there for a while, the worst thing you can do is slam on the brakes. If you come to a sudden stop, you put your heart at risk. When you stand or sit immediately after vigorous exercise, blood can pool in your legs. You need to keep moving at a slower pace to ensure an adequate supply of blood to your heart. Ideally, you should walk for 5 to 10 minutes at a comfortable pace before you end your workout session.

Cross-Training

Cross-training involves alternating two or more different types of fitness activities. The pioneers of contemporary cross-training were triathletes whose sport combines running, swimming, and cycling. Depending on the specific sports, cross-training can yield various benefits. Alternating aerobic workouts with weight lifting, for example, can increase speed and performance. Alternating running with a low-impact aerobic exercise, such as swimming, lessens the risk of knee, ankle, or shin injuries. Cross-training also offers the pleasures of variety and thus helps exercisers avoid boredom.

No one cross-training combination is right for everyone. To plan a program, first identify your fitness goals: Do you want to increase your cardiorespiratory endurance, control your weight, get stronger, improve your general health, or improve your performance in a particular competitive sport? Your unique fitness goals will dictate the cross-training program that's right for you.

Aerobic Interval Training

In aerobic activities, intensity training often is referred to as *interval training,* which intersperses small, manageable bouts of all-out effort with periods of low to moderate exertion. When the body works at its maximum, it quickly moves beyond aerobic to anaerobic and taps glycogen stored in the muscles for fuel. The combustion of this fuel leads to a buildup of lactate in the muscles and fatigue. The body slows down to a lower level of exertion and decreases intensity back into an aerobic training mode. Interval training helps improve overall fitness levels and also burns more calories than exercising at a steady rate.

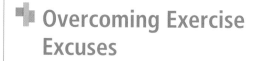

Overcoming Exercise Excuses

Why do you work out? Looking better and feeling better are two of the strongest motivators that pull college students to their feet.

Studies show that students with a greater sense of self-efficacy and an internal locus of control place greater value on health and fitness, are more conscious about living a healthy lifestyle, and are more likely to be actively involved in activities that maintain or enhance fitness.[6]

The primary motivators for students are a desire to increase their fitness, improve the way their bodies look, enhance muscle tone and strength, and gain a sense of personal accomplishment.

If you don't exercise regularly, why not? As studies have shown, sedentary college students perceive fewer benefits from exercise than their more active peers. They also cite more exercise barriers, things that get in the way of even the best intentions. The number one obstacle for students is lack of time. Others include feeling tired after exercise, thinking that exercise is hard work, and not getting encouragement from family to exercise.[7]

For every excuse not to exercise, there is an excuse buster. Here is a sampling of excuses from an Internet survey of college students—and some effective responses:

Excuse	Excuse-Buster
"Gym membership is too expensive."	You can get all the exercise you need on your own. Invest in a good pair of shoes and start walking or running. Select at-home strength and flexibility exercises from Chapter 5.
"The school gym is always crowded."	Try different times, for example, early morning or afternoon. Rather than standing in line for machines, work with free weights.
"I don't have time to spend an hour exercising."	Build activity into your day. Walk to classes or always take the stairs rather than the elevator in the dorms.
"I mean to exercise, but I get too busy."	Sign up for a fitness "class," such as spinning or cardiokick-boxing, so that exercise is built into your weekly schedule.
"I get to my room and just don't feel like leaving."	Arrange to meet friends at the gym. If you know they're waiting, you'll go out even if it's rainy and cold.
"I get bored."	Find a fun workout. If you hate the treadmill, try spinning, aerobic dance, or inline-skating.
"I forget why exercise is important."	Use humor to keep yourself motivated. One student put this sign on the wall: "You think flu season is scary? Wait till bathing suit season hits!"

▌ "Studying takes all my time."

Do double-duty. Some students read class notes while on a stairmaster or stationary bicycle. Others listen to required books through earphones as they work out.

⊞ Aerobic Options

You have lots of choices for aerobic exercise, so experiment. Focus on one for a few weeks; alternate different activities on different days; try something new every month. But don't believe the "pump fiction" that you can have instantaneous results—see Savvy Consumer: "Watch Out for 'Pump Fiction'."

Walking

More men and women are taking to their feet. Some are casualties of high-intensity sports and can no longer withstand the wear and tear of rigorous workouts. Others want to shape up, slim down, or ward off heart disease and other health problems. The good news for all is that walking is good exercise. Recent research has demonstrated that walking reduces the risk of cardiorespiratory disease, in some studies, as much as vigorous activity does.[8]

One major study of women, the Nurses' Health Study, found that women who walk briskly three hours a week are as well protected from heart disease as women who spend an hour and a half a week in more vigorous activities, such as aerobics or running. Women engaged in either form of exercise had a rate of heart attacks 30 to 40 percent lower than that of sedentary women.

Walking also protects men's hearts, whether they're healthy or have had heart problems. Men, who regularly engage in light exercise, including walking, have a significantly lower risk of premature death than their sedentary counterparts.

Walking has proved to be one of the safest and most effective ways of preventing bone and joint disorders in obese individuals.[9]

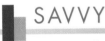

SAVVY
CONSUMER

WATCH OUT FOR "PUMP FICTION"

Shape up in seven days! Burn calories without breaking a sweat! A brand-new body in minutes a day!

Too good to be true? Absolutely. Advertisers promise no-sweat, no-effort ways to fitness with pills, potions, flab-melting belts, and thigh-slimming paddles. These claims amount to nothing more than what the American Council on Exercise calls "pump fiction." The benefits of fitness are real and well documented, but the only way to reap them is through regular exercise.

The Federal Trade Commission urges consumers to use common sense and good judgment when evaluating claims about exercise products. Here are some specific guidelines:

▌ Be wary of any program or product that promises "easy" or "effortless" results. Athletes in peak condition might use them without breaking

a sweat. Chances are that you, like most people, won't.

▌ Compared to what? Advertisers may claim that their exercise device burns calories faster or more efficiently. In general, aerobic exercises that work the whole body, like those described in this chapter, burn more calories than a product that works only the biceps, thighs, or gluteus.

▌ Watch out for "spot" reducers. You can't lose a "spare tire" or firm flabby thighs by targeting only that area of your body. You need to lose weight and tone your entire body.

▌ Read the fine print. Often it states that the results are based, not just on the device, but on dieting and exercise as well.

▌ Don't believe testimonials or celebrity endorsements. Just because one person had success with a particular type of fitness equipment doesn't mean that you will too. And slim, trim, smiling celebrities are paid well for their enthusiasm.

▌ Be skeptical of dramatic "before" and "after" photos. With today's technology, you never know if photos were doctored, or if the results lasted.

▌ Check the details on warranties, guarantees, and return policies. The ads may promise a "30-day, money-back guarantee" but fail to mention hefty shipping costs.

▌ If you have questions or complaints, check MedWatch, the FDA's voluntary reporting program at www.fda.gov/medwatch/how.htm. You also can file a complaint with the FTC by calling 1-877-FTC-HELP or going to www.ftc.gov/ftc/consumer.htm.

Here are some guidelines for putting your best foot forward:

▌ **Walk very slowly** for 5 minutes, and then do some simple stretches.

▌ **Maintain good posture.** Focus your eyes ahead of you, stand erect, and pull in your stomach.

▌ **Use the heel-to-toe method** of walking. The heel of your leading foot should touch the ground before the ball or toes of that foot do. When you push off with your trailing foot, bend your knee as you raise your heel. You should be able to feel the action in your calf muscles.

▌ **Pump your arms back and forth** to burn 5 to 10 percent more calories and get an upper-body workout as well.

▌ **End your walk the way you started it**—let your pace become more leisurely for the last 5 minutes.

Treadmills are a good alternative to outdoor walks—and not just in bad weather. They keep you moving at a certain pace, they're easier on the knees, and they allow you to exercise in a climate-controlled, pollution-free environment—a definite plus for many city dwellers. Holding onto the handrails while walking on a treadmill reduces both heart rate and oxygen consumption, so you burn fewer calories. Experts advise slowing the pace if necessary so you can let go of the handrails while working out.

Stepping Out

How many steps do you walk every day? The typical adult averages about 5,310 steps; a child from 11,000 to 13,000. According to the American College of Sports Medicine, college students who used a pedometer to count their daily steps took an average of 7,700 steps per day.[10] This falls short of the 10,000 steps recommended as part of the national "America on the Move" program.

How far is 10,000 steps? The average person's stride length is approximately 2.5 feet long. That means it takes just over 2,000 steps to walk 1 mile, and 10,000 steps is close to 5 miles. Wearing a pedometer is an easy way to track your steps each day. (See your Lab Booklet.) Start by wearing the pedometer every day for one week. Put it on when you get up in the morning and wear it until bedtime. Record your daily steps in your Wellness Journal. By the end of the week you can calculate your average daily steps. To increase your steps, add 500 daily steps every week until you reach 10,000.

Why 10,000 steps? According to researchers' estimates, you take about 5,000 steps just to accomplish your daily tasks. Adding about 2,000 steps brings you to a level that can improve your health and wellness. Another 3,000 steps can help you lose excess pounds and prevent weight gain. People who walk at least 10,000 steps a day are more likely to have healthy weights.[11] In addition,

10,000 steps generally translates into 30 minutes of activity, the minimum recommended by the U.S. Surgeon General.

Counting steps with a pedometer pays off, according to another report by the American College of Sports Medicine.[12] In the study, women who used a pedometer walked substantially more than those who simply tried to take a 30-minute brisk walk on most days.[13]

Jogging and Running

The difference between jogging and running is speed. You should be able to carry on a conversation with someone on a long jog or run; if you're too breathless to talk, you're pushing too hard.

If your goal is to enhance aerobic fitness, long, slow, distance running is best. If you want to improve your speed, try interval training—repeated hard runs over a certain distance, with intervals of relaxed jogging in between. Depending on what suits you and what your training goals are, you can vary the distance, duration, and number of fast runs, as well as the time and activity between them.

If you have been sedentary, it's best to launch a walking program before attempting to jog or run. Start by walking for 15 to 20 minutes three times a week at a comfortable pace. Continue at this same level until you no longer feel sore or unduly fatigued the day after exercising. Then increase your walking time to 20 to 25 minutes, speeding up your pace as well.

When you can handle a brisk 25-minute walk, alternate fast walking with slow jogging. Begin each session walking, and gradually increase the amount of time you spend jogging. If you feel breathless while jogging, slow down and walk. Continue to alternate in this manner until you can jog for 10 minutes without stopping. If you gradually increase your jogging time by 1 or 2 minutes with each workout, you'll slowly build up to 20 or 25 minutes per session. For optimal fitness, you should jog at least three times a week.

Here's how to be sure you're running right:

▌ **Always take time to warm up** and to stretch. Warm up with jumping jacks or running in place for 3 to 5 minutes. Spend at least one-fourth of the time that you plan to run on stretching exercises.

▌ **As you run, keep your back straight** and your head up. Run tall, with your buttocks tucked in. Look straight ahead. Hold your arms slightly away from your body. Your elbows should be bent slightly so that your forearms are almost parallel to the ground. Move your arms rhythmically to propel yourself along.

▌ **Have your heels hit the ground first.** Land on your heel, rock forward, and push off the ball of your foot. If this is difficult, try a more flat-footed style.

▌ **Avoid running on the balls of your feet;** this produces soreness in the calves because the muscles must contract for a longer time. To avoid shin splints (a dull ache in the lower shins), stretch regularly to strengthen the shin muscles and to develop greater flexibility in your ankles.

❙ **Avoid running on hard surfaces** and making sudden stops or turns.

❙ **Breathe through your nose and mouth** to get more volume. Learn to "belly breathe": when you breathe in, your belly should expand; when you breathe out, it should flatten. If your breathing becomes labored, try exhaling with resistance through pursed lips so that your body utilizes more oxygen per breath.

❙ **When you approach a hill, shorten your stride.** Lift your knees higher; pump your arms more. If the hill is really steep, lean forward. When you start down-hill, lean forward, and run as if you were on a flat surface. Don't lean back, because doing so could strain your knees and the muscles in your legs.

Swimming

More than 100 million Americans dive into the water every year. What matters for your heart's health, however, is getting a good workout, not just getting wet. Swimming is an excellent exercise for cardiorespiratory fitness and also rates fairly high for weight control, muscular function, and flexibility. However, it's not as effective for building strong bones and preventing osteoporosis as activities such as walking and running.

How Long Do I Have to Swim?

For aerobic conditioning, you have to swim laps, using the butterfly, breaststroke, backstroke, or crawl. (The sidestroke is too easy.) You've also got to be a good enough swimmer to keep churning through the water for at least 20 minutes. Your heart will beat more slowly in water than on land, so your heart rate while swimming is not an accurate guide to exercise intensity. You

should try to keep up a steady pace that's fast enough to make you feel pleasantly tired, but not completely exhausted, by the time you get out of the pool.

Swimming is good for people of all ages, particularly those over 50 or with physical handicaps. Swimming facilities are available in nearly all communities. Check your college gym; your local YWCA, YMCA, or JCC; your city recreation department; and other schools in your area.

Here are some guidelines for smart swimming:

❙ Start by swimming 50 yards and rest when you feel breathless.

❙ Try to swim 100 yards, rest for a minute, and then swim another 100 yards.

❙ Increase your distance slowly. See if you can work up to 700 yards in 18 minutes.

❙ Stick to the butterfly, breaststroke, backstroke, or crawl.

Cycling

Bicycling, indoors and out, can be an excellent cardiorespiratory conditioner, as well as an effective way to control weight—provided you aren't just along for the ride. If you coast down too many hills, you'll have to ride longer up hills or on level ground to get a good workout. Half of all bikes now sold in the United States are mountain bikes, sturdy cycles with knobby tires that allow bikers to climb up and zoom down dirt trails and explore places traditional racing bikes couldn't go. An 18-speed bike can make pedaling too easy, however, unless you choose gears carefully. To gain aerobic benefits, mountain bikers have to work hard enough to raise their heart rates to their target zone and keep up that intensity for at least 20 minutes.

Safety is an important concern for outdoor cyclists. Each year, bicycle crashes kill about 900 individuals; about 200 of those killed are children under age 15. About 567,000 people go to hospital emergency departments annually with bicycle-related injuries; 350,000 of the injured are children under 15. Safety helmets can reduce the risk of injury by 85 percent and could prevent one cyclist's death every day.

Another option is riding a stationary cycle indoors. Using a one-wheel stationary cycle with a tension-control knob, you can adjust the amount of effort required; start with low resistance, then increase the tension until you're working at your target heart rate. You can put the cycle in front of a television set or look out the window if you feel the need for some scenery—or you can read or simply meditate while pedaling.

Here's a guide to smart cycling:

❙ If you're not used to cycling, start slowly. Work up from 5 minutes of steady pedal-

© Stockbyte / PictureQuest

❙ If you choose to improve your cardiorespiratory fitness through swimming, you must swim laps for at least 20 minutes, using the butterfly, breaststroke, backstroke, or crawl.

ing (interrupted by rest periods if necessary) to 10, 15, 20, and 25 minutes. Limit your rides to 5 to 10 minutes the first week. Increase your time and speed gradually to avoid sore thigh muscles. Rest when you feel breathless.

▮ Keep your elbows slightly bent to allow for a more relaxed upper body. Change your hand positions periodically to avoid numbness.

▮ Monitor your heart rate to make sure you're working within your target range.

▮ When riding outdoors, be sure to wear a helmet. Look for proof that it conforms to either the Snell or the ANSI standard for head protection.

▮ Make yourself visible. Wear reflective clothing if you can. If you cannot, remember that drivers see bright pink, yellow, and orange most easily.

▮ Always follow the rules of the road—stick to the right, stop at stop signs, heed one-way signs, and so on.

Other Aerobic Activities

Because variety is the spice of an active life, many people prefer different forms of aerobic exercise. All can provide many health benefits. Among the popular options:

▮ **Spinning.™** Spinning is a cardiovascular workout for the whole body that utilizes a special stationary bicycle. Led by an instructor, a group of bikers listens to music, and modifies their individual bike's resistance and their own pace according to the rhythm. An average spinning class lasts 45 minutes.

In a recent study, participants at various fitness levels rated their levels of perceived exertion in the high

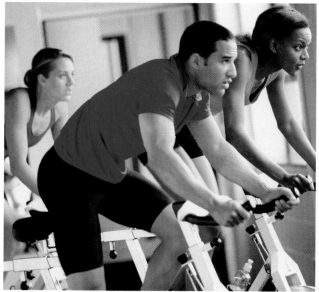

Spinning has become a popular option for aerobic exercise because people of different ages, skills, and fitness levels can participate in the same class.

teens through much of a typical spin class. However, the American Council on Exercise cautions that the intensity levels of many spin classes are far beyond what most beginners or part-time exercisers can achieve or maintain. You might want to train on a stationary bike before graduating to high-intensity spinning.[14]

▮ **Cardio kickboxing.** Also referred to as kickboxing or boxing aerobics, this hybrid of boxing, martial arts, and aerobics offers an intense cross-training and total-body workout. According to the American Council on Exercise, cardio kickboxing strengthens body and mind, decreases stress, sharpens reflexes, and increases cardiorespiratory endurance and power. An hour of kickboxing burns an average of 500 to 800 calories, compared to 300 to 400 calories in a typical step aerobics class.[15]

▮ **Rowing,** whether on water or a rowing machine, provides excellent aerobic exercise as well as working the upper and lower body. In addition to its benefits for the cardiorespiratory system, rowing tones the shoulders, back, arms, and legs. Correct rowing techniques are important to avoid back injury.

▮ **Skipping rope.** Essentially a form of stationary jogging with some extra arm action thrown in, skipping rope is excellent as both a heart conditioner and a way of losing weight. Always warm up before starting and cool down afterward.

▮ **Aerobic dancing.** This activity combines music with kicking, bending, and jumping. A typical class (you can also dance at home to a video or TV program) consists of stretching exercises and sit-ups, followed by aerobic dances and cool-down exercises. "Soft," or low-impact, aerobic dancing doesn't put as much strain on the joints as "hard," or high-impact, routines.

▮ **Step training or bench aerobics.** "Stepping" combines step, or bench, climbing with music and choreographed movements. Basic equipment consists of a bench 4 to 12 inches high. The fitter you are, the higher the bench—but the higher the bench, the greater the risk of knee injury.

▮ **Stair-climbing.** You could run up the stairs in an office building or dormitory, but most people use stair-climbing machines available in home models and at gyms and health clubs.

▮ **Inline skating.** Inline skating can increase aerobic endurance and muscular strength and is less stressful on joints and bones than running or high-impact aerobics. Skaters can adjust the intensity of their workout by varying the terrain.

▮ **Tennis.** As with other sports, tennis can be an aerobic activity—depending on the number of players and their skill level. In general, a singles match requires more continuous exertion than playing doubles.

▮ **Cross-country skiing.** One of the most effective forms of aerobic exercise is cross-country or Nordic skiing. Thanks to machines that simulate the moves of Nordic skiing, it's now possible to "ski" in any season.

Because almost every muscle in the body gets a workout, cross-country skiing is excellent for all-around conditioning. Another plus: The risk of joint and ligament injury while cross-country skiing is lower than for many other impact aerobic activities (and much lower than for downhill skiing).

✚ Exercising Outdoors

Prevention is the wisest approach to temperature and pollution problems. Always dress appropriately for the weather and be aware of the health risks associated with temperature extremes and with poor air quality.

Be Weather Wise

In hot weather, always wear as little as possible when exercising. Choose loose-fitting, lightweight, white or light-colored clothes. Never wear rubberized or plastic pants and jackets to sweat off pounds. Be sure to drink plenty of fluids while exercising (especially water), and watch for the earliest signs of heat problems, including cramps, stress, exhaustion, and heat stroke. (The next section provides more information on heat-related problems.)

In cool weather don't overdress. Excessive clothing can make you sweat more, which causes the body to lose heat rapidly. Dress in layers. The inner layer should be made of material that wicks perspiration away from the skin. The middle layers should provide insulation and absorb moisture. The outer layer should protect against wind and moisture.[16]

Start off feeling a little cool since your body temperature will increase when you start walking, running, or cycling. You are less likely to feel chilled if you start by heading into the wind and finish with the wind at your back. In cold weather, do not leave gaps of bare skin between your gloves and jacket. Wear a hat and cover your neck. Protect exposed areas, like your nose, with petroleum jelly.

Should I Run If It's Smoggy? ✚🔍

If you live in a large city, you may have to consider the risks of exercising in polluted air. On smoggy days, avoid a noontime workout. Exposure to ground-level ozone, produced as sunlight reacts with exhaust fumes, can irritate the lungs and constrict bronchial tubes. An ozone level of 0.12 part per million causes, on the average, a 13 percent decline in lung capacity. This level is the maximum considered safe under the Clean Air Act, but it is often surpassed in New York, Los Angeles, and other urban areas.

✚ Thinking of Temperature

Knowing what can go wrong is one of the keys to preventing problems related to heat or cold.

Heeding Heat

Two common heat-related maladies are **heat cramps** and **heat stress.** Heat cramps are caused by hard work and heavy sweating in the heat. Heat stress may occur simultaneously or afterward, as the blood vessels try to keep body temperature down. **Heat exhaustion,** a third such malady, is the result of prolonged sweating with inadequate fluid replacement. The first step in treating these three conditions is to stop exercising, move to a cool place, and drink plenty of water slowly. Don't resume work or activity until all the symptoms have disappeared; see a doctor if you're suffering from heat exhaustion.

Heat stroke is a life-threatening medical emergency caused by the breakdown of the body's mechanism for cooling itself. The treatment is to cool the body down: move to a cooler environment; sponge down with cool water, and apply ice to the back of the neck, armpits, and groin. Immersion in cold water could cause shock. Get medical help immediately. (Table 4-2 summarizes heat dangers.)

Coping with Cold

The tips of the toes, fingers, ears, nose, and chin and the cheeks are most vulnerable to exposure to high wind speeds and low temperatures, which can result in **frostnip.** Because frostnip is painless, you may not even be aware that it is occurring. Watch for a sudden blanching or lightening of your skin. The best early treatment is warming the area by firm, steady pressure with a warm hand; blowing on it with hot breath; holding it against your body; or immersing it in warm (not hot) water. As the skin thaws, it becomes red and starts to tingle. Be careful to protect it from further damage. Don't rub the skin vigorously or with snow, as you could damage the tissue.

TABLE 4-2 ❚ Heat Dangers

Illness	Symptoms	Treatment
Heat cramps	Muscle twitching or cramping; muscle spasms in arms, legs, and abdomen.	Stop exercising; cool off; drink water.
Heat stress	Fatigue, pale skin, blurred vision, dizziness, low blood pressure.	Stop exercising; cool off; drink water.
Heat exhaustion	Excessive thirst, fatigue, lack of coordination, increased sweating, elevated body temperature.	See a doctor.
Heat stroke	Lack of perspiration, high body temperature (over 105°F), dry skin, rapid breathing, coma, seizures, high pulse.	Cool the body; sponge down; get medical help.

the skin from further exposure to cold. See a doctor for further treatment. Deep frostbite, the freezing of skin, muscle, and even bone, requires medical treatment. It usually involves the tissues of the hands and feet, which appear pale and feel frozen. Keep the victim dry and as warm as possible on the way to a medical facility. Cover the frostbitten area with a dry, sterile dressing.

The center of the body may gradually cool at temperatures above, as well as below, freezing—usually in wet, windy weather. When body temperature falls below 95°F, the body is incapable of rewarming itself because of the breakdown of the internal system that regulates its temperature. This state is known as **hypothermia.** The first sign of hypothermia is severe shivering. Then the victim becomes uncoordinated, drowsy, listless, and confused and is unable to speak properly. Symptoms become more severe as body temperature continues to drop, and coma or death can result.

Hypothermia requires emergency medical treatment. Try to prevent any further heat loss. Move the victim to a warm place, cover him or her with blankets, remove wet clothing, and replace it with dry garments. If the victim is conscious, administer warm liquids, not alcohol.

Protect yourself in cold weather (or cold indoor gyms) by covering as much of your body as possible, but don't overdress. Wear one layer less than you would if you were outside but not exercising. Don't use warm-up clothes made of waterproof material, because they tend to trap heat and keep perspiration from evaporating. Make sure your clothes are loose enough to allow movement and exercise of the hands, feet, and other body parts, thereby maintaining proper circulation. Choose dark colors that absorb heat. And because 40 percent or more of your body heat is lost through your head and neck, wear a hat, turtleneck, or scarf. Make sure you cover your hands and feet as well; mittens provide more warmth and protection than gloves.

More severe is **frostbite.** There are two types of frostbite: *superficial* and *deep.* Superficial frostbite, the freezing of the skin and tissues just below the skin, is characterized by a waxy look and firmness of the skin, although the tissue below is soft. Initial treatment should be to slowly rewarm the area. As the area thaws, it will be numb and bluish or purple, and blisters may form. Cover the area with a dry, sterile dressing, and protect

MAKING HEALTHY CHOICES

For Living an Active Life

Rather than assuming you're working out only when you're on a track or treadmill, add movement to your day. If you don't have time for a full workout, schedule three 10-minute blocks to walk the dog, bike to the store, or walk around campus. If you have to wait for a delayed appointment, take a quick walk down the hall or up the stairs. Put extra oomph into your chores. Use wide, sweeping motions when you mop the floor. Turn on the radio and dance as you fold laundry or make a sandwich.

Here are some other suggestions for activating your lifestyle:

▪ **Occupy your mind.** If you're new to exercise, listening to music or watching TV while on the tread-

mill or stationary bike can distract you from the sheer effort you're putting in. As you adjust to exercise, you can try focusing on your breath or becoming "mindful" of other bodily sensations.

▪ **Recruit a coach.** A friend, mentor, or coach who exercises with you or simply checks on your progress periodically can keep you honest—and active.

▪ **Go for 10.** If you're feeling too whipped for your usual session, tell yourself you only have to exercise for 10 minutes. If you're still not feeling up for a longer workout, fine. Even 10 minutes of working out produces some benefits. Chances are, though, that once you get moving, you'll keep moving.

▪ **Join a group.** Even if you're an introvert, exercising at a place and a time where others are working out—

a park on Sunday afternoon or the gym on Wednesday evening—can motivate you to keep moving.

▍ **Talk to yourself.** Self-talk can be a powerful ally. Develop mantras to keep you moving: Every step counts. I'll feel great when I finish this lap. I can go the distance.

▍ **Include fun activities.** Rather than running, go inline-skating. In winter, substitute cross-country skiing for treadmill time. Or try aerobic dance classes.

▍ **If you're easily winded,** decrease intensity and increase duration. For example, slow your pace as you walk but extend the distance you cover.

▍ **Vary your routine.** Walk one day, bicycle the next. Go dancing. Mow the lawn. Learn how to play tennis.

SELF-SURVEY 1

Are You Ready for Aerobic Exercise?

Read each statement carefully and circle the number that best describes your feelings in each statement—be completely honest with your answers.

	Strongly Agree	Mildly Agree	Mildly Disagree	Strongly Disagree
1. I can walk, ride a bike (or a wheelchair), swim, or walk in a shallow pool.	4	3	2	1
2. I enjoy aerobic exercise.	4	3	2	1
3. I believe aerobic exercise can help decrease the risk for disease and premature death.	4	3	2	1
4. I believe aerobic exercise contributes to better health.	4	3	2	1
5. I have previously participated in an aerobic exercise program.	4	3	2	1
6. I have experienced the feeling of being physically fit.	4	3	2	1
7. I can envision myself doing an aerobic activity.	4	3	2	1
8. I am contemplating an aerobic exercise program.	4	3	2	1
9. I am willing to stop contemplating and give aerobic exercise a try for a few weeks.	4	3	2	1
10. I am willing to set aside time at least three times a week for aerobic exercise.	4	3	2	1
11. I can find a place for aerobic exercise (the streets, a park, a YMCA, the gym or rec center).	4	3	2	1
12. I can find other people who would like to exercise with me.	4	3	2	1
13. I will exercise when I am moody, fatigued, and even when the weather is bad.	4	3	2	1
14. I am willing to spend a small amount of money for adequate exercise clothing (shoes, shorts, leotards, swimsuit).	4	3	2	1
15. If I have any doubts about my present state of health, I will see a physician before beginning an exercise program.	4	3	2	1
16. Aerobic exercise will make me feel better and improve my quality of life.	4	3	2	1

Source: Hoeger and Hoeger, *Principles and Labs for Physical Fitness* 4e p. 181. Reprinted by permission of Thomson Higher Education, Belmont CA.

Scoring Your Test:

This questionnaire allows you to examine your readiness for exercise. You have been evaluated in four categories: mastery (self-control), attitude, health, and commitment. Mastery indicates that you can be in control of your exercise program. Attitude examines your mental disposition toward exercise. Health provides evidence of the wellness benefits of exercise. Commitment shows dedication and resolution to carry out the exercise program. Write the number you circled after each statement in the corresponding spaces below. Add the scores on each line to get your totals. Scores can vary from 4 to 16. A score of 12 and above is a strong indicator that that factor is important to you, and 8 and below is low. If you score 12 or more points in each category, your chances of initiating and adhering to an exercise program are good. If you fail to score at least 12 points in three categories, your chances of succeeding at exercise may be slim. You need to be better informed about the benefits of exercise, and a retraining process may be required.

Mastery:

1. ☐ + 5. ☐ + 6. ☐ + 9. ☐ = ☐

Attitude:

2. ☐ + 7. ☐ + 8. ☐ + 13. ☐ = ☐

Health:

3. ☐ + 4. ☐ + 15. ☐ + 16. ☐ = ☐

Commitment:

10. ☐ + 11. ☐ + 12. ☐ + 14. ☐ = ☐

SELF-SURVEY 2

How Much Do You Move Each Day?

For each question, circle the letter of your response and then add up the total points. Place this number in the space below and check your "movement" rating.

1. How often do you walk at least a mile for exercise each day?
   a. never   0 points
   b. sometimes   1 point
   c. usually   2 points
   d. always   3 points

2. When you play games outside, how often do they include running, jumping and throwing activities?
   a. never   0 points
   b. sometimes   1 point
   c. usually   2 points
   d. always   3 points

3. How many steps do you estimate you take in one day?
   a. 0–5,000   0 points
   b. 5001–7499   1 point
   c. 7500–10,000   2 points
   d. >10,000   3 points

4. Are you out of breath after walking up two flights of stairs?
   a. yes   0 points
   b. no   2 points

5. Walking at least 10,000 steps per day reduces your chances for:
   a. heart disease 1 points
   b. diabetes   2 point
   c. obesity   3 points
   d. all of the above 4 points

Total number of points:___

Rating:

0–5 points: You are sitting around too much and at higher risk for obesity. Start easy, but pick an activity and get up and get moving.

6–10 points: Good for you! You are somewhat active. Increase the number or the duration of the activities you do each day.

11–15 points: Congratulations! You are an active person and reaping the health benefits of your active lifestyle. Keep it up!

ACTION PLAN

Your Action Plan for Long-Term Fitness

One of the most common mistakes people make is to push too hard too fast. Often they end up injured or discouraged and quit entirely. If you are just starting an aerobic program, think of it as a series of phases: beginning, progression, and maintenance.

Beginning (4–6 weeks)

Start slow and low (in intensity). If you're walking, monitor your heart rate and aim for 55 percent of your maximum heart rate. Another good rule of thumb to make sure you're moving at the right pace: If you can sing as you walk, you're going too slow; if you can't talk, you're going too fast.

Progression (16–20 weeks)

Gradually increase the duration and/or intensity of your workouts. For instance, you might add 5 minutes every two weeks to your walking time. You also can gradually pick up your pace, using your target heart rate as your guide. Keep a log of your workouts so you can chart your progress until you reach your goal.

Maintenance (lifelong)

Once you've reached the stage of exercising for an hour every day, you may want to develop a repertoire of aerobic activities you enjoy. Combine or alternate activities to avoid monotony and keep up your enthusiasm. This is called cross-training.

SETTING GOALS

Personal Cardiorespiratory Fitness Goals

Your Personal Cardiorespiratory Fitness Goal:

Is it S.M.A.R.T?

　　Specific? _____

　　Measurable? _____

Achievable? _____

Rewarding? _____

Time Defined? _____

Strategies for Success

1. _____

2. _____

3. _____

Potential Obstacles

1. _____

2. _____

3. _____

Ways Around Them

1. _____

2. _____

3. _____

Daily Report

The Week That Was:

What went right?

What could I do better?

WELLNESS JOURNAL

Your Aerobic Workout Record

By utilizing this workout record, you will be able to monitor the intensity, mode, frequency, and duration of your workouts and also track improvements in your resting heart rate and aerobic capacity.

Cardiovascular Workout Record

NAME

Age:					Target Zone:		

Date	Cardiovascular Activity	Resting Heart Rate 15 Seconds × 4	Training Heart Rate 10 Seconds × 6	Recovery Heart Rate 10 Seconds × 6	Difference (Training − Recovery)/10	Time Duration	Perceived Exertion

1. Record the *date* of your workout in the first column. To see results, you need to work out at least three times a week.

2. Record the *type* of activity in the second column. Any mode of exercise that uses large muscle groups continuously for at least 20 minutes counts as an aerobic or cardiovascular workout (for example, jogging, walking, aerobics class, swimming, biking, step training, boxing).

3. Take your *resting heart rate* either for a full minute or for 15 seconds and multiply the number by 4. The best time to take your resting heart rate is in the morning before you get out of bed. That is when it is the lowest. Record the number in the third column. As your heart gets stronger, it will be able to pump more blood with each contraction. If you have a resting heart rate over 80 beats per minute, this number will most likely get lower as you improve your cardiovascular endurance.

4. Record your *age* at the upper left. Then use Figure 4-3 to compute your *target zone*. The target zone is the range of heart rates necessary to produce improved cardiovascular fitness. Record your *target zone* to the right of your age. This is your ideal intensity range. Change it only if your resting heart rate changes.

CHAPTER

4 Making This Chapter Work for You

1. The heart
   a. has four chambers, which are responsible for pumping blood into the veins for circulation through the body.
   b. pumps blood first to the lungs where it picks up oxygen and discards carbon dioxide.
   c. beats about 10,000 times and pumps about 75 gallons of blood per day.
   d. has specialized cells that generate electrical signals to control the amount of blood that circulates through the body.

2. Capillaries are tiny blood vessels that serve as transfer stations and
   a. are ten times the diameter of a single red blood cell.
   b. take up oxygen from the lungs and deliver carbon dioxide to the lungs.
   c. take up oxygen from body cells and deliver carbon dioxide to the lungs.
   d. drain into the heart from the body cells.

3. The greater your _____, the more efficiently your cardiorespiratory system is working.
   a. heart rate
   b. musculature
   c. oxygen uptake
   d. breathing rate

4. Which of the following best describes the primary benefit of aerobic exercise?
   a. It improves cardiorespiratory endurance.
   b. It helps condition your muscles, enabling them to work efficiently and reliably.
   c. It can enhance weight loss.
   d. It increases the range of motion of your joints.

5. To get cardiorespiratory benefits from your exercise, your target heart rate must be at least
   a. 40% of your maximum heart rate.
   b. 60% of your maximum heart rate.
   c. 80% of your maximum heart rate.
   d. 100% of your maximum heart rate.

6. Other ways to determine if you are exercising hard enough, besides target heart rate, are the RPE and the
   a. 1-mile run test.
   b. Karvonen formula.
   c. talk test.
   d. smell test.

7. When you design your aerobic workout, include these stages:
   a. stretching, aerobic activity, cool-down.
   b. stretching, aerobic activity, stretching, cool-down.
   c. warm-up, aerobic activity, stretching.
   d. warm-up, aerobic activity, cool-down.

8. Michael started a walking program two weeks ago. Which of these workouts would you recommend to him for aerobic exercise?
   a. 5 minutes of brisk walking, 30 minutes of flexibility exercises, 5 minutes of brisk walking.
   b. 5 minutes of stretching, 15 minutes of slow walking, 5 minutes of brisk walking, 15 minutes of slow walking.
   c. 10 minutes of slow walking, 35 minutes of brisk walking, 5 minutes of slow walking.
   d. 10 minutes of stretching, 45 minutes of slow walking.

9. To improve her cardiorespiratory fitness, Janelle is thinking of swimming laps at the Y. She will need to swim for at least _____ to get the benefits of aerobic exercise.
   a. 20 minutes
   b. 25 minutes
   c. 30 minutes
   d. 35 minutes

10. Jason has been practicing with the soccer team for 2 hours. He feels extraordinarily thirsty, extraordinarily sweaty, and thinks he has a temperature. Jason may be suffering from
    a. heat cramps
    b. heat stress
    c. heat exhaustion
    d. heat stroke

Answers to these questions can be found on page 376.

Critical Thinking

1. Your parents both work in offices all day long and get little exercise except for golfing. Your mother has put on weight, and your father complains about not having the energy he once did. How can you express your concern for the effects of their sedentary lifestyle on their hearts and lungs that might motivate them to get some aerobic exercise?

2. When he started working out, Jeff simply wanted to stay in shape. But he felt so pleased with the way his body looked and responded that he kept doing more. Now he runs 10 miles a day (longer on weekends), lifts weights, works out on exercise equipment almost every day, and plays racquetball or squash whenever he gets a chance. Is Jeff getting too much of a good thing? Is there any danger in his fitness program? What would be a more reasonable approach?

3. College athletes have died unexpectedly from heart-related problems. The American Heart Association has identified guidelines to screen competitive athletes. Does your school follow these guidelines? If not, what precautions are taken to protect young athletes?

Media Menu

Health⊗Now™

Don't forget to check out the wealth of resources on the HealthNow website at **http://healthnow.brookscole.com/itw** that will:
- Help you evaluate your knowledge of the material
- Allow you to take an exam-prep quiz
- Provide a Personalized Learning Plan targeting resources that address areas you should study
- Coach you through identifying target goals for behavior change and creating and monitoring your personal change plan throughout the semester.

INTERNET CONNECTIONS

American Council of Exercise—Cardiovascular Fitness Facts

www.acefitness.org/fitfacts/fitfacts_list.aspx#1
This site features information about a variety of cardiovascular forms of exercise, including walking, running, jumping rope, swimming, spinning, cross-training, interval training, and others.

Check Physical Activity and Heart IQ

http://www.nhlbi.nih.gov/health/public/heart/obesity/pa_iq_ab.htm
This site, sponsored by the National Heart, Lung, and Blood Institute, provides a true/false quiz to allow you to assess what you know about how physical activity affects your heart. The answers provided will uncover exercise myths and give you information on ways to improve your heart health.

The Cooper Institute

www.cooperinst.org
Founded in 1970 by Kenneth H. Cooper, M.D., M.P.H., the Cooper Institute for Aerobics Research has become widely acclaimed as a leader in preventive medicine research and education. As a nonprofit research organization, the Cooper Institute is dedicated to advancing the understanding of the relationship between living habits and health and to providing leadership in implementing these concepts to enhance people's physical and emotional well-being.

Exercise Your Heart: A Guide to Physical Activity

www.nhlbi.nih.gov/health/public/heart/obesity/lose_wt/phy_act.htm
Sponsored by the National Heart, Lung, and Blood Institute, this site discusses the advantages of physical activity and the effects of activity on the heart and provides practical guidelines for starting and staying on an exercise program as well as sample activity programs.

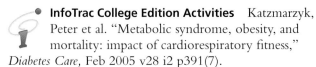 **InfoTrac College Edition Activities** Katzmarzyk, Peter et al. "Metabolic syndrome, obesity, and mortality: impact of cardiorespiratory fitness," *Diabetes Care,* Feb 2005 v28 i2 p391(7).

1. Why is it important to reduce the risk of metabolic syndrome?

2. Did this study show that obesity increases the risk of dying of cardiovascular disease in all men? Were those who were overweight or had metabolic syndrome at greater risk?

3. Does cardiorespiratory fitness reduce the risk of dying of cardiovascular disease in men who are overweight or have metabolic syndrome?

You can find additional readings related to personal health with InfoTrac College Edition, an online library of more than 900 journals and publications. Follow the instructions for accessing InfoTrac College Edition that were packaged with your textbook; then search for articles using a keyword search.

For additional links, resources, and suggested readings on the InfoTrac College Edition, visit our Health and Wellness Resource Center at **http://health .wadsworth.com.**

Key Terms

The terms listed are used on the page indicated. Definitions of the terms are in the Glossary at the end of the book.

aerobic exercise 66
alveoli 64

heat stress 76
heat stroke 76

anaerobic exercise 66
arteries 64
atrium 64
capillaries 64
**cardiorespiratory
   endurance** 66
cardiovascular system 64
cross-training 71
diastole 65
endothelium 67
frostbite 77
frostnip 76
heart rate 66
heat cramps 76
heat exhaustion 76

hypothermia 77
lactic acid 67
**maximal oxygen uptake
   (VO₂max)** 66
myocardium 65
oxygen uptake (VO₂) 66
**Rating of Perceived
   Exertion (RPE)** 69
respiratory system 64
resting heart rate 68
stroke volume 66
systole 65
target heart rate 68
veins 65
ventricles 64

Strengthening Your Muscles

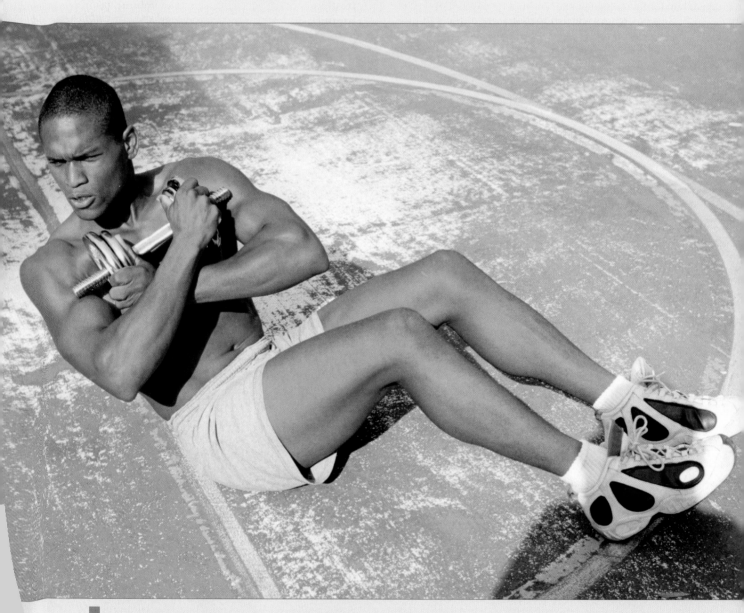

 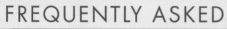

Yuko assumed she was in excellent condition. An energetic 19-year-old, she jogged four days a week, cycled around campus, and watched both her weight and what she ate. But when she tested the various components of fitness in her wellness class, the results surprised her. Her aerobic capacity was very good, but her performance on tests of muscle strength and endurance was poor. "You're not over-fat," her professor commented, "but you are under-muscled."

Many people who look and feel fit are in the same condition. According to a national survey, only 8.7 percent of adults work their muscles regularly. College-age men and women—those between ages 17 and 29—have the highest rate of exercising their muscles: 15.1 percent. (See Student Snapshot: "Working Up a Sweat.") This is half the 30 percent goal set by federal health officials in *Healthy People 2010*.[1]

Yet muscles are critically important: They set our bodies and our lives in motion. A ballerina's graceful pirouette, a baseball player's mighty swing, a runner's split-second sprint—all are made possible by well-trained muscles. Every day all of us, not just athletes and dancers, make use of the force supplied by the more than 600 muscles in the human body. Without them, we couldn't rise from our chairs, lift a backpack, walk across a room, inhale a breath of air, or digest our food.

Your muscles never stay the same. If you don't use them, they weaken or break down. If you use them rigorously and regularly, they grow stronger. The only way to develop muscular fitness is to demand more of your muscles than you usually do.

This chapter provides a detailed understanding of how muscles work, discusses the benefits of muscular fitness, describes methods of assessing and developing muscular strength and endurance, and offers guidelines for making the most of muscle workouts.

After studying the material in this chapter, you should be able to:

▐ **Explain** how muscles work.

▐ **List** the benefits of muscular training.

▐ **Describe** methods for assessing and developing muscular strength and endurance.

▐ **Discuss** the elements involved in designing a muscle workout.

▐ **List** the advantages and disadvantages of working with free weights and on strength-training machines.

▐ **Discuss** safety techniques for avoiding injuries in a weight-training program.

Health⊗Now™

Don't forget to check out the wealth of resources on the HealthNow website at **http://healthnow.brookscole.com/itw** that will:

• Help you evaluate your knowledge of the material

• Allow you to take an exam-prep quiz

• Provide a Personalized Learning Plan targeting resources that address areas you should study

• Coach you through identifying target goals for behavior change and creating and monitoring your personal change plan throughout the semester.

◼ Building Muscular Fitness

Although aerobic workouts condition your insides (heart, blood vessels, and lungs), they don't exercise many of the muscles that shape your outsides and provide power when you need it. Strength workouts are important because they enable muscles to work more efficiently and reliably. Conditioned muscles function more smoothly and contract somewhat more vigorously and with less effort. With exercise, muscle tissue becomes firmer and can withstand much more strain—the result of toughening the sheath protecting the muscle and developing more connective tissue within it (**Figure 5-1**).

The two dimensions of muscular fitness are strength and endurance. **Muscular strength** is the maximal force that a muscle or group of muscles can generate for one movement. **Muscular endurance** is the capacity to sustain repeated muscle actions. Both are important. You need strength to hoist a shovelful of snow—and endurance so you can keep shoveling the entire driveway.

Prolonged exercise prepares the muscles for sustained work by improving the circulation of blood in the tissue. The number of **capillaries** increases by as much as 50 percent in regularly exercised muscles, and existing capillaries open wider so that the total circulation increases by as much as 400 percent, thus providing the muscles with a much greater supply of nutrients (Figure 5-1). This increase occurs after about 8 to 12 weeks in young persons, but takes longer in older individuals. Inactivity reverses the process, gradually shutting down the extra capillaries that have developed.

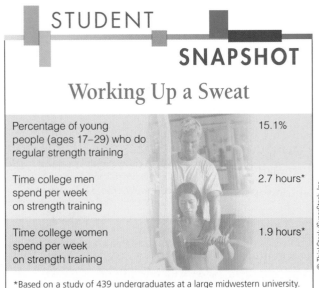

STUDENT SNAPSHOT

Working Up a Sweat

Percentage of young people (ages 17–29) who do regular strength training	15.1%
Time college men spend per week on strength training	2.7 hours*
Time college women spend per week on strength training	1.9 hours*

*Based on a study of 439 undergraduates at a large midwestern university.
Source: Buckworth, Janet and Claudio Nigg. "Physical Activity, Exercise, and Sedentary Behavior in College Students." *Journal of American College Health*, Vol. 53, No. 1, July/August 2004, p. 28.

© ThinkStock/SuperStock, Inc.

Muscles at Work

There are three types of muscles: **skeletal muscles** (those attached to the bones or skeleton), **cardiac** (heart) **muscle,** and **smooth muscle** (which primarily lines hollow internal structures such as the stomach and arteries). Together, they make up about half of total body weight, with skeletal muscles accounting for about 40 percent and the smooth muscles of the circulatory and digestive systems about 10 percent.

Muscles all perform the same general function: they cause movement. The contraction of our skeletal muscles allows us to move our limbs. But movement also occurs in less visible places and ways. Internal organs, such as the heart, stomach, lungs, and blood vessels, move—once again, through the action of muscles. Only the skeletal muscles are "voluntary," however; that is, they contract as the result of conscious or voluntary control. The functioning of cardiac and smooth muscles is considered "involuntary" because we cannot consciously control their contractions.

All muscles have common properties, including:

▮ *Contractibility.* This quality, which distinguishes muscle from other tissues, refers to the ability of a muscle to contract or shorten on receiving a stimulus from the nervous system.

▮ *Elasticity.* This refers to the ability of muscle tissue to return to its normal resting length and shape after being stretched. If a muscle were not elastic, it would remain at whatever length to which it was stretched.

▮ *Excitability.* This is the ability of muscle tissue to respond to a stimulus from the nervous system.

▮ *Extensibility.* This refers to the ability of muscle tissue to stretch. If our muscles were not capable of stretching, we would not be as mobile or enjoy the range of motion that we do.

▮ *All-or-nothing principle.* A muscle contracts completely or not at all. If a stimulus for contraction is too weak, no contraction occurs. If the stimulus meets or surpasses a certain threshold, there is a complete contraction.

The Structure of Skeletal Muscle

The individual cells in a muscle are called **muscle fibers.** A muscle consists of many bundles of muscle fibers covered by layers of connective tissue that hold the fibers together. Skeletal muscle fibers are generally long and relatively small in diameter. Within each muscle fiber are long, threadlike structures called **myofibrils** that run lengthwise through the muscle fiber. Each myofibril consists of many **sarcomeres,** the basic contractile units of muscle tissue, attached end to end (**Figure 5-2**). Within a sarcomere are myofilaments. The thinner myofilaments are called **actin;** the thicker ones, **myosin.**

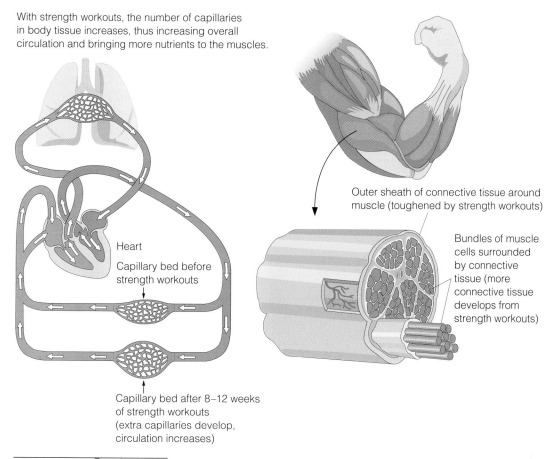

With strength workouts, the number of capillaries in body tissue increases, thus increasing overall circulation and bringing more nutrients to the muscles.

Heart

Capillary bed before strength workouts

Capillary bed after 8–12 weeks of strength workouts (extra capillaries develop, circulation increases)

Outer sheath of connective tissue around muscle (toughened by strength workouts)

Bundles of muscle cells surrounded by connective tissue (more connective tissue develops from strength workouts)

FIGURE 5-1 ▍ **Benefits of Strength Training on the Body**
Strength training increases blood circulation and oxygen supply to body tissues and develops muscles.

All skeletal muscles have connective tissue both through and around them. The skeletal muscles move bones by pulling on **tendons,** the connective tissues that attach muscle to bone.

Weight training causes the size of individual muscle fibers to increase by increasing the number of myofibrils. Larger muscle fibers mean a larger and stronger muscle.

Muscle Contraction

Muscles can do only two things: contract or relax. As they do so, skeletal muscles either pull on bones or stop pulling on bones. All exercise involves muscles pulling on bones across a joint. The movement that takes place depends upon the structure of the joint and the position of the muscle attachments involved.

According to the **"sliding filament" theory** of muscle contraction, myosin filaments have cross-bridges that contract the actin filaments. The length of the actin and myosin filaments does not change, but the myosin cross-bridges pull the actin filaments toward the center of the sarcomere (Figure 5-2). Because the actin filaments are attached to the ends of the sarcomere, the sarcomere becomes shorter as the actin filaments are pulled toward the center.

Isometric Contraction *Iso* means equal or uniform, and *metric* refers to length or measure. In an **isometric contraction** the muscle applies force while maintaining the same length. The muscle contracts and tries to shorten but cannot overcome the resistance. In an isometric exercise, you push or pull against an immovable object, with each muscle contraction held for 5 to 8 seconds and repeated five to ten times daily. An example is pushing against an immovable object, like a wall, or tightening an abdominal muscle while sitting. The muscle contracts but there is no movement.

Isotonic Contraction *Tonic* refers to tone or tension. An **isotonic contraction** involves movement, but the muscle tension remains the same. In isotonic exercises, the muscle moves a moderate load several times, as in weight lifting or calisthenics. Isotonic exercises that involve high resistance and a low number of repetitions are best for producing muscular

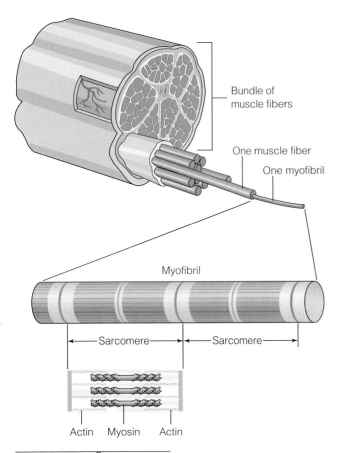

FIGURE 5-2 | Structure of Skeletal Muscle

Labels in figure:
Bundle of muscle fibers
One muscle fiber
One myofibril
Myofibril
Sarcomere
Sarcomere
Actin Myosin Actin

strength, whereas those that incorporate lower resistance and frequent repetitions develop the greatest flexibility, coordination, and endurance. We will talk about isometric and isotonic contractions later, under "Static and Dynamic Training" on page 91.

There are two types of isotonic contractions: concentric and eccentric. In a **concentric contraction,** the muscle becomes shorter and applies force. An example is the contracting of the bicep as it lifts a barbell toward the shoulder. In an **eccentric contraction,** the muscle contracts and tries to shorten but is overcome by the resistance. Eccentric contractions occur when the muscle applies force as it lengthens. They allow you to lower things smoothly and slowly, for example, lowering a barbell in a controlled manner.

Isokinetic Contraction *Kinetic* refers to motion, and true **isokinetic contraction** is a constant-speed contraction. Isokinetic exercises require special machines that provide resistance to overload muscles throughout the entire range of motion.

Muscle Fibers

Most muscles contain a combination of slow-twitch and fast-twitch fibers. Muscle fibers are classified as fast twitch or slow twitch according to their strength, speed of contraction, and energy source. **Slow-twitch oxida-**

tive fibers are relatively resistant to fatigue, but they don't contract as rapidly or as strongly as fast-twitch fibers. **Fast-twitch fibers,** which contract more rapidly and forcefully than slow-twitch fibers, tire more quickly. Although oxygen is important in the energy system that fuels fast-twitch fibers, they rely more on anaerobic metabolism than slow-twitch fibers do.

The type of fiber that acts depends on the type of work required. Endurance activities like jogging tend to use slow-twitch fibers, whereas strength and power activities use fast-twitch fibers.

The Muscle-Brain Connection

How does your brain tell your muscles to move? A motor nerve coming from the brain or spinal cord carries the message and sends impulses to muscle fibers. A motor unit consists of a single motor nerve and all the muscle fibers it sends impulses to. Although a motor nerve is connected to many muscle fibers, each muscle fiber is controlled by only one motor nerve. A motor nerve that is responsible for very fine movements may be connected to very few muscle fibers, such as those responsible for eye movements. In contrast, a motor nerve that is responsible for large or heavy movements may be connected to many muscle fibers, such as those responsible for hip extension.

Each muscle contains hundreds of motor units. The force a muscle exerts is determined primarily by the size and number of motor units recruited for the task. If only a small amount of force is necessary, only one motor unit may be used. If more force is needed, several motor units might be employed.

Power

Power is the explosive aspect of strength. While muscular strength is fundamental for performance, some sports, such as football, require speed as well as strength, and these are the two components of power. If two individuals have equal strength, the one who can lift or move an identical load the same distance in less time has greater power. Most increases in power come through gains in strength.

Gender and Strength

In absolute terms, men are the stronger gender, but gender differences in absolute strength do not apply to all muscle groups. Women have about 40 to 60 percent of the upper-body strength of men but 70 to 75 percent of the lower-body strength.

When other measures are used, the strength of men and women is nearly equal. If the amount of lean body mass is taken into consideration, women are about equal in strength to men. When strength is calculated per cross-sectional area of muscle, there are no significant gender differences.

Sex hormones, particularly testosterone, play a role in strength development in men and women, but their exact influence is complex. Though women on average have about one-tenth the testosterone of men, the level of this sex hormone varies greatly among women and influences their strength development more than is typical in men. Women with higher testosterone levels may have greater potential strength than others, but most likely hormones do not account for the gender differences in absolute strength. These are thought to stem more from physiological differences such as size and body structure.

Men typically have taller, wider frames that support more muscle, as well as broader shoulders that provide a greater strength advantage. With training, however, a woman's leg strength, compared pound for pound, can equal or surpass a man's. Women in a muscle-conditioning program will increase their strength and then plateau after 4 to 6 months, when they approach the limits of their genetic potential for improvement. Men continue to make progress for 8 to 12 months.

Although biological gender differences in strength exist, resistance training programs should be based on individual needs and goals, rather than on preconceptions about gender. Women and men who train their muscles in the same ways, using the same program design, exercises, and intensities, relative to their body size and level of strength, can and do benefit equally. Both increase their lean body mass, decrease their body fat, and enhance their self-confidence.

✚ Benefits of Muscular Training

Building muscular strength and endurance can enhance health and fitness in many ways, including:

▮ **Healthier muscles.** With regular exercise, muscles function more efficiently. Muscle tissue becomes firmer and can withstand much more strain—the result of toughening the sheath protecting the muscle and developing more connective tissue within it.

▮ **More lean body mass, less body fat.** The latest research on fat-burning shows that the best way to reduce your body fat is to add muscle-strengthening exercise to your workouts. Muscle tissue is your very best calorie-burning tissue, and the more you have, the more calories you burn, even when you are resting.

▮ **Stronger bones.** High-intensity strength training can enhance bone modeling, increase bone formation, and lower the risk of osteoporosis. In studies of women with weak resistance training slowed and even reversed the deterioration of their bones. Weight training is one of several strategies that college students can employ to preserve bone health throughout life.

▮ **Reduced risk of cardiovascular disease.** Weight training two or three times a week can reduce blood pressure, improve circulation, decrease body fat, and enhance glucose metabolism, thereby reducing the likelihood of heart disease.

▮ **Reduced risk of diabetes.** Weight training can boost glucose utilization in the body and lower the likelihood of developing diabetes.

▮ **Lower risk of injury.** Stronger connective tissues increase joint stability and help lower the danger of falls or exercise injuries. According to the American College of Sports Medicine, resistance training reduces low-back injuries and muscular-skeletal injuries caused by balance problems.

▮ **Improved physical performance.** Muscle training increases the storage of fuel in muscles and the size of muscle fibers, which builds muscular strength and power and delays fatigue. Whatever your sport, strength training may improve proficiency and decrease risk of injury.

▮ **Enhanced mood.** Weight training relieves depression and reduces anxiety, even in persons not accustomed to regularly performing such exercise. It also improves self-esteem and confidence. In women, strength training often fosters a sense of personal power, especially for those who have been abused or sexually victimized.

▮ **Less pain.** In various studies, strengthening the low-back muscles had up to an 80 percent success rate in eliminating or alleviating low-back pain. Weight training also can ease arthritis pain and strengthen joints, so you feel fewer aches.

▮ **Feel younger.** Even men and women in their eighties and nineties can make significant gains in strength and mobility with weight training.

Regular resistance training—lifting handheld weights or working on weight machines for at least ten minutes three times a week—can maintain muscle mass, prevent bone loss, and help control weight throughout the aging process.

WELLNESS COACH

✚ Behavioral Change and Muscular Fitness

Most fitness-related studies of the stages of change and of change processes (discussed in depth in Chapter 2) have focused on cardiorespiratory activity. However, researchers have found that recognizing your current stage of change for muscular-fitness-promoting behaviors, using appropriate processes of change, and boosting your self-efficacy (your belief in your ability to manage prospective situations) can motivate you to strengthen your muscles.[2]

To identify your current stage of change, take the brief Self-Survey on page 100. If you are in the pre-contemplation or contemplation stages, you're most likely to respond to cognitive processes of change, such as learning about the benefits of muscular fitness or finding places with strength-training equipment. If you are in the action or maintenance changes, you might try a different cognitive approach, such as subscribing to a fitness magazine, which would help maintain your commitment to exercise. However, behavioral processes, such as signing a contract committing yourself to a muscle-training program or using reminders (such as Post-it Notes) so you remember your gym bag, may be more effective once you've begun training.[3]

You can boost your self-efficacy by planning your training program to ensure success. For example, start with simple exercises and move to more complicated ones as your mastery improves. Increase the amount of weight you press or lift slowly. Look for a supportive, well-qualified instructor for stretching, Yoga, or Pilates classes.

Table 5-1 may help you choose the most effective tools for changing your muscular fitness behavior.

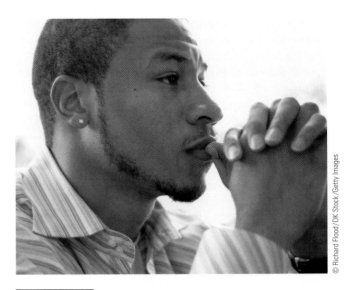

When you think about muscular fitness, in which stage of readiness for change are you? Are you more likely to respond to cognitive or behavioral approaches?

Assessing Muscular Fitness

Muscular strength is the maximum amount of force a muscle can produce in a single effort, for example, the maximum amount of weight a person can lift one time. This is called **1 repetition maximum (1 RM).** To develop strength, you increase the load, object, or weight your muscles move and do a few repetitions with this heavy load. You can use the tests in your Lab Booklet to assess the strength of your major muscle groups.

To assess muscular endurance, the ability of a muscle to exert force repeatedly or continuously over time, count

TABLE 5-1 ▌ Cognitive and Behavioral Change Processes: Tools for Improving Muscular Fitness

Change Process	Definition	Example
Cognitive:		
Consciousness-raising	Seeking information on options for muscular training	Reading about the benefits of conditioning your muscles
Emotional arousal	Emotional responses to change	Feeling concerned about not having enough muscular strength
Self-reevaluation	Assessing your values with respect to your lifestyle	Getting frustrated with yourself when you don't train with weights
Social liberation	Awareness and acceptance of available alternative lifestyle choices	Understanding that society is changing in ways that make it easier for you to train with weights
Behavioral:		
Countering	Substituting alternative behaviors	Lifting weights when you feel stressed to relieve tension
Reward	Changing conditions that encourage sedentary living	Rewarding yourself when you weight train
Helping relationships	Getting support from others	Finding a weight-training "buddy"
Environmental control	Taking charge of situations that support inactivity	Blocking out time to weight train
Self-liberation, or commitment	Believing, choosing, and committing to change	Signing a written contract to develop your muscular fitness

Source: Cardinal, Bradley, and Maria Kosma. "Self-efficacy and the Stages and Process of Change Associated with Adopting and Maintaining Muscular Fitness-Promoting Behaviors." *Research Quarterly for Exercise and Sport,* Vol. 78, No. 2, June 2004, p. 186.

the maximum number of repetitions of a muscular contraction that you can do or the maximum amount of time you can sustain a muscle contraction. The tests in your Lab booklet can assess your muscular endurance. Record your results in your Wellness Journal and use them to set goals for your training program.

Muscular Training Fundamentals

You need to exercise differently for strength than for endurance. *To develop strength,* do a few repetitions with heavy loads. As you increase the weight your muscles must move, you increase your strength. *To increase endurance,* you do many more repetitions with lighter loads. If your muscles are weak and you need to gain strength in your upper body, you may have to work for weeks to do a half-dozen regular push-ups. Then you can start building endurance by doing as many push-ups as you can before collapsing in exhaustion.

Overload

The only way to develop muscles is by demanding more of them than you usually do. This is called **overloading.** (Remember the overload principle?) As you train, you have to gradually increase the number of repetitions or the amount of resistance and work the muscle to temporary fatigue. That's why it's important not to quit when your muscles start to tire. Progressive overload—steadily increasing the stress placed on the body—builds stronger muscles.[4]

Specificity

Muscle training is highly specific, which means that you have to exercise certain muscles or muscle groups for certain results. If you want to build up your leg muscles to run a marathon, push-ups won't help— just as running a marathon won't develop your upper body. If you're training with a specific goal in mind, you have to tailor your muscle workouts to make sure you meet it.

Hypertrophy and Atrophy

Muscles that are forced to work harder than normal generally undergo **hypertrophy;** that is, they increase in size. Transient hypertrophy is the pumping up of the muscle that happens during a single exercise bout; chronic hypertrophy refers to the increase in muscle size that occurs with long-term resistance training. Permanent muscle growth

is much more visible and pronounced in men than in women. The hormone testosterone and the larger number of muscle fibers in a man's muscle are thought to account for this difference. Some women have doubled their strength without any observable change in muscle size. Only women with a genetic predisposition for hypertrophy who participate in high-intensity training experience any significant increase in muscle size.

Muscles that are not used shrink, or **atrophy,** to a size that is adequate for the demands placed upon them. For example, if you break your leg and it is immobilized in a cast, the broken leg will become much smaller than the other. The same happens to the muscles of people who do not exercise.

Can I Train to Look Toned, Not Bulky?

It takes a lot of hard training for most men and almost all women to increase their muscle size. If you want to be sure to increase muscle tone but not size, however, you should work at light-to-moderate resistance (60 to 80 percent of your 1 RM) for a relatively high number of repetitions (12 to 15) and relatively few sets (one or two) of relatively few exercises (one exercise per muscle group) performed relatively few days per week (two or three days).

Static and Dynamic Training

The two basic approaches to working the muscles are static, in which isometric contractions produce little or no movement, and dynamic, in which muscle contractions produce movements. **Static,** or isometric, **training** has significant limitations because it doesn't develop strength throughout a joint's range of motion. Nevertheless, it can be useful in strengthening muscles after an injury or surgery and in overcoming weak points in an individual's range of motion so that more weight can be lifted during dynamic exercise. Isometric exercise seems to raise blood pressure in some people, which can be dangerous.

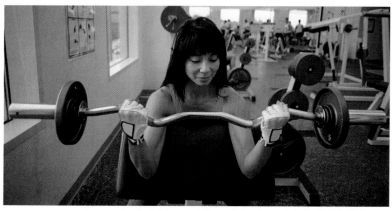

▮ Specificity means that you get certain results when you exercise certain muscles or muscle groups.

Dynamic training, the most popular approach to conditioning the muscles, involves isotonic and isokinetic exercises and uses a variety of equipment, including free weights, fixed-resistance machines, variable-resistance machines, and isokinetic equipment. *Free weights* refers to barbells and dumbbells. Strength-training equipment, found in most gyms and health clubs, uses the principle of progressive resistance. Some equipment involves a system of valves, pulleys, and weights. Other machines have a special cam (a pulley with an off-center axis) that adjusts the resistance for exercise in all positions.

Designing a Muscle Workout

A workout with weights should exercise your body's primary muscle groups: the *deltoids* (shoulders), *pectorals* (chest), *triceps* and *biceps* (back and front of upper arms), *quadriceps* and *hamstrings* (front and back of thighs), *gluteus maximus* (buttocks), *trapezius, rhomboids,* and *latissimus dorsi* (back), and *abdomen* (**Figure 5–3**). Various machines and free-weight routines focus on each muscle group, but the principle is always the same: Muscles contract as you raise and lower a weight, and you repeat the lift-and-lower routine until the muscle group is tired.

A weight training program is made up of **reps** (the single performance, or **repetition,** of an exercise, such as lifting 50 pounds one time) and **sets** (a *set* number of repetitions of the same movement, such as a set of 20 push-ups). You should allow your breath to return to normal before moving on to each new set. Pushing yourself to the limit builds strength. Although the ideal number of sets in a strength training program remains controversial, recent evidence suggests that multiple sets lead to additional benefits in short- and long-term training in young and middle-aged adults.[5] The number of reps depends on your goal (**Table 5–2**).

Maintaining proper breathing during weight training is crucial. To breathe correctly, inhale when muscles are relaxed and exhale when you push or lift. Don't ever hold your breath, because oxygen flow helps prevent muscle fatigue and injury.

Warming Up

As with cardiovascular workouts, a warm-up is critical to prevent injuries and improve performance. The American College of Sports Medicine recommends 5 to 7 minutes.[6] You can warm up with an aerobic activity, such as walking or low-intensity jogging. Another option is to perform light strength exercises. Most competitive lifters warm up in this fashion. For instance, they perform at least one set of bench presses slowly and smoothly. (Note: This may be dangerous for beginners.) This warms up the same muscles and joints that they will use when performing heavier sets of this exercise. At the same time, it focuses the mind on the exercise and improves concentration.

Some people include stretching in their warm-up routine, but as noted in Chapter 6, this is controversial. Little scientific evidence backs up the premise that stretching prevents injuries or improves performance, particularly in sports like jogging or cycling.[7] And vigorous stretching of cold, stiff muscles may itself be dangerous. If you want to stretch before a muscle workout, be sure to warm up beforehand and start with light, gentle stretching exercises.

Range of Motion

Whenever possible, you should exercise a muscle through its entire range of motion, that is, from full extension to full contraction and back to full extension. This works a muscle through the two phases of range of motion: concentric, when the muscle shortens to overcome the resistance and lift a weight, and eccentric, when the muscle lengthens to lower the weight.

The eccentric phase of an exercise should take 1 or 2 seconds; the concentric phase should be at least as long. In some cases, it may be twice as long (2 to 4 seconds). If you simply allow a weight to drop after lifting it, you complete only half of the exercise. Similarly, if you jerk or throw a weight upward, your muscles receive less benefit, and the risk of injury rises.

Frequency

As explained earlier, a muscle-conditioning workout consists of both sets and reps. The American College of Sports Medicine recommends a minimum of one set (8 to 15 repetitions) of eight to ten different exercises two days per week. Individuals younger than 50 should work major muscle groups two to three days a week with weight loads that permit 8 to 12 repetitions. Older individuals should exercise with weight loads that allow one set of 10 to 15 repetitions.

The conventional recommendation has been to aim for three sets, but some argue that one set of 10 repetitions provides most of the improvement afforded by three. A single training session a week can prevent losses in muscle strength and endurance.

Resistance

Resistance, or weight lifted, determines the intensity of a muscle workout. The amount of resistance depends on your muscular fitness goals. To increase strength, the re-

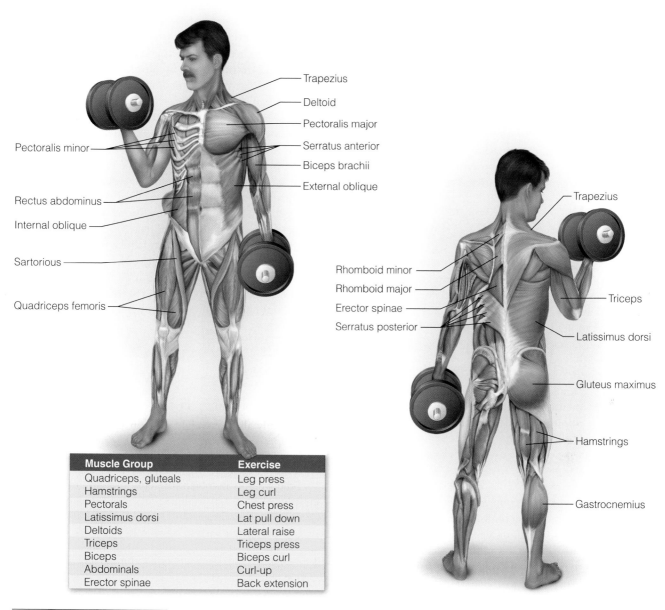

Muscle Group	Exercise
Quadriceps, gluteals	Leg press
Hamstrings	Leg curl
Pectorals	Chest press
Latissimus dorsi	Lat pull down
Deltoids	Lateral raise
Triceps	Triceps press
Biceps	Biceps curl
Abdominals	Curl-up
Erector spinae	Back extension

FIGURE 5-3 ▮ Core Curriculum

Exercise each muscle group at least two times per week, with a minimum of two days of rest between workouts.

TABLE 5-2 ▮ Using Free Weights

The American College of Sports Medicine recommends different routines for different goals:

For muscle strength: 5–8 reps, 1–3 sets

For muscle endurance: 15–20 reps, 1–3 sets

For muscle power: 3–5 reps, 1–3 sets

Source: "Selecting and Effectively Using Free Weights." American College of Sports Medicine, www.acsm.org

sistance should be about 80 percent of maximum capacity (1 RM). Rather than repeatedly trying to determine an individual's maximum capacity on each lift, most coaches recommend performing from 3 to 12 maximum repetitions. If you cannot lift a weight or load more than 12 times, the resistance is high enough to ensure that you are increasing muscle strength. Once you can lift a weight more than 12 times, you can increase resistance and again build up to 12 repetitions. To build endurance, you would work with a resistance of less than 80 percent. This would translate into a weight that you can lift more than 12 times. (See your Lab Booklet for specific exercises.)

Your personal goals will determine the resistance you choose. Body-builders who primarily want to increase the size of their muscles usually work with moderate resistance (60 to 85 percent of 1 RM) and perform 8 to 20 repetitions to near fatigue. Athletes who want maximum strength often work with very high resistance of what they can lift for up to 5 repetitions. For health and fitness, performing about 10 repetitions of your maximum usually is best for improving strength and endurance. (Check these recommendations with your instructors.)

Duration

Resistance and frequency are more important for muscle training than how long a workout lasts. In general, it takes about 20 minutes to complete one set of weight-training exercises (number may vary) and 50 minutes to complete three sets. Although more frequent training and additional sets and repetitions may produce larger gains in strength, the difference in improvement is usually small in the average healthy adult. Therefore, don't assume that more reps or a longer workout is necessarily better. In addition, more intense resistance training may increase the risk of injury or cardiovascular symptoms in middle-aged and older participants.

Progression

Weight training can be very intense, and beginners often make the mistake of trying to do too much too soon. The result is delayed-onset muscle soreness (DOMS), discussed in Chapter 3. To avoid soreness and injuries, it's important to start slowly and build up your muscle workouts gradually.

Start with light weights. Focus on learning how to perform each exercise correctly and on breathing smoothly throughout the exercise. For the first two weeks, perform up to 20 repetitions in each set (different programs recommend slightly different numbers of repetitions). Once you can complete 20 repetitions while maintaining the correct position and technique, you can increase the resistance for the next session. If the weight feels light and the repetitions are extremely easy, you can try a larger increase. If the weight feels moderately difficult, try a small increase. By the end of six training sessions over a two-week period, you should be working with a weight that challenges you to complete 20 repetitions. If you can complete 15 repetitions but not 20, keep the weight the same, but try to increase the number of repetitions at your next session. If you complete fewer than 15 repetitions, reduce the weight for your next session. If you cannot fol-

low the correct lifting technique, stop after that repetition and either use a lighter weight for the next set or choose a lighter weight for your next session.

In your third and fourth weeks of training, keep trying to find the heaviest weight you can lift 20 times on the first set. After resting 1 or 2 minutes, perform a second set of 10 repetitions. If you can complete 10 repetitions in the second set, use a heavier weight at your next exercise session. Gradually work toward the heaviest weight you can lift 20 times in the first set and the heaviest you can lift 10 times in the second set while maintaining correct form. If you cannot complete at least 8 repetitions in the second set, reduce the weight for the next session.

During the fifth and sixth week of your training program, perform one set of 20 repetitions first, one set of 10 repetitions, and one set of 5 reps. Continue to try to find the heaviest weight you can handle in this routine.

If you have not been working out, you should see fairly rapid increases in strength within about 6 to 8 weeks. In young people, 8 to 12 weeks of training will bring about changes in circulation and muscle size.

Should I Work with Free Weights or Strength-Training Machines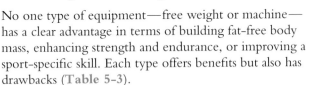

No one type of equipment—free weight or machine—has a clear advantage in terms of building fat-free body mass, enhancing strength and endurance, or improving a sport-specific skill. Each type offers benefits but also has drawbacks (**Table 5–3**).

Free weights involve more core muscles, offer great versatility for strength training, and develop strength and coordination faster. With dumbbells, for example, you can perform a variety of exercises to work specific muscle groups, such as the chest and shoulders. Simply by altering your grip, that is, by holding a dumbbell with palms facing forward, facing the thighs, or facing the rear or placing your hands closer or farther apart on a barbell, you can get the benefit of several different exercises. Machines, in contrast, are much more limited; most allow only one exercise. Barbells and dumbbells are relatively inexpensive, although accessories such as benches and racks add to the cost.

Many strength coaches believe that free weights offer greater benefits than machines for athletes in sports like football because lifting heavy barbells helps to promote explosive bursts of power. By contrast, strength-training machines tend to control movements and to discourage explosiveness. Free-weight exercises that involve several major muscle groups at the same time—lifting a barbell from the floor to the chest, for example, then pressing it overhead—also help in transferring strength from the gym to athletics. Athletes themselves often prefer free weights because of the additional challenge of gaining

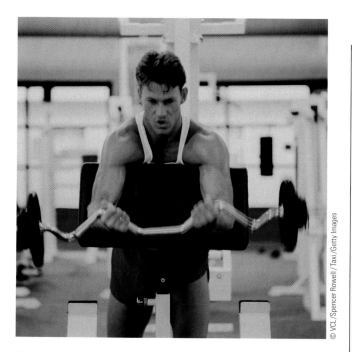

▌ As you begin a strengthening program, remember the principle of progressive overloading: Start slowly and build up your workouts gradually.

control of a barbell and maintaining balance. Many report that lifting a loaded barbell offers a greater sense of accomplishment than working against a given resistance on a machine.

Free weights also have drawbacks, however. They require a good sense of balance, cause more blisters and calluses, and require a spotter to ensure safety.

Strength-training machines (Cybex, Nautilus, Universal, Technogym, etc.) have several advantages. They ensure correct movement for a lift, which helps protect against injury. They isolate specific muscles, which is good for rehabilitating an injury or strengthening a specific body part. They make it easy to move from one exercise to the next and often provide support for the back.

Disadvantages include the high cost of purchasing home resistance equipment, the inconvenience of going to a gym or fitness center, and the limited number of exercises that can be done with most equipment. In general, novices often prefer to work with exercise machines because of their convenience, safety, and ease of operation. As the individuals become stronger, they can add free-weight exercises to their routines.

Ideally, a comprehensive strength-training program should incorporate both free weights and machines. Both offer advantages in terms of promoting lean tissue growth, increasing strength and endurance, and enhancing a certain sport-specific skill. Remember, however, that successful strength training depends more on proper technique than on equipment.

STRATEGIES for PREVENTION

Working with Weights

If you plan to work with free weights, here are some guidelines for using them safely and effectively:

▌ Don't train alone—for safety's sake. Work with a partner so you can serve as spotters for each other and help motivate each other as well.

▌ Always warm up before weight training; also be sure to stretch after training.

▌ Breathe! Holding your breath during exertion can produce a dangerous rise in blood pressure. Exhale during concentric contractions, when muscles are shortening, and inhale during eccentric contractions, when muscles are lengthening.

▌ Begin with relatively light weights (50 percent of the maximum you can lift), and increase the load slowly until you find the weight that will cause muscle failure at anywhere from 8 to 12 repetitions. (Muscle failure is the point during a workout at which you can no longer perform or complete a repetition through the entire range of motion.)

▌ In the beginning, don't work at maximum intensity. Increase your level of exertion gradually over two to six weeks to allow your body to adapt to new stress without soreness.

▌ Always train your entire body, starting with the larger muscle groups. Don't focus only on specific areas, although you may want to concentrate on your weakest muscles.

▌ Always use proper form. Unnecessary twisting, lurching, lunging, or arching can cause serious injury. Remember, quality matters more than quantity. One properly performed set of lifts can produce a greater increase in strength and muscle mass than many sets of improperly performed lifts.

▌ Work through the full range of motion. Be careful not to hyperextend or overextend.

Circuit Resistance Training

A circuit usually consists of 8 to 15 exercise stations. Exercisers typically select a weight of 40 to 60 percent of 1 RM and do as many repetitions as possible for 15 to 30 seconds at each station. The rest interval between stations equals the time spent exercising at each station. As training progresses, exercisers can apply the

TABLE 5-3 ❚ Free Weights vs. Strength-Training Machines

Equipment	Advantages	Disadvantages
Free weights	Inexpensive, portable, don't take up much space	Risk of injury if you don't use proper technique, especially when lifting weights overhead
	Extremely "user-friendly"	
	More versatile, can work different muscles in different ways	Difficult to isolate specific muscles
	Work the body in ways that more closely match the movement patterns needed for specific sports	Swinging with momentum is less effective in working the muscles than lifting slowly and steadily
	May be more effective in producing overall muscular strength	
Machines	With instruction, easier to use, which is an advantage for beginners	Less effective in strengthening the stabilizing muscles
	More efficient in isolating a specific muscle or muscle group	Limited to only one or two exercises for a muscle or muscle group per machine
	Ensure correct movements for a lift, which helps prevent cheating when muscles become fatigued	Geared to average-size person, so some machines may be difficult to use for very short or very tall individuals
		Bulky and expensive, usually available only at a gym or health club

overload principle by increasing the amount of weight at each station, increasing the amount of time exercising at each station, and/or decreasing rest intervals between stations. Exercisers may repeat the circuit two or three times.

Both free weights and machines can be used as stations. The risk of injury is low because relatively light weights are used. A key advantage of circuit training is that it develops several fitness dimensions at the same time.

Safety Basics

Safety is an important consideration in muscle workouts. When you are working with weights or machines, you have to be aware of the people and equipment around you as well as your own body movements. Stay clear of weight machines when someone is working with them. Train with a partner who can help you load and change weights and move equipment. Store all dumbbells, barbells, and weight plates properly.

When lifting a barbell or dumbbell, always use collars, the devices that secure weights to the bar. Lifting weights without collars is dangerous because you could easily lose your balance or raise one side of the weight faster than the other. Without collars, the weights on one side of the bar will slip off.

A spotter can help you get ready for a lift and provide help or additional resistance during a lift. When working with a spotter, talk before the lift so that you both know which exercise will be performed, how much help you expect, how many repetitions you'll attempt, and whether you'll need help guiding the weight into position or onto a rack after a set. If you're spotting for someone else, be sure you know what signs or signals the lifter will use to communicate with you. Give the lifter your full attention, do not look away or carry on a conversation with someone else, stay close and in proper position so that you can help immediately if needed, and provide whatever help is needed to complete the lift.

STRATEGIES for CHANGE

Working with Exercise Machines

❚ **Be sure to position your body correctly.** Make all available adjustments for height, weight, and size. Wear seat belts on machines that have them.

❚ **Go slowly.** Most machines are not designed for speed. You're more likely to injure yourself or damage the machine by lifting with a fast, jerky motion.

❚ **Work through the full range of motion.** You will get better muscle development and maintain more flexibility if you work through the range of motion.

❚ **Pay attention to the equipment.** If something seems loose or needs adjustment, report it immediately. If many people use the same machines, be courteous. Always wipe your perspiration off the machine with a towel when you finish.

Recovery

The American College of Sports Medicine recommends a minimum of eight to ten exercises involving the major muscle groups two to three days a week.

Remember that your muscles need sufficient time to recover from a weight-training session. Never work a sore muscle because soreness may indicate that too-heavy weights have caused tiny tears in the fibers.

Allow no less than 48 hours, but no more than 96 hours, between training sessions, so your body can recover from the workout and you avoid overtraining. Workouts on consecutive days do more harm than good because the body can't recover that quickly. Strength training twice a week at greater intensity and for a longer duration can be as effective as working out three times a week. However, your muscles will begin to atrophy if you let more than three or four days pass without exercising them.

Will I Put on Weight by Lifting Weights?

You may weigh a little more because lean muscle mass is denser and weighs more than fat and because of a shift in the volume of body fluids. However, you may lose weight in the long run. Muscle burns three times more calories than fat, so the more muscle mass you have, the more efficiently your metabolism works.[9] Your muscles

---

SAVVY CONSUMER

THE PERILS OF PERFORMANCE-BOOSTING DRUGS

Professional athletes aren't the only ones who use and abuse performance-enhancing drugs. Teenage boys and young men are the heaviest users. As the American College of Sports Medicine has reported, they face serious risks to their hearts, liver, reproductive systems, and psychological well-being. Here's what we know—and don't know—about the most widely used performance boosters.

▪ **Androstenedione** ("andro") is a testosterone precursor normally produced by the adrenal glands and gonads. Manufacturers claim that androstenedione improves testosterone concentration, increases muscular strength and mass, helps reduce body fat, enhances mood, and improves sexual performance. However, most studies contradict these claims and raise serious concerns about potential dangers of long-term use.

▪ **Anabolic steroids** are synthetic derivatives of the male hormone testosterone that have been reported to increase lean muscle mass, strength, and ability to train longer and harder. They pose serious health hazards, including liver tumors, jaundice (yellowish pigmentation of skin, tissues,

and body fluids), fluid retention, high blood pressure, and severe acne. Men may experience shrinking of the testicles, reduced sperm count, infertility, baldness, and development of breasts. Women may experience growth of facial hair, acne, changes in or cessation of the menstrual cycle, enlargement of the clitoris, deepened voice, and decreased immune function. In women, these changes are irreversible. In men, side effects may be reversible once abuse stops.[8] In adolescents, steroids may bring about a premature halt in skeletal maturation.

Anabolic steroid abuse may lead to aggression and other psychiatric side effects. Many users report feeling good about themselves while on anabolic steroids, but researchers report that anabolic steroid abuse can cause wild mood swings including manic-like symptoms leading to violent, even homicidal episodes.

▪ **Creatine** is an amino acid made by the body and stored predominantly in skeletal muscle. Creatine serves as a reservoir to replenish adenosine triphosphate (ATP), a substance involved in energy production. While some studies show creatine may

increase strength and endurance, other effects on the body remain unknown.

Muscle cramping, diarrhea, and dehydration have been reported in creatine users, as well as a few cases of kidney dysfunction. Some experts are concerned that creatine may damage internal organs, but there is no evidence of this so far.

▪ **GBL (gamma butyrolactone)** is an unapproved drug that is being studied as a treatment for narcolepsy, a disabling sleep disorder. Nevertheless, it is marketed on the Internet and in some professional gyms as a muscle-builder and performance-enhancer. The Food and Drug Administration has warned consumers to avoid any products containing GBL, which has been associated with at least one death and several incidents in which users became comatose or unconscious.

▪ **Designer steroid substances,** such as tetrahydrogestrinone (THG), that are undetectable through existing testing procedures also are serious threats, although their health risks compared to anabolic steroids are not currently known.

use energy even at rest, not just while you are working out. For each pound of muscle you gain, you will be burning 35 to 50 more calories a day. Strength training may prevent the slowing of metabolism associated with aging—and with weight gain over time.

Regardless of the numbers on the scale, you're likely to look slimmer. That's because muscle is denser and takes up less space than fat. In addition, particularly when combined with aerobic exercise, strength training decreases fatty tissue around muscle fibers themselves so you may lose inches rather than pounds.

✚ Other Forms of Training

Most individuals interested in developing muscle strength and endurance can achieve their goals with progressive resistance training. There are other approaches, however.

Functional Strength Exercises

Certain exercises train our bodies in ways that enhance our ability to perform daily functions or tasks, such as lifting, reaching, climbing stairs, or balancing. Three of the simplest and most effective are:

▪ Push-ups, which firm your chest, arms, abdominals, and back. Start with standing push-ups against a wall. Progress to pushing against something lower, such as a kitchen counter or heavy dresser.

▪ Squats or lunges, which strengthen your knees, quadriceps, and hips. Don't let your knees go farther forward than your toes. (This may not be possible if you are extremely tall.)

▪ Lifts, which strengthen your arms. At a gym, use free weights, pulleys, or machines to work the biceps and triceps. At home lift a heavy grocery bag or laundry basket several times.

Core Strength Conditioning

"Core strength," a popular trend in exercise and fitness, refers to the ability of the muscles to support your spine and keep your body stable and balanced. When you have good core stability, the muscles in your pelvis, lower back, hips, and abdomen work in harmony. This improves your posture, breathing, appearance, and performance in sports, while reducing your risk of muscle strain. When your core is weak, you become more susceptible to lower back pain and injury.

The major muscles of your core (**Figure 5-4**) include the transverse abdominis, the deepest of the abdominal muscles; the external and internal obliques on the side and front of the abdomen around your waist; and the rectus abdominis, a long muscle that extends along the front of the abdomen. Strengthening all of your core muscles provides stability, improves balance, and protects you from injury.

One popular approach to core strength conditioning is Pilates, which we discuss in Chapter 6.

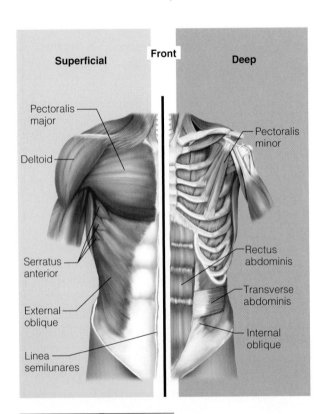

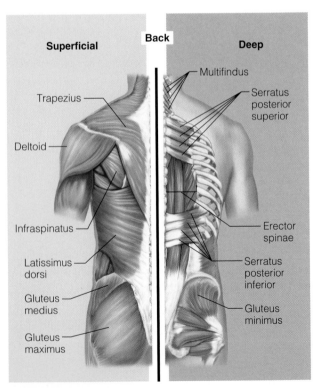

FIGURE 5-4 ▌ Major Muscles in Your Body's Core

Other Options for Resistance Training

You can also build muscle strength by working with a "stability" or fitness ball, elastic bands and tubing, or a partner.

Stability Balls

A large inflatable rubber ball can be a fun, effective way of building core strength, improving posture, and increasing balance. When performing standard exercises like crunches and abdominal curls, the ball provides an additional challenge: maintaining a stable trunk throughout each exercise. You also can sit on the ball while working with hand weights to build core strength and balance. Introductory videos and DVDs are available for rental or purchase.

Resistance Tubing

Developed by physical therapists for rehabilitation after injuries, elastic bands and tubing come in different strengths, based on the thickness of the plastic. If you're a beginner, start with a thin band, particularly for the upper body. As shown in your Lab Booklet, you can use tubes and bands to work your entire body. The lightweight, inexpensive, and easy-to-carry bands aren't particularly risky, but you should check for holes or worn spots, choose a smooth surface, maintain good posture, and perform the exercises in a slow, controlled manner.

STRATEGIES for CHANGE

Hitting a Plateau

People typically experience the greatest gains in strength in the first few weeks of training as their bodies respond to new challenges. As you adapt, you may feel that your strength training is running out of steam. If so:

■ **Try new exercises.** Different exercises for a particular muscle group may stimulate further strength development.

■ **Be sure you aren't overtraining.** If you're working the same muscle groups more than three times a week, they may not be getting enough time to recover.

■ **Vary the load, number of repetitions, or number of sets.** You might increase the load and do fewer repetitions, decrease the load and do more repetitions, or do an additional set or two.

Partner Resistance

As in all cooperative endeavors, communication is critical. Your partner cannot—and shouldn't be expected to—guess your strength level or degree of fatigue. You also need to work together to vary resistance for different muscle groups and increase resistance during the eccentric part of each contraction. As shown in your Lab Booklet, you don't need any special equipment.

■ MAKING HEALTHY CHOICES

For Strong Muscles

By some estimates, as many as half of all people who start an exercise program drop out within a year. You are more likely to keep up a healthy level of physical activity if you:

■ **Believe that you will benefit from exercise.** Once you start working out regularly, you'll feel the physical benefits. Until you do, reread "The Benefits of Exercise" in Chapters 3, 4, and 6 to remind yourself of what exercise can do for you.

■ **Try to remain flexible with your training.** Be prepared to change your workouts to accommodate personal circumstances such as illness, mood, or injuries.

■ **Aim to do half a workout.** Once you get started, you may find you want to keep going.

■ **Show up.** Once you're at the gym, you're more likely to be in the mood to exercise.

■ **If you're embarrassed about your body,** remind yourself that you're more concerned about your appearance than anyone else is. Look around: people come in all different shapes and sizes.

■ **Make sure you can fit the activities into your daily schedule.** If you don't have time to get to the gym, change, work out, shower, and get dressed, walk, jog, or bicycle close to home.

■ **Don't blow your budget.** If a health club membership is too expensive, check out your school's fitness facility (see your Lab Booklet) or buy a set of free weights to use in your room or home.

SELF-SURVEY

What's Your Muscular Fitness Level?

For each of following questions circle Yes or No to determine your stage of change for behaviors that promote muscular fitness:

1. Do you presently perform at least one set of 8–12 repetitions of muscular development activities (e.g., callisthenics, weight lifting) on 8–10 different major muscle groups of the body, 2 or more days per week?

   No   Yes

   A. If yes, have you been doing this consistently for 6 or more months?

   No   Yes

   B. If no, have you recently made plans to start such a program (e.g., joined a fitness center, bought some equipment)?

   No   Yes

   C. If no, do you think you would like to start a muscular development exercise program, such as the one described, between now and 1 month from now?

   No   Yes

Scoring: Yes to question 1 and Yes to question A = Maintenance; Yes to question 1 and No to question A = Action; No to question 1 and Yes to question B = Preparation; No to question 1, No to question B, and Yes to question C = Contemplation; No to all questions = Precontemplation.

Source: Cardinal, Bradley, and Maria Kosma. "Self-Efficacy and the Stages and Process of Change Associated with Adopting and Maintaining Muscular Fitness-Promoting Behavior," *Research Quarterly for Exercise and Sport,* Vol. 78, No. 2, June 2004, p. 186.

ACTION PLAN

Your Action Plan for Muscular Fitness

Now that you have completed the basic muscular strength and endurance fitness tests and developed goals and strategies for improvement, it is time to put your plan into action. Here are some suggestions to get you started:

1. Investigate the fitness facilities you have in your area. For convenience, start with your campus recreation center and see what is offered there. Ask friends that workout off campus, such as at the local Y or in other facilities, to bring you as a guest so you can get a feel for the place. If that isn't possible, most fitness facilities will allow you to workout for a day or two as a courtesy to attracting a new member. Schedule a tour and talk with the person in charge of new members. Go at different times to see if the clientele is what you are looking for. Many facilities have special discounts for students so don't forget to ask about that. Make sure the hours of operation, cleanliness, type and amount of equipment, locker room, staff service, and schedule of group activities or classes is what you are looking for. Be hesitant to sign a long-term (1 year or more) contract, as you may end up having to pay even if the fitness center closes.

2. Find a workout buddy. Exercising is a social activity and working out with friends can make it more enjoyable. This also will increase the chances of you staying on course and working toward your goals. There will be times when you may not feel like working out but knowing that your workout partner or group is expecting you can be a motivator toward more consistent participation.

3. Vary your intensity and volume. Your muscles need to be progressively challenged (overloaded) and doing the same thing over and over will not accomplish this. Your chapter discusses how to develop a muscular fitness program that incorporates this concept and will keep you steadily improving.

4. Vary the types of "lifts" you do. There are a number of exercises to do for each muscle group and it is a good idea to use different ones on occasion. Your chapter shows a variety of lifts for each muscle group. Placing a different demand on your muscles will help challenge them to adapt and grow.

5. Be a safe lifter. Lifting weights can be dangerous to yourself and others if safety precautions aren't followed. Make sure you get a good warm-up with some light stretching. A few minutes on an exercise bike or NordicTrack ski machine can get your heart and muscles ready to go. Learn techniques for proper lifting and breathing and ask for a spotter if attempting to lift heavy weights. Re-rack your weights and dumbbells to keep the floor area clear and decrease the chance of accidents. Don't eat or chew gum while lifting. Keep your eyes and ears open for potential accidents that others may cause.

6. Anticipate lapses and lazy days. Missing a workout or two is healthy for your body and your mind. However, if you find yourself not wanting to workout for several days in a row you may be guilty of trying to do too much too soon, or overtraining. Developing muscular fitness takes time as the body adapts to the new loads placed upon it. You will reach your goals with consistency and commitment, but you will most likely take a little longer than you originally thought.

7. Keep accurate records. This can help you review past lifting accomplishments and serve as a motivator. It also allows you to critique your lifting to help determine why you may not have achieved the results you feel you should have within a certain time period.

8. Reward yourself and have fun. Getting in better shape can be fun, exciting and provide you with a tremendous sense of accomplishment. But don't forget to reward yourself along the way for a job well done. Rewards don't have to be expensive, but should provide a personal incentive to stick to the workout program and enjoyed when goals are achieved.

9. Be good to your body. Beginning and maintaining a fitness program requires your body to go through a number of changes. In order for optimum results to occur, a plan for improving muscular fitness should also include a well-rounded diet, with sufficient nutrients from all food categories to support muscular growth. Getting adequate rest and sleep is vitally important, since the muscle grows during the period be-tween workouts in response to the stimulation provided in the previous workout. Creating a healthier lifestyle will not only benefit your muscular fitness but your overall health and wellness, too.

Weight Training Plan

Use the chart below to help you create a weight training program. Refer to Figure 5-3 to see which exercises are used to train a particular muscle group. A general lifting program for muscular fitness should work each of the nine major muscle groups in the body 2–3 times per week. Training intensity should be maintained between 60%–75% of one repetition maximum (the most weight you can lift in a particular exercise, using proper form), for 8–12 repetitions, over 2–3 sets.

Muscle Group Developed	Exercise Performed	1 RM (pounds)	Desired Intensity (1 RM × %)	Starting Weight	# of Reps	# of Sets
Quadriceps						
Hamstrings						
Pectorals						
Latissimus Dorsi						
Deltoids						
Calves						
Biceps						
Triceps						
Erector Spinae						

SETTING GOALS

Setting Personal Muscular Strength Goals

Your Personal Muscular Strength Goal:

Is it S.M.A.R.T?
Specific? _____
Measurable? _____
Achievable? _____
Rewarding? _____
Time Defined? _____

Strategies for Success
1. _____
2. _____
3. _____

Potential Obstacles
1. _____
2. _____
3. _____

Ways Around Them
1. _____
2. _____
3. _____

Daily Report

The Week That Was:

What went right?
What could I do better?

WELLNESS JOURNAL

Assess Your Muscular Fitness Program

Starting and/or maintaining a program for muscular fitness takes commitment and time management to be successful. Is weight lifting a priority for you, or is it something you just hope works into your schedule? Have you had certain problems in the past that are still affecting your workouts? Are there time management issues that you need to resolve in order to consistently get to the gym?

Plan to lift weights 2–3 times this coming week. Monitor this workout schedule and note any reasons that keep you from working out. In your Wellness Journal, explore these issues and write about what you need to do to overcome them.

CHAPTER 5

Making This Chapter Work for You

1. Which of these statements is *false?*
   a. Muscles can do only two things: contract or shorten.
   b. Myofibrils are long structures inside a muscle fiber.
   c. Exercise toughens the muscle sheath protecting the muscle.
   d. Skeletal muscles are those attached to the bones.

2. Which statement is true about isometric, isotonic, and isokinetic exercises?
   a. Isokinetic exercises usually involve pushing on an object; isotonic exercises involve pulling on an object; and isometric exercises involve lifting an object.
   b. Isometric and isokinetic exercises can be done with free weights, but isotonic exercises require special resistance machines.
   c. Weight lifting is an isotonic exercise; pushing against the wall is an isometric exercise; and isokinetic exercises require special machines that move muscles through their range of motion.
   d. Isotonic exercises are much more effective at contracting muscles than isometric or isokinetic.

3. Gender differences in strength are thought to stem mostly from
   a. testosterone levels.
   b. physically challenging games played as children.
   c. physiological differences in size and body structure.
   d. distribution of fast-twitch and slow-twitch muscle fibers.

4. Muscle training has these benefits:
   a. improved circulation, more lean body mass, more body fat
   b. stronger connective tissues, stronger bones, stronger kidneys
   c. more efficient muscles, less risk of diabetes, less risk of cancer
   d. more efficient muscles, less risk of diabetes, less risk of injury

5. Understanding and using cognitive and behavioral change processes can help you change your muscular fitness behavior. Rewarding yourself with a stop at the coffee shop after your weight training session is an example of which change process?
   a. emotional arousal
   b. reward
   c. environmental control
   d. countering

6. To develop your muscles, you must exert yourself overloading the muscles. To develop muscular endurance when working out,
   a. do a few repetitions with lighter loads.
   b. do a few repetitions with heavy loads.
   c. do many repetitions with lighter loads.
   d. do many repetitions with heavy loads.

7. Your muscle workout should exercise your primary muscle groups. Which of these descriptions is *incorrect?*
   a. Your triceps and biceps are the muscles in the back and front of your upper arms.
   b. Your latissimus dorsi are back muscles that can be exercised using the lat pulldown.
   c. Your "quads" are the muscles in the back of your thighs.
   d. Your "glutes" are the muscles in your buttocks.

8. In your muscle workout,
   a. exercise a muscle through its full range of motion.
   b. breathe after every set.
   c. stretch rather than warming up.
   d. the amount of resistance is not important.

9. In your muscle workout, if you cannot lift a weight more than 12 times, the resistance is high enough
   a. that you will suffer DOMS.
   b. to ensure that you are increasing muscle strength.
   c. to ensure that you are increasing muscle endurance.
   d. that your workout will be shorter than usual.

10. Your muscles need time to recover from muscle workouts—how many hours should you allow between training sessions?
    a. 12
    b. 24
    c. 36
    d. 48

Answers to these questions can be found on page 376.

Critical Thinking

1. Jenna wants to be strong but doesn't want to look bulked up. You have read that women typically don't gain size from strength training because women have so much less testosterone, which makes muscles bulky. Besides this physiological reason, what advice can you give Jenna about designing her workout to allay her fear?

2. Unlike Jenna, Jerry wanted to bulk up and look muscular, so he trained seven days a week, started with weights he could barely lift, and lifted as fast as he could. Jerry now has a pulled hamstring and DOMS. Explain the concept of progression—and what Jerry did wrong.

3. Steroids are controlled substances (like heroin), but some argue that professional athletes should be allowed to take steroids if they don't mind damaging their own bodies. The counterargument is that if one professional athlete uses steroids, then others must also take them—or they may lose their competitive edge. As a result, sports organizations would be condoning or even silently encouraging players (their employees) to ingest substances known to be harmful. What is your view on steroid use in professional sports and why?

Media Menu

Health ⊗ Now ™

Don't forget to check out the wealth of resources on the HealthNow website at **http://healthnow.brookscole.com/itw** that will:
- Help you evaluate your knowledge of the material
- Allow you to take an exam-prep quiz
- Provide a Personalized Learning Plan targeting resources that address areas you should study
- Coach you through identifying target goals for behavior change and creating and monitoring your personal change plan throughout the semester.

INTERNET CONNECTIONS

Muscle and Fitness Magazine—Training

www.muscleandfitness.com/training/
This comprehensive site features information on intermediate and advanced training techniques, with photographs and informative articles on the use of dietary supplements, as well as the importance of mind-body activities to enhance your workout.

Strength Training Muscle Map and Explanation

www.global-fitness.com/strength/s_musclemap.php
This site provides an anatomical map of the body's muscles. Click on the muscle for exercises designed to specifically strengthen that particular muscle, complete with a video and safety information.

American Council on Exercise: Strength and Resistance Training

www.acefitness.org/fitfacts/fitfacts_list.aspx#7
This site features tips on strength training, crunches, plyometrics, and an article on how women build muscle.

Sport Fitness Advisor

www.sport-fitness-advisor.com
This site includes a battery of fitness tests and information about general and sport-specific training programs.

InfoTrac College Edition Activities Harne, Amanda and Bixby, Walter. "The benefits of and barriers to strength training among college-age women," *Journal of Sport Behavior,* June 2005 v28 i2 p151(16)

1. What are some of the benefits of strength training for women?

2. Do women who do strength training differ from those who don't in their perceptions of these benefits?

3. What do women in this study see as the biggest barrier to strength training? How do you think they can overcome it?

You can find additional readings related to personal health with InfoTrac College Edition, an online library of more than 900 journals and publications. Follow the instructions for accessing InfoTrac College Edition that were packaged with your textbook; then search for articles using a keyword search.

For additional links, resources, and suggested readings on the InfoTrac College Edition, visit our Health and Wellness Resource Center at **http://health.wadsworth.com.**

Key Terms

The terms listed are used on the page indicated. Definitions of the terms are in the Glossary at the end of the book.

actin 86	**1 repetition maximum**
atrophy 91	**(1 RM)** 90
capillaries 86	**overloading** 91
cardiac muscle 86	**repetition** 93
concentric contraction 88	**reps** 93
dynamic training 91	**resistance** 94
eccentric contraction 88	**sarcomeres** 86
fast-twitch fibers 88	**sets** 93
hypertrophy 91	**"sliding filament"**
isokinetic contraction 88	**theory** 87
isometric contraction 87	**skeletal muscle** 86
isotonic contraction 87	**slow-twitch oxidative**
muscle fibers 86	**fibers** 88
muscular endurance 86	**smooth muscle** 86
muscular strength 86	**static training** 91
myofibrils 86	**tendons** 87
myosin 86	

Staying Flexible

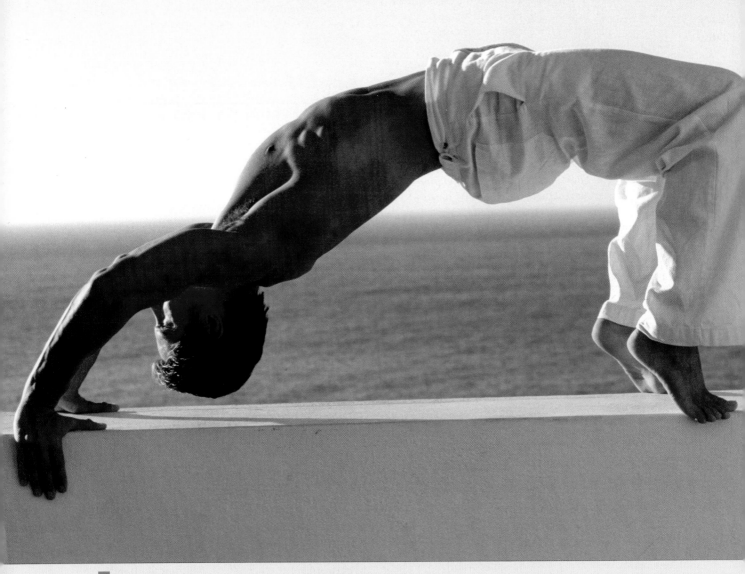

Tyler went to his girlfriend's yoga class on a dare. Even though he'd played varsity basketball in high school and worked out regularly with weights, she claimed that even basic yoga postures would be too challenging for him. Tyler didn't believe her—until he tried to raise his legs over his head in a classic yoga plow, a challenging position that can be dangerous for novices. "How do you bend like that?" he whispered to his girlfriend. "You've got to be flexible," she answered, "and practice."

Like Tyler, many people who are strong and aerobically fit ignore flexibility, even though it is an essential component of physical fitness. Every day you reach and bend, twist and turn, raise your head and lift your arms dozens of times. How easily, smoothly, and painlessly you do so depends on your flexibility.

Regardless of age, sex, general health, or overall fitness, everyone needs to be flexible. Being able to move with ease and comfort depends on your ability to go through the complete range of motion—the fullest extent of possible movements—that is possible for any given joint.

If muscles aren't stretched regularly, they shorten and tighten. The result can be muscle strain and chronic pain. If you spend a lot of time sitting in front of a computer, for instance, the hamstring muscles in your legs get shorter, and you may develop low-back pain, the most common cause of disability among men and women under age 45.

This chapter describes the anatomy of a stretch, the types of stretching, and the physical benefits of flexibility; indicates ways of stretching safely; describes yoga and other practices that increase flexibility; and offers suggestions for preventing and managing low-back pain.

© Royalty-Free/Corbis

After studying the material in this chapter, you should be able to:

▌ **Define** flexibility and **list** the physical benefits of flexibility training.

▌ **Explain** the different forms of stretching exercises.

▌ **Design** a safe and injury-free flexibility program.

▌ **List** ways to avoid back injuries.

▌ **Describe** how yoga can improve flexibility.

Health Now™

Don't forget to check out the wealth of resources on the HealthNow website at **http://healthnow.brookscole.com/itw** that will:

• Help you evaluate your knowledge of the material
• Allow you to take an exam-prep quiz
• Provide a Personalized Learning Plan targeting resources that address areas you should study
• Coach you through identifying target goals for behavior change and creating and monitoring your personal change plan throughout the semester.

✚ Becoming More Flexible

Stretching, if done right, not only does good but feels good. Like a body yawn, it loosens you up and relieves tension. Even a brief stretch break during the day can be relaxing. But it is important to know how to stretch properly so that you don't end up hurting rather than helping yourself.

What Is Flexibility?

Flexibility is the characteristic of body tissues that determines the range of motion achievable without injury at a joint or group of joints. There are two types of flexibility: static and dynamic. **Static flexibility**—the type most people think of as flexibility—refers to the ability to assume and maintain an extended position at one end point in a joint's range of motion. **Dynamic flexibility,** by comparison, involves movement. It is the ability to move a joint quickly and fluidly through its entire range of motion with little resistance. The static flexibility in the hip joint determines whether you can do a split; dynamic flexibility is what would enable you to perform a split leap.

Static flexibility depends on many factors, including the structure of a joint and the tightness of the muscles, tendons, and ligaments attached to it. Dynamic flexibility is influenced by static flexibility but also depends on additional factors, such as strength, coordination, and resistance to movement.

Genetics, age, gender, and body composition all influence how flexible you are. Girls and women tend to be more flexible than boys and men, to a certain extent because of hormonal and anatomical differences. The way females and males use their muscles and the activities they engage in can also have an effect. Over time, the natural elasticity of muscles, tendons, and joints decreases in both genders, resulting in stiffness.

Joints and Muscles

The **joints**—the parts of the body where bones meet—enable us to move. Good flexibility assures full range of motion through each of our joints. If the muscles, ligaments, and other tissues that support a joint are tight, they can cause abnormal pressure on, for example, a knee or shoulder. Poor flexibility in the joints can also lead to inadequate lubrication within a joint, which can cause the cartilage cells lining the joint to deteriorate. This produces pain and often leads to more extensive damage to the joint.

The structure and nature of a joint determine its flexibility. For example, the structure of the finger and knee joints limits their **range of motion.** The fingers and knees work like hinges and allow only limited forward and backward motion. In contrast, the hip and

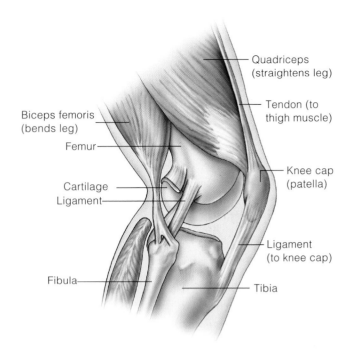

FIGURE 6-1 ▍ The knee joint is the largest and most complex joint in the body.

shoulder are ball-and-socket joints that allow movement in many different directions and have a greater range of motion. Each major joint is surrounded by a joint capsule, a semi-elastic structure made up of connective tissues that provide strength and stability but limit movement (**Figure 6-1**).

The flexibility of a joint also depends on soft tissues, that is, skin, muscles, tendons, and ligaments. As discussed in Chapter 5, muscle is composed of contractile fibers (actin and myosin) wrapped in a web of connective tissue, which accounts for about 30 percent of muscle mass and provides structure, elasticity, and bulk. Muscle fibers are relatively elastic because of one type of connective tissue.

What Is Connective Tissue?

The two principal types of connective tissue are **collagen,** white fibers that provide support and structure and are not elastic, and **elastin,** yellow fibers that are elastic and flexible. Because collagen and elastin are closely intertwined in muscles, muscle tissue exhibits the properties of both types.

The "stretchability" of connective tissue is limited. If the tissue is stretched too far, it becomes brittle and more vulnerable to a tear or rupture. This is why a stretching program should be designed to elongate connective tissue but not push to the extent of possible damage. Quick, jerky stretching is less effective and can lead to injury.

Flexibility improves best when muscles are warm (from heat or warm-up exercises) and the stretch is gradual. Hyaluronic acid, the viscous medium of connective tissue, has the consistency of Vaseline at room temperature when the muscles are "cold" and becomes more fluid as the temperature of a muscle increases.

∎ The Benefits of Flexibility

Just as cardiorespiratory fitness benefits the heart and lungs and muscular fitness builds endurance and strength, a stretching program produces unique benefits, including enhancement of the ability of the respiratory, circulatory, and neuromuscular systems to cope with the stress and demands of our high-pressure world. Flexibility makes everyday tasks, like bending over to tie a shoe or reaching up to a high shelf, easier and safer. It can also prevent and relieve the ankle, knee, back, and shoulder pain that many people feel as they get older. If you do other forms of exercise, flexibility lowers your risk of injury and may improve your performance.

Among the other benefits of flexibility are:

∎ **Prevention of injuries.** Flexibility training stretches muscles and increases the elasticity of joints. Strong, flexible muscles resist stress better than weak or inflexible ones. Adding flexibility to a training program for sports such as soccer, football, or tennis can reduce the rate of injuries by as much as 75 percent.

∎ **Relief of muscle strain.** Muscles tighten as a result of stress or prolonged sitting. If you study or work in one position for several hours, you'll often feel stiffness in your back or neck. Stretching helps relieve this tension and enables you to work more effectively.

∎ **Relaxation.** Flexibility exercises are great stress-busters that reduce mental strain, slow the rate of breathing, and reduce blood pressure.

∎ **Relief of soreness after exercise.** Many people develop delayed-onset muscle soreness (DOMS) one or two days after they work out. This may be the result of damage to the muscle fibers and supporting connective tissue.

∎ **Improved posture.** Bad posture can create tight, stressed muscles. If you slump in your chair, for instance, the muscles in the front of your chest may tighten, causing those in the upper spine to overstretch and become loose.

∎ **Better athletic performance.** Good flexibility allows for more efficient movement and exertion of more force through a greater range of motion, a special benefit for any activity, from gymnastics to golf, where positions beyond the normal range of motion are necessary to perform certain skills.

∎ Stretching

When you stretch a muscle, you are primarily stretching the connective tissue. The stretch must be intense enough to increase the length of the connective tissue without tearing it.

Static and Passive Stretching

Static stretching involves a gradual stretch held for a short time (10 to 30 seconds). A shorter stretch provides little benefit; a longer stretch does not provide additional benefits. Since a slow stretch provokes less of a reaction from the stretch receptors, the muscles can safely stretch farther than usual. Fitness experts most often recommend static stretching because it is both safe and effective. An example of such a stretch is letting your hands slowly slide down the front of your legs (keeping your knees in

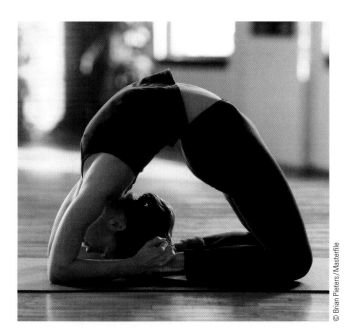

Not everyone can become as flexible as a dancer, but regular stretching can increase your flexibility.

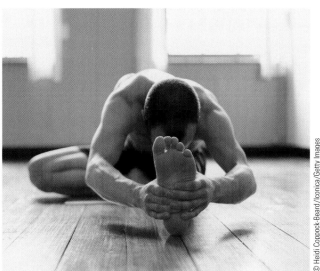

A gradual stretch held for about 20 seconds is static stretching.

a soft, unlocked position) until you reach your toes and holding this final position for several seconds before slowly straightening up. You should feel a pull, but not pain, during this stretch.

In **passive stretching,** your own body, a partner, gravity, or a weight serves as an external force or resistance to help your joints move through their range of motion. You can achieve a more intense stretch and a greater range of motion with passive stretching. There is a greater risk of injury, however, because the muscles themselves are not controlling the stretch. If working with a partner, it's very important that you communicate clearly so as not to force a joint outside its normal functional range of motion.

Research on stretching demonstrates a 5 to 20 percent increase in static flexibility within four to six weeks of stretching. Much of this long-term increase in range of motion is due to an increased "stretch tolerance," or ability to tolerate the discomfort of a stretched position.

Active Stretching

Active stretching involves stretching a muscle by contracting the opposing muscle (the muscle on the opposite side of the limb). In an active seated hamstring stretch, for example, the stretch occurs by actively contracting the muscles on top of the shin, which produces a reflex that relaxes the hamstring. This method allows the muscle to be stretched farther with a low risk of injury.

The disadvantage of active stretching is that a person may not be able to produce enough of a stretch to increase flexibility only by means of contracting opposing muscle groups. Although active stretching is the safest and most convenient approach, an occasional passive assist can be helpful.

A variation of this approach, active isolated (AI) stretching, is based on a principle called Sherrington's law of reciprocal inhibition in muscular contraction. This means that when a muscle on one side of a joint is contracted, the muscle on the opposite side of the joint is sent a neurological signal to relax or release. Using this law in combination with slow, controlled rhythmic stretches, AI stretching increases flexibility in a relatively short time with little or no harmful effect.

In this method, you isolate a specific muscle, such as the hamstring, and reduce the load it bears by lying on your back. To activate the opposite muscle group—in this example, the quads—you raise the leg until you feel the stretch. You then intensify the stretch with gentle pressure from a rope or yoga strap, hold for three to five seconds, and gently return the leg to the floor. At least in theory, these slow rhythmic stretches could be used in the midst of competition to relieve cramping and tightness because they would increase, rather than decrease, blood flow in the muscle.

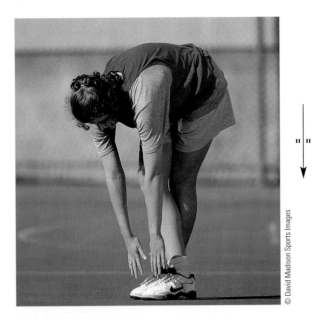

▮ Be wary of the rapid bouncing movements of ballistic stretching.

Ballistic Stretching

Ballistic stretching is characterized by rapid bouncing movements, such as a series of up-and-down bobs as you try again and again to touch your toes with your hands. These bounces can stretch the muscle fibers too far, causing the muscle to contract rather than stretch. They also can tear ligaments and weaken or rupture tendons, the strong fibrous cords that connect muscles to bones. The heightened activity to stretch receptors caused by the rapid stretches can continue for some time, possibly causing injuries during any physical activities that follow. Because of its potential dangers, fitness experts generally recommend against ballistic stretching.

Proprioceptive Neuromuscular Facilitation

Strong muscle contractions produce a reflex that causes the muscles to relax and keeps them from contracting too hard. This inverse stretch reflex can be used to improve flexibility. Contracting a muscle prior to stretching causes it to relax, allowing it to stretch farther. This technique, called **proprioceptive neuromuscular facilitation (PNF),** is being studied to determine the extent to which it can cause muscle relaxation and help develop flexibility. PNF stretching consists of alternating isometric muscle contraction and passive stretching. The technique is sometimes described as active/assisted, contract/relax, or hold/relax.

PNF uses reflexes initiated by muscle and joint receptors to cause greater training effects. The most popular PNF stretching technique is the contract-relax stretching method, in which a muscle is contracted before it is stretched. In a seated calf muscle stretch, you first contract the calf muscles for about 6 seconds. After a brief relaxation period, you stretch the calf muscles by pulling the tops of the feet toward the body for 10 to 30 seconds. While PNF may allow more effective stretching, it tends to cause more muscle stiffness and soreness than static stretching. It also usually requires more time and a partner to provide resistance.

Doing each stretching exercise several times in a row can "reset" the sensitivity of muscle stretch receptors. Stretching a muscle, relaxing, and then stretching it again cause the stretch receptors to become slightly less sensitive, thereby enabling the muscle to stretch farther. In theory, prolonged flexibility training may induce neural changes to help increase flexibility, but research has not yet proved this effect.

What Is the Difference Between Stretching and Warming Up?

Warming up means getting the heart beating faster, raising your core body temperature, and readying the body for more vigorous activity. Stretching is a specific activity intended to elongate the muscles and keep joints limber, not simply a prelude to a game of tennis or a three-mile run. According to a review of recent studies, the value of stretching varies with different activities. While it does not prevent injuries from jogging, cycling, or swimming, stretching may be beneficial in sports, like soccer and football, that involve bouncing and jumping.[1]

For aerobic activities, one of the best times to stretch is after an aerobic workout. Your muscles will be warm, more flexible, and less prone to injury. In addition, stretching after aerobic activity can help a fatigued muscle return to its normal resting length and possibly help reduce delayed muscle soreness.

✚ Designing a Flexibility Program

There are various approaches to improving flexibility through stretching. These include static stretching, active stretching, and proprioceptive neuromuscular facilitation (PNF). The American College of Sports Medicine advocates a modest flexibility program that includes a variety of dynamic and static range-of-motion stretches of all major muscle and tendon groups two to three days per week.

Before beginning to design a flexibility program, you need to know how flexible you are. Although dynamic flexibility is important both for daily activities and for sports, most assessments focus on static flexibility. The most widely used flexibility test is the sit and reach exercise, which rates the flexibility in the muscles in the

lower back and hamstrings. These muscles may play a role in preventing low-back pain. See your Lab Booklet for this test and several others.

Intensity and Duration

For each exercise, your own body is the best guide to how intensely you should work. Slowly stretch your muscles to the point of slight tension or mild discomfort, then hold the stretch for 10 to 30 seconds. Do not stretch to the point of experiencing pain. As you hold the stretch, the slight tension should subside, and at that point you can try to stretch a bit farther. Throughout the stretch, remember to relax and breathe easily. Rest for 30 to 60 seconds between stretches, and do at least four repetitions of each stretch. A complete flexibility workout usually takes 20 to 30 minutes.

STRATEGIES for PREVENTION

How to Avoid Stretching Injuries

Before you begin, increase your body temperature by slowly marching or running in place. Sweat signals that you're ready to start stretching.

▌ Don't force body parts beyond their normal range of motion. Stretch to the point of tension, back off, and hold for 10 seconds to a minute.

▌ Do a minimum of four repetitions of each stretch, with equal repetitions on each side.

▌ Don't hold your breath. Continue breathing slowly and rhythmically throughout your stretching routine.

▌ Don't attempt to stretch a weak or injured muscle.

▌ Start small. Work the muscles of the smaller joints in the arms and legs first and then work the larger joints like the shoulders and hips.

▌ Stretch individual muscles before you stretch a group of muscles, for instance, the ankle, knee, and hip before a stretch that works all three.

▌ Don't make any quick, jerky movements while stretching. Stretches should be gentle and smooth.

▌ Certain positions can be harmful to the knees and lower back. In particular, avoid stretches that require deep knee bends or full squats because they can harm your knees and lower back.

Frequency

The American College of Sports Medicine recommends that stretching exercises be performed a minimum of two to three days a week, although many people do flexibility training three to five days for even greater benefits. It's best to stretch when your muscles are warm, so try to incorporate stretching into your cool-down after cardio-respiratory endurance exercise or weight training.

Specificity

Flexibility is specific to each joint. You may have excellent flexibility in your shoulders but poor hip flexibility —or vice versa. That's why it's important to follow a well-rounded program that works all the major joints of the body by stretching their associated muscles. If you don't, stiffness in one area (the shoulders, for instance) can increase the risk of injury in others (such as the knees and ankles during a run).

If you exercise regularly, make sure to focus on different parts of the body. For instance, if you're a swimmer, flexible shoulders are critical. For tennis and golf, the lower back has to be limber. Cyclists should be sure to stretch their quadriceps (front thigh muscles) and calves, while runners should be sure to stretch their hamstring muscles and feet. A personal trainer can help you design a program to meet your specific needs. (see "Savvy Consumer: Selecting a Personal Trainer").

Safety Basics

While stretching yields many benefits, it also poses some risks. The danger of injury from stretching is greatest when stretches are performed with poor technique, when individuals are in poor overall condition, or when stretches are performed before muscles are properly warmed.

One way to understand what happens when you stretch is to think of Silly Putty. If you tug at Silly Putty slowly and gently, it elongates gradually. If you pull at it quickly, the putty has greater stiffness and usually breaks after minimal elongation. Alternatively, you can think of muscle as a rubber band. If you abruptly stretch it out and release it, a rubber band snaps back. If you stretch it too hard or too far, it can break. But if you pull it gently, hold it, and gently release it, the rubber band stretches with far less strain. The same principles apply to what are called the "viscoelastic properties" of human muscle. This is why static stretching is safer in theory than ballistic stretching, which creates significantly greater muscle stiffness and is much more likely to result in injury to the muscle than slower stretching techniques.

Always move slowly into a stretch position. You should never feel pain, although you will feel a slight tugging as you extend your stretch. Reach to this point of discomfort and then back off slightly, relaxing and allowing your muscles to adjust. You should hold this stretch until the feeling of tension diminishes. Concentrate on

SAVVY

CONSUMER

SELECTING A PERSONAL TRAINER

A personal trainer can help you design a workout that will meet your needs or work with you regularly, motivating you through each workout and ensuring that you use proper technique (especially important for flexibility training) and avoid injury. Here are some factors to consider in choosing a trainer:

▪ Does the trainer have a solid background in exercise physiology, anatomy, injury prevention, and monitoring of exercise intensity? Ideally, a trainer should have a degree in a related medical or physical science field or certification through a nationally recognized organization, such as the American College of Sports Medicine.

▪ Does the trainer have experience?

▪ Does he or she keep current with research through associations and educational programs and publications?

▪ Is the trainer certified in CPR and first aid?

▪ Can the trainer provide you with references from other clients?

▪ Does the trainer keep a record of your workouts and update your medical history periodically?

▪ Does the trainer provide clear-cut written statements of his or her policies on cancellation and billing?

▪ Is the trainer within your budget? Trainers charge a broad range of fees

depending on the length of the workout, the location, and the trainer's experience.

▪ Does the trainer listen to what you want and communicate well with you?

▪ Is the trainer willing to put his or her workout methods in writing and explain the reasoning behind the exercise program?

▪ Do you feel you will get along well with the trainer? Are your personalities compatible?

▪ Is the trainer interested in helping you maintain a balanced, healthy lifestyle in addition to exercise?

the feeling of the stretch itself, not on the flexibility you want to attain. Perform stretching exercises regularly. "Use it or lose it" is the motto to keep in mind when it comes to flexibility.

WELLNESS COACH

✚ Mind-Body Approaches

As discussed in Chapter 3, physical fitness can contribute to every dimension of wellness. However, some specific approaches, which are increasingly popular on campuses and throughout the country, emphasize total wellness and incorporate body, mind, and spirit. Wellness Coach encompasses yoga, Pilates, and t'ai chi, described in the following pages, can help reduce stress, enhance health and wellness, and improve physical fitness.

Yoga

One of the most ancient of mind-body practices, "yoga" comes from the Sanskrit word meaning *union*. Traditionally associated with religion, yoga consists of various breathing and stretching exercises that unite all aspects of a person. According to a national poll, 16.5 million Americans—7.5 percent of the population—practice yoga.[2] The fastest-growing segment consists of young adults between ages 18 and 34. (See Student Snapshot: "Getting Flexible.")

The best way to get started is to find a class that appeals to you and learn a few yoga moves and breathing techniques. Once you have mastered these, you can easily integrate yoga into your total fitness program.

The types of yoga include:

■ Hatha Yoga, the most practiced form, described as the yoga of "balanced body energy."[3] Its practices include breath control, concentration, and gentle stretching and strengthening exercise. (See your Lab Booklet for some basic hatha yoga postures that help reduce stress.)

■ Ashtanga yoga, also called power yoga. A series of postures flow together to create constant movement. The emphasis is on muscular endurance as well as flexibility, and even very fit individuals may find it difficult to complete every pose in the first few sessions. If you have wrist or shoulder problems, avoid the poses that put much of your body weight on these joints.

■ Bikram yoga, an athletic workout conducted in temperatures of 80 to 100 degrees or higher. This can be dangerous if you are not accustomed to extreme heat.

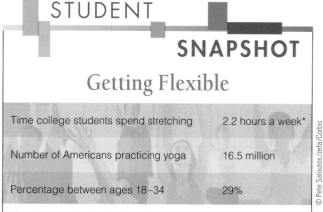

© Pete Saloutos/zefa/Corbis

STUDENT SNAPSHOT

Getting Flexible

Time college students spend stretching	2.2 hours a week*
Number of Americans practicing yoga	16.5 million
Percentage between ages 18–34	29%

*Based on a study of 439 undergraduates at a large midwestern university. *Source:* Buckworth, Janet, and Claudio Nigg. "Physical Activity, Exercise, and Sedentary Behavior in College Students." *Journal of American College Health,* Vol. 53, No. 1, July/August 2004, p. 28. "Yoga Becomes Big Business." *Sporting Good Business,* Vol. 38, No. 3, March 2005, p. 16.

■ Sivanada, a gentle meditative form of yoga ideal for relieving stress. (The use of yoga for stress management is discussed in Chapter 7.)

■ Iyengar, which focuses more on skeletal alignment. Iyengar is often used for rehabilitation after injury.

Once considered an exotic pursuit, yoga has gained acceptance as part of a comprehensive stress management and fitness program. Scientific studies have demonstrated its benefits, which include:

■ Improved flexibility, which may offer protection from back pain and injuries.

■ Protection of joints because yoga postures take joints through their full range of motion, providing a fresh supply of nutrients to joint cartilage.

■ Stronger, denser bones from yoga's weight-bearing postures.

■ Enhanced circulation, which also boosts the supply of oxygen throughout the body.

■ Lower blood pressure.

■ Lower levels of the stress hormone cortisol, which, as discussed in Chapter 7, can affect the immune system, interfere with memory, and increase the risk of depression and osteoporosis.

■ Lower blood sugar in people with diabetes, which reduces the risk of complications.

■ Reduced pain in people with back problems, arthritis, carpal tunnel syndrome, fibromyalgia, and other chronic problems.[4]

The American College of Sports Medicine cautions that yoga should help, not hurt. To prevent injuries to your knees, back, neck, shoulders, wrists, or ankles, avoid forcing your body into difficult postures. Proper technique is essential to safety. With the lotus position, for instance, forcing your legs apart can damage cartilage in the knees. However, a skilled instructor can teach you how to redirect the force away from the knees.[5] (See Savvy Consumer on page 110.)

Pilates

Used by dancers for deep body conditioning and injury rehabilitation, Pilates (pronounced Pilah-teez), was developed more than seven decades ago by German immigrant Joseph Pilates. Increasingly used to complement aerobics and weight training, Pilates exercises improve flexibility and joint mobility and strengthen the core by developing pelvic stability and abdominal control.

Pilates-trained instructors offer "mat" or "floor" classes that stress the stabilization and strengthening of the back and abdominal muscles. Fitness centers also may offer training on Pilates equipment, primarily a device called the Reformer, a wooden contraption with various cables, pulleys, springs, and sliding boards attached that is used for a series of progressive, range-of-motion exercises. Instructors typically work one-on-one or with small groups of two or three participants and tailor exercise sessions to individual flexibility and strength limitations. Unlike exercise techniques that emphasize numerous repetitions in a single direction, Pilates exercises involve very few, but extremely precise, repetitions in several planes of motion.

According to research from the American College of Sports Medicine, Pilates can enhance flexibility as well as muscular endurance, particularly for intermediate and advanced practitioners. However, its potential to increase cardiorespiratory fitness and reduce body weight is limited. The intensity of a Pilates workout increases from basic to intermediate to advanced levels, as does the number of calories burned.

For intermediate practitioners, a 30-minute session burns 180 calories, with each additional quarter-hour burning another 90 calories. A single weekly session enhances flexibility but has little impact on body composition.[6]

Whether you work out at a studio or home, Pilates exercises can refresh and relax you in addition to making you stronger and more flexible. The mind-body connection associated with yoga and meditation also plays an integral part in Pilates.

T'ai Chi

This ancient Chinese practice, designed to exercise body, mind, and spirit, gently works muscles, focuses concentration, and improves the flow of "qi" (often spelled "chi"), the vital life energy that sustains health. Popular with all ages, from children to seniors, t'ai chi is easy to learn and perform. Because of its focus on breathing and flowing gestures, t'ai chi is sometimes described as "meditation in motion."

Classes are available on campuses and in fitness centers, community centers, and some martial arts schools. Physicians may recommend t'ai chi for those with musculoskeletal disorders like arthritis to improve flexibility and build muscle strength gently and gradually. As the American College of Sports Medicine reports, t'ai chi has proved effective in reducing falls in the elderly and those with balance disorders.[7]

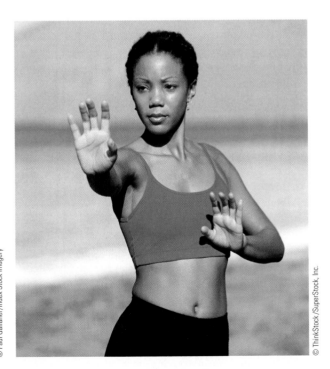

Pilates exercises strengthen the body's core muscles and improve flexibility.

© Paul Gallaher/Index Stock Imagery

T'ai chi improves flexibility, focuses concentration, and gently builds muscle strength.

© ThinkStock/SuperStock, Inc.

Keeping Your Back Healthy

The average person has an 80 percent chance of experiencing low-back pain in the course of a lifetime.[8] Back pain strikes slightly more women than men and is most common between the ages of 20 and 55. You are at greater risk if you smoke or if you're overstressed, overweight, or out of shape. Back pain, which accounts for 40 percent of sickness absences, causes more lost workdays and costs the country more than any other malady.

Anyone, from a young athlete to a middle-aged executive, can suffer a back injury. About one in three intercollegiate rowers develop back pain during their college career, and they often worry that they will continue to have back problems throughout life. This is not the case. In a study of 1561 former competitive rowers who had graduated a mean of 13 years previously, rowers—even those who develop back pain during college—are no more likely than the general population to have episodic back pain or to miss work because of back pain.

Usually, the source of back pain isn't the spine itself but its supporting structures. Deeper muscles, hamstrings, and tendons become less resilient and less elastic. After age 40 or so, they are more susceptible to strain with any unusual stress. Yet age itself is rarely the only culprit in a disabling back attack.

Extra pounds, particularly if stuffed into a pot belly, tug at the back, causing constant strain. And without exercise, the muscles supporting the spine are less capable of doing their job. Slouching in front of a computer, slumping on overstuffed cushions, sleeping on a soft mattress, and bending from the waist to hoist a heavy load further jeopardize a back's well-being.

Though workers whose jobs demand heavy lifting are at greatest risk of back injury, desk jockeys also are vulnerable because sitting weakens and strains muscles. If you rush onto the tennis court or softball field after a week off your feet, your stiff, underused muscles may become so painful you won't be able to move on Monday. After years of bad posture and general wear and tear, even the slightest movement—sometimes just a cough or sneeze—can trigger a muscle spasm so excruciating that any movement is impossible.

Low-Back Pain

The lower, or lumbar, part of the back, which bears the greatest pressure during lifts and bends, is the most vulnerable. Five to 10 percent of back problems involve the disks. Most common is the protrusion (or herniation) of the soft center of a disk through the casing so that it presses on spinal nerves. Another 10 percent of back problems involve structural defects, which may be the result of injuries, tumors, arthritis, congenital malformations, osteoporosis (weakening of the bones), or scoliosis (side-to-side curving of the spine). Sometimes a sore

STRATEGIES for PREVENTION

Back Talk

▪ When standing, shift your weight from one foot to the other. If possible, place one foot on a stool, step, or railing 4 to 6 inches off the ground. Hold in your stomach, tilt your pelvis toward your back, and tuck in your buttocks to provide crucial support for the lower back.

▪ Because sitting places more stress on the lower back than standing, try to get up from your seat at least once an hour to stretch or walk around. Whenever possible, sit in a straight chair with a firm back. Avoid slouching in overstuffed chairs or dangling your legs in midair. When driving, keep the seat forward so that your knees are raised to hip level; your right leg should not be fully extended. A small pillow or towel can help support your lower back.

▪ Sleep on a flat, firm mattress. The best sleep position is on your side, with one or both knees bent at right angles to your torso. The pillow should keep your head in line with your body so that your neck isn't bent forward or to the side.

▪ When lifting, bend at the knees, not from the waist. Get close to the load. Tighten your stomach muscles, but don't hold your breath. Let your leg muscles do the work.

▪ Don't smoke. Smoking may interfere with circulation to the lower back; and a chronic smoker's cough can be so irritating that it provokes a back spasm.

back is a symptom of diseases of other organs, such as the kidneys, gallbladder, heart, or stomach.

Most severe back pain lasts only a few days, although less severe symptoms may persist for many months, and most patients have intermittent recurrences of back pain. More than 90 percent of individuals with back pain recover within three months.

Once bedrest was the primary treatment for back pain, but now doctors urge patients to avoid it. Even two to seven days of bedrest may provide little, if any benefit. Acetaminophen (Tylenol) is the first-line therapy for pain relief. If it is not effective, doctors recommend nonsteroidal anti-inflammatory drugs, such as ibuprofen (Motrin or Advil). Muscle relaxants seem to be effective for a spasm in the lower back. The sooner that back patients return to normal activity, the less pain medication they require and the less long-term disability they suffer.[9]

So many people with back pain have been disappointed with the treatments provided by their doctors that an entire industry of alternative therapies has sprung up. Many patients swear by chiropractic manipulation (discussed in Chapter 12), but studies have not shown that it works better than other approaches.[10] Popular treatments involving ice, heat, and ultrasound are probably harmless but have never been shown to be effective in scientific studies. There is no hard evidence that phys-ical therapy, biofeedback, shoe insoles and shoe lifts, or special corsets and supports make any difference in easing back pain. Spinal surgery has not proved more effective than rehabilitation for chronic low-back pain. Less than 1 percent of patients with chronic low-back pain benefit from surgery.[11]

✚ MAKING HEALTHY CHOICES

for Greater Flexibility

Becoming flexible is a crucial step toward total fitness and wellness. Staying flexible requires an ongoing commitment to regular stretching exercises. Incorporate flexibility routines into your weekly exercise schedule. To keep yourself motivated for the long haul, try the following:

▮ **Avoid boredom.** Try a new activity such as yoga or Pilates to avoid monotony and add more variety to your flexibility routine.

▮ **Find a flexibility role model.** Do you know someone who's an outstanding gymnast, dancer, or yoga practitioner? Ask that person's advice. Or collect articles or books about real-life folks who credit their success or well-being to flexibility training. Examine their secrets of success, and try those that you think might work for you.

▮ **Reward yourself.** Put a dime or a quarter in a jar every time you do your stretches. When it starts to add up, buy yourself a new water bottle, visor, or a tee shirt. You've earned it!

▮ **If an injury knocks you off your feet, start over like a beginner.** Get specific advice from a qualified professional on stretches to avoid during recovery.

▮ **Remember that tomorrow really is another day.** If you don't stretch as planned today, get back on track tomorrow. Take setbacks in stride, and don't delay getting back into your program.

SELF-SURVEY

Proper Form

Proper form usually refers to your posture as you're doing an exercise or lifting weights. There are, however, certain things you can do while standing during the day that will reduce your chances of developing chronic pain as a result of poor posture. When you are standing, proper posture aligns your body so that the pull of gravity is evenly distributed.

Good posture includes

> A straight line from your ears, shoulders, hips, knees and ankles
> Head centered and not leaning to one side or the other

Some of the most common posture mistakes include

> Forward head
> Rounded shoulders
> Arched lower back
> Excessive anterior pelvic tilt (protruding buttocks)
> Excessive posterior pelvic tilt (protruding abdomen/pelvis)

Test Your Posture

To check if you have good posture, take the following posture tests.

The Wall Test Stand with the back of your head touching the wall and your heels six inches from the baseboard.

With your buttocks touching the wall, stick your hand between your lower back and the wall, and then between your neck and the wall. If you can get within an inch or two at the low back and two inches at the neck, you are close to having excellent posture.

The Mirror Test Circle *yes* or *no* after you stand *facing* a full length mirror and check:

1. Is your head straight?	Yes	No
2. Are your shoulders level?	Yes	No
3. Are your hips level?	Yes	No
4. Do your kneecaps face the front?	Yes	No
5. Are your ankles straight?	Yes	No

Now look at yourself *from the side* (or have someone else check your form) and look for the following:

6. Is your head straight rather than slumped forwards or backwards?	Yes	No
7. Is your chin parallel to the floor?	Yes	No
8. Are your shoulders in line with your ears?	Yes	No
9. Are your knees straight and not hyperextended?	Yes	No

10. Is there a slight forward curve to your lower back?   Yes   No

Rating (based upon the number of yes responses):

9–10   Great! You can balance your books on your head while walking to class.

7–8   Good for you. You're generally walking tall but should consider posture improvements.

<7   You're heading for back pain and misery. Take steps now to improve your posture.

How did you do? Are there posture areas in which you can improve? What can you do <u>now</u> to help improve in this area?

ACTION PLAN

Your Action Plan for Staying Flexible

Improving and maintaining flexibility can often be a tough battle. With our time-conscious society, we don't have enough time to stretch, even though we know how beneficial it can be to our overall health and well-being. So how *does* one find the time to stretch?

1. Review your schedule daily and see if there is any extra time to devote to stretching. An extra 10–15 minutes per day in this area can result in a big improvement.

2. Instead of just socializing at the end (or beginning) of your workout, combine it with a stretching program. Ask friends to join you on the mats while you catch up with each other's lives.

3. Stretch while watching TV. Sitcoms last for 30 minutes, so pick out a show each night and stretch during it. Even if you only do it during commercials, there are so many of them that you'll be surprised how much time is devoted to stretching. Work up to an hour drama show!

4. Stretch with your dog or cat. Animals love to stretch. You'll have so much fun playing this game (and so will your pet) that you may want to turn it into a nightly event.

5. Check with your Campus Rec, local Parks Department or YMCA for classes in yoga, Pilates or t'ai chi. Paying for a class will motivate you to stick with it, as well as help you learn more about the proper way to improve flexibility.

SETTING GOALS

Personal Flexibility

Your Personal Flexibility Goal:

Is it S.M.A.R.T.?
Specific? _____
Measurable? _____
Achievable? _____
Rewarding? _____
Time Defined? _____

Strategies for Success
1. _____
2. _____
3. _____

Potential Obstacles
1. _____
2. _____
3. _____

Ways Around Them
1. _____
2. _____
3. _____

Daily Report

The Week That Was:

What went right?
What could I do better?

WELLNESS JOURNAL

How's My Posture?

Improving and maintaining flexibility promotes joint health, decreases the potential for painful, chronic lower back soreness, helps prevent injuries during sports participation and enhances posture. Our increasingly sedentary lifestyle, however, does not lend itself to becoming more flexible, as we find ourselves sitting for long periods of time in positions that lead to numerous muscular aches and pains. Over time, this may affect one's quality of life by causing a reduction in mobility and an avoidance of those day-to-day activities that once provided fun and satisfaction.

The first step to improving posture is to be aware of not practicing good posture and making a conscious effort to correct it. There are most likely many times throughout the day that you may be exhibiting poor posture and not even realize it. Over the next few days, see how often you notice yourself having any of the following "posture problems" and write an assessment in your wellness journal.

Walking across campus

▮ Do you hang your head down and have your chin toward your chest?
▮ Is your backpack too heavy, making you lean to one side and/or causing pain in your shoulder?
▮ When standing in line, does your pelvic area tilt down, resulting in your abdomen protruding and causing an exaggerated curve of your lower back?

Sitting in class and/or reading

▮ Is the base of your spine more toward the front of the seat than the rear?
▮ Are your shoulders rounded inward with elbows against the sides of your abdomen?

Eating meals and/or watching TV

▮ Are you sitting up straight in the chair at a table or are you hunched over your food?
▮ Are your feet on the floor or over the arm of the couch?

Working on a computer

▮ Are you hunched over the keyboard, with your head forward trying to view the monitor?
▮ Do you feel a tightness or cramping in your neck and shoulders?

Comments from other people

▮ Do people mention you are "slouching" or not "standing up straight"?

CHAPTER 6 Making This Chapter Work for You

1. Our flexibility determines our range of motion at a joint and is influenced by
   a. genetics and body weight.
   b. genetics and gender.
   c. age and ethnicity.
   d. genetics and the environment.

2. The connective tissue in the muscle fibers that makes muscles "stretchable" is
   a. collagen
   b. lubrication
   c. elastin
   d. myosin

3. A regular flexibility program provides which of these benefits?
   a. stronger heart and lungs
   b. relief of muscle strain and soreness
   c. increased strength and endurance
   d. increased bone mass and leaner muscles

4. Most of your flexibility workout will be static stretching, in which you hold a gradual stretch for
   a. 5 to 10 seconds
   b. 10 to 20 seconds
   c. 30 to 40 seconds
   d. 1 minute

5. There is a greater risk of injury in passive stretching than in static stretching because
   a. you hold the stretch longer.
   b. of the bouncing movements.
   c. the rhythm is different.
   d. your muscles are not controlling the stretch.

6. In your flexibility workout,
   a. stretch until you feel pain.
   b. stretch until you feel mild discomfort.
   c. stretch for exactly 20 minutes.
   d. stretch when your muscles are cold.

7. The benefits of yoga include all of the following except
   a. improved flexibility
   b. lower blood pressure
   c. lower risk of cancer
   d. lower levels of stress hormones

8. Pilates exercises stress the strengthening of
   a. the back and abdominal muscles.
   b. the shoulders and pectoral muscles.
   c. the abs and the quads.
   d. the quads and the glutes.

9. Strengthening the muscles that support the back can help prevent the likelihood of back pain. Other lifestyle choices that can help are
   a. getting up every hour and walking around when you are sitting for long periods.
   b. bending at the knees, not from the waist, when lifting something.
   c. not smoking.
   d. all of the above.

10. The primary treatment for back pain is
    a. bedrest.
    b. acetaminophen.
    c. chiropractic manipulation.
    d. ultrasound.

Answers to these questions can be found on page 376.

Critical Thinking

1. Research is mixed on whether stretching can decrease delayed-onset muscle soreness. Do you think a placebo effect can occur in studies on exercise and training as it does in research on medications? Why?

2. Suzanne had glanced into a yoga class and seen the students with eyes closed and hands pressed together as if in prayer, so she concluded that some religious practice was part of yoga. What can you tell her to enlighten her about yoga as a means of improving her flexibility?

3. Darrell's dad had a back spasm while building a patio and now suffers from low-back pain. When his dad mentioned surgery, Darrell decided to look into some less invasive alternatives. What might Darrell recommend that his dad try first?

Media Menu

Health Now™

Don't forget to check out the wealth of resources on the HealthNow website at **http://healthnow.brookscole.com/itw** that will:
- Help you evaluate your knowledge of the material
- Allow you to take an exam-prep quiz
- Provide a Personalized Learning Plan targeting resources that address areas you should study
- Coach you through identifying target goals for behavior change and creating and monitoring your personal change plan throughout the semester.

INTERNET CONNECTIONS

Stretching and Flexibility: Everything You Never Wanted to Know
www.cmcrossroads.com/bradapp/docs/rec/stretching/
This very comprehensive and academic site describes the physiology of muscles, types of flexibility, types of stretching, and factors limiting flexibility. It includes how to stretch and specific exercises, as well as references.

Yoga.com
www.yoga.com
This site features information on the techniques of yoga, pilates, and other forms of stretching exercises.

Stretching to Increase Flexibility
http://k2.kirtland.cc.mi.us/~balbachl/flex.htm
In addition to a comprehensive description of the health benefits of regular stretching, this site features a series of exercises tailored to one of three levels of fitness based on the frequency that you perform stretching exercises.

The Basics of Stretching
www.bodybuilding.com/fun/davidslon2.htm
This site describes the fundamentals of what stretching means, what it can achieve, the advantages to improving flexibility, and exercise tips.

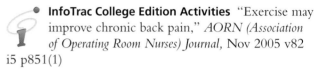 **InfoTrac College Edition Activities** "Exercise may improve chronic back pain," *AORN (Association of Operating Room Nurses) Journal,* Nov 2005 v82 i5 p851(1)

1. What types of exercises were used to improve flexibility in this study?

2. What was the major cause of back injuries in the participants in this study?

3. Describe the improvements patients reported after participating in this study.

You can find additional readings related to personal health with InfoTrac College Edition, an online library of more than 900 journals and publications. Follow the instructions for accessing InfoTrac College Edition that were packaged with your textbook; then search for articles using a keyword search.

For additional links, resources, and suggested readings on the InfoTrac College Edition, visit our Health and Wellness Resource Center at **http://health.wadsworth.com.**

Key Terms

The terms listed are used on the page indicated. Definitions of the terms are in the Glossary at the end of the book.

active stretching 108
ballistic stretching 108
collagen 106
dynamic flexibility 106
elastin 106
joints 106
passive stretching 108
proprioceptive neuromuscular facilitation (PNF) 108
range of motion 106
static flexibility 106
static stretching 107

Surviving and Thriving

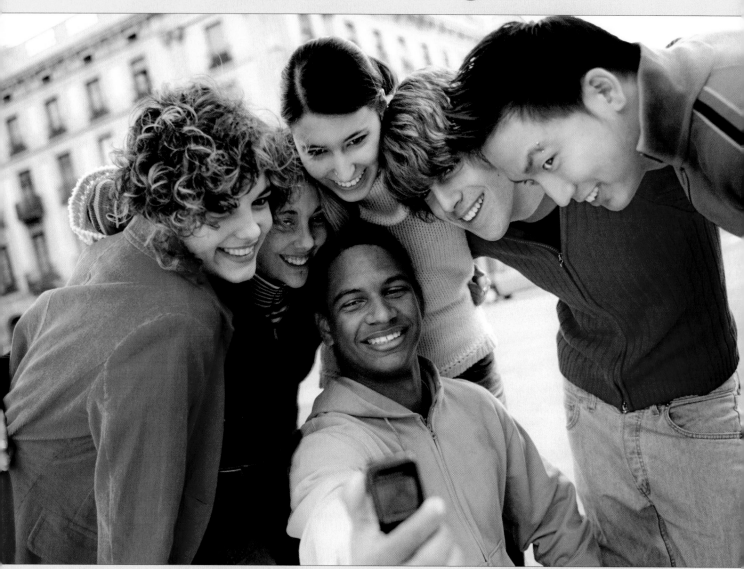

Two months into her freshman year, Maria feels as if a tornado has torn through her life. She is living thousands of miles from her family and the friends who share her culture and ethnic background. Her dormmates range from different to downright difficult. Her professors expect her to read and learn more in a week than in an entire month of high school. After blowing her budget decorating her room, she took on a part-time job—only to end up so exhausted that she dozes off in lectures.

Like Maria, you face challenges every day, whether you're studying for exams, meeting people, facing new experiences, or figuring out how to live on a budget. You're not alone. Everyone, regardless of age, gender, race, or income, has to deal with stress and psychological difficulties—as an individual and as a member of society.

Your state of mind has profound effects, both immediate and long-term, on your body. An ever growing number of studies has implicated stress as a culprit in medical problems that range from insomnia and infections to potentially deadly heart disorders.

Yet even though stress and challenge are inevitable, you don't have to be their victim. By developing positive attitudes and coping skills, you can take control of your psychological wellness. As you organize your time, manage day-to-day hassles, cultivate optimism and gratitude, and prevent stress overload, you can stop endlessly running on a treadmill of alarm, panic, and exhaustion. You can do more than survive: You can thrive. This chapter can show you how.

© Randy Faris/Corbis

After studying the material in this chapter, you should be able to:

- **Define** stress and stressors and **describe** how the body responds to stress according to the general adaptation syndrome theory.
- **Discuss** how stress can affect aging and the cardiovascular, immune, and digestive systems.
- **Describe** some personal causes of stress, especially those experienced by students, and **discuss** how their effects can be prevented or minimized.
- **Describe** some techniques to help manage stress.
- **Identify** ways of managing time more efficiently.
- **Describe** the values and other self-esteem components of psychological wellness.
- **Describe** the wellness benefits of spirituality.
- **Describe** some of the physical problems associated with or exacerbated by depression.

HealthNow™

Don't forget to check out the wealth of resources on the HealthNow website at **http://healthnow.brookscole.com/itw** that will:

- Help you evaluate your knowledge of the material
- Allow you to take an exam-prep quiz
- Provide a Personalized Learning Plan targeting resources that address areas you should study
- Coach you through identifying target goals for behavior change and creating and monitoring your personal change plan throughout the semester.

⬛ Surviving, Thriving, and the Dimensions of Wellness

As you'll see in this chapter, it is impossible to separate issues of body, mind, and spirit. Daily living challenges us in every way—physically, mentally, spiritually. Learning skills to manage stress not only enhances psychological wellness but also affects other dimensions of wellness:

- **Physical.** As discussed later in this chapter, stress can take a toll on physical wellness, including our cardiovascular and immune systems. Yet one of the best ways of becoming stress-resilient is to stay in good physical shape through regular exercise, adequate sleep, healthy habits, and good nutrition.
- **Emotional.** Being able to identify, experience, and express emotions is key, not just to emotional and mental health but to total wellness. No one can avoid emotional upsets, but you can learn to deal with them in positive ways.
- **Social.** Ironically, the people who matter most to us—our families and friends—can cause the greatest worry and stress. On the other hand, social support can bolster us just when we need others most.
- **Intellectual.** Stress and psychological difficulties make it harder to focus on studies and work productively. However, your mind is your best resource for acquiring information, organizing your time, and finding help if needed.
- **Spiritual.** As described in this chapter, spirituality has proved beneficial for mind, body, and soul. Expanding your spiritual experiences can reduce stress and conflict in your life as well as contribute to other dimensions of wellness.
- **Occupational.** Regardless of what you do or hope to do, stress comes with the territory. However, by gaining skills to manage stress and cope with challenges, you can perform at a higher level—and feel less anxious about your job.
- **Environmental.** A chaotic, noisy, threatening environment creates stress and undermines wellness. By working to create order, calm, safety, and peace, you can lower stress and raise life satisfaction for both yourself and others.

⬛ What Is Stress?

People use the word *stress* in different ways: as an external force that causes a person to become tense or upset, as the internal state of arousal, and as the physical response of the body to various demands. Dr. Hans Selye, a pioneer in studying physiological responses to challenge, defined **stress** as "the nonspecific response of the body to any demand made upon it." In other words, the body reacts to **stressors**—the things that upset or excite us—in the same way, regardless of whether they are positive or negative.

Based on nearly 300 studies over four decades, researchers have distinguished five categories of stressors:

- **Acute time-limited stressors** include anxiety-provoking situations, such as having to give a talk in public or work out a math problem like calculating a tip or dividing a bill under pressure.
- **Brief naturalistic stressors** are more serious challenges, such as taking SATs or meeting a deadline for a big project.
- **Stressful event sequences** are the difficult consequences of a natural disaster or another traumatic

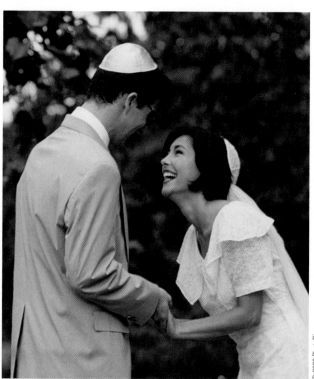

An automobile accident is an acute, negative stressor. Getting married is an example of a positive stressor that triggers both joy and apprehension.

occurrence, such as the death of a spouse. The individuals involved recognize that these difficulties will end at some point in the future.

▮ **Chronic stressors** are ongoing demands caused by life-changing circumstances, such as permanent disability following an accident or caregiving for a parent with dementia, that do not have any clear end point.

▮ **Distant stressors** are traumatic experiences that occurred long ago, such as child abuse or combat, yet continue to have an emotional and psychological impact.[1]

Not all stressors are negative. Some of life's happiest moments—births, reunions, weddings—are enormously stressful. We weep with the stress of frustration or loss; we weep, too, with the stress of love and joy. Selye coined the term **eustress** for positive stress in our lives (*eu* is a Greek prefix meaning "good"). Eustress challenges us to grow, adapt, and find creative solutions in our lives. **Distress** refers to the negative effects of stress that can deplete or even destroy life energy. Ideally, the level of stress in our lives should be just high enough to motivate us to satisfy our needs and not so high that it interferes with our ability to reach our fullest potential.

✚ What Causes Stress?

Of the many biological theories of stress, the best known may be the **general adaptation syndrome (GAS),** developed by Hans Selye. He postulated that our bodies constantly strive to maintain a stable and consistent physiological state, called **homeostasis.** Stressors, whether in the form of physical illness or a demanding job, disturb this state and trigger a nonspecific physiological response. The body attempts to restore homeostasis by means of an **adaptive response.**

Selye's general adaptation syndrome, which describes the body's response to a stressor—whether threatening or exhilarating—consists of three distinct stages:

1. **Alarm.** When a stressor first occurs, the body responds with changes that temporarily lower resistance. Levels of certain hormones may rise; blood pressure may increase (**Figure 7-1**). The body quickly makes internal adjustments to cope with the stressor and return to normal activity.

2. **Resistance.** If the stressor continues, the body mobilizes its internal resources to try to sustain homeostasis. For example, if a loved one is seriously hurt in an accident, we initially respond intensely and feel great anxiety. During the subsequent stressful period of recuperation, we struggle to carry on as normally as possible, but this requires considerable effort.

3. **Exhaustion.** If the stress continues long enough, we cannot keep up our normal functioning. Even a small amount of additional stress at this point can cause a breakdown.

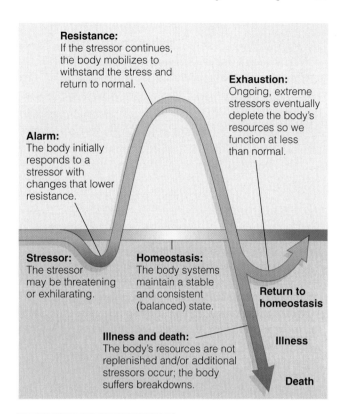

FIGURE 7-1 ▮ General Adaptation Syndrome (GAS)

The three stages of Hans Selye's General Adaptation Syndrome are alarm, resistance, and exhaustion.

Among the nonbiological theories is the cognitive-transactional model of stress, developed by Richard Lazarus, which looks at the relation between stress and health. As he sees it, stress can have a powerful impact on health. Conversely, health can affect a person's resistance or coping ability. Stress, according to Lazarus, is "neither an environmental stimulus, a characteristic of the person, nor a response, but a relationship between demands and the power to deal with them without unreasonable or destructive costs."[2] Thus, an event may be stressful for one person but not for another, or it may seem stressful on one occasion but not on another. For instance, one student may think of speaking in front of the class as extremely stressful, while another relishes the chance to do so—except on days when he's not well prepared.

"Perceived" stress—an individual's view of how challenging life is—undermines a sense of well-being in people of all ages and circumstances, including urban African-American women and healthy young adults.[3] However, good self-esteem, social support, and internal resources buffer the impact of perceived stress.[4]

✚ How Does Stress 🔖 Affect Wellness?

While stress alone doesn't cause disease, it triggers molecular changes throughout the body that make us more susceptible to many illnesses. Severe emotional distress—whether caused by a divorce, the loss of a job, or caring for an ill child or parent—can have such a powerful effect on the DNA in body cells that it speeds up aging, adding the equivalent of a decade to biological age.[5]

Stress triggers complex changes in the body's endocrine, or hormone-secreting, system. When you confront a stressor, the adrenal glands, two triangle-shaped glands that sit atop the kidneys, respond by producing stress hormones, including catecholamines, cortisol (hydrocortisone), and epinephrine (adrenaline), that speed up heart rate, raise blood pressure, and prepare the body to deal with the threat. This "fight-or-flight" response prepares you for quick action: Your heart works harder to pump more blood to your legs and arms. Your muscles tense, your breathing quickens, and your brain becomes extra alert. Because it's nonessential in a crisis, your digestive system practically shuts down (**Figure 7-2**).

Cortisol speeds the conversion of proteins and fats into carbohydrates, the body's basic fuel, so we have the energy to fight or flee from a threat. However, stress increases the amount of time required to clear triglycerides, a type of fat linked to heart disease, from the bloodstream.

Cortisol can cause excessive central or abdominal fat, which heightens the risk of diseases such as diabetes, high blood pressure, and stroke. Even slender, premenopausal women faced with increased stress and lacking good coping skills are more likely to accumulate excess weight around their waists, thereby increasing their risk of heart disease and other health problems.

In one study, African-American college students who scored low in coping skills had higher levels of cortisol than those better equipped to cope with stress.[6] Challenges that seem uncontrollable or unpredictable have a greater impact on cortisol than others.[7]

Figure 7-2 illustrates how persistent or repeated increases in the stress hormones can be hazardous throughout the body. In the brain, stress hormones linked to powerful emotions may help create long-lasting memories of

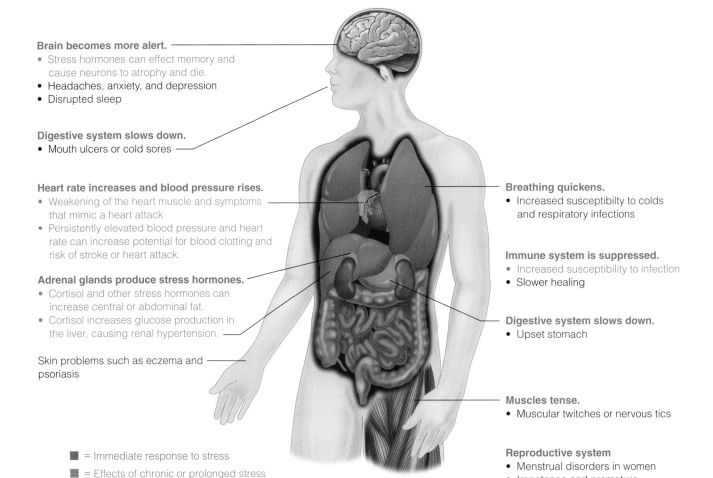

Brain becomes more alert.
- Stress hormones can effect memory and cause neurons to atrophy and die.
- Headaches, anxiety, and depression
- Disrupted sleep

Digestive system slows down.
- Mouth ulcers or cold sores

Heart rate increases and blood pressure rises.
- Weakening of the heart muscle and symptoms that mimic a heart attack
- Persistently elevated blood pressure and heart rate can increase potential for blood clotting and risk of stroke or heart attack.

Adrenal glands produce stress hormones.
- Cortisol and other stress hormones can increase central or abdominal fat.
- Cortisol increases glucose production in the liver, causing renal hypertension.

Skin problems such as eczema and psoriasis

Breathing quickens.
- Increased susceptibilty to colds and respiratory infections

Immune system is suppressed.
- Increased susceptibility to infection
- Slower healing

Digestive system slows down.
- Upset stomach

Muscles tense.
- Muscular twitches or nervous tics

Reproductive system
- Menstrual disorders in women
- Impotence and premature ejaculation in men

■ = Immediate response to stress
■ = Effects of chronic or prolonged stress
■ = Other possible effects of chronic stress

FIGURE 7-2 ▮ The Effects of Stress on the Body

events such as the collapse of the World Trade Center towers. But very prolonged or severe stress can damage the brain's ability to remember and can actually cause brain cells, or neurons, to atrophy and die.

Stress and the Heart

Stress may be the most significant inherited risk factor in people who develop heart disease at a young age. According to behavioral researchers, family transmission of emotional and psychosocial stress, specifically anger in males, greatly increases the likelihood of early heart disease.[8] Young adults whose blood pressure spikes in response to stress may be at risk of hypertension as they get older.[9]

In the 1970s, cardiologists Meyer Friedman, M.D., and Ray Rosenman, M.D., compared their patients to individuals of the same age with healthy hearts and developed two general categories of personality: Type A and Type B. Hardworking, aggressive, and competitive, Type A's never have time for all they want to accomplish, even though they usually try to do several tasks at once. Type B's are more relaxed, though not necessarily less ambitious or successful.

The degree of danger associated with Type-A behavior remains controversial. Of all the personality traits linked with Type-A behavior, the most sinister are anger and chronic hostility.[10] People who are always mistrustful, cynical, and suspicious are twice as likely to suffer blockages of their coronary arteries. Social isolation, depression, and stress may be even stronger risk factors for men.[11]

A tragic or shocking event can stun the heart and produce classic heart attack–like symptoms, including chest pain, shortness of breath, and fluid in the lungs. Triggered by stress hormones, "broken heart syndrome" can cause severe weakness in the heart. Unlike a heart attack, the condition is reversible. Patients typically recover within days and suffer no permanent damage to their hearts.[12]

Stress and Immunity

The immune system is the network of organs, tissues, and white blood cells that defend against disease. Impaired immunity makes the body more susceptible to many diseases, including infections (from the common cold to tuberculosis) and disorders of the immune system itself.

A recent "meta-analysis"—a study of studies in peer-reviewed scientific journals—confirmed earlier findings that stress alters immunity, but the effects differ between short-term and long-term stress. Short term stress "revs up" the immune system, a way of preparing for injury or infection. Acute, time-limited stressors, the type that produce a "fight-or-flight" response, prompt the immune system to ready itself for the possibility

of infections resulting from bites, punctures, or other wounds.[13]

However, long-term, or chronic, stress creates excessive wear and tear, and the system breaks down. Chronic stressors, so profound and persistent that they seem endless and beyond a person's control, suppress immune responses the most. The longer the stress, the more the immune system shifts from potentially adaptive changes to potentially harmful ones, first in cellular immunity and then in broader immune function. Traumatic stress, such as losing a loved one through death or divorce, can impair immunity for as long as a year.

Minor hassles that aren't related to trauma do take a toll. Under exam stress, students experience a dip in immune function and a higher rate of infections. Ohio State University researchers found that during exam periods, there is a significant drop in the immune cells that normally ward off infection and cancer in medical students.

Age and overall health also affect immune response. The immune systems of individuals who are elderly or ill are more vulnerable to acute and chronic stressors, possibly because their bodies find it more difficult to regulate their reactions.

Stress and Digestion

Do you ever get butterflies in your stomach before giving a speech in class or before a big game? The digestive system is, as one psychologist quips, "an important stop on the tension trail." To avoid problems, pay attention to how you eat: Eating on the run, gulping food, or overeating results in poorly chewed foods, an overworked stomach, and increased abdominal pressure.

Some simple strategies can help you avoid stress-related stomachaches. Many people experience dry mouth or sweat more under stress. By drinking plenty of water, you replenish lost fluids and prevent dehydration. Fiber-rich foods counteract common stress-related problems, such as cramps and constipation. Do not skip meals. If you do, you're more likely to feel fatigued and irritable.

Be wary of overeating under stress. Some people eat more because they scarf down meals too quickly. Others reach for snacks to calm their nerves or comfort themselves. In a study of college women, higher stress increased the risk of binge eating.[14]

Watch out for caffeine. Coffee, tea, and cola drinks can make your strained nerves jangle even more. Also avoid sugary snacks. They'll send your blood sugar levels on a roller coaster ride—up one minute, down the next.

✚ Stress on Campus

You've probably heard that these are the best years of your life, but being a student—full-time or part-time, in your late teens, early twenties, or later in life—can be extremely stressful. You may feel pressure to perform well to qualify for a good job or graduate school. To meet steep tuition payments, you may have to juggle part-time work and coursework. You may feel stressed about choosing a major, getting along with a difficult roommate, passing a particularly hard course, or living up to your parents' and teachers' expectations. If you're an older student, you may have children, housework, and homework to balance. Your days may seem so busy and your life so full that you worry about coming apart at the seams. One thing is for certain: You're not alone.

After a steady surge upward in the 1990s, the percentage of students who say they are "frequently overwhelmed by all they have to do" has declined from the peak of 30.7 percent in 1999 to 27.4 percent in 2004.[15] However, women are more than twice as likely to report stress as men. (See Student Snapshot: "Stressed Out on Campus.") According to surveys of students at colleges and universities around the country and the world, stressors are remarkably similar. Among the most common are:

▮ Test pressures.
▮ Financial problems.
▮ Frustrations, such as delays in reaching goals.
▮ Problems in friendships and dating relationships.
▮ Daily hassles.
▮ Academic failure.
▮ Pressures as a result of competition, deadlines, and the like.
▮ Changes, which may be unpleasant, disruptive, or too frequent.
▮ Losses, whether caused by the breakup of a relationship or the death of a loved one.

Many students bring complex psychological problems with them to campus, including learning disabilities and mood disorders like depression and anxiety. "Students arrive with the underpinnings of problems that are brought out by the stress of campus life," says one counselor. Some have grown up in broken homes and bear the scars of family troubles. Others fall into the same patterns of alcohol abuse that they observed for years in their families or suffer lingering emotional scars from childhood physical or sexual abuse.

Students and Stress

Stress, according to the students surveyed in the ACHA-National College Health Assessment (sponsored by the American College Health Association), ranks as the highest impediment to academic success.[16] The sources of student stress are many: relocation, separation from family, academic challenges, relationships, finances, chronic illness, depression, anxiety, sleep problems, and the day-to-day rigors of college life. Women typically experience stress more often than men, and U.S. citizens are more stressed than non-citizens.[17]

Your stress level may depend on where you live. In a recent study of students living in residence halls at a midwestern university, various factors influenced how stressed the undergraduates felt. Those who were unable to study in their dorms, often because of noise, loud music, or a roommate's behavior, experienced higher levels of stress. Roommate conflict was another significant source of stress. Living in a residence where residents respected each other and each others' beliefs reduced stress.[18]

More than a quarter of freshmen feel overwhelmed by all they have to do at the beginning of the academic year; by the year's end, 44 percent feel overwhelmed.[19] In a study of students at three universities, underclassmen were most vulnerable to negative life events, perhaps because they lacked experience in coping with stressful situations. Freshmen had the highest levels of depression; sophomores had the most anger and hostility. Seniors may handle life's challenges better because they have developed better coping mechanisms. In the study, more seniors reported that they faced problems squarely and took action to resolve them, while younger students were more likely to respond passively, for instance, by trying not to let things bother them.[20]

First-generation college students—those whose parents never experienced at least one full year of college—encounter more difficulties with social adjustment than freshmen whose parents attended college. Second-generation students may have several advantages: more knowledge of college life, greater social support, more preparation for college in high school, a greater focus on college activities, and more financial resources.[21]

The percentage of students seeking psychological help because of stress or anxiety has risen dramatically in the last 15 years. Excessive levels of stress can lead to increased headaches, sleep disturbances, and colds. Students

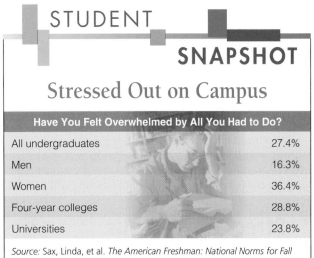

STUDENT

SNAPSHOT

Stressed Out on Campus

Have You Felt Overwhelmed by All You Had to Do?	
All undergraduates	27.4%
Men	16.3%
Women	36.4%
Four-year colleges	28.8%
Universities	23.8%

Source: Sax, Linda, et al. *The American Freshman: National Norms for Fall 2004.* Los Angeles: University of California, Los Angeles Higher Education Research Institute, 2004.

© Purestock /Alamy

say they react to stress in various ways: physiologically (by sweating, stuttering, trembling, or developing physical symptoms); emotionally (by becoming anxious, fearful, angry, guilty, or depressed); behaviorally (by crying, eating, smoking, being irritable or abusive); or cognitively (by thinking about and analyzing stressful situations and strategies that might be useful in dealing with them).

A supportive network of friends and family makes a difference. Undergraduates with higher levels of social support and self-efficacy reported feeling less stressed and more satisfied with life than others.

Does stress increase drinking among college students? Many assume so, since life stress is a recognized risk for alcohol use in general. In a recent study of 137 undergraduates, however, the relationship between drinking and stress turned out to be more complex. For some, drinking occasions were times to discuss problems with friends, regardless of the day's stress. On average, students tended to drink more on days when they were feeling good—possibly because of what the researchers called the "celebratory and social" nature of college drinking. Drinking—and positive emotions—also peaked on weekends.[22] (See Chapter 13 for more on student drinking.)

Campuses are providing more frontline services than they have in the past, including career-guidance workshops, telephone hot lines, and special social programs for lonely, homesick freshmen. In one study of 128 undergraduates, those who learned relaxation and stress-reduction techniques in a six-week program reported less stress, anxiety, and psychological distress than a control group of students. The participants—who had described themselves as "extremely stressed" before the intervention—also began to increase health-promoting behaviors.

How Can I Cope with Test Stress?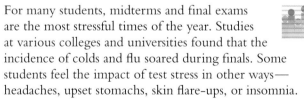

For many students, midterms and final exams are the most stressful times of the year. Studies at various colleges and universities found that the incidence of colds and flu soared during finals. Some students feel the impact of test stress in other ways—headaches, upset stomachs, skin flare-ups, or insomnia.

Because of stress's impact on memory, students with advanced skills may perform worse under exam pressure than their less skilled peers.[23] Sometimes students become so preoccupied with the possibility of failing that they can't concentrate on studying. Others, including many of the best and brightest students, freeze up during tests and can't comprehend multiple-choice questions or write essay answers, even if they know the material.

The students most susceptible to exam stress are those who believe they'll do poorly and who see tests as extremely threatening. Unfortunately, such negative thoughts often become a self-fulfilling prophecy. As they study, these students keep wondering: What good will studying do? I never do well on tests. As their fear

---

STRATEGIES for PREVENTION

Defusing Test Stress

▮ **Plan ahead.**
A month before finals, map out a study schedule for each course. Set aside a small amount of time every day or every other day to review the course materials.

▮ **Be positive.**
Picture yourself taking your final exam. Imagine yourself walking into the exam room feeling confident, opening up the test booklet, and seeing questions for which you know the answers.

▮ **Take regular breaks.**
Get up from your desk, breathe deeply, stretch, and visualize a pleasant scene. You'll feel more refreshed than you would if you chugged another cup of coffee.

▮ **Practice.**
Some teachers are willing to give practice finals to prepare students for test situations, or you and your friends can test each other.

▮ **Talk to other students.**
Chances are that many of them share your fears about test taking and may have discovered some helpful techniques of their own. Sometimes talking to your adviser or a counselor can also help.

▮ **Be satisfied with doing your best.**
You can't expect to ace every test; all you can and should expect is your best effort. Once you've completed the exam, allow yourself the sweet pleasure of relief that it's over.

---

increases, they try harder, pulling all-nighters. Fueled by caffeine, munching on sugary snacks, they become edgy and find it harder and harder to concentrate. By the time of the test, they're nervous wrecks, scarcely able to sit still and focus on the exam.

Can you do anything to reduce test stress and feel more in control? Absolutely. One way is to defuse stress through relaxation. Students taught relaxation techniques—such as controlled breathing, meditation, progressive relaxation, and guided imagery (visualization)—a month before finals tend to have higher levels of immune cells during the exam period and feel in better control during their tests.

Minorities and Stress

Regardless of your race or ethnic background, college may bring culture shock. You may never have encountered such a degree of diversity in one setting. You probably

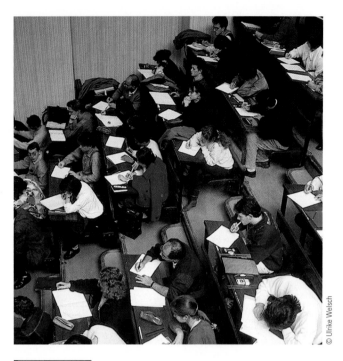

© Ulrike Welsch

▌ You can take control of your stress responses by practicing relaxation techniques, avoiding cramming, and being positive about your performance on the test.

will meet students with different values, unfamiliar customs, entirely new ways of looking at the world—experiences you may find both stimulating and stressful.

Mental health professionals have long assumed that minority students may feel a double burden of stress. Racism has indeed been shown to be a source of stress that can affect health and well-being.[24] In the past, some African-American students have described predominately white campuses as hostile, alienating, and socially isolating and have reported greater estrangement from the campus community and heightened estrangement in interactions with faculty and peers.[25] However, the generalization that all minority students are more stressed may not be valid.

A study conducted at a racially diverse university in a large metropolitan area in the Northeast evaluated 595 freshmen. The study group was made up of both genders and students of various racial and ethnic backgrounds, including Asians, African Americans, and Hispanics.[26] Fewer than 15 percent of these students—whether Asian, African American, Hispanic, white, or another ethnic minority—reported clinically significant levels of anger, anxiety, and depression, and there was no correlation between these stress-linked symptoms and ethnicity or race.

"Diversity, in and of itself, is unlikely to be related to higher levels of reported psychological symptoms on campus," the researchers concluded, theorizing that minority students "may have developed strengths while growing up within their particular cultures, subcommunities, and families that have often gone unrecognized or

unnoted.[27] And some coping mechanisms, especially spirituality, can buffer the negative effects of racism.[28]

All minority students do share some common stressors. In one study of minority freshmen entering a large, competitive university, Asian, Filipino, African-American, and Native-American students all felt more sensitive and vulnerable to the college social climate, to interpersonal tensions between themselves and nonminority students and faculty, to experiences of actual or perceived racism, and to racist attitudes and discrimination. Despite scoring above the national average on the SAT, the minority students in this study did not feel accepted as legitimate students and sensed that others viewed them as unworthy beneficiaries of affirmative action initiatives. While most said that overt racism was rare and relatively easy to deal with, they reported subtle pressures that undermined their academic confidence and their ability to bond with the university. Balancing these stressors, however, was a strong sense of ethnic identity, which helped buffer some stressful effects.

Hispanic students have identified three major types of stressors in their college experiences: academic (related to exam preparation and faculty interaction), social (related to ethnicity and interpersonal competence), and financial (related to their economic situation). Some Asian students who recently immigrated to the United States report feeling ostracized by students of similar ancestry who are second- or third-generation Americans. While they take pride in being truly bicultural and bilingual, the newcomers feel ambivalent about mainstream American culture. "My parents stress the importance of traditions; my friends tell me to get with it and act like an American," says one Asian-born student who

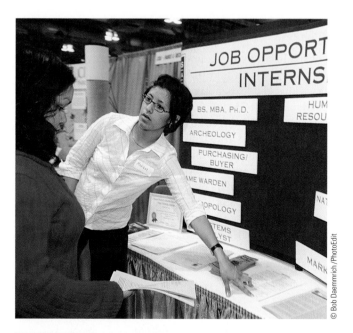

© Bob Daemmrich/PhotoEdit

▌ Minority students can often find support services and other resources on campus.

has spent five years in the United States. "I feel trapped between cultures."

Gender and Stress

Women, who make up 56 percent of today's college students, also shoulder the majority of the stress load. In a nationwide survey of students in the class of 2008, more women (36.4 percent) described themselves as "overwhelmed by all I have to do," compared with just 16.3 percent of men. More women than men reported feeling depressed, insecure about their physical and mental health, and worried about paying for college. More men —57.1 percent, compared with 45.8 percent of women— considered themselves above average or in the top 10 percent of people their age in terms of emotional health.[29]

Gender differences in lifestyle may help explain why women feel so stressed. College men, the survey revealed, spend significantly more time doing things that are fun and relaxing: exercising, partying, watching TV, and playing video games. Women, on the other hand, tend to study more, do more volunteer work, and handle more household and child-care chores.

The stress gender gap, which appeared in the mid-1980s, is "one of the ironies of the women's movement," says Alexander Astin of UCLA, founder of the annual American Freshman Survey, which has tracked shifting student attitudes for 35 years. By adding more commitments and responsibilities on top of all the other things they have to cope with, he believes that college women are experiencing an early version of the stress that "supermoms" feel later in life when they pursue a career, care for children, and maintain a household.

Where can stressed-out college women turn for support? The best source, according to University of California research, is other women. In general, the social support women offer their friends and relatives seems more effective in reducing the blood-pressure response to stress than that provided by men.

At all ages, women and men tend to respond to stress differently. While males (human and those of other species) react with the classic fight-or-flight response, females under attack try to protect their children and seek help from other females—a strategy dubbed *tend-and-befriend*. When exposed to experimental stress (such as a loud, harsh noise), women show more affection for friends and relatives; men show less. When working mothers studied by psychologists had a bad day, they coped by concentrating on their children when they got home. Stressed-out fathers were more likely to withdraw.

Other Personal Stressors

At every stage of life, you will encounter challenges and stressors. Among the most common are those related to work and overwork. More people are caught up in an exhausting cycle of overwork, which causes stress, which makes work harder, which leads to more stress. Yet work in itself is not hazardous to health. Attitudes about work and habits related to how we work are the true threats. In facts, a job—stressful or not, enjoyable or not—can be therapeutic.

A common source of stress for college students is a learning disability, which may affect one of every ten Americans. Most learning-disabled have average or above-average intelligence, but they rarely live up to their abilities in school. Some have only one area of difficulty, such as reading or math. Others have problems with attention, writing, communicating, reasoning, coordination, and social skills.

Not all students with learning disabilities experience greater stress. In one in-depth study comparing 34 undergraduates with and without learning disabilities, the learning-disabled (LD) students reported significantly fewer college stressors and demonstrated a higher need for achievement. The LD students also scored significantly higher in resiliency and initiative in solving problems and working toward goals.[30]

WELLNESS COACH

Managing Stress

The key to coping with stress is realizing that your *perception* of and *response* to a stressor are crucial. Changing the way you interpret events or situations—a skill called *reframing*—makes all the difference. An event, such as a move to a new city, is not stressful in itself. A move becomes stressful if you see it as a traumatic upheaval rather than an exciting beginning of a new chapter in your life.

In times of stress, the following simple exercises can stop the stress buildup inside your body and help you regain a sense of calm and control.

▪ **Breathing.** Deep breathing relaxes the body and quiets the mind. Draw air deeply into your lungs, allowing your chest to fill with air and your belly to rise and fall. You will feel the muscle tension and stress begin to melt away. When you're feeling extremely stressed, try this calming breath: Sit or lie with your back straight and place the tip of your tongue on the roof of your mouth behind your teeth. Exhale completely through the mouth, then inhale through the nose for 4 seconds. Hold the breath for 7 seconds, then exhale audibly through the mouth for 8 seconds. Repeat four times.

▪ **Refocusing.** Thinking about a situation you can't change or control only increases the stress you feel. Force your mind to focus on other subjects. If you're stuck in a long line, distract yourself. Check out what other people are buying or imagine what they do for a living. Imagine that you're in a hot shower and a wave of relaxation is washing your stress down the drain.

▍ **Serenity breaks.** Build moments of tranquility into your day. For instance, while waiting for your computer to start up or a file to download, look at a photograph of someone you love or a poster of a tropical island. If none is available, close your eyes and visualize a soothing scene, such as walking in a meadow or along a beach.

▍ **Stress signals.** Learn to recognize the first signs that your stress load is getting out of hand: Is your back bothering you? Do you have a headache? Do you find yourself speeding or misplacing things? Whenever you spot these early warnings, force yourself to stop and say, I'm under stress. I need to do something about it.

▍ **Reality checks.** To put things into proper perspective, ask yourself: Will I remember what's made me so upset a month from now? If I had to rank this problem on a scale of 1 to 10, with worldwide catastrophe as 10, where would it rate?

▍ **Stress inoculation.** Rehearse everyday situations that you find stressful, such as speaking in class. Think of how you might make the situation less tense, for instance, by breathing deeply before you talk or jotting down notes beforehand. Think of these small "doses" of stress as the psychological equivalent of allergy shots: They immunize you so you feel less stressed when bigger challenges come along.

▍ **Rx: Laughter.** Humor counters stress by focusing on comic aspects of difficult situations and may, as various studies have shown, lessen harmful effects on the immune system and overall health. However, humor may have different effects on stress in men and women. In a study of 131 undergraduates, humor buffered stress-related physical symptoms in men and women. However, it reduced stress-linked anxiety only in men. The researchers theorized that men may prefer humor as a more appropriate way of expressing emotions such as anxiety, whereas women are more likely to use self-disclosure, that is, to confide in friends.

▍ **Spiritual coping.** Saying a prayer under stress is one of the oldest and most effective ways of calming yourself. Other forms of spiritual coping, such as putting trust in God and doing for others (for instance, by volunteering at a shelter for battered women) also can provide a different perspective on daily hassles and stresses.

▍ **Sublimation.** This term refers to the redirection of any drives considered unacceptable into socially acceptable channels. Outdoor activity is one of the best ways to reduce stress through sublimation. For instance, if you're furious with a friend who

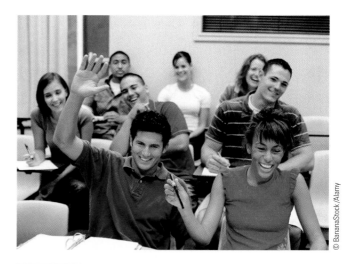

▍ Shared laughter is a powerful antidote to stress.

betrayed your trust or frustrated because your boss rejects all of your proposals, you might go for a long run or hike to sublimate your anger.

▍ **Exercise.** Regular physical activity can relieve stress, boost energy, lift mood, and keep stress under control. Young adults who adopt and continue regular aerobic exercise show less intense cardiovascular responses to stress, which may protect them against coronary heart disease as they age.[31] Strength training may have similar benefits.

In one study, college students who engaged in an eight-week weight training reported lower stress levels than those who participated in an aerobic dance program.

▍ **Journaling.** One of the simplest, yet most effective, ways to work through stress is by putting your feelings into words that only you will read. The more honest and open you are as you write, the better. College students who wrote in their journals about traumatic events felt much better afterward than those who wrote about superficial topics. Focus on intense emotional experiences and "autopsy" them to try to understand why they affected you the way they did. Rereading and thinking about your notes may reveal the underlying reasons for your response. (See your Wellness Journal.)

▍ **Focusing.** Take a strain inventory of your body every day to determine where things aren't feeling quite right. Ask yourself, What's keeping me from feeling terrific today? Focusing on problem spots, such as stomach knots or neck tightness, increases your sense of control over stress.

▍ **Reconstructing stressful situations.** Think about a recent episode of distress; then write down three ways it could have gone better and three ways it could have gone worse. This should help you see that the situation wasn't as disastrous as it might have been and help you find ways to cope better in the future.

Recognize the Warning Signals of Stress Overload

▐ Experiencing physical symptoms, including chronic fatigue, headaches, indigestion, diarrhea, and sleep problems.

▐ Having frequent illness or worrying about illness.

▐ Self-medicating, including nonprescription drugs.

▐ Having problems concentrating on studies or work.

▐ Feeling irritable, anxious, or apathetic.

▐ Working or studying longer and harder than usual.

▐ Exaggerating, to yourself and others, the importance of what you do.

▐ Becoming accident-prone.

▐ Breaking rules, whether it's a curfew at home or a speed limit on the highway.

▐ Going to extremes, such as drinking too much, overspending, or gambling.

✚ Learning to Relax

Relaxation is the physical and mental state opposite that of stress. Rather than gearing up for fight or flight, our bodies and minds grow calmer and work more smoothly. We're less likely to become frazzled and more capable of staying in control. The most effective relaxation techniques include progressive relaxation, visualization, meditation, mindfulness, and biofeedback.

Progressive relaxation works by intentionally increasing and then decreasing tension in the muscles. While sitting or lying down in a quiet, comfortable setting, you tense and release various muscles, beginning with those of the hand, for instance, and then proceeding to the arms, shoulders, neck, face, scalp, chest, stomach, buttocks, genitals, and so on, down each leg to the toes. Relaxing the muscles can quiet the mind and restore internal balance.

Visualization, or **guided imagery,** involves creating mental pictures that calm you down and focus your attention. Some people use this technique to promote healing when they are ill. Visualization skills require practice and, in some cases, instruction by qualified health professionals.

Meditation has been practiced in many forms over the ages, from the yogic techniques of the Far East to the Quaker silence of more modern times. Although many studies have documented the benefits of meditation for overall health, it may be particularly helpful for people dealing with stress-related medical conditions such as high blood pressure.

In a study of African Americans with atherosclerosis, or hardening of the arteries, those who meditated showed a marked decrease in the thickness of their artery walls, while the nonmeditators showed an increase. This benefit is particularly important because African Americans are twice as likely to die from cardiovascular disease as are whites.

Meditation helps a person reach a state of relaxation, but with the goal of achieving inner peace and harmony. There is no one right way to meditate, and many people have discovered how to meditate on their own, without even knowing what it is they are doing.

Among college students, meditation has proved especially effective in increasing relaxation. Most forms of meditation have common elements: sitting quietly for 15 to 20 minutes once or twice a day, concentrating on a word or image, and breathing slowly and rhythmically. If you wish to try meditation, it often helps to have someone guide you through your first sessions. Or try tape recording your own voice (with or without favorite music in the background) and playing it back to yourself, freeing yourself to concentrate on the goal of turning the attention within.

Mindfulness is a modern form of an ancient Asian technique that involves maintaining awareness in the present moment. You tune in to each part of your body,

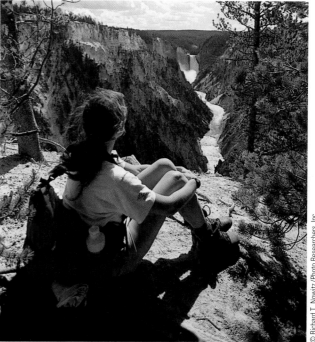

▍ Spending time outdoors is a great way to leave behind daily tensions and gain a new perspective.

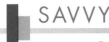

SAVVY CONSUMER

CAN STRESS-RELIEF PRODUCTS HELP?

You're stressed out, and you see an ad for a product—an oil, candle, cream, herbal tea, pill, or potion—that promises to make all your cares disappear. Should you soak in an aromatic bath, have a massage, try kava, squeeze foam balls? In most cases, you're probably not doing yourself much harm, but you aren't necessarily doing yourself much good either. Keep these considerations in mind:

■ Be wary of instant cures. Regardless of the promises on the label, it's unrealistic to expect any magic ingredient or product to make all your problems disappear.

■ Focus on stress-reducing behavior, rather than a product. An aromatic candle may not bring instant serenity,

but if you light a candle and meditate, you may indeed feel more at peace. A scented pillow may not be a cure for a stress, but if it helps you get a good night's sleep, you'll cope better the next day.

■ Experiment with physical ways to work out stress. Exercise is one of the best ways to lower your stress levels. Try walking, running, swimming, cycling, kick-boxing—anything physical that helps you release tension.

■ Don't make matters worse by smoking (the chemicals in cigarettes increase heart rate, blood pressure, and stress hormones), consuming too much caffeine (it speeds up your system for hours), eating snacks high in sugar (it

produces a quick high followed by a sudden slump), or turning to drugs or alcohol (they can only add to your stress when their effects wear off).

■ Be cautious when trying "alternative" products. "Natural" products, such as herbs and enzymes, claim to have psychological effects. However, because they are not classified as drugs, these products have not undergone the rigorous scientific testing required of psychiatric medications, and little is known about their safety or efficacy. "Natural" doesn't mean risk-free. Opium and cocaine are "natural" substances that have dramatic and potentially deadly effects on the mind.

scanning from head to toe, noting the slightest sensation. You allow whatever you experience—an itch, an ache, a feeling of warmth—to enter your awareness. Then you open yourself to focus on all the thoughts, sensations, sounds, and feelings that enter your awareness. Mindfulness keeps you in the here and now, thinking about what is rather than about *what if* or *if only.*

STRATEGIES for CHANGE

"Mini-Relaxation"

Here is a quick deep-breathing exercise from Harvard psychologist Alice Domar:

■ Sit upright or lie on your back.

■ Place your hand just beneath your navel so you can feel the rise and fall of your belly as you breathe deeply through your nose.

■ As you inhale, count slowly, saying to yourself, one, two, three, four. Exhale slowly, counting back down from four to one.

■ Do this for one minute or longer.

Biofeedback is a method of obtaining feedback, or information, about some physiological activity occurring in the body. An electronic monitoring device attached to the body detects a change in an internal function and communicates it back to the person through a tone, light, or meter. By paying attention to this feedback, most people can gain some control over functions previously thought to be beyond conscious control, such as body temperature, heart rate, muscle tension, and brain waves.

Organizing Your Time

We live in what some sociologists call hyperculture, a society that moves at warp speed. Information bombards us constantly. The rate of change seems to accelerate every year. Our "time-saving" devices—pagers, cell phones, modems, faxes, palm-sized organizers, laptop computers—have simply extended the boundaries of where and how we work.

As a result, more and more people are suffering from "timesickness," a nerve-racking feeling that life has become little more than an endless to-do list. The best antidote is time management, and hundreds of books, seminars, and experts offer training in making the most of the hours in the day. Yet these well-intentioned methods often fail, and sooner or later most of us find ourselves caught in a time trap.

How Can I Better Manage My Time?

Time management involves skills that anyone can learn, but they require commitment and practice to make a difference in your life. It may help to know the techniques that other students have found most useful:

- **Schedule your time.** Use a calendar or planner. Beginning the first week of class, mark down deadlines for each assignment, paper, project, and test scheduled that semester. Develop a daily schedule, listing very specifically what you will do the next day, along with the times. Block out times for working out, eating dinner, calling home, and talking with friends as well as for studying.
- **Develop a game plan.** Allow at least two nights to study for any major exam. Set aside more time for researching and writing papers. Make sure to allow time to revise and print out a paper—and to deal with emergencies like a computer breakdown. Set daily and weekly goals for every class. When working on a big project, don't neglect your other courses. Whenever possible, try to work ahead in all your classes.
- **Identify time robbers.** For several days keep a log of what you do and how much time you spend doing it. You may discover that disorganization is eating away at your time or that you have a problem getting started. (See the following section on "Overcoming Procrastination.")
- **Make the most of classes.** Read the assignments before class rather than waiting until just before you have

a test. By reading ahead of time, you'll make it easier to understand the lectures. Go to class yourself. Your own notes will be more helpful than a friend's or those from a note-taking service. Read your lecture notes at the end of each day or at least at the end of each week.

- **Develop an efficient study style.** Some experts recommend studying for 50 minutes, then breaking for 10 minutes. Small incentives, such as allowing yourself to call or visit a friend during these 10 minutes, can provide the motivation to keep you at the books longer. When you're reading, don't just highlight passages. Instead, write notes or questions to yourself in the margins, which will help you retain more information. Even if you're racing to start a paper, take a few extra minutes to prepare a workable outline. It will be easier to structure your paper when you start writing.
- **Focus on the task at hand.** Rather than worrying about how you did on yesterday's test or how you'll ever finish next week's project, focus intently on whatever you're doing at any given moment. If your mind starts to wander, use any distraction—the sound of the phone ringing or a noise from the hall—as a reminder to stay in the moment.
- **Turn elephants into hors d'oeuvres.** Cut a huge task into smaller chunks so it seems less enormous. For instance, break down your term paper into a series of steps, such as selecting a topic, identifying sources of research information, taking notes, developing an outline, and so on.
- **Keep your workspace in order.** Even if the rest of your room is a shambles, try to keep your desk clear. Piles of papers are distracting, and you can end up wasting lots of time looking for notes you misplaced or an article you have to read by morning. Try to spend the last ten minutes of the day getting your desk in order so you get a fresh start on the new day.
- See the time-management lab in your Lab Booklet.

Overcoming Procrastination

Putting off until tomorrow what should be done today is a habit that creates a great deal of stress for many students. It also takes a surprising toll. In studies with students taking a health psychology course, researchers found that although procrastinating provided short-term benefits, including periods of low stress, the tendency to dawdle had long-term costs, including poorer health and lower grades. Early in the semester, the procrastinators reported less stress and fewer health problems than students who scored low on procrastination. However, by the end of the semester, procrastinators reported more health-related symptoms, more stress, and more visits to health-care professionals than nonprocrastinators. Students who procrastinate also get poorer grades in courses with many deadlines.

The three most common types of procrastination are putting off unpleasant things, putting off difficult tasks, and putting off tough decisions. Procrastinators are most

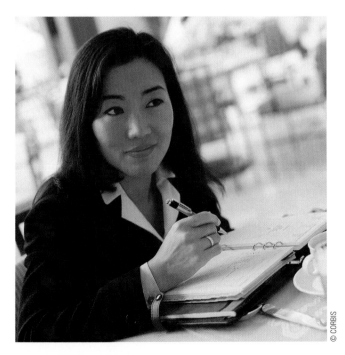

© CORBIS

A calendar or planner is an important tool in time management. You can use it to keep track of assignment due dates, class meetings, and other "to do's."

likely to delay by wishing they didn't have to do what they must or by telling themselves they "just can't get started," which means they never do.

To get out of the procrastination trap, keep track of the tasks you're most likely to put off, and try to figure out why you don't want to tackle them. Think of alternative ways to get tasks done. If you put off library readings, for instance, is the problem getting to the library or the reading itself? If it's the trip to the library, arrange to walk over with a friend whose company you enjoy.

Do what you like least first. Once you have it out of the way, you can concentrate on the tasks you enjoy. Learn to live according to a three-word motto: Just do it!

✚ Defense Mechanisms

Sometimes we respond to stress or challenge with self-destructive behaviors, such as drinking or using drugs. These responses can lead to psychological problems, such as anxiety or depression, and physical problems, including psychosomatic illnesses.

Defense mechanisms, such as those described in **Table 7-1,** are another response to stress. These psychological devices are mental processes that help us cope with personal problems. Such responses also are not the answer to stress—and learning to recognize them in yourself will enable you to deal with your stress in a healthier way.

✚ What Is Psychological Wellness?

Unlike physical health, psychological well-being cannot be measured, tested, X-rayed, or dissected. Yet psychologically healthy men and women generally share certain characteristics: They value themselves and strive toward happiness and fulfillment. They establish and maintain

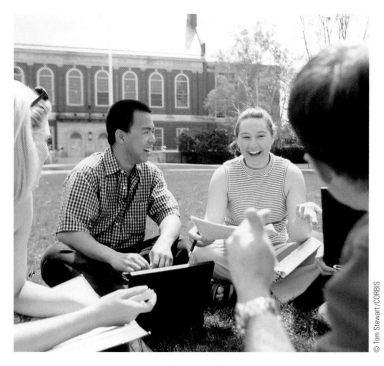

▌ Psychologically healthy people have compassion for others and form strong and deep relationships. They adapt to a variety of circumstances and strive to achieve their full potential.

close relationships with others. They accept the limitations as well as the possibilities that life has to offer. And they feel a sense of meaning and purpose that makes the gestures of living worth the effort required.

Psychological wellness encompasses both our emotional and mental states—that is, our feelings and our thoughts. **Emotional wellness** generally refers to feelings and moods, both of which are discussed later in this chapter. Characteristics of emotionally healthy persons, identified in an analysis of major studies of emotional wellness, include the following:

▌ **Determination and effort** to be healthy.
▌ **Flexibility and adaptability** to a variety of circumstances.

TABLE 7-1 ▌ Common Defense Mechanisms Used to Alleviate Anxiety and Eliminate Conflict

Defense Mechanism	Example
Denial: the refusal to accept a painful reality.	You don't accept as true the news that a loved one is seriously ill.
Displacement: the redirection of feelings from their true object to a more acceptable or safer substitute.	Instead of lashing out at a coach or a teacher, you snap at your best friend.
Projection: the attribution of unacceptable feelings or impulses to someone else.	When you want to end a relationship, you project your unhappiness onto your partner.
Rationalization: the substitution of "good," acceptable reasons for the real motivations for our behavior.	You report a classmate who has been mean to you for cheating on an exam and explain that cheating is unfair to other students.
Reaction formation: adopting attitudes and behaviors that are the opposite of what you feel.	You lavishly compliment an acquaintance whom you really despise.
Repression: the way we keep threatening impulses, fantasies, memories, feelings, or wishes from becoming conscious.	You don't "hear" the alarm after a late night, or you "forget" to take out the trash.

▌ **Development of a sense of meaning** and affirmation of life.

▌ **An understanding** that the self is not the center of the universe.

▌ **Compassion** for others.

▌ **The ability to be unselfish** in serving or relating to others.

▌ **Increased depth and satisfaction** in intimate relationships.

▌ **A sense of control** over the mind and body that enables the person to make health-enhancing choices and decisions.[32]

Mental wellness describes our ability to perceive reality as it is, to respond to its challenges, and to develop rational strategies for living (**Figure 7-3**). The mentally healthy person doesn't try to avoid conflicts and distress but can cope with life's transitions, traumas, and losses in a way that allows for emotional stability and growth. The characteristics of mental health include:

▌ **The ability to function** and carry out responsibilities.

▌ **The ability to form** relationships.

▌ **Realistic perceptions** of the motivations of others.

▌ **Rational, logical thought** processes.

▌ **The ability to adapt** to change and to cope with adversity.[33]

There is considerable overlap between psychological and **spiritual wellness,** which involves our ability to identify our basic purpose in life and to experience the fulfillment of achieving our full potential. In one study, more than half of individuals with mental disorders, including

depression, turned to spiritual readings or practices to increase calmness, find inner strength and meaning, improve self-awareness, and increase their sense of well-being.[34] Religious support has also been shown to help lower depression and increase life satisfaction beyond the benefits of social support from friends and family.[35]

In addition, **culture** helps to define psychological health. In one culture, men and women may express feelings with great intensity, shouting in joy or wailing in grief, while in another culture such behavior might be considered abnormal or unhealthy. In our diverse society, many cultural influences affect Americans' sense of who they are, where they came from, and what they believe. Cultural rituals help bring people together, strengthen their bonds, reinforce the values and beliefs they share, and provide a sense of belonging, meaning, and purpose.

Knowing Your Needs

Newborns are unable to survive on their own. They depend on others for the satisfaction of their physical needs for food, shelter, warmth, and protection, as well as their less tangible emotional needs. In growing to maturity, children take on more responsibility and become more independent. No one, however, becomes totally self-sufficient. As adults, we easily recognize our basic physical needs, but we often fail to acknowledge our emotional needs. Yet they, too, must be met if we are to be as fulfilled as possible.

The humanist theorist Abraham Maslow believed that human needs are the motivating factors in personality development. First, we must satisfy basic physiological needs, such as those for food, shelter, and sleep. Only then can we pursue fulfillment of our higher needs—for safety and security, love and affection, and self-esteem. Few individuals reach the state of **self-actualization,** in which one functions at the highest possible level and derives the greatest possible satisfaction from life (**Figure 7-4**).

Clarifying Your Values

Your **values** are the criteria by which you evaluate things, people, events, and yourself; they represent what's most important to you. In a world of almost dizzying complexity, values can provide guidelines for making decisions that are right for you. If understood and applied, they help give life meaning and structure.

There can be a large discrepancy between what people say they value and what their actions indicate about their values. That's why it's important to clarify your own values, making sure you understand what you believe so that you can live in accordance with your beliefs. To do so, follow these steps:

1. Carefully consider the consequences of each choice.
2. Choose freely from among all the options.

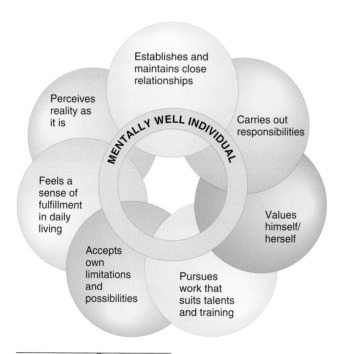

FIGURE 7-3 ▌ The Mentally Well Individual
Mental well-being is a combination of many factors.

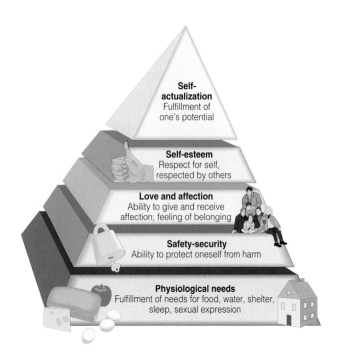

FIGURE 7-4 ▮ The Maslow Pyramid
To attain the highest level of psychological health, you must first satisfy your needs for safety and security, love and affection, and self-esteem.

Source: A. Maslow. *Motivation and Personality,* 3rd ed., © 1997. Reprinted by permission of Pearson Education, Inc.

3. Publicly affirm your values by sharing them with others.
4. Act out your values.

Values clarification is not a once-in-a-lifetime task, but an ongoing process of sorting out what matters most to you. If you believe in protecting the environment, do

STRATEGIES for CHANGE

Being True to Yourself

▮ Take the tombstone test: What would you like to have written on your tombstone? In other words, how would you like to be remembered? Your honest answer should tell you, very succinctly, what you value most.

▮ Describe yourself, as you are today, in a brief sentence. Ask friends or family members for their descriptions of you. How would you have to change to become the person you want to be remembered as?

▮ Try the adjective test: Choose three adjectives that you'd like to see associated with your reputation. Then list what you've done or can do to earn such descriptions.

you shut off lights, or walk rather than drive, in order to conserve energy? Do you vote for political candidates who support environmental protection? Do you recycle newspapers, bottles, and cans? Values are more than ideals we'd like to attain; they should be reflected in the way we live day by day.

Building Self-Esteem

Each of us wants and needs to feel significant as a human being with unique talents, abilities, and roles in life. A sense of **self-esteem,** of belief or pride in ourselves, gives us confidence to dare to attempt to achieve at school or work and to reach out to others to form friendships and close relationships. Self-esteem is the little voice that whispers, "You're worth it. You can do it. You're okay."

Self-esteem is based, not on external factors like wealth or beauty, but on what you believe about yourself. It's not something you're born with; self-esteem develops over time. It's also not something anyone else can give to you, although those around you can either help boost or diminish your self-esteem.

The seeds of self-esteem are planted in childhood when parents provide the assurance and appreciation youngsters need to push themselves toward new accomplishments: crawling, walking, forming words and sentences, learning control over their bladder and bowels.

Adults, too, must consider themselves worthy of love, friendship, and success if they are to be loved, to make friends, and to achieve their goals. Low self-esteem is more common in people who have been abused as children and in those with psychiatric disorders, including depression, anxiety, alcoholism, and drug dependence. Feeling a lack of love and encouragement as a child can also lead to poor self-esteem. Adults with poor self-esteem may unconsciously enter relationships that reinforce their self-perceptions and may prefer and even seek out people who think poorly of them.

In the last decade, self-esteem became a major cultural preoccupation, with thousands of articles and books published and hundreds of programs developed to boost self-esteem. As demonstrated in study after study, people with high self-esteem see themselves as intelligent, attractive, and popular, typically have greater self-confidence than others, believe they are superior to others in many ways, and expect their futures to be rosy.

Yet, although high self-esteem produces pleasant feelings, a review of the psychological literature shows that it does not cause high academic achievement, good job performance, or leadership; nor does poor self-esteem cause violence, smoking, drinking, drug abuse, or early sexual activity. What may matter more than levels of self-esteem is its pursuit, that is, on how people strive to obtain a sense of self-worth.[36]

People whose sense of self-esteem is based on academics, for instance, might take challenging courses, strive for high grades, or apply for graduate school simply

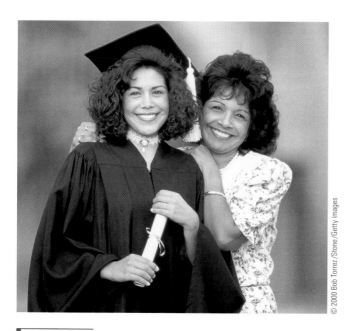

▌ Self-esteem, which is based on what you believe about yourself, tends to increase when you experience success.

to prove their competence, not necessarily to expand their intellectual horizons. They may end up sabotaging their own success. In a study of college students, those who were striving to demonstrate their intelligence in a difficult course did not do well initially showed a downward spiral in performance.[37]

In other research on college students, those who base their self-esteem on appearance or on acceptance by others use more alcohol and drugs and are more likely to have unprotected sex. External criteria for self-worth—appearance, other people's acceptance, competition, academic performance—are associated with more problems during freshman year, while students whose standards for self-worth are internal, such as virtue or religious faith, have fewer problems at college.[38]

✚ Positive Wellness

Psychology, a field that traditionally concentrated on what goes wrong in our lives and in our minds, has shifted its focus to the study of human strengths, virtues, and positive emotions. The three pillars of positive psychology are the study of positive emotions, such as hope and trust; positive traits, such as wisdom and courage; and positive institutions, such as strong families and democracy.[39]

According to psychologist Martin Seligman, the "father" of positive psychology, everyone, regardless of genes or fate, can achieve a happy, gratifying, meaningful life. The goal is not simply to feel good momentarily or to avoid bad experiences, but to build positive strengths and virtues that enable us to find meaning and purpose

in life.[40] The traits that may well protect us from physical and mental illness include courage, optimism, hope, interpersonal skills, a work ethic, responsibility, future-mindedness, honesty, and perseverance.

Happy Mind, Healthy Body

According to a growing number of studies, mental attitude may be just as important a risk factor for certain diseases as age, race, gender, education, habits, and health history.[41] Positive states like happiness and optimism have been linked with longer lifespans as well as lower risk of cardiovascular and lung disease, stroke, diabetes, colds, and upper respiratory infections. People who rate high in happiness develop more antibodies in response to flu vaccine than glummer individuals.

Using brain imaging techniques, scientists have pinpointed areas of the brain that light up when individuals are feeling hopeful or happy. Certain brain chemicals, such as the neurotransmitter dopamine, may play a role. Several studies suggest that happy folks have lower levels of the damaging stress hormone cortisol.

Happy people also take better care of their bodies. According to longitudinal studies, they spend more time exercising, get regular checkups, and take preventive steps like using sunscreen. Those who rate high in gratitude (discussed later in this chapter) view good health as a gift worth maintaining and describe themselves as more energetic, more enthusiastic, and more alert than others.

How Can I Find Happiness?

A joke, a chocolate, a compliment, or a back rub can make us happy—briefly. The more such happy moments we experience, the more pleasant life feels. But according to positive psychologist Martin Seligman, picture-perfect Hollywood happiness represents the lowest level of gratification. The second category is the good life, which consists of applying core virtues and character strengths daily in relationships, studies, work, and leisure. The third and highest is the meaningful life, in which individuals commit their abilities to the service of some larger purpose.[42]

Many factors influence individual happiness, including genetics. Research on twins raised separately and apart suggest that each of us may have an innate "set point" for happiness. Although this set point may fluctuate, it rarely changes radically.

Having an unhappy childhood does not doom anyone to a lifetime of misery, but it does increase the likelihood of unhappiness in adulthood. In a study of community college students, the vast majority reported a happy or very happy childhood. The risk of having an unhappy adulthood was two and a half times greater for those who'd been unhappy as children.

Life events, such as illness, unemployment, or marriage, can have a temporary impact on happiness. In general, people react to events, whether positive or negative, but quickly adapt back to baseline levels of subjective well-being. Setbacks such as being laid off, achievements such as being promoted, or thrills like winning the lottery lose their impact on happiness levels within a few months. However, a 15-year longitudinal study of the impact of marital transitions on more than 24,000 individuals found significant individual differences. A major loss, such as the death of a loved one, can continue to undermine happiness for many years.[43]

Wealth and health have different and often surprising effects on happiness. Rich people are, on average, only slightly happier than poor ones. Good health is not a prerequisite for happiness. Even seriously ill cancer patients and individuals with serious disabilities differ only slightly in life satisfaction from healthier people.

Life satisfaction goes up slightly with age, and emotions become less intense and more stable. Education, intelligence, gender, and race do not matter much for happiness. African Americans and Hispanics have lower rates of depression than white Americans, but they do not report greater happiness. Neither gender is clearly happier, but in different studies women are both happier and sadder than men.

What does make a difference? Love and faith. Married people consistently rank as happier than single or divorced ones. And religious people are usually happier than nonreligious ones. Relationships are key to happiness among undergraduates. In a survey of 222 college students, psychologists found that the "happiest" 10 percent, as determined by six different rating scales, shared one distinctive characteristic: a rich and fulfilling social life. Almost all were involved in a romantic relationship as well as in rewarding friendships. The happiest students spent the least time alone, and their friends rated them as highest on good relationships.[44]

Becoming More Optimistic

The dictionary defines **optimism** as "an inclination to anticipate the best possible outcome." For various reasons—because they believe in themselves, because they trust in a higher power, because they feel lucky—optimists expect positive experiences from life. When bad things happen, they tend to see setbacks or losses as specific, temporary incidents. In their eyes, a disappointment is "one of those things" that happens every once in a while, rather than the latest in a long string of disasters. And rather than blaming themselves ("I always mess things up," pessimists might say), optimists look at all the different factors that may have caused the problem.[45]

Individuals aren't born optimistic or pessimistic; in fact, researchers have documented changes over time in the ways that individuals view the world and what they expect to experience in the future. The key is disputing the automatic negative thoughts that flood our brains and choosing to believe in our own possibilities.

Positive psychologist Martin Seligman provides "optimism training" to freshmen at the University of Pennsylvania. Those trained to look on the bright side suffered fewer illnesses throughout college than those who did not. Optimism may even help people live longer, healthier lives. In a 40-year Mayo Clinic study, the longevity of optimists was 19 percent greater compared to pessimists. On average, people with positive attitudes regarding aging live about 7.5 years longer.[46]

Looking on the Light Side

Humor, which enables us to express fears and negative feelings without causing distress to ourselves or others, is one of the healthiest ways of coping with life's ups and downs. Laughter stimulates the heart, alters brain wave patterns and breathing rhythms, reduces perceptions of pain, decreases stress-related hormones, and strengthens the immune system. In psychotherapy, humor helps channel negative emotions toward a positive effect. Even in cases of critical or fatal illnesses, humor can relieve pain and help people live with greater joy until they die.[47]

Joking and laughing are ways of expressing honest emotions, of overcoming dread and doubt, and of connecting with others. They also can defuse rage. After all, it's almost impossible to stay angry when you're laughing. To tickle your funny bone, try keeping a file of favorite cartoons or jokes. Go to a comedy club instead of a movie. And when you see or hear something that makes you laugh out loud, don't keep it to yourself—multiply the mirth by sharing it with a friend.

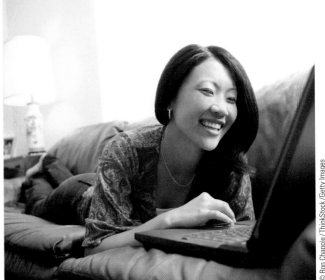

© Ron Chapple/ThinkStock/Getty Images

▌ Laughter enhances wellness physically and emotionally. Don't throw away those e-mail jokes—send them on!

STRATEGIES for CHANGE

How to Be Happy

- Make time for yourself. It's impossible to meet the needs of others without recognizing and fulfilling your own.

- Invest yourself in closeness. Give your loved ones the gift of your time and caring.

- Work hard at what you like. Search for challenges that satisfy your need to do something meaningful.

- Be upbeat. If you always look for what's wrong about yourself or your life, you'll find it—and feel even worse.

- Organize but stay loose. Be ready to seize an unexpected opportunity to try something different.

How Can I Get Out of a Bad Mood?

Feelings come and go within minutes. A **mood** is a more sustained emotional state that colors our view of the world for hours or days. According to surveys by psychologist Randy Larsen, of the University of Michigan, bad moods descend upon us an average of three out of every ten days. "A few people—about 2 percent—are happy just about every day," he says. "About 5 percent report bad moods four out of every five days." [48]

There are gender differences in mood management: Men typically try to distract themselves (a partially successful strategy) or use alcohol or drugs (an ineffective tactic). Women are more likely to talk to someone (which can help) or to ruminate on why they feel bad (which doesn't help). Learning effective mood-boosting, mood-regulating strategies can help both men and women pull themselves up and out of an emotional slump.

The most effective way to banish a sad or bad mood is by changing what caused it in the first place—if you can figure out what made you upset and why. "Most bad moods are caused by loss or failure in work or intimate relationships," says Larsen. "The questions to ask are What can I do to fix the failure? What can I do to remedy the loss? Is there anything under my control that I can change? If there is, take action and solve it." Rewrite the report. Ask to take a makeup exam. Apologize to the friend whose feelings you hurt. Tell your parents you feel bad about the argument you had.

If there's nothing you can do, accept what happened and focus on doing things differently next time. "In our studies, resolving to try harder actually was as effective in improving mood as taking action in the present," says Larsen. You also can try to think about what happened in

a different way and put a positive spin on it. This technique, known as *cognitive reappraisal,* or "reframing," helps you look at a setback in a new light: What lessons did it teach you? What would you have done differently? Could there be a silver lining or hidden benefit?

If you can't identify or resolve the problem responsible for your emotional funk, the next-best solution is to concentrate on altering your negative feelings. For example, try setting a quick, achievable goal that can boost your spirits with a small success. Clean out a drawer; sort through the piles of paper on your desk; send an e-mail or instant message to an old friend.

Another good option is to get moving. In studies of mood regulation, exercise consistently ranks as the single most effective strategy for banishing bad feelings. Numerous studies have confirmed that aerobic workouts, such as walking or jogging, significantly improve mood. Even nonaerobic exercise, such as weight lifting, can boost spirits; improve sleep and appetite; reduce anxiety, sadness, irritability, and anger; and produce feelings of mastery and accomplishment.

Taking your mind off your troubles, rather than mulling over what's wrong, is one of the most often used mood boosters, but it's only partly successful. Simple distractions—watching television, for instance, or reading—work only temporarily. Activities that engage the imagination, on the other hand, seem to have more lasting effects. Listening to music, for instance, is one of the most popular and effective ways of distracting people from their troubles and changing their bad moods.

✚ Spirituality

Whatever your faith, whether or not you belong to any formal religion, you are more than a body of a certain height and weight occupying space on the planet. You have a mind that equips you to learn and question. And you have a spirit that animates everything you say and do. Spiritual wellness refers to this breath of life.

Spirituality is a belief in what some call a higher power, in someone or something that transcends the boundaries of self. It gives rise to a strong sense of purpose, values, morals, and ethics. Throughout life you make choices and decide to behave in one way rather than another because your spirituality serves as both a compass and a guide.

The term "religiosity" refers to various spiritual practices. That definition may seem vague, but one thing is clear. According to thousands of studies on the relationship between religious beliefs and practices and health, religious individuals are less depressed, less anxious, and better able to cope with crises such as illness or divorce than nonreligious ones. The more that a believer incorporates spiritual practices, such as prayer, meditation, or attending services, into daily life, the greater their sense of satisfaction with life.

STRATEGIES for CHANGE

Enhancing Spiritual Wellness

▍ **If you are religious**
Deepen your spiritual commitment through prayer, more frequent church attendance, or joining a prayer group.

▍ **If you are not religious**
Keep an open mind about the value of religion or spirituality. Consider visiting a church or synagogue. Read the writings of inspired people of deep faith, such as Rabbi Harold Kushner and Rev. Martin Luther King, Jr.

▍ **If you are not ready to consider religion**
Try nonreligious meditation or relaxation training. In decades of research, Dr. Herbert Benson of Harvard University has shown that focusing the mind on a single sound or image can slow heart rate, respiration, and brain waves; relax muscles; and lower stress-rated hormones—responses similar to those induced by prayer.

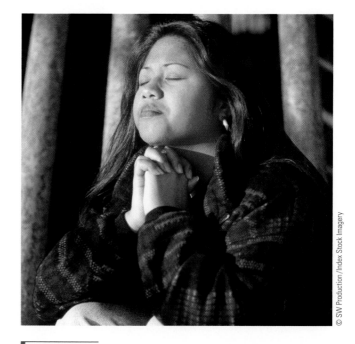

▍ Prayer provides benefits for physical health as well as spiritual well-being.

Even when age, health, habits, demographics, and other factors are considered, individuals who pray regularly and attend religious services stay healthier and live longer than those who rarely or never do. In studies at several medical centers, prayer and faith speeded recovery from alcoholism, hip surgery, drug addiction, stroke, rheumatoid arthritis, heart attacks, and bypass surgery.[49]

In one study, researchers assessed religiosity and symptoms of depression in 104 intercollegiate athletes at a public university in the Southeast. The greater the athletes' intrinsic religiosity, the less likely they were to suffer depressive symptoms.

"Perhaps intrinsic religious beliefs provide a sense of hope and security that protect against distressing events," the researchers speculated. "It may also be that unconditional love by one's God provides a stable sense of self-worth" that buffers against stress.[50]

Can Prayer Make Us Well? FAQ

Prayer, a spiritual practice of millions, is the most commonly used form of complementary and alternative medicine. However, only in recent years has science launched rigorous investigations of the healing power of prayer.

Petitionary prayer—praying directly to a higher power—affects both the quality and quantity of life, says Dr. Harold Koenig, director of Duke University's Center for the Study of Religion/Spirituality and Health. "It boosts morale, lowers agitation, loneliness, and life dissatisfaction and enhances ability to cope in men, women, the elderly, the young, the healthy, and the sick."[51]

People who pray regularly have significantly lower blood pressure and stronger immune systems than the less religious, says Dr. Koenig. They're also less prone to alcoholism, less likely to smoke heavily, and are hospitalized less often. Science cannot explain the physiological mechanisms for what happens in human beings when they pray, but in cultures around the world throughout recorded history, when people or their loved ones are sick, they pray.

The impact of prayer for others—called "intercessory prayer" or distant healing—has not been proved, but it may help those who pray, if not the individuals for whom they pray.[52]

In a national survey, 35 percent of Americans prayed for health concerns, with 75 percent of these praying for wellness and 22 percent praying for alleviation of specific medical conditions, such as chronic headaches, depression, back or neck pain, and digestive problems. Among those who prayed because of a medical condition, 69 percent found prayer very helpful. Only 11 percent of patients using prayer discussed it with their physicians.[53]

Some scientists speculate that prayer may foster a state of peace and calm that could lead to beneficial changes in the cardiovascular and immune systems. Sophisticated brain imaging techniques have shown that prayer and meditation cause changes in blood flow in particular regions of the brain that may lead to lower blood pressure, slower heart rate, decreased anxiety, and an enhanced sense of well-being. Membership in a faith community provides an identity as well as support, although individuals vary in their religious practices and observances.[54]

Will science ever be able to prove the power of prayer? No one is certain. "While I personally believe that God heals people in supernatural ways, I don't think science can shape a study to prove it," says Duke's Dr. Koenig. "But we now know enough, based on solid scientific research, to recommend prayer, much like exercise and diet, as one of the best and most cost-effective ways of protecting and enhancing health."

Expressing Gratitude

A grateful spirit brightens mood, boosts energy, and infuses daily living with a sense of glad abundance. Although giving thanks is an ancient virtue, only recently have researchers focused on the "trait" of gratitude—appreciation, not just for a special gift, but for everything that makes life a bit better.

"Gratitude is an emotional and intellectual phenomenon that rises out of recognition that someone has treated you benevolently," says psychologist Michael McCullough of Southern Methodist University, a pioneer in gratitude research. "It's not feeling happy because something good happens, but realizing that someone who didn't have to deliberately did something of value to you."[55]

Since gratitude is not just a feeling but a mental outlook, we can consciously become more grateful—with practice. "Volunteers on college campuses who are asked to list things they're grateful for every day report more positive feelings," says McCullough. "They have more energy. They sleep better. They feel richer, regardless of how much money they have. Even their families notice visible, positive changes."

How can you help your gratitude grow? Here are some suggestions:

- Train yourself to pay attention to good things, large and small.
- Build a time for thankfulness into your day. Some people write nightly in a gratitude journal or log.
- Develop a "good" memory, one that stores the kindnesses and comforts that have come your way.
- Pass on simple kindnesses. Open the door for a student juggling a backpack and an umbrella. Flash a smile at a server in the cafeteria. Pitch in on a beach or park clean-up. Give others a reason to savor a moment of gratitude.

Forgiveness

While "I forgive you" may be three of the most difficult words to say, they are also three of the most powerful—and the most beneficial for the body as well as the soul. Being angry, harboring resentments, or reliving hurts over and over again is bad for your health in general and your heart in particular. The word *forgive* comes from the Greek for letting go, and that's what happens when you forgive: You let go of all the anger and pain that have been demanding your time and wasting your energy.

STRATEGIES for CHANGE

How to Forgive

▮ **Compose an apology letter.**
Address it to yourself, and write it from someone who's hurt you. This simple task enables you to get a new perspective on a painful experience.

▮ **Leap forward in time.**
In a visualization exercise, imagine that you are very old, meet a person who hurt you long ago, and sit down together on a park bench on a beautiful spring day. You both talk until everything that needs to be said finally is. This allows you to benefit from the perspective time brings without having to wait for years to achieve it.

▮ **Talk with "safe" people.**
Vent your anger or disappointment with a trusted friend or a counselor without the danger of saying or doing anything you'll regret later. And if you can laugh about what happened with a friend, the laughter helps dissolve the rage.

▮ **Forgive the person, not the deed.**
In themselves, abuse, rape, murder, or betrayal are beyond forgiveness. But you can forgive people who couldn't manage to handle their own suffering, misery, confusion, and desperation.

▮ **Write a letter to the person who hurt you.**
Spell out the truth of what happened as you experienced it without blaming or judging. If the person is dead or incapable of hearing what you have to say, some counselors suggest burning the letter—a symbolic way of letting old angers go up in smoke.

To some people, forgiveness seems a sign of weakness or submission. People may feel more in control, more powerful, when they're filled with anger, but forgiving instills a much greater sense of power. When you forgive, you reclaim your power to choose. It doesn't matter whether someone deserves to be forgiven; you deserve to be free.

However, forgiveness isn't easy. It's not a one-time thing but a process that takes a lot of time and work. Most people pass through several stages in their journey to forgiveness. The initial response may involve anger, sadness, shame, or other negative feelings. Later, there's a reevaluation of what happened, then reframing to try to make sense of it or to take mitigating circumstances into account. This may lead to a reduction in negative feelings, especially if the initial hurt turns out to be accidental rather than intentional.

Forgiveness can occur without anyone else's involvement or even awareness. The people you forgive may never realize they wronged you or never know you forgave them. They may be dead. They may be alcoholics who cannot hear what you're trying to say. They may deny anything bad ever happened. What's important is that you embrace the idea of forgiveness, let go of your anger, and open up your heart to a deeper understanding.

Doing Good

Altruism—helping or giving to others—enhances self-esteem, relieves physical and mental stress, and protects psychological well-being. Hans Selye, the father of stress research, described cooperation with others for the self's sake as altruistic egotism, whereby we satisfy our own needs while helping others satisfy theirs. This concept is essentially an updated version of the golden rule: Do unto others as you would have them do unto you. The important difference is that you earn your neighbor's love and help by offering them love and help.

Many colleges offer students an opportunity to practice altruism in "service learning" experiences, which combine community service with classroom instruction and personal reflection. In a recent survey of students at 504 colleges and universities, an average of one in three reported doing some form of community service. More than half of the schools surveyed noted an increase in student involvement in community service.[56] Various studies have shown that students find service learning personally and professionally enriching and are more likely to continue volunteer work after college.

The options for giving of yourself are limitless: Volunteer to serve a meal at a homeless shelter. Collect donations for a charity auction. Teach in an illiteracy program. Perform the simplest act of charity: Pray for others.

✚ Feeling in Control

Although no one has absolute control over destiny, we can do a great deal to control how we think, feel, and behave. By assessing our life situations realistically, we can make plans and preparations that allow us to make the most of our circumstances. By doing so, we gain a sense of mastery. In nationwide surveys, Americans who feel in control of their lives report greater psychological well-being than those who do not, as well as extraordinarily positive feelings of happiness.

Developing Autonomy

One goal that many people strive for is **autonomy,** or independence. Both family and society influence our ability to grow toward independence. Autonomous individuals are true to themselves. As they weigh the pros and cons of any decision, whether it's using or refusing drugs or choosing a major or career, they base their judgment on their own values, not those of others. Their ability to draw on internal resources and cope with challenges has a positive impact on both their psychological well-being and their physical health, including recovery from illness.

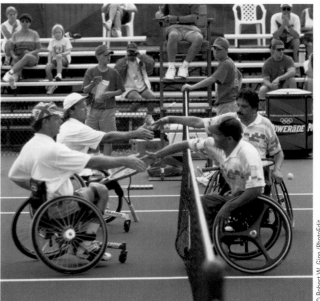

You may not have complete control over your destiny, but you can control how you respond to challenges. Even under the most difficult of circumstances, individuals can gain a sense of mastery and personal fulfillment.

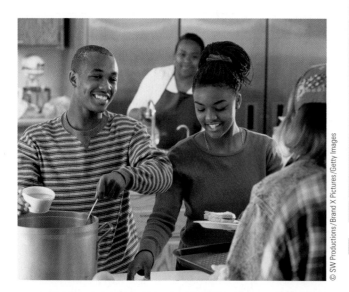

Helping others makes us feel better about ourselves.

Those who've achieved autonomy may seek the opinions of others, but they do not allow their decisions to be dictated by external influences. For autonomous individuals, their **locus of control**—that is, where they view control as originating—is *internal* (from within themselves) rather than *external* (from others).

Asserting Yourself

Being **assertive** means recognizing your feelings and making your needs and desires clear to others. Unlike aggression, a far less healthy means of expression, assertiveness usually works. You can change a situation you don't like by communicating your feelings and thoughts in non-provocative words, by focusing on specifics, and by making sure you're talking with the person who is directly responsible.

Becoming assertive isn't always easy. Many people have learned to cope by being passive and not communicating their feelings or opinions. Sooner or later they become so irritated, frustrated, or overwhelmed that they explode in an outburst—which they think of as being assertive. However, such behavior is so distasteful to them that they'd rather be passive. But assertiveness doesn't mean screaming or telling someone off. You can communicate your wishes calmly and clearly. Assertiveness is a behavior that respects your rights and the rights of other people even when you disagree.

Even at its mildest, assertiveness can make you feel better about yourself and your life. The reason: When you speak up or take action, you're in the pilot seat. And that's always much less stressful than taking a back seat and trying to hang on for dear life.

✚ Connecting with Others

At every age, people who feel connected to others tend to be healthier physically and psychologically. College students are no exception: Those who have a supportive, readily available network of relationships are less psychologically distressed and more satisfied with life.

The opposite of *connectedness* is **social isolation,** a major risk factor for illness and early death. Individuals with few social contacts face two to four times the mortality rate of others. The reason may be that their social isolation weakens the body's ability to ward off disease. Medical students with higher-than-average scores on a loneliness scale had lower levels of protective immune cells. The end of a long-term relationship—through separation, divorce, or death—also dampens immunity.

It is part of our nature as mammals and as human beings to crave relationships. But invariably we end up alone at times. Solitude is not without its own quiet joys—time for introspection, self-assessment, learning from the past, and looking toward the future. Each of us can cultivate the joy of our own company, of being alone without crossing the line and becoming lonely.

Overcoming Loneliness

More so than many other countries, we are a nation of loners. Recent trends—longer work hours, busy family schedules, frequent moves, high divorce rates—have created even more lonely people. Only 23 percent of Americans say they're never lonely. Loneliest of all are those who are divorced, separated, or widowed and those who live alone or solely with children. Among single adults who have never been married, 42 percent feel lonely at least sometimes. However, loneliness is most likely to cause emotional distress when it is chronic rather than episodic.

To combat loneliness, people may join groups, fling themselves into projects and activities, or surround themselves with superficial acquaintances. Others avoid the effort of trying to connect, sometimes limiting most of their personal interactions to chat groups on the Internet.

The true keys to overcoming loneliness are developing resources to fulfill our own potential and learning to reach out to others. In this way, loneliness can become a means to personal growth and discovery.

Facing Shyness and Social Anxiety

Many people are uncomfortable meeting strangers or speaking or performing in public. In some surveys, as many as 40 percent of people describe themselves as shy, or socially anxious. Some shy people—an estimated 10 to 15 percent of children—are born with a predisposition to shyness. Others become shy because they don't learn proper social responses or because they experience rejection or shame.

Some people are "fearfully" shy; that is, they withdraw and avoid contact with others and experience a high degree of anxiety and fear in social situations. Others are "self-consciously" shy. They enjoy the company of others but become highly self-aware and anxious in social situations.

In one study of college students, men reported somewhat more shyness than women. African-Americans were less shy than either Asian Americans or Caucasians.[57] Students may develop symptoms of shyness or social anxiety when they go to a party or are called on in class. Some experience symptoms when they try to perform any sort of action in the presence of others, even such everyday activities as eating in public, using a public restroom, or writing a check.

About 7 percent of the population could be diagnosed with a severe form of social anxiety, called **social phobia,** in which individuals typically fear and avoid various social situations. Adolescents and young adults with severe social anxiety are at increased risk of major depression. The key difference between these problems and normal shyness and self-consciousness is the degree of distress and impairment that individuals experience.

If you're shy, you can overcome much of your social apprehensiveness on your own, in much the same way as you might set out to stop smoking or lose weight. For example, you can improve your social skills by pushing yourself to introduce yourself to a stranger at a party or to chat about the weather or the food selections with the person next to you in a cafeteria line. Gradually, you'll acquire a sense of social timing and a verbal ease that will take the worry out of close encounters with others.

✚ The Role of Sleep

You stay up late cramming for a final. You drive through the night to visit a friend at another campus. You get up for an early class during the week but stay in bed until noon on weekends. And you wonder: "Why am I so tired?" The answer: You're not getting enough sleep.

Whenever we fail to get adequate sleep, we accumulate what researchers call a *sleep debt*. With each night of too little rest, our body's need for sleep grows until it becomes irresistible. The only solution to sleep debt is

the obvious one: paying it back. College students who extended their nightly sleep time were more alert, more productive, and less likely to have accidents.[58] And because sleepy people tend to be irritable and edgy, those who get more rest also tend to be happier, healthier, and easier to get along with.

Why Sleep Matters

Sleep problems, as medical scientists now recognize, are hazardous to health. Breathing-related sleep disorders, such as chronic snoring and obstructive sleep apnea, increase the risk of high blood pressure, heart attacks, and stroke. Individuals with insomnia, the most common sleep complaint, become irritable and depressed, get into more traffic accidents, develop memory problems, and have difficulties concentrating and doing their jobs. According to recent research, inadequate sleep affects growth hormone secretion, increasing the likelihood of obesity, and impairs the body's ability to use insulin, which can lead to diabetes.[59] Individuals chronically deprived of enough sleep may become more susceptible to certain sicknesses, and researchers speculate that disturbed sleep may be the reason why individuals under stress—such as students taking exams or grieving widows and widowers—may have lower levels of certain infection-fighting cells than normal.[60]

More than half of Americans report difficulty falling or staying asleep a few nights a week. Yet effective treatments for sleep problems could help three of every four poor sleepers.

Medications can help in the short run but lose their effectiveness over time and interfere, to varying degrees, with the normal stages of sleep. One of the most promising alternatives is cognitive-behavior training, which combines cognitive therapy with specific strategies to improve sleep habits, such as avoiding daytime naps and limiting time in bed.

How Much Sleep Do I Need?

Over the last century, we have cut our average nightly sleep time by 20 percent. According to the National Commission on Sleep Disorder, more than 70 million men and women have problems sleeping. More than half of us try to get by with fewer than seven hours of shut-eye a night.[61]

College students are no exception. In a recent study of 212 undergraduates, their average sleep time was slightly less than seven hours, with little difference between men and women. Those who slept the least reported the lowest life satisfaction.[62] Short-sleepers also have poorer psychological health, less creativity, and lower academic performance.[63]

No formula can say how long a good night's sleep should be. Normal sleep times range from five to ten hours; the average is seven and a half. About one or two people in a hundred can get by with just five hours; another small minority needs twice that amount. Each of us seems to have an innate sleep *appetite* that is as much a part of our genetic programming as hair color and skin tone.

To figure out your sleep needs, keep your wake-up time the same every morning and vary your bedtime. Are you groggy after six hours of shut-eye? Does an extra hour give you more stamina? What about an extra two hours? Since too much sleep can make you feel sluggish, don't assume that more is always better. Listen to your body's signals, and adjust your sleep schedule to suit them.

✚ The Mind-Wellness Connection

Mental problems affect not just the mind but also the body. **Anxiety** can lead to intensified asthmatic reactions, skin conditions, and digestive disorders. Stress can play a role in hypertension, heart attacks, sudden cardiac death, and immune disorders in the young as well as in older individuals.

Depression has increasingly been recognized as a serious risk factor for physical illness. According to a review of large-scale studies on depression, of more than 36,000 men and women, depressed individuals were 1.5 to 4 times more likely to develop heart problems.[64] In still unknown ways, depression may increase risk factors for heart disease, such as high blood pressure, and for premature death.[65] Together, depression and heart disease worsen a patient's prognosis more than either condition alone.

Depressed individuals are more likely to suffer heart attacks and chest pain than others and to die of heart disease. Between 15 to 20 percent of patients experience major depression following a heart attack, and the incidence of depression is three times higher in people with heart disease than in the general public.[66]

Major depression is associated with lower bone density in young men, but not in women.[67] A history of depression increases the risk of physical problems such as headache and shoulder and neck pain in women as they reach middle age.[68]

By some estimates, as many as 60 percent of those who seek help from physicians suffer primarily from a psychological problem. Treating mental health problems leads not only to improved health but also to lower health-care costs. Psychiatric treatment reduces hospitalizations, cuts medical expenses, and reduces work disability.

Emotional Wellness on Campus

About 15 percent of students seek counseling during college.[69] The emotional difficulties of college students have become more complex and more severe than in the past. In one national survey, more than 80 percent of directors of counseling centers reported an increase in the number of students with serious psychological disorders.[70]

Undergraduates are more likely to seek psychological counseling as they progress through college. Those with A and B averages are more likely to seek help than those with averages of C or below.[71]

According to the American College Health Association's survey—the National College Health Assessment—the incidence of depression among college students increased by 4.6 percent over the four-year period from 2000 to 2004. In a survey of 47,202 students from 74 campuses across the country, 15 percent reported having ever been diagnosed with depression, up from 10 percent in 2000. Of those diagnosed with depression, 28 percent were currently in therapy for depression, and 38 percent were taking medication for depression. Roughly 40 percent of men and 50 percent of women reported having experienced debilitating incidences of depression (**Table 7-2**).[72]

Researchers at the University of Michigan have identified three key contributors to depression in college

TABLE 7-2 ❚ Depression Among College Students

Have you ever felt so depressed it was difficult to function?	Male	Female	Total
Never	60.9	51.7	54.9
1–10 times	32.8	40.4	37.7
11 or more times	6.3	8.0	7.4

Based on the American College Health Association's National College Health Assessment survey of 47,202 students from 74 campuses around the country, www.acha.org.

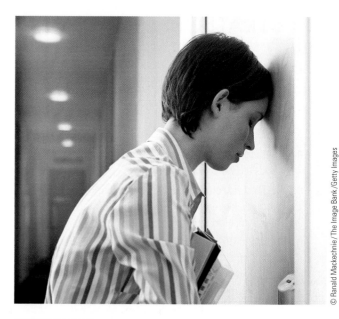

Factors that can contribute to depression in college include stress, poor academic performance, loneliness, and relationship problems.

students: stress, substance abuse, and sleep loss. As they adjust to campus life, undergraduates face the ongoing stress of forging a new identity and finding a place for themselves in various social hierarchies. This triggers the release of the stress hormones discussed earlier, which can change brain activity. Drugs and alcohol, widely used on campus, also affect the brain in ways that make stress even harder to manage.

In a sample of Canadian freshmen, those who maintained or increased their levels of physical activity in their first months of college reported greater levels of vigor and less fatigue and tension than those who exercised less than before.[73]

The few studies that have looked into ethnic and gender differences in psychological health have yielded conflicting or inconclusive results: Some found no differences; others suggested higher rates of depression among Korean and South Asian students.

Why Are So Many Young People Depressed?

Once young people were considered immune to sadness. Now mental health professionals know better. An estimated 5 to 10 percent of American teenagers suffer from a serious depressive disorder; girls are twice as susceptible as boys. Prior to puberty, girls and boys are equally likely to develop depression.

The risks of depression in the young are high. Four in ten depressed adolescents think about killing themselves; two in ten actually try to do so. Every year an estimated 11 to 13 in every 100,000 teens take their own lives, twice as many as the number who die from all natural causes combined.

"Depression is the most common emotional problem in adolescence and the single greatest risk factor for teen suicide," says child psychiatrist Peter Jensen, M.D., director for the Center for the Advancement of Children's Mental Health at Columbia University, who notes that depression rates have been rising over the last half century.

No one knows the reason for this steady surge in sadness, but experts point to the breakdown of families, the pressures of the information age, and increased isolation.

A family history of depression greatly increases a young person's vulnerability. A mother's anxiety and depression during early childhood can increase the risk that adolescents will develop symptoms of anxiety and depression.[74]

However, the strongest predictor of depression is cigarette smoking. Depressed teens may smoke because they think smoking will make them feel better, but nicotine alters brain chemistry and actually worsens symptoms of depression.

The link between tobacco and depression continues during college. Students who had been diagnosed with or treated for depression were 7.5 times as likely as other students to use tobacco, possibly because of nicotine's stimulating effects.[75] In another study of college smokers, young women with symptoms of depression and those who did not feel connected with a peer group were more likely to smoke.[76]

According to various studies, 5 to 7 percent of college students take antidepressant medications. Direct-to-consumer advertisements for antidepressant drugs can influence students' perceptions of what is wrong with them. In one study, college women were more likely to rate themselves as having mild-to-moderate depression as a result of reading pharmaceutical company information for popular antidepressants. The researchers cautioned that students should try alternative treatments for mild depression, including simple changes such as reduced class load, increased exercise, and more sleep, before starting medication.[77]

© Ranald Mackechnie / The Image Bank / Getty Images

Getting Help

As a student, your best contact for identifying local services may be your health education instructor or department. The health instructors can tell you about general and mental health counseling available on campus, school-based support groups, community-based programs, and special emergency services. On campus, you can also turn to the student health services or the office of the dean of student services or student affairs.

Within the community, you may be able to get help through the city or county health department and neighborhood health centers. Local hospitals often have special clinics and services, and there are usually local branches of national service organizations, such as United Way or Alcoholics Anonymous, other 12-step programs, and various support groups. You can call the psychiatric or psychological association in your city or state for the names of licensed professionals. (Check the telephone directory for listings.) Your primary physician may also be able to help.

▌ MAKING HEALTHY CHOICES

To Lower Stress and Feel Good

College is a perfect time to learn and practice the skills of psychological wellness. You can start applying the techniques and concepts outlined in this chapter immediately. You may want to begin by doing some relaxation or awareness exercises. They can give you the peace of mind you need to focus more effectively on larger issues, goals, and decisions.

Like physical health, psychological well-being is not a fixed state of being, but a process. The way you live every day affects how you feel about yourself and your world. Here are some basic guidelines that you can rely on to make the most of the process of living:

- **Accept yourself.** As a human being, you are, by definition, imperfect. Come to terms with the fact that you are a worthwhile person despite your mistakes.
- **Respect yourself.** Recognize your abilities and talents. Acknowledge your competence and achievements, and take pride in them.
- **Trust yourself.** Learn to listen to the voice within you, and let your intuition be your guide.
- **Love yourself.** Be happy to spend time by yourself. Learn to appreciate your own company and to be glad you're you.
- **Stretch yourself.** Be willing to change and grow, to try something new and dare to be vulnerable.
- **Look at challenges as opportunities for personal growth.** "Every problem brings the possibility of a widening of consciousness," psychologist Carl Jung once noted. Put his words to the test.
- **Think of not only where but also who you want to be a decade from now.** The goals you set, the decisions you make, the values you adopt now will determine how you feel about yourself and your life in the future.
- **Seek new horizons.** When your life feels out of control, turn to a new challenge. You might try volunteering at a nursing home, going for a long-distance bike trip, or learning a foreign language. As you work toward your new goal, you'll realize that you still can cope and achieve.

You also may be able to find help through support groups or counseling. Your school may provide counseling services or referrals to mental health professionals; ask your health instructor or the campus health department for this information. Remember that each day of distress robs you of energy, distracts you from life's pleasures, and interferes with achieving your full potential.

SELF-SURVEY

Physical Stress Symptoms Scale

The first signs of stress are often physical and show up as little aches and pains, an uneasy feeling that is hard to explain, or a distinct health-related problem. Some people are too busy (and often too stressed!) to take a step back to determine why these things are happening. By recognizing the signs and symptoms of physical stress you can respond to your stress more quickly and manage it more effectively.

Identify how often each of the following effects happens to you either while you are experiencing stress or after exposure to a significant stressor. Respond to each item with a number between 0 and 5, using the following scale:

0 = Never	1 = Once or twice a year	2 = Every few months
3 = Every few weeks	4 = Once or more each week	5 = Daily

Cardiovascular symptoms

_____ heart pounding   _____ heart racing or beating erratically

_____ cold, sweaty hands   _____ headaches (throbbing pain)   Subtotal _____

Gastrointestinal symptoms

_____ upset stomach, nausea, or vomiting   _____ constipation

_____ diarrhea   _____ sharp abdominal pains   Subtotal _____

Immunity symptoms

_____ allergy flare-up   _____ common cold

_____ influenza   _____ skin rash   Subtotal _____

Metabolic symptoms

_____ increased appetite   _____ increased craving for tobacco or sweets

_____ thoughts racing or difficulty sleeping   _____ feelings of anxiety or nervousness   Subtotal _____

Muscular symptoms

_____ headaches (steady pain)   _____ back or shoulder pains

_____ muscle tremors or hands shaking   _____ arthritis   Subtotal _____

Respiratory symptoms

_____ rapid, erratic, or shallow breathing   _____ shortness of breath

_____ asthma attack   _____ difficulty in speaking because of poor breathing control   Subtotal _____

Skin symptoms

_____ acne   _____ dandruff

_____ perspiration   _____ excessive dryness of skin, hair or nails   Subtotal _____

Overall symptomatic total (add all seven subtotals): _____

What Does Your Score Mean?

0–35
Moderate physical stress symptoms

A score in this range indicates a low level of physical stress manifestations, hence minimal overall future probability of encounter with diseases that have no basic physical cause.

36–75
Average physical stress symptoms

Most people in this range experience physical stress symptoms. It is representative of an increased predisposition to diseases having no basic physical cause, but not an immediate threat to health.

76–140
Excessive physical stress symptoms

If your score falls in this range, you are experiencing a serious number and frequency of stress symptoms. It is a clear indication that you may be headed toward one or more diseases having no basic physical cause, but a very real threat to your health sometime in the future. You should take a deliberate course of action to reduce your level of stress.

Adapted from: Allen, R.J., and D. Hyde. *Investigations in Stress Control*, pp. 101–105. Minneapolis: Burgess, 1980.

ACTION PLAN

Your Action Plan for Stress Management and Psychological Wellness

Stress can manifest itself in many ways, including physical, behavioral and emotional outcomes. Just as you can improve your physical well-being, you can enhance the state of your mind. Making small changes to counteract stress and have a more positive attitude can affect every aspect of your life, and reduce both physical and mental manifestations of stress. Here are some suggestions:

- Recognize and express your feelings. Pent-up emotions tend to fester inside, building into anger or depression.
- Don't brood. Rather than merely mulling over a problem, try to find solutions that are positive and useful.
- Take one step at a time. As long as you're taking some action to solve a problem, you can take pride in your ability to cope.
- Spend more time doing those activities you know you do best. For example, if you are a good cook, prepare a meal for someone.
- Separate what you do, especially any mistakes you make, from who you are. Instead of saying, "I'm so stupid," tell yourself, "That wasn't the smartest move I ever made, but I'll learn from it."
- Use affirmations, positive statements that help reinforce the most positive aspects of your personality and experience. Every day, you might say, "I am a loving, caring person," or "I am honest and open in expressing my feelings." Write some affirmations of your own on index cards and flip through them occasionally.
- List the things you would like to have or experience. Construct the statements as if you were already enjoying the situations you list, beginning each sentence with "I am." For example, "I am feeling great about doing well in my classes."
- When your internal critic—the negative inner voice we all have—starts putting you down, force yourself to think of a situation that you handled well.
- Set a limit on self-pity. Tell yourself, "I'm going to feel sorry for myself this morning, but this afternoon, I've got to get on with my life."
- Volunteer. A third of Americans—some 89 million people—give of themselves through volunteer work. By doing the same, you may feel better too.
- Exercise. In various studies around the world, physical exertion ranks as one of the best ways to change a bad mood, raise energy, and reduce tension.
- When change occurs, think about its meaning and your feelings about it. Try to come up with different ways of adjusting to the change.
- Pace yourself. Even if you have a lot to do, stick to a reasonable schedule that allows you some time off to relax.
- Look at each change as a part of life's natural flow, rather than as a disruption in the way things should be.

SETTING GOALS

Stress-Reducing Goals

Your Personal Stress-Reducing Goal:

Is It S.M.A.R.T.?
  Specific? _____
  Measurable? _____
  Achievable? _____
  Rewarding? _____
  Time Defined? _____

Strategies for Success
  1. _____
  2. _____
  3. _____

Potential Obstacles
  1. _____
  2. _____
  3. _____

Ways Around Them
  1. _____
  2. _____
  3. _____

Daily Report

The Week that Was:

What Went Right?
What Could I Do Better?

WELLNESS JOURNAL

Your Stress-Busting Strategies

Make a list of all the ways you can lower your stress level. Include everything from a long shower to listening to music to a brisk walk. For a week, record every time you engage in one of these stress-relieving activities and how you feel afterward. For example:

Activity	When	Effect
A deep, lung-filling breath	Just before a midterm	Felt more clear-headed
Singing a song in my head	Coming back from library	Started to smile

CHAPTER

7

Making This Chapter Work for You

1. Stress can be defined as:
   a. a negative emotional state related to fatigue and similar to depression.
   b. the physiological and psychological response to any event or situation that either upsets or excites us.
   c. the end result of the general adaptation syndrome.
   d. a motivational strategy for making life changes.

2. Over time, increased levels of stress hormones have been shown to increase a person's risk for which of the following conditions?
   a. diabetes, high blood pressure, memory loss, and skin disorders
   b. stress fractures, male pattern baldness, and hypothyroidism
   c. hemophilia, AIDS, and hay fever
   d. none of the above

3. Stress levels in college students
   a. may be high due to stressors such as academic pressures, financial concerns, learning disabilities, and relationship problems.
   b. are usually low because students feel empowered, living independently of their parents.
   c. are typically highest in seniors because their self-esteem diminishes during the college years.
   d. are lower in minority students because they are used to stressors such as a hostile social climate and actual or perceived discrimination.

4. If you are stuck in a traffic jam, which of the following actions will help reduce your stress level?
   a. deep slow breathing
   b. honking your horn
   c. berating yourself for not taking a different route
   d. getting on your cell phone to reschedule appointments

5. A relaxed, peaceful state of being can be achieved with which of the following activities?
   a. an aerobic exercise class
   b. playing a computer game
   c. meditating for 15 minutes
   d. attending a rap concert

6. To effectively manage your time, which of these techniques should you try?
   a. Use a calendar or planner.
   b. Keep a log of your activities for a week.
   c. Tackle a large task by breaking it down into a series of smaller tasks.
   d. All of the above.

7. Psychological health is influenced by all of the following *except:*
   a. spiritual health
   b. physical agility
   c. culture
   d. a firm grasp on reality

8. Which of the following activities can contribute to a lasting sense of personal fulfillment?
   a. becoming a Big Sister or Big Brother to a child from an inner city, single-parent home
   b. volunteering at a local soup kitchen on Thanksgiving
   c. being a regular participant in an Internet chat room
   d. going on a shopping spree

9. Individuals who have developed a sense of mastery over their lives are
   a. skilled at controlling the actions of others.
   b. usually passive and silent when faced with a situation they don't like.
   c. aware that their locus of control is internal, not external.
   d. aware that their locus of control is external, not internal.

10. Which of the following statements about psychological health is *incorrect?*
    a. Individuals with social phobia typically fear and avoid various social situations.
    b. Mentally healthy individuals value themselves, accept their limitations, and carry out their responsibilities.
    c. In one study, fewer than 15 percent of college students reported high levels of anger, anxiety, and depression.
    d. Depressed individuals are less likely to develop heart problems.

Answers to these questions can be found on page 376.

Critical Thinking

1. Identify three stressful situations in your life and determine whether they are examples of eustress or distress. Describe both the positive and negative aspects of each situation.

2. Can you think of any ways in which your behavior or attitudes might create stress for others? What changes could you make to avoid doing so?

3. What advice might you give an incoming freshman at your school about managing stress in college? What techniques have been most helpful for you in dealing with stress? Suppose that this student is from a different ethnic group than you. What additional suggestions would you have for this student?

4. Would you say that you view life positively or negatively? Would your friends and family agree with your assessment? Ask two of your closest friends for feedback about what they perceive are your typical responses to a problematic situation. Are these indicative of positive attitudes? If not, what could you do to become more psychologically positive?

Media Menu

Health⊗Now™

Don't forget to check out the wealth of resources on the HealthNow website at **http://healthnow.brookscole.com/itw** that will:
- Help you evaluate your knowledge of the material
- Allow you to take an exam-prep quiz
- Provide a Personalized Learning Plan targeting resources that address areas you should study
- Coach you through identifying target goals for behavior change and creating and monitoring your personal change plan throughout the semester.

INTERNET CONNECTIONS

Stress Management: A Review of Principles
www.unl.edu/stress/mgmt/
This is an online series of lectures on stress management presented by Wesley E. Sime, Ph.D., M.P.H., Professor of Health and Human Performance at the University of Nebraska—Lincoln. It features information on the psychobiology of stress and relaxation as well as the pathophysiology of stress.

How to Survive Unbearable Stress
www.teachhealth.com
This comprehensive website is written specifically for college students by Steven Burns, M.D. It features the following topics: signs of how to recognize stress, two stress surveys for adults and college students, information on the pathophysiology of stress, the genetics of stress and stress tolerance, and information on how to best manage and even treat stress.

Mind Tools
www.mindtools.com/smpage.html
This site covers a variety of topics on stress management, including recognizing stress, exercise, time management, coping mechanisms, and more. The site also features a free comprehensive personal self-assessment with questions pertaining to work and home stressors, physical

and behavioral signs and symptoms, as well as personal coping skills and resources.

InfoTrac College Edition Activities Dusselier, Laurie et al. "Personal, health, academic, and environmental predictors of stress for residence hall students," *Journal of American College Health,* July-August 2005 v54 i1 p15(10)

1. Which students reported greater levels of stress? Why do you think this is so?
2. What were the most frequent predictors of chronic stress?
3. What is the relationship between depression and stress?

You can find additional readings related to personal health with InfoTrac College Edition, an online library of more than 900 journals and publications. Follow the instructions for accessing InfoTrac College Edition that were packaged with your textbook; then search for articles using a keyword search.

For additional links, resources, and suggested readings on the InfoTrac College Edition, visit our Health and Wellness Resource Center at **http://health .wadsworth.com.**

Key Terms

The terms listed are used on the page indicated. Definitions of the terms are in the Glossary at the end of the book.

adaptive response 121
altruism 140
anxiety 143
assertive 141
autonomy 140
biofeedback 130
culture 133
defense mechanisms 132
depression 143
distress 121
emotional wellness 132
eustress 121
general adaptation syndrome (GAS) 121
guided imagery 129
homeostasis 121
locus of control 141
meditation 129
mental wellness 133
mindfulness 129
mood 137
optimism 136
progressive relaxation 129
self-actualization 133
self-esteem 134
social isolation 141
social phobia 141
spiritual wellness 133
stress 120
stressors 120
values 133
visualization 129

Making Healthy Food Choices

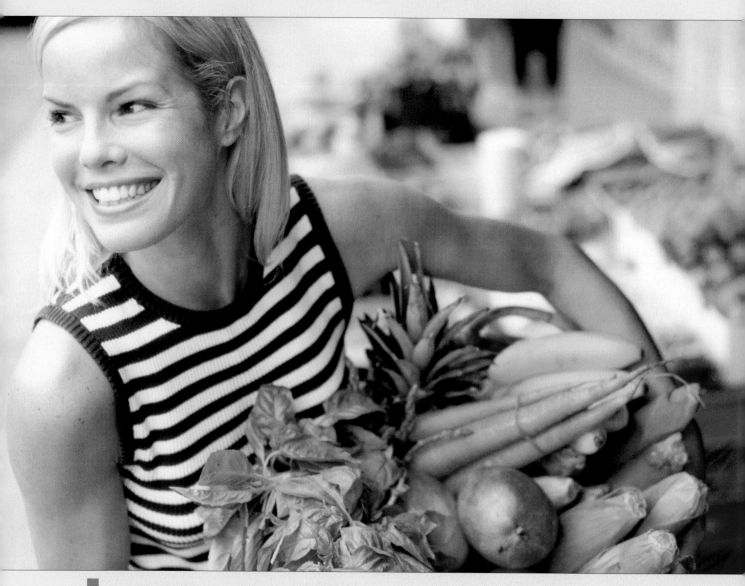

The freshmen on the fifth floor of a university dormitory decided to test a dubious premise: that man—and woman—can live on pizza alone. For a month, they vowed to eat nothing but pizza in all its savory varieties—mushroom, pepperoni, sausage, anchovies, extra cheese, thin crust, double crust. In less than a week, most cringed at the very sight of yet another cardboard delivery box. It wasn't just the boredom of having the same meal that got to them. Some felt bloated. Others had stomachaches. A few complained of headaches and fatigue. One was convinced she had scurvy, a vitamin deficiency disease caused by a lack of fruit and vegetables. None of them managed to stick with pizza for an entire month.

As these students discovered, the foods we choose to eat have an enormous impact on how we feel—and not just in the short term. As demonstrated by the science of **nutrition,** the field that explores the connections between our bodies and the foods we eat, our daily diet affects how long and how well we live. Sensible eating can provide energy for our daily tasks, protect us from many chronic illnesses, and may even extend longevity. A high-quality diet also enhances day-to-day vitality, energy, and sense of well-being.

This chapter can help you make better food choices. It translates the latest information on good nutrition, based on the *2005 Dietary Guidelines for Americans,* into specific advice that you can use to nourish yourself as well as enjoy the pleasure of eating well.

After studying the material in this chapter, you should be able to:

▌ **List** the basic nutrients necessary for a healthy body and **describe** their functions.

▌ **Describe** the key themes of the USDA MyPyramid System.

▌ **List** five specific messages in the 2005 Dietary Guidelines.

▌ **Explain** how to interpret the nutritional information provided on food labels.

▌ **List** the food safety hazards and describe prevention measures.

Health Now™

Don't forget to check out the wealth of resources on the HealthNow website at **http://healthnow.brookscole.com/itw** that will:

• Help you evaluate your knowledge of the material
• Allow you to take an exam-prep quiz
• Provide a Personalized Learning Plan targeting resources that address areas you should study
• Coach you through identifying target goals for behavior change and creating and monitoring your personal change plan throughout the semester.

⬛ What You Need to Know About Nutrients

Every day your body needs certain **essential nutrients** that it cannot manufacture for itself. They provide energy, build and repair body tissues, and regulate body functions. The six classes of essential nutrients, which are discussed in this section, are water, protein, carbohydrates, fats, vitamins, and minerals (**Table 8-1**).

Water makes up about 60 percent of the body and is essential for health and survival. Besides water, we also need energy to live, and we receive our energy from the carbohydrates, proteins, and fats in the foods we eat. The digestive system (**Figure 8-1**) breaks down food into these **macronutrients.** They are the nutrients required by the human body in the greatest amounts. The amount of energy that can be derived from the macronutrients is measured in **calories.** There are 9 calories in every gram of fat and 4 calories in every gram of protein or carbohydrate. The other two essential nutrients —the vitamins and minerals—are called **micronutrients** because our bodies need them in only very small amounts.

Your need for macronutrients depends on how much energy you expend. Because fats, carbohydrates, and protein can all serve as sources of energy, they can, to some extent, substitute for one another in providing calories. Adults, according to federal standards, should get 45 to 65 percent of calories from carbohydrates, 20 to 35 percent from fat, and 10 to 35 percent from protein. Children's fat intake should be slightly higher: 25 to 40 percent of their caloric intake.[1]

To eat well without overeating, choose foods that are "nutrient-dense," that is, foods that provide the most nutritional value. For example, both a cup of nonfat milk and an ounce and a half of cheddar cheese provide about 300 mg of calcium, but the milk offers the same amount of calcium for half the calories. Foods that are extremely low in nutrient density—such as potato chips, candy, and soft drinks—are "empty," delivering only calories with few, if any, nutrients.

How Many Calories Do I Need?

Calories are the measure of the amount of energy that can be derived from food. How many calories you need depends on your gender, age, body-frame size, weight, percentage of body fat, and your **basal metabolic rate (BMR)**—the number of calories needed to sustain your body at rest. Your activity level also affects your calorie requirements. Regardless of whether you consume fat, protein, or carbohydrates, if you take in more calories than required to maintain your size and don't work them off in some sort of physical activity, your body will convert the excess to fat. (See Chapter 9.)

TABLE 8-1 ▌ The Essential Nutrients

	Sources	Functions
Water	Liquids, fruits, and vegetables	Carries nutrients and removes waste; dissolves amino acids, glucose, and minerals; cleans body by removing toxins; regulates body temperature
Proteins	Meat, poultry, fish, eggs, beans, nuts, cheese, tofu, vegetables, cottage cheese, some fruits, pastas, breads, cereal, and rice	Help build new tissue to keep hair, skin, and eyes healthy; build antibodies, enzymes, hormones, and other compounds; provide fuel for body
Carbohydrates	Grains, cereal, pasta, fruits and vegetables, nuts, milk, and sugars	Provide energy
Fats		
Saturated Fats	Red meat, dairy products, egg yolks, and coconut and palm oils; shortening; stick margarine; commercial baked goods	Provide energy; trigger production of cholesterol (see Chapter 10)
Unsaturated Fats	Some fish; nuts; avocados; olive, canola, and peanut oils	Also provide energy, but trigger more "good" cholesterol production and less "bad" cholesterol production (see Chapter 10)
Vitamins	Fruits, vegetables, grains, some meat and dairy products	Facilitate use of other nutrients; involved in regulating growth, maintaining tissue, and manufacturing blood cells, hormones, and other body components
Minerals	Many foods	Help build bones and teeth; aid in muscle function and nervous system activity; assist in various body functions including growth and energy production

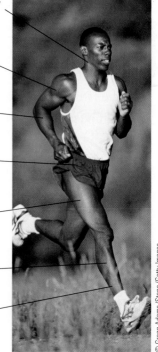

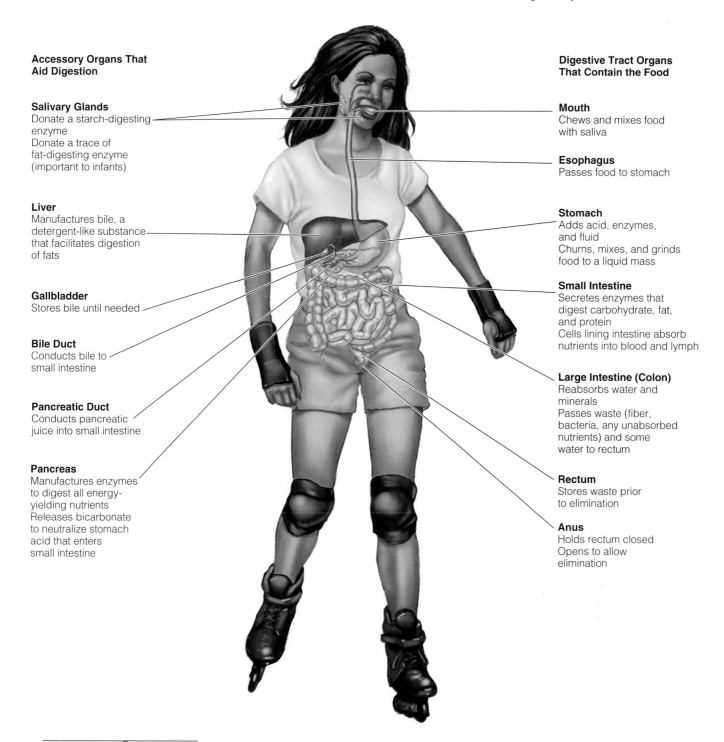

Accessory Organs That Aid Digestion

Salivary Glands
Donate a starch-digesting enzyme
Donate a trace of fat-digesting enzyme (important to infants)

Liver
Manufactures bile, a detergent-like substance that facilitates digestion of fats

Gallbladder
Stores bile until needed

Bile Duct
Conducts bile to small intestine

Pancreatic Duct
Conducts pancreatic juice into small intestine

Pancreas
Manufactures enzymes to digest all energy-yielding nutrients
Releases bicarbonate to neutralize stomach acid that enters small intestine

Digestive Tract Organs That Contain the Food

Mouth
Chews and mixes food with saliva

Esophagus
Passes food to stomach

Stomach
Adds acid, enzymes, and fluid
Churns, mixes, and grinds food to a liquid mass

Small Intestine
Secretes enzymes that digest carbohydrate, fat, and protein
Cells lining intestine absorb nutrients into blood and lymph

Large Intestine (Colon)
Reabsorbs water and minerals
Passes waste (fiber, bacteria, any unabsorbed nutrients) and some water to rectum

Rectum
Stores waste prior to elimination

Anus
Holds rectum closed
Opens to allow elimination

FIGURE 8-1 ▮ The Digestive System
The organs of the digestive system break down food into nutrients that the body can use.

On average, daily calorie needs are:

▮ Most women, some older adults, children ages two to six: 1,600
▮ Average adult: 2,000
▮ Most men, active women, teenage girls, older children: 2,200
▮ Active men, teenage boys: 2,800

Water

Water, which makes up 85 percent of blood, 70 percent of muscles, and about 75 percent of the brain, performs many essential functions: It carries nutrients, maintains temperature, lubricates joints, helps with digestion, rids the body of waste through urine, and contributes to the production of sweat, which evaporates from the skin to

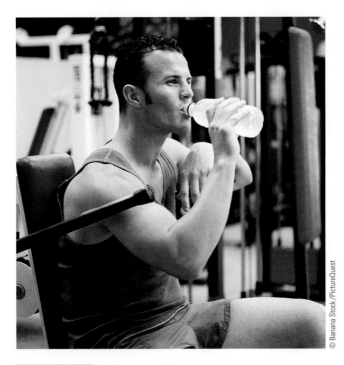

▌Water is an essential nutrient. Remember: each day you must replace the amount you use.

cool the body. Research has correlated high fluid intake with a lower risk of kidney stones, colon cancer, and bladder cancer.

You lose about 64 to 80 ounces of water a day—the equivalent of eight to ten 8-ounce glasses—through perspiration, urination, bowel movements, and normal exhalation. You lose water more rapidly if you exercise, live in a dry climate or at a high altitude, drink a lot of caffeine or alcohol (which increase urination), skip a meal, or become ill. To assure adequate water intake, nutritionists advise drinking a minimum of 64 ounces, enough so that your urine is not dark in color. Healthy individuals can get adequate hydration from beverages other than plain water, including juice and soft drinks.[2]

Protein

Critical for growth and repair, **proteins** form the basic framework for our muscles, bones, blood, hair, and fingernails. Supplying 4 calories per gram, they are made of combinations of 20 **amino acids,** 9 of which we must get from our diet because the human body cannot produce them. These are called *essential amino acids.*

Animal proteins—meat, fish, poultry, and dairy products—are **complete proteins** that provide the nine essential amino acids. Grains, dry beans, and nuts are **incomplete proteins** that may have relatively low levels of one or two essential amino acids but fairly high levels of others. Combining incomplete proteins, such as beans and rice, ensures that the body gets sufficient protein. The recommended level of protein intake is 0.8 gram per kilogram of body weight for adults.

Carbohydrates

Carbohydrates are organic compounds that provide our brains and bodies with *glucose,* their basic fuel. The major sources of carbohydrates are plants—including grains, vegetables, fruits, and beans—and milk. There are two types: *simple carbohydrates* (sugars) and *complex carbohydrates* (starches and fiber). All provide 4 calories per gram. Both adults and children should consume at least 130 grams of carbohydrates each day, the minimum needed to produce enough glucose for the brain to function.

Forms of Carbohydrates

Simple carbohydrates include *natural sugars,* such as the lactose in milk and the fructose in fruit, and *added sugars* that are found in candy, soft drinks, fruit drinks, pastries, and other sweets. Those whose diets are higher in added sugars typically have lower intakes of other essential nutrients.

Complex carbohydrates include grains, cereals, vegetables, beans, and nuts. Americans, however, get most of their complex carbohydrates from refined grains, which have been stripped of fiber and many nutrients.[3]

Far more nutritious are whole grains, which are made up of all components of the grain: the *bran* (or fiber-rich outer layer), the *endosperm* (middle layer), and the *germ* (the nutrient-packed inner layer). Increasing whole-grain consumption has become a public health priority, and the 2005 Dietary Guidelines recommend that Americans increase their consumption of whole-grain foods.[4] Individuals who eat whole-grain products each day have about a 15 to 25 percent reduction in death from all causes, including heart disease and cancer.[5]

Should I Switch to Low-Carb Foods?

The popularity of diets that restrict carbohydrate intake, such as the Atkins diet discussed in Chapter 9, prompted an explosion in products touted as "low-carb." You can get low-carb versions of everything from beer to bread. However, the Food and Drug Administration (FDA), which regulates health claims on food labels in the United States, hasn't defined what *low-carb* means. Words like *low-carb, carb-wise,* or *carb-free* are marketing terms created by manufacturers to sell their products.

Although many people may buy low-carbohydrate foods because they believe that they're healthier, that isn't necessarily the case. A low-carb nutrition bar, for instance, may be high in saturated fat and calories. Since low-carb food products are relatively new on grocery shelves, no one knows their long-term hazards. Some cause digestive symptoms because food companies often replace the carbohydrates in a cookie or cracker with substances such as the sweetener sorbitol, which can cause diarrhea or stomach cramps.

Dieters often buy low-carb products in order to lose weight. According to proponents of low-carbohydrate diets, if carbohydrates raise blood sugar and insulin levels and cause weight gain, a decrease in carbs should result in lower blood sugar and insulin levels—and weight loss. With limited carbohydrates in the diet, the body would break down fat to provide needed energy.[6]

Some people do lose weight when they switch to low-carb foods, but the reasons are probably that they consumer fewer calories, lose water weight, and have decreased appetite because of a buildup of ketones (a by-product of fat metabolism) in the blood.[7] As discussed in Chapter 9, a low-carb diet can lead to fairly rapid weight loss but is no easier to maintain over the long run than any other diet.[8]

Glycemic Index and Glycemic Load

The glycemic index is a ranking of carbohydrates, gram for gram, based on their immediate effect on blood glucose (sugar) levels. Carbohydrates that break down quickly during digestion and trigger a fast, high glu-cose response have the highest glycemic index rating. Those that break down slowly, releasing glucose gradu-ally into the blood stream, have low glycemic index ratings. Potatoes, which raise blood sugar higher and faster than apples, for instance, earn a higher glycemic-index rating than apples. Glycemic index does not ac-count for the amount of food you typically eat in a serving.

Glycemic load is a measure of how much a typical serving size of a particular food raises blood glucose. For example, the glycemic index of table sugar is high, but you use so little to sweeten your coffee or tea that its glycemic load is low.[9]

Some diets are based on the theory that high-glycemic-index foods raise blood sugar and insulin levels and cause weight gain, while low-glycemic-index foods lower your blood sugar and insulin levels so you'll lose weight. Although some people do lose weight on low-glycemic diets, this theory has not been scientifically proved. Experts are dubious because many factors play a role in how much blood glucose rises, including age and weight. And people typically don't eat single foods at a meal, but a combination of foods that affect blood sugar differently.

Fiber

Dietary fiber is the nondigestible form of complex carbohydrates occurring naturally in plant foods, such as leaves, stems, skins, seeds, and hulls. **Functional fiber** consists of isolated, nondigestible carbohydrates that may be added to foods and that provide beneficial effects in humans. Total fiber is the sum of both.

The various forms of fiber enhance health in dif-ferent ways: They slow the emptying of the stomach, which creates a feeling of fullness and aids weight con-trol. They interfere with absorption of dietary fat and cholesterol, which lowers the risk of heart disease and

stroke in both middle-aged and elderly individuals.[10] In addition, fiber helps prevent constipation, diverticulosis (a painful inflammation of the bowel), and diabetes.[11] The link between fiber and colon cancer is complex. Some studies have indicated that increased fiber intake reduces risk; a large-scale study of almost 90,000 women found no such correlation.[12]

The Institute of Medicine has set the first-ever rec-ommendations for daily intake levels of total fiber (di-etary plus functional fiber): 38 grams of total fiber for men and 25 grams for women. For men and women over 50 years of age, who consume less food, the recommen-dations are, respectively, 30 and 21 grams. The American Dietetic Association recommends 25 to 35 grams of di-etary fiber a day, much more than the amount Americans typically consume.[13]

Good fiber sources include wheat and corn bran (the outer layer); leafy greens; the skins of fruits and root vegetables; oats, beans, and barley; and the pulp, skin, and seeds of many fruits and vegetables, such as apples and strawberries (**Table 8-2**). Because sudden increases in fiber can cause symptoms like bloating and gas, experts recommend gradually adding more fiber to your diet with an additional serving or two of vegetables, fruit, or whole wheat bread.

Fats

Fats carry the fat-soluble vitamins A, D, E, and K; aid in their absorption in the intestine; protect organs from injury; regulate body temperature; and play an impor-tant role in growth and development. They provide 9 calories per gram—more than twice the amount in carbohydrates or proteins.

Both high- and low-fat diets can be unhealthy. When people eat very low levels of fat and very high levels of carbohydrates, their levels of high-density lipoprotein, the so-called *good cholesterol,* declines. On the other hand, high-fat diets can lead to obesity and its related health dangers, discussed in Chapter 9.

Forms of Fat

Saturated fats and **unsaturated fats** are distinguished by the type of fatty acids in their chemical structures. Unsaturated fats can be divided into monounsaturated or polyunsaturated, again depending on their chemical struc-ture. All dietary fats are a mix of saturated and unsaturated fats but are predominantly one or the other.[14] Unsaturated fats, like oils, are likely to be liquid at room temperature and saturated fats, like butter, are likely to be solid. In general, vegetable and fish oils are unsaturated and animal fats are saturated.

Olive, soybean, canola, cottonseed, corn, and other vegetable oils are unsaturated fats. Used for thousands of years, olive oil, a staple of the Mediterranean diet, dis-cussed later in this chapter, has been correlated with a

TABLE 8-2 ❚ Putting Fiber into Meals and Snacks

High-Fiber Options for Breakfast

Whole-grain toast		2 g per slice
Bran cereal:		
Bran flakes	1 cup	7 g
All bran	1/3 cup	10 g
Raisin bran	3/4 cup	5 g
Oat bran	1/3 cup	5 g
Bran muffin, with fruit	1 small	3 g
Strawberries	10	2 g
Raspberries	1/2 cup	3 g
Banana	1 medium	2 g

Lunches that Include Fiber

Whole-grain bread		2 g per slice
Baked beans	1/2 cup	10 g
Carrot	1 medium	2 g
Raisins	1/4 cup	2 g
Peas	1/2 cup	6 g
Peanut butter	2 tablespoons	2 g

Fiber on the Menu for Supper

Brown rice	1/2 cup	2 g
Potato	1 medium	3 g
Dried cooked beans	1/2 cup	8 g
Broccoli	1/2 cup	3 g
Corn	1/2 cup	5 g
Tomato	1 medium	2 g
Green beans	1/2 cup	3 g

Fiber-Filled Snacks

Peanuts	1/4 cup	3 g
Apple	1 medium	2 g
Pear	1 medium	4 g
Orange	1 medium	3 g
Prunes*	3	2 g
Sunflower seeds	1/4 cup	2 g
Popcorn	2 cups	2 g

* Prunes contain fiber, but their laxative effect is primarily due to a naturally occurring chemical substance that causes an uptake of fluid into the intestines and the contraction of muscles that line the intestines.

Source: Judith E. Brown. *Nutrition Now,* 3rd ed. Belmont, CA: Wadsworth, 2002.

lower incidence of heart disease, including strokes and heart attacks.

Fish oils are rich in omega-3 fatty acids, which make molecules such as prostaglandins that enhance cardiovascular health. Fish oils also improve healthy blood lipid levels (fats), prevent blood clots, ward off the age-related vision problem called macular degeneration, and may lower blood pressure, especially in people with hypertension or atherosclerosis.[15] However, most college students do not consume the recommended amount of omega-3 fatty acids.[16]

In contrast, saturated fats can increase the risk of heart disease and should be avoided as much as possible. In response to consumer and health professionals' demand for less saturated fat in the food supply, many manufacturers switched to partially hydrogenated oils.

The process of hydrogenation creates unsaturated fatty acids called **trans fat.** They are found in some margarine products and most foods made with partially hydrogenated oils, such as baked goods and fried foods. Even though trans fats are unsaturated, they appear similar to saturated fats in terms of raising cholesterol levels. Epidemiological studies have suggested a possible link between cardiovascular disease risk and high intakes of trans fats, and researchers have concluded that they are, gram for gram, twice as damaging as saturated fat. There is no safe level for trans fats, which occur naturally in meats as well as in foods prepared with partially hydrogenated vegetable oils.

To cut down on both saturated and trans fats, choose soybean, canola, corn, olive, safflower, and sunflower oils. Look for reduced-fat, low-fat, fat-free, and trans fat–free versions of baked goods, snacks, and other processed foods. **Table 8-3** compares saturated fat content and calories for some typical foods.

TABLE 8-3 ❚ Comparing Saturated Fat and Calorie Content

Food	Saturated Fat Content (grams)	Calories
Cheese (1 oz.)		
Regular cheddar cheese	6.0	114
Low-fat cheddar cheese	1.2	49
Ground Beef (3 oz. cooked)		
Regular ground beef (25% fat)	6.1	236
Extra lean ground beef (5% fat)	2.6	148
Milk (1 cup)		
Whole milk (3.24%)	4.6	146
Low-fat (1%) milk	1.5	102
Breads (1 medium)		
Croissant	6.6	231
Bagel, oat bran (4")	0.2	227
Frozen desserts (1/2 cup)		
Regular ice cream	4.9	145
Frozen yogurt	2.0	110
Table spreads (1 tsp)		
Butter	2.4	34
Trans fat–free soft margarine	0.7	25
Chicken (3 oz. cooked)		
Fried chicken (leg)	3.3	212
Chicken breast	0.9	140
Fish (3 oz.)		
Fried fish	2.8	195
Baked fish	1.5	129

Source: ARS Nutrient Database for Standard Reference, 2005 Dietary Guidelines Advisory Committee Report.

Do Men and Women Have Different Nutritional Needs?

Men and women do not need to eat different foods, but their nutritional needs are different. Because most men are bigger and taller than most women, they consume more calories. Eating more means it's easier for them to get the nutrients they need, even though many don't make the wisest food choices.

Women, particularly those who restrict their caloric intake or are chronically dieting, are more likely to develop specific deficiencies. Calcium is one example. Women drink less milk than men, and many do not consume the recommended 800 to 1,200 milligrams of calcium daily. This deficiency increases the risk of bone-weakening osteoporosis.

Many women also get too little iron. Even in adolescence, girls are more prone to iron deficiency than boys; some suffer memory and learning impairments as a result. In adult women, menstrual blood loss and poor eating habits can lead to low iron stores, which puts them at risk for anemia. According to U.S. Department of Agriculture research, most women consume only 60 percent of the recommended 15 milligrams of iron per day. (The recommendation for men is 10 milligrams.) Regular blood tests can monitor a woman's iron status.

Here are some gender-specific strategies for better nutrition:

▌ Men should cut back on fat and meat in their diets, two things they eat too much.

▌ Women should increase their iron intake by eating meat (iron from animal sources is absorbed better than that from vegetable sources) or a combination of meat and vegetable iron sources together (for example, a meat and bean burrito). Those with iron deficiencies should consult a physician. Because large doses of iron can be toxic, iron supplements should be taken only with medical supervision.

▌ Women should consume more calcium-rich foods, including low-fat and nonfat dairy products, leafy greens, and tofu. Women who cannot get adequate amounts of calcium from their daily diet should take calcium supplements. This is not advised for all men because of a possible connection between calcium and prostate cancer.

▌ Women who could become pregnant should take a multivitamin with 400 *micro*grams (mcg) of **folic acid,** which helps prevent neural tube defects such as spina bifida. Folic acid is also useful to men because it may cut the risk of heart disease, stroke, and colon cancer.

▌ Both genders should increase their fruit and vegetable intake to ensure that they are getting adequate amounts of vitamins and fiber in their daily diet.

Vitamins and Minerals

Vitamins, which help put proteins, fats, and carbohydrates to use, are essential to regulating growth, maintaining tissue, and releasing energy from foods. Together with the enzymes in the body, they help produce the right chemical reactions at the right times. They're also involved in the manufacture of blood cells, hormones, and other compounds.

The body produces some vitamins, such as vitamin D, which is manufactured in the skin after exposure to sunlight. Other vitamins must be ingested.

Vitamins A, D, E, and K are fat-soluble; they are absorbed through the intestinal membranes and stored in the body.

The B vitamins and vitamin C are water soluble; they are absorbed directly into the blood and then used up or washed out of the body in urine and sweat. They must be replaced daily.

Antioxidants are substances that prevent the harmful effects caused by oxidation within the body. They include vitamins C, E, and beta-carotene (a form of vitamin A), as well as compounds like carotenoids and

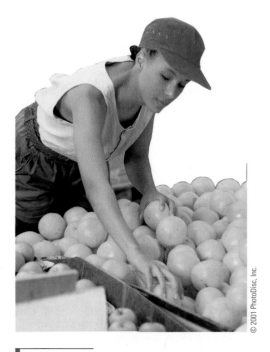

© 2001 PhotoDisc, Inc.

▌ Antioxidants are found in vegetables and fruit. By eating an orange at breakfast and half a carrot for lunch, you will have all the antioxidants you need for the day.

flavonoids. All share a common enemy: renegade oxygen cells called *free radicals* released by normal metabolism, as well as by pollution, smoking, radiation, and stress.

Diets high in antioxidant-rich fruits and vegetables have been linked with lower rates of esophageal, lung, colon, and stomach cancer. Nevertheless, scientific studies have not proved conclusively that any specific antioxidant, particularly in supplement form, can prevent cancer.

Carbon, oxygen, hydrogen, and nitrogen make up 96 percent of our body weight. The other 4 percent consists of **minerals** that help build bones and teeth, aid in muscle function, and help our nervous system transmit messages. Every day we need about a tenth of a gram (100 milligrams, or mgs) or more of the major minerals: sodium and potassium chloride, calcium, phosphorus, magnesium, and sulfur. We also need about a hundredth of a gram (10 milligrams) or less of each of the trace minerals: iron (although premenopausal women need more), zinc, selenium, molybdenum, iodine, copper, manganese, fluoride, and chromium.

Americans get adequate amounts of most nutrients. However, the 2005 Advisory Committee for Dietary Guidelines reported that intakes of several nutrients are low enough to be of concern (**Table 8-4**):

❚ **For adults:** vitamins A, C, and E, calcium, magnesium, potassium, and fiber
❚ **For children:** vitamin E, calcium, magnesium, potassium, and fiber

Among the groups at highest risk of nutritional deficiencies are:

❚ **Teenage girls**
❚ **Women of child-bearing age** (iron and folic acid)
❚ **Persons over age 50** (vitamin B_{12})
❚ **The elderly, persons with dark skin,** and those who do not get adequate exposure to sunshine (vitamin D)[17]

Calcium

Calcium, the most abundant mineral in the body, builds strong bone tissue throughout life and plays a vital role in blood clotting and muscle and nerve functioning. Pregnant or nursing women need more calcium to meet the additional needs of their babies' bodies. Calcium may also help control high blood pressure, prevent colon cancer in adults, and promote weight loss.

Adequate calcium intake during childhood, adolescence, and young adulthood is crucial to prevent **osteoporosis,** the bone-weakening disease that strikes one of every four women over the age of 60. National health organizations are promoting greater calcium consumption among college students, particularly women, to increase bone density and safeguard against osteoporosis.

TABLE 8-4 ❚ Are You Getting Enough of These Nutrients?	
Nutrient	**Function**
Vitamin A	Vitamin A plays a significant role in vision, gene expression, cellular differentiation, growth, immune function, and maintenance of healthy bones, teeth, and hair.
Vitamin C	As a dietary antioxidant, vitamin C counteracts the oxidative damage to biomolecules; additionally, vitamin C helps strengthen blood vessels and maintain healthy gums and aids in the absorption of iron.
Vitamin E	As a dietary antioxidant, vitamin E counteracts the oxidative damage to biomolecules; in addition, vitamin E helps in the formation of red blood cells and muscles.
Calcium	Calcium is the key nutrient in the development and maintenance of bones; additionally, calcium aids in blood clotting and muscle and nerve functioning.
Magnesium	Magnesium plays a key role in the development and maintenance of bones, and activates enzymes necessary for energy release.
Potassium	Potassium assists in muscle contraction, maintaining fluid and electrolyte balance in cells, transmitting nerve impulses, and releasing energy during metabolism. Diets rich in potassium lower blood pressure, blunt the adverse effects of salt on blood pressure, may reduce the risk of developing kidney stones, and may decrease bone loss.
Dietary fiber	Fiber helps maintain the health of the digestive tract and promotes proper bowel functioning.

In a study of college athletes, the most common food sources of calcium for both white and black students were mixed dishes and dairy products. There were no racial differences in calcium consumption levels, but male athletes consumed significantly more calcium than females.

In both men and women, bone mass peaks between the ages of 25 and 35. Over the next 10 to 15 years, bone mass remains fairly stable. At about age 40, bone loss equivalent to 0.3 to 0.5 percent per year begins in both men and women. Women may experience greater bone loss, at a rate of 3 to 5 percent, at the time of menopause. This decline continues for approximately five to seven years and is the primary factor leading to postmenopausal osteoporosis.

The higher an individual's peak bone mass, the longer it takes for age- and menopause-related bone losses to increase the risk of fractures. Osteoporosis is less common in groups with higher peak bone mass—men versus women, blacks versus whites. A combination of calcium and exercise can boost bone mineral density in teenage girls, which may prevent or delay osteoporosis later in life.[18]

Dietary calcium, according to recent clinical trials, can significantly reduce body fat in obese men and women, even if they are not dieting, and can accelerate weight loss for those on a reduced-calorie diet.[19]

Calcium is a special concern for African Americans who, as a group, have a higher risk for high blood pressure and obesity than the rest of the population but, on average, consume less than one serving of dairy foods a day. In fact, more than 80 percent of African Americans fail to get their daily recommended amount of calcium.[20]

Sodium

Sodium helps maintain proper fluid balance, regulates blood pressure, transmits muscle impulses, and relaxes muscles. Excess sodium isn't a problem for most healthy people, but for those who are sodium-sensitive—as many as 30 percent of the population—too much sodium contributes to high blood pressure.

The National Heart, Lung, and Blood Institute recommends less than 2.4 grams (2,400 milligrams) of sodium a day, the equivalent of about one teaspoon of table salt a day. For someone with high blood pressure, a daily intake of less than 1,500 mg of sodium is better for lowering blood pressure.

Blacks, who have higher rates of high blood pressure and diseases related to hypertension, such as stroke and kidney failure, tend to be more sensitive to salt than nonblacks. African Americans also have lower intakes of calcium and potassium—both of which can protect against heart disease.[21]

STRATEGIES

for CHANGE

Building Stronger Bones

┃ Make calcium-rich foods part of your daily diet. These include dairy products, leafy green vegetables, canned fish, and tofu. Also look for products fortified with calcium and vitamin D, which aids in calcium absorption.

┃ Avoid cigarette smoking, which has been linked with bone loss.

┃ Drink alcohol only in moderation. Prolonged or heavy use of alcohol may decrease bone metabolism.

┃ Be wary of high-protein diets. Excess protein intake may increase the rate of calcium loss from the body.

┃ Do weight-bearing exercises. Activities such as walking, running, doing push-ups and sit-ups, and lifting weights all contribute to the development and maintenance of bone mass.

Phytochemicals

Phytochemicals, compounds that exist naturally in plants, serve many functions, including helping a plant protect itself from bacteria and disease. Some phytochemicals such as solanine, an insect-repelling chemical found in the leaves and stalks of potato plants, are natural toxins, but many are beneficial to humans. Flavonoids, found in apples, strawberries, grapes, onions, green and black tea, and red wine, may decrease atherosclerotic plaque and DNA damage related to cancer development. Phytochemicals are associated with a reduced risk of heart disease, certain cancers, age-related macular degeneration, adult-onset diabetes, stroke, and other diseases. However, in Western societies, research has shown neither an increase nor decrease in breast cancer with consumption of phytochemicals.[22]

Should I Take Dietary Supplements?

Many health experts feel that the best way to make sure your body gets the vitamins and minerals it needs is to eat a wide variety of foods. Nonetheless, 52 percent of adults report taking a dietary supplement in the past month; 35 percent take a multivitamin/multimineral. More than 5 percent of adults take vitamin C, vitamin E, B-complex vitamins, calcium, or calcium-containing antacids. Individuals who use supplements are more likely to be female, older, more educated, white, physically active, normal- or underweight, in good or excellent health, former smokers, and more frequent drinkers of wine or spirits. About half take just one supplement.[23]

Marketed as foods, supplements do not have to undergo the same rigorous testing required of drugs. They can carry *structure/function claims*—claims that a product may affect the structure or functioning of the body—but not claims that they can treat, diagnose, cure, or prevent a disease. For example, statements such as "helps maintain a healthy cholesterol level" are acceptable, while statements like "lowers cholesterol levels" are not.

The FDA has issued rules for nutritional supplement labeling. Labels must include an information panel titled Supplement Facts (similar to the Nutrition Facts panel that appears on processed foods), a clear identity statement, and a complete list of ingredients.

Scientists note that most health benefits and dangers stem from more than one source, so it's unlikely that changing any one nutrient will in itself produce great benefits—and may, by interfering with the complex balance of nutrients, do harm. In particular, the fat-soluble vitamins, primarily A and D, can build up in our bodies and cause serious complications, such as damage to the kidneys, liver, or bones. Large doses of water-soluble vitamins, including the B vitamins, may also be harmful.

Excessive intake of vitamin B_6 (pyridoxine), often used to relieve premenstrual bloating, can cause neurological damage, such as numbness in the mouth and tingling in the hands. (An excessive amount in this case is 250 to 300 times the recommended dose.) High doses of vitamin C can produce stomachaches and diarrhea. Niacin, often taken in high doses to lower cholesterol, can cause jaundice, liver damage, and irregular heartbeats as well as severe, uncomfortable flushing of the skin.

▮ Using the MyPyramid System to Eat Smarter

Making healthy choices about what and how to eat isn't easy. However, the federal government is trying to help. In its most recent edition of *Nutrition and Your Health: Dietary Guidelines for Americans,* the Department of Health and Human Services and the U.S. Department of Agriculture provides science-based advice both to promote wellness and to reduce the risk of major chronic diseases. The MyPyramid Food Guidance System (**Figure 8–2**) translates the Guidelines into a personalized, balanced, total diet.

The key themes of MyPyramid are:

▮ **Variety:** eating foods from all food groups and subgroups

▮ **Proportionality:** eating more of some foods (fruits, vegetables, whole grains, fat-free or low-fat milk products) and less of others (foods high in saturated or trans fats, added sugars, cholesterol, salt, and alcohol)

▮ **Moderation:** choosing forms of foods that limit intake of saturated or trans fats, added sugars, cholesterol, salt, and alcohol

▮ **Activity:** being physically active every day

▮ **Personalization:** finding the kinds and amounts of food to eat each day at www.MyPyramid.gov (See your Lab Booklet.)

The following guidelines, based on the MyPyramid system, can help you eat smart—and stay well.

Consume a Variety of Foods

The six colors on the MyPyramid graphic represent the five food groups—grains, vegetables, fruits, milk, and meat and beans—and oils. The greater the variety of colors and of foods you choose, the more likely you are to obtain the nutrients you need (**Table 8–5**). In general, the USDA recommends a diet that is high in fruits and vegetables, whole grains, and nonfat or low-fat milk products that provides amounts of nutrients (including potassium and fiber) that can help reduce the risk of chronic disease and is low in saturated fat, cholesterol, added sugars, trans fat, and sodium.

Manage Your Weight

As discussed in Chapter 9, you must expend as much energy (calories) as you take in to stay at the same weight. Among the best ways to balance this energy equation are limiting portion sizes (discussed later in this chapter), substituting nutrient-rich foods (such as raw vegetables or low-fat soups) for nutrient-poor foods (such as candy and cake), and limiting added sugars, solid fats, and alcoholic beverages.

Get Physical Every Day

As discussed in Chapter 3, regular physical activity helps maintain a healthy weight and reduces risk for several chronic diseases. While 30 minutes of moderate physical activity (such as walking at a pace of three or four miles an hour) on most days provides important benefits, exercising more often and more intensely yields additional health dividends. Many adults need up to 60 minutes of moderate to vigorous physical activity—the equivalent of 150 to 200 calories, depending on body size, daily to prevent unhealthy weight gain. Men and women who have lost weight may need 60 to 90 minutes to keep off excess pounds. Children and teenagers require at least 60 minutes of moderate physical activity every day.[24]

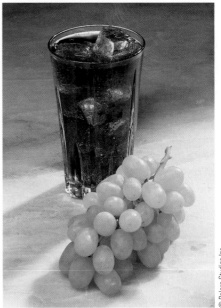

▮ This cola and bunch of grapes each provide about 150 calories, but the nutrient-rich grapes offer a trace of protein, some vitamins, minerals, and fiber. The cola beverage offers only "empty" calories from sugar without any other nutrients.

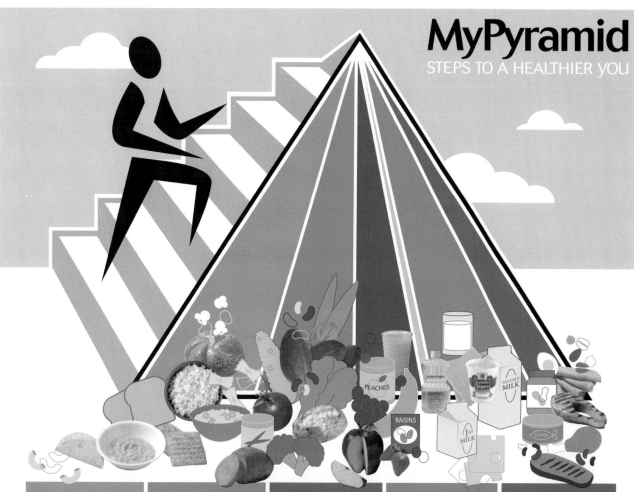

MyPyramid
STEPS TO A HEALTHIER YOU

GRAINS	VEGETABLES	FRUITS	MILK	MEAT & BEANS
Make half your grains whole	Vary your veggies	Focus on fruits	Get your calcium-rich foods	Go lean with protein
Eat at least 3 oz. of whole-grain cereals, breads, crackers, rice, or pasta every day 1 oz. is about 1 slice of bread, about 1 cup of breakfast cereal, or ½ cup of cooked rice, cereal, or pasta	Eat more dark-green veggies like broccoli, spinach, and other dark leafy greens Eat more orange vegetables like carrots and sweet potatoes Eat more dry beans and peas like pinto beans, kidney beans, and lentils	Eat a variety of fruit Choose fresh, frozen, canned, or dried fruit Go easy on fruit juices	Go low-fat or fat-free when you choose milk, yogurt, and other milk products If you don't or can't consume milk, choose lactose-free products or other calcium sources such as fortified foods and beverages	Choose low-fat or lean meats and poultry Bake it, broil it, or grill it Vary your protein routine — choose more fish, beans, peas, nuts, and seeds

For a 2,000-calorie diet, you need the amounts below from each food group. To find the amounts that are right for you, go to MyPyramid.gov.

Eat 6 oz. every day	Eat 2½ cups every day	Eat 2 cups every day	Get 3 cups every day; for kids aged 2 to 8, it's 2	Eat 5½ oz. every day

Find your balance between food and physical activity
- Be sure to stay within your daily calorie needs.
- Be physically active for at least 30 minutes most days of the week.
- About 60 minutes a day of physical activity may be needed to prevent weight gain.
- For sustaining weight loss, at least 60 to 90 minutes a day of physical activity may be required.
- Children and teenagers should be physically active for 60 minutes every day, or most days.

Know the limits on fats, sugars, and salt (sodium)
- Make most of your fat sources from fish, nuts, and vegetable oils.
- Limit solid fats like butter, stick margarine, shortening, and lard, as well as foods that contain these.
- Check the Nutrition Facts label to keep saturated fats, *trans* fats, and sodium low.
- Choose food and beverages low in added sugars. Added sugars contribute calories with few, if any, nutrients.

MyPyramid.gov
STEPS TO A HEALTHIER YOU

FIGURE 8-2 | The MyPyramid Food Guidance System

Source: U.S. Department of Agriculture, www.MyPyramid.gov.

TABLE 8-5 Nutrient Contributions of Each Food Group

Food group	Major contribution(s)[1]	Substantial contribution(s) (>10% of total)[2]		
Fruit Group	Vitamin C	Thiamin Vitamin B$_6$ Folate	Copper Potassium Carbohydrate	Magnesium Fiber
Vegetable Group	Vitamin A Potassium	Vitamin E Vitamin C Thiamin Niacin Vitamin B$_6$	Magnesium Iron Zinc Copper Carbohydrate	Folate Calcium Phosphorus Fiber Alpha-linolenic acid
Vegetable Subgroups:				
Dark green vegetables		Vitamin A Vitamin C		
Orange vegetables	Vitamin A			
Legumes		Folate Copper	Fiber	
Starchy vegetables		Vitamin B$_6$ Copper		
Other vegetables			Vitamin C	
Grain Group	Thiamin Folate Magnesium Iron Copper Carbohydrate Fiber	Vitamin A Riboflavin Niacin Vitamin B$_6$ Vitamin B$_{12}$ Calcium	Phosphorus Zinc Potassium Protein Linoleic acid Alpha-linolenic acid	
Grain Subgroups:				
Whole grains	Folate (tie) Magnesium Iron Copper Carbohydrate (tie) Fiber	Thiamin Riboflavin Niacin Vitamin B$_6$	Vitamin B$_{12}$ Phosphorus Zinc Protein	
Enriched grains	Folate (tie) Thiamin Carbohydrate (tie)	Riboflavin Niacin	Iron Copper	
Meat, Poultry, Fish, Eggs, and Nuts Group	Niacin Vitamin B$_6$ Zinc Protein	Vitamin E Thiamin Riboflavin Vitamin B$_{12}$ Phosphorus	Magnesium Iron Copper Potassium Linoleic acid	
Milk Group	Riboflavin Vitamin B$_{12}$ Calcium Phosphorus	Vitamin A Thiamin Vitamin B$_6$ Magnesium	Zinc Potassium Carbohydrate Protein	
Oils and Soft Margarines	Vitamin E Linoleic acid Alpha-linolenic acid			

1. *Major contribution* means that the food group or subgroup provides more of the nutrient than any other single food group, averaged over all calorie levels. When two food groups or subgroups provide equal amounts, it is noted as a tie.

2. A *substantial contribution* means that the food group or subgroup provides 10% or more of the total amount of the nutrient in the food patterns, averaged over all calorie levels.

Source: 2005 Dietary Guidelines Advisory Committee. *Report of the Dietary Guidelines Advisory Committee on the Dietary Guidelines for Americans, 2005.* Washington, DC: Health and Human Services and U.S. Department of Agriculture, 2004, www.health.gov/dietaryguidelines/dga2005/report.

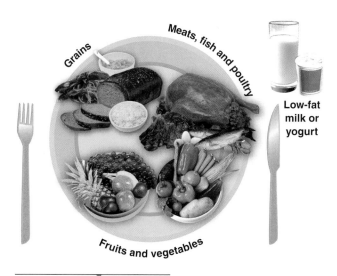

FIGURE 8-3 ▌ Make Fruits and Vegetables Half Your Plate . . . Every Meal

Increase Foods from Certain Food Groups

Greater consumption of fruits and vegetables (5 to 13 servings or 2½ to 6½ cups per day, depending on how many calories you burn) may reduce the risk of stroke, certain cancers, and type 2 diabetes (vegetables more so than fruit) as well as helping reach and maintain a healthy weight (**Figure 8–3**). The more fruits and vegetables men and women consume, the lower their levels of harmful low-density lipoprotein (LDL) cholesterol.[25] Plant-based foods also reduce the risk of rectal cancer in both men and women (**Table 8–6**).[26]

Among the ways to increase your fruit and vegetable intake:

▌ **Toss fruit into a green salad** for extra flavor, variety, color, and crunch.

▌ **Start the day with a daily double:** a glass of juice and a banana or other fruit on cereal.

▌ **Buy pre-cut vegetables** for snacking or dipping (instead of chips).

▌ **Make or order sandwiches** with extra tomatoes or other vegetable toppings.

Consuming at least three servings (the equivalent of 3 ounces) of whole grains per day can reduce the risk of diabetes and coronary heart disease and maintain a healthy weight. To increase your intake of grains:

▌ **Check labels of rolls and bread,** and choose those with at least 2 to 3 grams of fiber per slice.

▌ **Add brown rice or barley** to soups.

▌ **Choose whole-grain** ready-to-eat cereals.

As noted earlier, eating at least three servings of milk, cheese, or yogurt a day may reduce your risk for high blood pressure, obesity, and osteoporosis. Dairy products do not seem to have an effect on breast cancer risk.[27]

TABLE 8-6 ▌ Which Fruits and Vegetables[1] Provide the Most Nutrients?

Sources of Vitamin A (carotenoids)

Bright orange vegetables like carrots, sweet potatoes, and pumpkin

Dark green leafy vegetables such as spinach, collards, and turnip greens

Bright orange fruits like mango, cantaloupe, and apricots

Sources of Vitamin C

Citrus fruits and juices, kiwi fruit, strawberries, and cantaloupe

Broccoli, peppers, tomatoes, cabbage, and potatoes

Leafy greens such as romaine, turnip greens, and spinach

Sources of Folate

Cooked dried beans and peas

Oranges and orange juice

Deep green leaves like spinach and mustard greens

Sources of Potassium

Baked white or sweet potatoes, cooked greens (such as spinach), winter (orange) squash

Bananas, plantains, many dried fruits, and orange juice

1. Often, the fruits and vegetables with brighter colors have the higher content of vitamins and minerals.

Source: Dietary Guidelines for Americans 2005, U.S. Department of Health and Human Services, U.S. Department of Agriculture, **www.healthierus.gov/dietaryguidelines.**

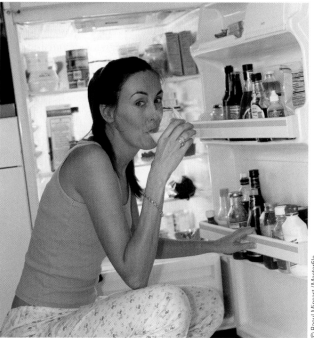

▌ Three servings from the Milk Group each day may reduce the risk of high blood pressure and osteoporosis and can help with weight loss.

To get more dairy products with less fat, try the following:

▮ **Substitute fat-free sour cream** or nonfat, plain yogurt for sour cream.
▮ **Add low-fat milk** instead of water to oatmeal and hot cereals.
▮ **Eat cereals with added calcium** and with milk.
▮ **Top salads or soups with low-fat shredded cheese.**

Be Finicky About Fats

Reducing saturated fat, trans fat, and cholesterol can lower harmful LDL cholesterol and your risk of heart disease. You should keep saturated fat below 10 percent of total calories, trans fat as low as possible, and cholesterol intake below 300 mg per day. Your total fat intake should make up no more than 20 to 35 percent of calories. For children ages 2 and 3, recommended minimum fat intake is 30 percent of calories; for those between ages 4 and 18, it is 25 percent.

To keep within these limits:

▮ **Restrict animal fats** (such as those in cheese, milk, butter, ice cream, and other full-fat dairy products, fatty meat, bacon, sausage, and poultry skin and fat).
▮ **Cut back** on foods made with partially hydrogenated vegetable oils.
▮ **Limit your intake** of eggs and organ meats.

As noted, other fats, particularly the omega-3 fatty acids found in certain fish, can boost your heart's health and reduce your risk of dying of heart disease. The new guidelines recommend two servings of fish high in omega-3 fatty acids every week. Pregnant or nursing women and children should avoid fish with a high mercury content and limit consumption of fish with a moderate mercury content.

Choose Carbohydrates Wisely

Eating more fruits, vegetables, whole grains, and nonfat or low-fat milk and dairy products is a healthful way to get the carbohydrates you need. Fiber-rich choices—an apple rather than apple juice, for example—have the added benefit of promoting digestive health and reduce the risk of type 2 diabetes and heart disease.

The new guidelines do not include a specific message about sugar but caution against "added" sugars, those added to foods during processing or preparation or at the table. Recent research has implicated sugar-sweetened beverages as a culprit in weight gain.[28] Carbohydrates (including sucrose, glucose, fructose, lactose, and starch) also can increase the risk of dental cavities. Drinking fluoridated water and/or using fluoride-containing dental hygiene products can protect your teeth.

Limit Salt

Reducing salt in your diet is one way to lower your blood pressure and reduce your risk of stroke, heart disease, and kidney disease. Another effective strategy is to eat more foods rich in potassium, which blunts the effects of salt on blood pressure, may decrease bone loss, and reduces the risk of kidney stones.

The guidelines recommend less than 2,300 mg of sodium per day. Many people, including those with hypertension, blacks, and older adults, should reduce their salt intake even more and increase potassium to at least 4,700 mg.

To reduce sodium intake:

▮ **Look for labels that say "low sodium."** They contain 140 mg or less of sodium per serving.
▮ **Learn to use spices and herbs rather than salt** to enhance the flavor of food.
▮ **Go easy on condiments** such as soy sauce, pickles, olives, ketchup, and mustard, which can add a lot of salt to your food.
▮ **Always check the amount of sodium** in processed foods, such as frozen dinners, packaged mixes, cereals, salad dressings, and sauces. The amount in different types and brands can vary widely.

If You Drink Alcoholic Beverages, Do So in Moderation

As discussed in Chapter 13, alcohol has different effects on health for different age groups. In middle-aged and older adults, one to two drinks a day seem to lower the risk of dying, primarily because moderate alcohol consumption protects against heart disease. Compared with nondrinkers, however, women who consume one alcoholic beverage per day appear to have a slightly higher risk of breast cancer. For younger people, alcohol provides little, if any, health benefits and increases the risk of traumatic injury and death. At any age, heavy drinking contributes to automotive accidents and deaths, assaults, liver disease, and other health problems.

Keep Food Safe to Eat

See the section "Food Safety" later in the chapter for an in-depth discussion of this topic. The key steps you can take to ensure food safety and prevent a problem with foodborne illnesses are:

▮ **Thoroughly wash hands,** contact surfaces, and fruits and vegetables (but not meat and poultry).
▮ **Separate raw, cooked, and ready-to-eat foods** while shopping, preparing, or storing.
▮ **Cook foods to a safe temperature.**
▮ **Chill (refrigerate) perishable foods promptly.**

✚ The Way We Eat

Just as there is no one perfect food, there is no one eating pattern than suits all people of all ages and backgrounds at all times. Your ethnic background and family makeup influenced the way you ate as a child. In college, you probably will find yourself eating in different—and not necessarily better—ways. Because the United States is so diverse, you also will have the opportunity to sample the cuisines of many cultures.

Nutrition 101: The Eating Habits of College Students

Often on their own for the first time, college students typically change their usual eating patterns. In one recent survey, 59 percent of freshmen said their diet had changed since they began college. (See Student Snapshot: "What's on an Undergraduate's Plate?") Two-thirds reported that they did not eat five fruits or vegetables daily; one-third no longer ate red meat.[29] In other studies, students of different ethnic backgrounds typically ate far less than the recommended amount of fruits and vegetables. Even college athletes, bombarded with nutrition information from coaches, trainers, and popular sports magazines, often do not know the role of various nutrients or which foods or fluids can boost their performance.[30]

Unfortunately, if undergraduates were graded on their nutritional know-how, many would receive poor grades. Perhaps because they don't get five daily servings of fruit and vegetables, students also fall short in fiber intake. When 144 undergraduates at a four-year university completed three-day food intake reports, only 19 met the recommended 20 to 35 grams per day of dietary fiber: 13 percent of the women and 16 percent of the men.[31]

The same holds true for consumption of healthful omega-3 polyunsaturated fats, such as fish oils. In a recent study of 51 college-aged women, 84 percent failed to meet the recommended levels for adequate intake. Only the small percentage consuming higher-than-recommended levels for total fat intake met or exceeded the recommended amounts of beneficial fats.[32]

Snacking has become more widespread on campuses, as in other places. College students snack primarily "to satisfy hunger"; the second most common reason is "no time for meals." Other reasons for munching between meals: "for energy," "to be sociable," and "to relieve stress." One-third snack at 9:00 p.m. or later.

Most college students do not calculate portion sizes accurately. One of the best ways to improve such estimates is by using three-dimensional food models. In a study of 380 undergraduates enrolled in an introductory nutrition course, students first estimated the amount of food in three dinners, each with varying portions of five foods (starchy food, cooked vegetables, salad, milk, and

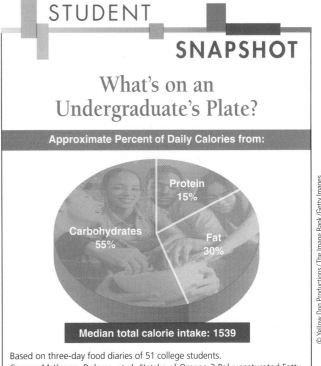

STUDENT SNAPSHOT

What's on an Undergraduate's Plate?

Approximate Percent of Daily Calories from:

Protein 15%

Carbohydrates 55%

Fat 30%

Median total calorie intake: 1539

Based on three-day food diaries of 51 college students.
Source: McKenna, Dolores, et al. "Intake of Omega-3 Polyunsaturated Fatty Acids Among College-Age Women." *Topics in Clinical Nutrition,* Vol. 19, No. 2, April–June 2004, p. 107.

meat). After correcting their own estimates, students were asked to estimate portion sizes on a new display with different foods and amounts after one week, and then again after four weeks. Each day between these two tests, different food models were passed around in class. The accuracy of the students' estimates improved significantly afterward.

Dietary Diversity

Whatever your cultural heritage, you have probably sampled Chinese, Mexican, Indian, Italian, and Japanese foods. If you belong to any of these ethnic groups, you may eat these cuisines regularly. Each type of ethnic cooking has its own nutritional benefits and potential drawbacks.

Mediterranean Diet

Several years ago epidemiologists noticed something unexpected in the residents of regions along the Mediterranean Sea: a lower incidence of deaths from heart disease. Scientists have identified antioxidants in red wine and olive oil that may account for the beneficial effects on the heart of the Mediterranean diet, which features lots of fruits and vegetables, legumes, nuts, and grains. Meat is used mainly as a condiment rather than as a main course, and fish, yogurt, and low-fat feta cheese are the predominant animal foods. The diet is relatively high in fat, but the main source is olive oil, an unsaturated fat.

Ethnic Cuisines

The cuisine served in Mexico features rice, corn, and beans, which are low in fat and high in nutrients. However, the dishes Americans think of as Mexican are far less healthful. Burritos, especially when topped with cheese and sour cream, are very high in fat. Although guacamole has a high fat content, it contains mostly monounsaturated fatty acids, a better form of fat.

African-American cuisine traces some of its roots to food preferences from west Africa (for example, peanuts, okra, and black-eyed peas), as well as to traditional American foods, such as fish, game, greens, and sweet potatoes. It uses many nutritious vegetables, such as collard greens and sweet potatoes, as well as legumes. However, some dishes include high-fat food products such as peanuts and pecans or involve frying, sometimes in saturated fat.

The mainland Chinese diet, which is plant-based, high in carbohydrates, and low in fats and animal protein, is considered one of the healthiest in the world. However, Chinese restaurants here serve more meat and sauces than are generally eaten in China. According to laboratory tests of typical take-out dishes from Chinese restaurants, many have more fats and cholesterol than hamburger or egg dishes from fast-food outlets.

Traditional French cuisine, which includes rich, high-fat sauces and dishes, has never been considered healthful. Yet, nutritionists have been stumped to explain the so-called French paradox. Despite a diet high in saturated fats, the French have had one of the lowest rates of coronary artery disease in the world. The French diet increasingly resembles the American diet, but French portions tend to be one-third to one-half the size of American portions.

Many Indian dishes highlight healthful ingredients such as vegetables and legumes (peas and beans). However, many also use *ghee* (a form of butter) or coconut oil; both are rich in harmful saturated fats. The best advice in an Indian restaurant is to ask how each dish is prepared. Good choices include *daal* or *dal* (lentils), *karbi* or *karni* (chickpea soup), and *chapati* (tortilla-like bread).

The traditional Japanese diet is very low in fat, which may account for the low incidence of heart disease in Japan. Dietary staples include soybean products, fish, vegetables, noodles, and rice. A variety of fruits and vegetables are also included in many dishes. However, Japanese cuisine is high in salted, smoked, and pickled foods. Watch out for deep-fried dishes such as tempura and salty soups and sauces.

What Should I Know About Vegetarian Diets?

Not all vegetarians avoid all meats. Some, who call themselves *lacto-ovo-pesco-vegetarians,* eat dairy products, eggs, chicken, and fish, but not red meat. **Lacto-vegetarians** eat dairy products as well as grains, fruits, and vegetables; **ovo–lacto–vegetarians** also eat eggs. Pure vegetarians, called **vegans,** eat only plant foods; often they take vitamin B_{12} supplements because that vitamin is normally found only in animal products. If they select their food with care, vegetarians can get sufficient amounts of protein, vitamin B_{12}, iron, and calcium without supplements.

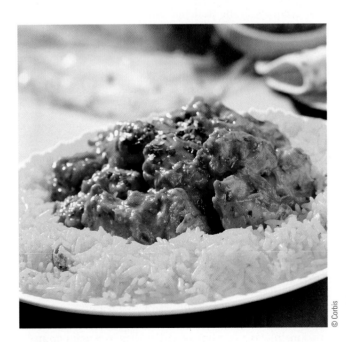

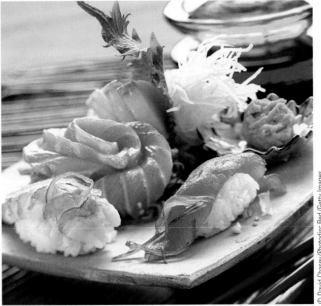

In today's ethnically diverse United States, all-American food ranges from Indian to Japanese. The vegetables and legumes in the Indian diet are healthy and high in protein, but too much saturated fat can cancel some of the benefits. The Japanese diet is high in seafood and rice and low in fats, cheese, and meat.

The key to getting sufficient protein from a vegetarian diet is understanding the concept of **complementary proteins.** Meat, poultry, fish, eggs, and dairy products are *complete proteins* that provide the nine essential amino acids—substances that the human body cannot produce itself. *Incomplete proteins,* such as legumes or nuts, may have relatively low levels of one or two essential amino acids but fairly high levels of others. By combining complementary protein sources, you can make sure that your body makes the most of the nonanimal proteins you eat. Many cultures rely heavily on complementary foods for protein. In Middle Eastern cooking, sesame seeds and chickpeas are a popular combination; in Latin American dishes, beans and rice or beans and tortillas; in Chinese cuisine, soy and rice.

According to the 2005 Dietary Guidelines, vegetarians can best meet their nutrient needs by paying special attention to protein, iron, vitamin B_{12}, calcium, and vitamin D. Instead of a 6-ounce serving of meat, they can substitute one egg, 1.5 ounces of nuts, or two-thirds cup of legumes. Those who avoid milk because of its lactose content may obtain all the nutrients of milk by using lactose-reduced milk, calcium-fortified orange juice or fortified soy milk.[33]

Vegetarian diets have proven health benefits. Studies show that vegetarians' cholesterol levels are low, and vegetarians are seldom overweight. As a result, they're less apt to be candidates for heart disease than those who consume large quantities of meat. Vegetarians also have lower incidences of breast, colon, and prostate cancer; high blood pressure; and osteoporosis.

Fast Food: Nutrition on the Run

On any given day, about 25 percent of adults in the United States go to a fast-food restaurant. The typical American consumes three hamburgers and four orders of french fries every week.[34] Not all fast foods are junk foods—that is, high in calories, sugar, salt, and fat and low in beneficial nutrients. But while it's not all bad, fast food has definite disadvantages. A meal in a fast-food restaurant may cost twice as much as the same meal prepared at home and may provide half your daily calorie needs. The fat content of many items is extremely high. A Burger King Whopper with cheese contains 723 calories and 48 grams of fat, 18 grams from saturated fat. A McDonald's Sausage McMuffin with egg has 517 calories and 33 grams of fat, 13 grams from saturated fat. Many fast-food chains have switched from beef tallow or lard to unsaturated vegetable oils for frying, but the total fat content of the foods remains the same. Some consumer advocacy groups have sued fast-food restaurant chains, asserting that because of their aggressive marketing, particularly to children, they should bear responsibility for the costs of the nation's obesity epidemic.

STRATEGIES *for* PREVENTION

A Guide to Fast Foods

▪ For breakfast, avoid croissants or muffins stuffed with eggs or meat; they pack as many as 700 calories. Better options include plain scrambled eggs (150–180 calories), pancakes without butter or syrup (400 calories), and English muffins (185 calories each).

▪ For lunch or dinner, if you want meat, go for plain hamburgers (no cheese), which average 275 to 350 calories. An even better choice is roast beef, which is lower in fat and calories.

▪ Be wary of fast-food fish. With frying oil trapped in the breading and creamy tartar sauce on top, fried-fish sandwiches supply more calories (425–500) and fat than regular hamburgers.

▪ Avoid fried chicken; the coatings tend to retain grease. If you want bite-sized chicken, select bites made of chicken breast, not processed chicken (which contains fatty, ground-up skin).

▪ Ask for unsalted items, they are available. (Many chains also have reduced the amount of sodium used in cooking.)

▪ If you sample the salad bar, steer clear of mayonnaise, bacon bits, oily vegetable salads, and rich dressings.

WELLNESS COACH

✚ Taking Charge of What You Eat

You can't control what you don't know. Because of the Nutrition Labeling and Education Act, food manufacturers must provide information about fat, calories, and ingredients in large type on packaged food labels, and they must show how a food item fits into a daily diet of 2,000 calories. The law also restricts nutritional claims for terms such as *healthy, low-fat,* and *high-fiber.*

In evaluating food labels and product claims, keep in mind that while individual foods vary in their nutritional value, what matters is your total diet. If you eat too much of any one food—regardless of what its label states—you may not be getting the variety and balance of nutrients that you need.

TABLE 8-7 ▌ Supersizing Portions

Food Item	Calories per Portion	
	20 Years Ago	Today
Bagel	140 Calories (3-in. diameter)	350 calories (6-in. diameter)
Fast food cheeseburger	333 calories	590 calories
Spaghetti and meatballs	500 calories (1 cup of spaghetti with sauce and 3 small meatballs)	1,025 calories (2 cups of spaghetti and 3 large meatballs)
Bottle of soda	85 calories (6.5 oz.)	250 calories (20 oz.)
Fast food french fries	210 calories (2.4 oz.)	610 calories (6.9 oz.)
Turkey sandwich	320 calories	820 calories (10-in. sub)

Source: Dietary Guidelines for Americans 2005, U.S. Department of Health and Human Services, U.S. Department of Agriculture, www.healthierus.gov/dietaryguidelines. Adapted from the Portion Distortion Quiz, National Heart, Lung, and Blood Institute, www.nhlbi.nih.gov.

Portions and Servings

Consumers often are confused by what a *serving* actually is, especially since many American restaurants have super-sized the amount of food they put on their customers' plates. The average bagel has doubled in size in the last ten to fifteen years (**Table 8-7**). A standard fast-food serving of french fries is larger in the United States than in the United Kingdom.

A food-label *serving* is a specific amount of food that contains the quantity of nutrients described on the Nutrition Facts label. A *portion* is the amount of a specific food that an individual eats at one time. Portions can be bigger or smaller than the servings on food labels. According to nutritionists, "marketplace portions" —the actual amounts served to customers—are two to

eight times larger than the standard serving sizes defined by the USDA. In fast-food chains, today's portions are two to five times larger than the original sizes. As studies have shown, people presented with larger portions eat 30 to 50 percent more than they otherwise would.[35]

If you are trying to balance your diet or control your weight, it's important to keep track of the size of your portions so that you do not exceed the recommended serving. For instance, a 3-ounce serving of meat is about the size of a pack of playing cards—see **Figure 8-4**. If you eat a larger amount, count it as more than one serving.

What Should I Look for on Nutrition Labels?

As **Figure 8-5** shows, the Nutrition Facts on food labels present a wealth of information—if you know what to look for. The label focuses on those nutrients most clearly associated with disease risk and health: total fat, saturated fat, cholesterol, sodium, total carbohydrate, dietary fiber, sugar, and protein.

▌ **Calories.** Calories are the measure of the amount of energy that can be derived from food. Science defines a *calorie* as the amount of energy required to raise the temperature of 1 gram of water by 1 degree Celsius. In the laboratory, the caloric content of food is measured in 1,000-calorie units called *kilocalories*. The calorie referred to in everyday usage is actually the equivalent of the laboratory kilocalorie.

The Nutrition Facts label lists two numbers for calories: calories per serving and calories from fat per serving. This allows consumers to calculate how many calories they'll consume and to determine the percentage of fat in an item.

▌ **Serving size.** Rather than the tiny portions manufacturers sometimes used in the past to keep down the number of calories per serving, the new labels

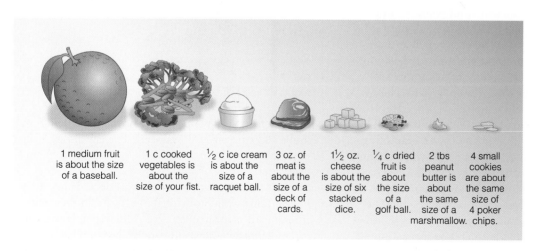

1 medium fruit is about the size of a baseball.

1 c cooked vegetables is about the size of your fist.

½ c ice cream is about the size of a racquet ball.

3 oz. of meat is about the size of a deck of cards.

1½ oz. cheese is about the size of six stacked dice.

¼ c dried fruit is about the size of a golf ball.

2 tbs peanut butter is about the same size of a marshmallow.

4 small cookies are about the same size of 4 poker chips.

FIGURE 8-4 ▌ Quick and Easy Estimates of Portion Sizes

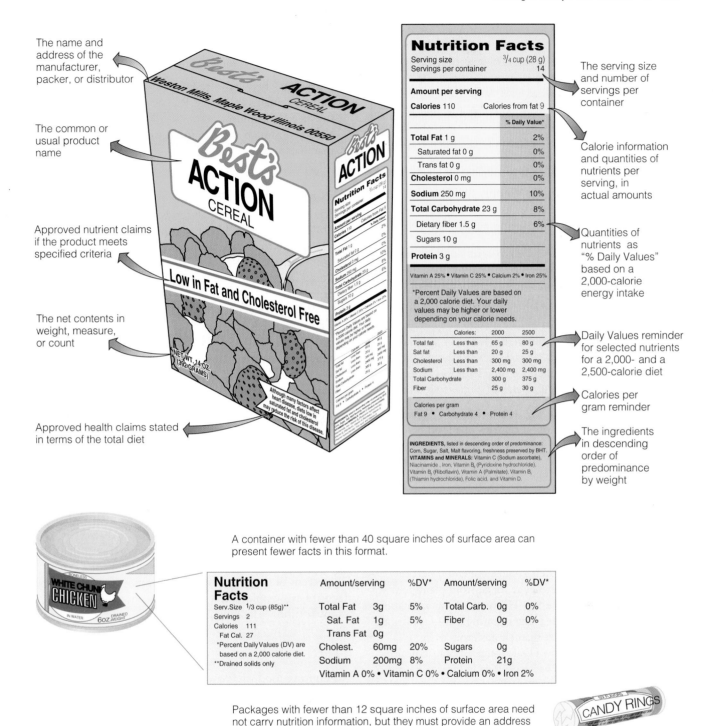

Nutrition Facts

Serving size ¾ cup (28 g)
Servings per container 14

Amount per serving

Calories 110   Calories from fat 9

	% Daily Value*
Total Fat 1 g	2%
Saturated fat 0 g	0%
Trans fat 0 g	0%
Cholesterol 0 mg	0%
Sodium 250 mg	10%
Total Carbohydrate 23 g	8%
Dietary fiber 1.5 g	6%
Sugars 10 g	
Protein 3 g	

Vitamin A 25% • Vitamin C 25% • Calcium 2% • Iron 25%

*Percent Daily Values are based on a 2,000 calorie diet. Your daily values may be higher or lower depending on your calorie needs.

	Calories:	2000	2500
Total fat	Less than	65 g	80 g
Sat fat	Less than	20 g	25 g
Cholesterol	Less than	300 mg	300 mg
Sodium	Less than	2,400 mg	2,400 mg
Total Carbohydrate		300 g	375 g
Fiber		25 g	30 g

Calories per gram
Fat 9 • Carbohydrate 4 • Protein 4

INGREDIENTS, listed in descending order of predominance: Corn, Sugar, Salt, Malt flavoring, freshness preserved by BHT. **VITAMINS and MINERALS:** Vitamin C (Sodium ascorbate), Niacinamide , Iron, Vitamin B₆ (Pyridoxine hydrochloride), Vitamin B₂ (Riboflavin), Vitamin A (Palmitate), Vitamin B₁ (Thiamin hydrochloride), Folic acid, and Vitamin D.

Label callouts (left side):

- The name and address of the manufacturer, packer, or distributor
- The common or usual product name
- Approved nutrient claims if the product meets specified criteria
- The net contents in weight, measure, or count
- Approved health claims stated in terms of the total diet

Label callouts (right side):

- The serving size and number of servings per container
- Calorie information and quantities of nutrients per serving, in actual amounts
- Quantities of nutrients as "% Daily Values" based on a 2,000-calorie energy intake
- Daily Values reminder for selected nutrients for a 2,000- and a 2,500-calorie diet
- Calories per gram reminder
- The ingredients in descending order of predominance by weight

Box text: Best's ACTION CEREAL — Weston Mills, Maple Wood Illinois 00550 — Low in Fat and Cholesterol Free — NET WT. 14 OZ. (392 GRAMS) — Although many factors affect heart disease, diets low in saturated fat and cholesterol may reduce the risk of this disease.

A container with fewer than 40 square inches of surface area can present fewer facts in this format.

Nutrition Facts

Serv.Size ⅓ cup (85g)**
Servings 2
Calories 111
  Fat Cal. 27
*Percent Daily Values (DV) are based on a 2,000 calorie diet.
**Drained solids only

Amount/serving		%DV*	Amount/serving		%DV*
Total Fat	3g	5%	Total Carb.	0g	0%
Sat. Fat	1g	5%	Fiber	0g	0%
Trans Fat	0g				
Cholest.	60mg	20%	Sugars	0g	
Sodium	200mg	8%	Protein	21g	

Vitamin A 0% • Vitamin C 0% • Calcium 0% • Iron 2%

WHITE CHUNK CHICKEN — IN WATER — 6 OZ. DRAINED WEIGHT

Packages with fewer than 12 square inches of surface area need not carry nutrition information, but they must provide an address or telephone number for obtaining information.

CANDY RINGS

FIGURE 8-5 ▌ Understanding Nutrition Labels

The Nutrition Facts label lists the essential nutrient content of packaged food as well as the amount of potentially harmful substances such as fat and sodium.

---

reflect more realistic portions. Serving sizes, which have been defined for approximately 150 food categories, must be the same for similar products (for example, different brands of potato chips) and for similar products within a category (for example, snack foods such as pretzels, potato chips, and pop-corn). This makes it easier to compare the nutritional content of foods.

▌ **Daily Values (DVs).** DVs refer to the total amount of a nutrient that the average adult should aim to get or not exceed on a daily basis. The DVs for cholesterol, sodium, vitamins, and minerals are the same for

all adults. The DVs for total fat, saturated fat, carbohydrate, fiber, and protein are based on a 2,000-calo-
rie daily diet—the amount of food ingested by many
American men and active women.

- **Percent Daily Values (%DVs).** The goal for a
  full day's diet is to select foods that together add up
  to 100 percent of the DVs. The %DVs show how a
  particular food's nutrient content fits into a 2,000-
  calorie diet. Individuals who consume (or should
  consume) fewer than 2,000 total calories a day have
  to lower their DVs for total fat, saturated fat, and
  carbohdrates. For example, if their caloric intake
  is 10 percent less than 2,000 calories, they would
  lower the DV by 10 percent. Similarly, those who
  consume more than 2,000 calories should adjust the
  DVs upward.
- **Calories per gram.** The bottom of the food label
  lists the number of calories per gram for fat, carbohydrates, and protein.

People zero in on different figures on the food
label—for example, calories if they're watching their
weight, specific ingredients if they have food allergies.
Among the useful items to check are the following:

- **Calories from fat.** Get into the habit of calculating the percentage of fat calories in a food before
  buying or eating it.
- **Total fat.** Since the average person munches on 15
  to 20 food items a day, it's easy to overload on fat.
  Saturated fat and trans fat numbers deserve special
  attention because of their reported link to several
  diseases.
- **Cholesterol.** Cholesterol is made by and contained
  in products of animal origin only. Many high-fat
  products, such as potato chips, contain 0 percent
  cholesterol because they're made from plants and are
  cooked in vegetable fats. However, if the vegetable
  fats are hydrogenated, the resulting trans fat is more
  harmful to the heart than cholesterol.
- **Sugars.** There is no DV for sugars because health
  experts have yet to agree on a daily limit. The figure
  on the label includes naturally present sugars, such as
  lactose in milk and fructose in fruit, as well as those
  added to the food, such as sucrose, corn syrup, or
  dextrose.
- **Fiber.** A "high-fiber" food has 5 or more grams of
  fiber per serving. A "good" source of fiber provides
  at least 2.5 grams. "More" or "added" fiber means at
  least 2.5 grams more per serving than similar foods
  —10 percent more of the DV for fiber.
- **Calcium.** "High" equals 200 mg or more per serving. "Good" means at least 100 mg, while "more"
  indicates that the food contains at least 100 mg more
  calcium—10 percent more of the DV—than the
  item usually would have.
- **Sodium.** Most of us routinely get more sodium
  than we need. Read labels carefully to avoid excess
  sodium, which can be a health threat.

- **Vitamins.** A DV of 10 percent of any vitamin makes
  a food a "good" source; 20 percent qualifies it as
  "high" in a certain vitamin.

Nutrition labeling for fresh produce, fish, meat, and
poultry remains voluntary. Packages too small for a
full-sized label must provide an address or phone number so consumers can obtain information from the
manufacturer.

Functional Foods

As the ADA has noted, all foods are functional at some
physiological level. However, the term *functional* generally applies to a food specifically created to have health-
promoting benefits. The International Food Information Council defines functional foods as those "that
provide health benefits beyond basic nutrition."

Some manufacturers are adding herbs, such as the
cold-fighter echinacea, to food products and promoting them as functional foods. However, the amounts
added are often too low to have any effect, and many
herb-sprinkled foods are high-sugared drinks and snack
foods. These products have other dangers, including
the use of low-quality or contaminated herbs and adverse drug and food interactions.

✚ Food Safety

Foodborne illnesses cause an estimated 76 million illnesses, 325,000 hospitalizations, and 5,000 deaths in the
United States every year. Three organisms—*Salmonella,
Listeria,* and *Toxoplasma*—are responsible for more than
75 percent of these deaths. Although most foodborne infections cause mild illness, severe infections and serious
complications—including death—do occur.

Fight BAC!

To improve food safety awareness and practices, government and private agencies have developed the Fight Bac!
campaign, identifying four key culprits in foodborne illness:

- **Improper cooling**
- **Improper hand washing**
- **Inadequate cooking**
- **Failure to avoid cross-contamination.**[36]

What Causes Food Poisoning?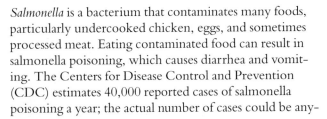

Salmonella is a bacterium that contaminates many foods,
particularly undercooked chicken, eggs, and sometimes
processed meat. Eating contaminated food can result in
salmonella poisoning, which causes diarrhea and vomiting. The Centers for Disease Control and Prevention
(CDC) estimates 40,000 reported cases of salmonella
poisoning a year; the actual number of cases could be any-

where from 400,000 to 4 million. The FDA has warned consumers about the dangers of unpasteurized orange juice because of the risk of salmonella contamination.

Another bacterium, *Campylobacter jejuni,* may cause even more stomach infections than salmonella. Found in water, milk, and some foods, campylobacter poisoning causes severe diarrhea and has been implicated in the growth of stomach ulcers.

Bacteria can also cause illness by producing toxins in food. *Staphylococcus aureus* is the most common culprit. When cooked foods are cross-contaminated with the bacteria from raw foods and not stored properly, staph infections can result, causing nausea and abdominal pain anywhere from thirty minutes to eight hours after ingestion.

Even many healthy foods can pose dangers. The FDA has urged consumers to avoid eating raw sprouts because of the risk of getting sick. Sprouts, particularly alfalfa and clover, can be contaminated by salmonella or *E. coli* bacteria, which can cause nausea, diarrhea, and cramping in healthy adults. Children and senior citizens can experience serious symptoms that lead to kidney failure and compromised immune systems. The FDA advises people to either cook sprouts before eating them or request that they be left off sandwiches and other food ordered in restaurants. Homegrown sprouts can also present a risk if they come from contaminated seeds.

An uncommon but sometimes fatal form of food poisoning is **botulism,** caused by the *Clostridium botulinum* organism. Improper home-canning procedures are the most common cause of this potentially fatal problem.

There have been several outbreaks of listeriosis, caused by the bacteria **listeria,** commonly found in deli meats, hot dogs, soft cheeses, raw meat, and unpasteurized milk. Although rare, listeriosis can be life-threatening. At greatest risk are pregnant women, infants, and those with weakened immune systems. You can reduce your risk by cooking meats and leftovers thoroughly and by washing everything that may come into contact with raw meat.

"Hamburger Disease"/ Barbecue Syndrome

Barbecue syndrome is the common name for a type of food poisoning caused by the bacteria *verotoxigenic E. coli,* or VTEC. People who develop this syndrome frequently report that they ate ground beef hamburgers prior to getting sick. Other kinds of undercooked meat and poultry and unpasteurized milk and unchlorinated water also are culprits.

As shown in **Figure 8-6**; a higher percentage of students eat pink hamburger meat, while fewer read or remember the labels on raw meat or poultry and change food preparation because of the information on the label.

Symptoms, which can range from mild to life-threatening, usually develop within two to ten days and include severe stomach cramps, vomiting, and a mild fever. Most people recover within seven to ten days. Proper handling and cooking of food can practically eliminate hamburger disease.

Pesticides and Irradiation

Plants and animals naturally produce compounds that act as pesticides to aid in their survival. The vast majority of the pesticides we consume are therefore natural, not

---

STRATEGIES
for PREVENTION

Protecting Yourself from Food Poisoning

▪ Always wash your hands with liquid or clean bar soap before handling food. Rub your hands vigorously together for 10 to 15 seconds; the soap combined with the scrubbing action dislodges and removes germs.

▪ When preparing fresh fruits and vegetables, discard outer leaves, wash under running water, and when possible, scrub with a clean brush or hands. Do not wash raw meat or poultry.

▪ To avoid the spread of bacteria to other foods, utensils or surfaces, do not allow liquids to touch or drip onto other items. Wipe up all spills immediately.

▪ Clean out your refrigerator regularly. Throw out any leftovers stored for three or four days.

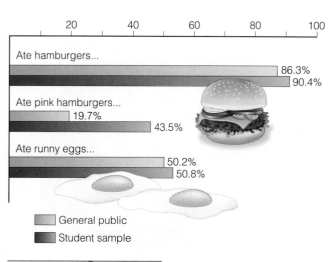

FIGURE 8-6 | Comparing the Food Safety Behavior of Students to the General Public

Source: Data from Morrone, Michele, and Ann Rathbun. "Health Education and Food Safety Behavior in the University Setting." *Journal of Environmental Health,* Vol. 65, No. 7, March 2003, p. 9.

added by farmers or food processors. *Commercial pesticides* save billions of dollars of valuable crops from pests, but they also may endanger human health and life.

Fearful of potential risks in pesticides, many consumers are purchasing **organic** foods. The term *organic* refers to foods produced without the use of commercial chemicals at any stage. Independent groups now certify foods before they can be labeled *organic*. Foods that are truly organic are cleaner and have much lower levels of residues than standard commercial produce. There's no guarantee that the organic produce you buy at a grocery or health-food store is more nutritious than other pro-duce. However, buying organic foods is one way in which you can work toward a healthier environment.

Irradiation is the use of radiation, either from radioactive substances or from devices that produce X rays, on food. It doesn't make the food radioactive. Its primary benefit is to prolong the shelf life of food. Like the heat in canning, irradiation can kill all the microorganisms that might grow in a food, and the sterilized food can then be stored for years in sealed containers at room temperature without spoiling. Are irradiated foods safe to eat? The best available answer is a qualified yes, because we don't have complete data yet.

SAVVY CONSUMER

SPOTTING NUTRITION MISINFORMATION

▮ Don't believe everything you read. A quick way to spot a bad nutrition self-help book is to look in the index for a diet to prevent or treat rheumatoid arthritis (none exists). If you find one, don't buy the book.

▮ Before you try any new nutritional approach, check with your doctor or a registered dietitian or call the American Dietetic Association's consumer hot line, (800)366-1655.

▮ Don't believe ads or advisers basing their nutritional recommendations on hair analysis, which is not accurate in detecting nutritional deficiencies.

▮ Be wary of anyone who recommends megadoses of vitamins or nutritional supplements, which can be dangerous. High doses of vitamin A, which some people take to clear up acne, can be toxic.

▮ Question personal testimonies about the powers of some magical-seeming pill or powder, and be wary of "scientific articles" in journals that aren't reviewed by health professionals.

▮ Be wary of any nutritional supplements sold in health stores or through health and body-building magazines. These products may contain ingredients that have not been tested and proved safe.

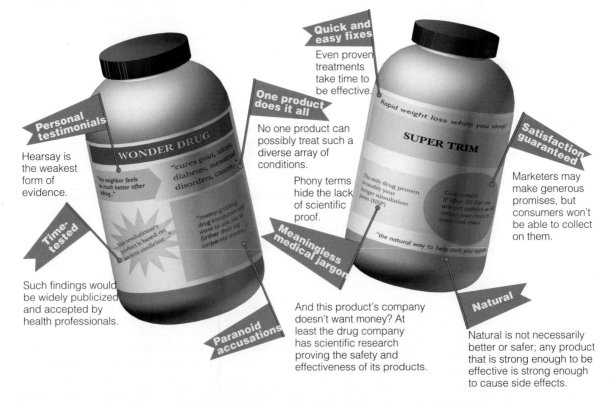

Personal testimonials
Hearsay is the weakest form of evidence.

Time-tested
Such findings would be widely publicized and accepted by health professionals.

One product does it all
No one product can possibly treat such a diverse array of conditions.

Phony terms hide the lack of scientific proof.

Meaningless medical jargon
And this product's company doesn't want money? At least the drug company has scientific research proving the safety and effectiveness of its products.

Paranoid accusations

Quick and easy fixes
Even proven treatments take time to be effective.

Satisfaction guaranteed
Marketers may make generous promises, but consumers won't be able to collect on them.

Natural
Natural is not necessarily better or safer; any product that is strong enough to be effective is strong enough to cause side effects.

Nutritional Quackery

The American Dietetic Association describes nutritional quackery as a growing problem for unsuspecting consumers. Because so much nutritional nonsense is garbed in scientific-sounding terms, it can be hard to recognize bad advice when you get it. One basic rule: If the promises of a nutritional claim sound too good to be true—they probably are. (See Savvy Consumer: "Spotting Nutrition Misinformation.")

If you seek the advice of a nutrition consultant, carefully check his or her credentials and professional associations. Because licensing isn't required in all states, almost anyone can use the label "nutritionist," regardless of qualifications. Be wary of diplomas from obscure schools and organizations that allow anyone who pays dues to join. (One physician obtained a membership for his dog!) A registered dietitian (R.D.), who has a bachelor's degree and specialized training (including an internship), and who passed a certification examination, is usually a member of the American Dietetic Association (ADA), which sets the standard for quality in diets. A nutrition expert with an M.D. or Ph.D. generally belongs to the ADA, the American Institute of Nutrition, or the American Society of Clinical Nutrition; all have stringent membership requirements.

MAKING HEALTHY CHOICES

For Personal Nutrition

As nutritional knowledge expands and evolves, it's easy to be confused by changing advice on which foods to avoid and which to eat. But even though research may challenge or change thinking on a specific food, some basic principles always apply. At the very least, keep in mind the American Dietetic Association's ABCs.

- **Aim for fitness.** In order to maintain a healthy weight, build physical activity into your daily routine.
- **Build a healthy base.** Select a variety of foods to help you get all the nutrients and fiber you need.
- **Choose sensibly.** Put together a diet that is low in saturated fat and cholesterol and moderate in total fat.

Here are some other guidelines that never go out of style:

- **Eat breakfast.** Easy to prepare breakfasts include cold cereal with fruit and low-fat milk, whole-wheat toast with peanut butter, yogurt with fruit, or whole-grain waffles.
- **Snack smart.** Choose snacks from different food groups—a glass of low-fat milk and a few graham crackers, an apple or celery sticks with peanut butter and raisins, or some dry cereal.
- **Don't eat too much of one thing.** Your body needs protein, carbohydrates, fat, and many different vitamins and minerals such as vitamins C and A, iron, and calcium from a variety of foods.
- **Eat more grains, fruits, and vegetables.** These foods give you carbohydrates for energy, plus vitamins, minerals, and fiber. Try breads such as whole-wheat, bagels, and pita. Spaghetti and oatmeal are also in the grain group.
- **Don't ban any food.** Fit in a higher-fat food, like pepperoni pizza, at dinner by choosing lower-fat foods at other meals. And don't forget about moderation. If two pieces of pizza fill you up, don't eat a third.
- **Make every calorie count.** Load up on nutrients, not on big portions. Choosing foods that are nutrient dense will help protect against disease and keep you healthy.

SELF SURVEY

How Healthy Is Your Diet?

Step 1

For a week, write down everything you eat and drink for meals and snacks. Include the approximate amount eaten (for example, ½ cup, 1 large, 12-oz. can, and so on).

	Mon	Tues	Wed	Thurs	Fri	Sat	Sun
Grains							
Vegetables							
Fruits							
Milk, yogurt, cheese							
Meat, poultry, dry beans, eggs, nuts							
Fats, oil, sweets, cheese							

Step 2: Are You Getting Enough Vegetables, Fruits, and Grains?

How often do you eat:	Seldom/never	1–2 times a week	3–5 times a week	Almost daily
At least three servings of vegetables a day?				
Starchy vegetables like potatoes, corn, or peas?				
Foods made with dry beans, lentils, or peas?				
Dark green or deep yellow vegetables (broccoli, spinach, collards, carrots, sweet potatoes, squash)?				
At least two servings of fruit a day?				
Citrus fruits and 100% fruit juices (oranges, grapefruit, tangerines)?				
Whole fruit with skin or seeds (berries, apples, pears)?				
At least six servings of breads, cereals, pasta, or rice a day?				

The best answer for each is "almost daily." Use your food diary to see which foods you should be eating more often.

Step 3: Are You Getting Too Much Fat?

How often do you eat:	Seldom/never	1–2 times a week	3–5 times a week	Almost daily
Fried, deep-fat fried, or breaded food?				
Fatty meats, such as sausages, luncheon meat, and fatty steaks or roasts?				
Whole milk, high-fat cheeses, or ice cream?				
Pies, pastries, or rich cakes?				
Rich cream sauces and gravies?				
Oily salad dressings or mayonnaise?				
Butter or margarine on vegetables, rolls, bread, or toast?				

Ideally, you should be eating these foods no more than one or two times a week. If your food diary indicates that you're eating them more frequently, your fat intake may well be too high.

Step 4: Are You Getting Too Much Sodium?

How often do you eat:	Seldom/never	1–2 times a week	3–5 times a week	Almost daily
Cured or processed meats, such as ham, sausage, frankfurters, or luncheon meats?				
Canned vegetables or frozen vegetables with sauce?				
Frozen TV dinners, entrees, or canned or dehydrated soups?				
Salted nuts, popcorn, pretzels, corn chips, or potato chips?				
Seasoning mixes or sauces containing salt?				
Processed cheese?				
Salt added to table foods before you taste them?				

Ideally, you should be eating these high-sodium items no more than one or two times a week. If your food diary indicates that you're eating them more frequently, your sodium intake may well be too high.

ACTION PLAN

Your Health Action Plan for Better Nutrition

- **Eat five servings of fruits and vegetables per day.** For breakfast, have 100% juice or add raisins, berries, or sliced fruit to cereal, pancakes, or waffles. For lunch, have vegetable soup or salad with your meal or pile vegetables on your sandwich. For dinner, choose vegetables that are green, orange (such as carrots or squash), and red (such as tomatoes or bell peppers).

- **Include three servings of whole-grain foods every day.** To identify whole-grain products, check the ingredient list. The first ingredient should be a whole grain, such as "whole-grain oats," "whole-grain wheat," or "whole wheat."

- **Consume a calcium-rich food at each meal.** Good options include low-fat and nonfat milk, cheese, or yogurt; tofu; broccoli; dried beans; spinach; and fortified soy milk.

- **Eat less meat.** Rather than making meat the heart of a meal, think of it as a flavoring ingredient.

- **Avoid high-fat fast foods.** Hot dogs, fried foods, packaged snack foods, and pastries are most likely to be laden with fat.

- **Check the numbers.** When buying prepared foods, choose items that contain no more than 3 grams of fat per 100 calories.

- **Think small.** A dinner-size serving of meat should be about the size of a deck of cards; half a cup is the size of a woman's fist; a pancake is the diameter of a CD.

- **Read labels carefully.** Remember that "cholesterol-free" doesn't necessarily mean fat-free. Avoid products that contain saturated coconut oil, palm oil, lard, or hydrogenated fats.

- **Switch to low-fat and no-fat dairy products.** Rather than buying whole-fat dairy products, choose skim milk, fat-free sour cream, and low- or nonfat yogurt.

- **The brighter the better.** When selecting fruits and vegetables, choose the most intense color. A bright orange carrot has more beta-carotene than a pale one. Dark green lettuce leaves have more vitamins than lighter ones. Orange sweet potatoes pack more vitamin A than yellow ones.

SETTING GOALS

Healthy Eating

Your Personal Healthy Eating Goal

Is It S.M.A.R.T.?

Specific? _____

Measurable? _____

Achievable? _____

Rewarding? _____

Time Defined? _____

Strategies for Success

1. _____
2. _____
3. _____

Potential Obstacles

1. _____
2. _____
3. _____

Ways Around Them

1. _____
2. _____
3. _____

Daily Report

The Week That Was:

What went right?

What could I do better?

WELLNESS JOURNAL

Why Do You Choose the Foods You Do?

Nutrition is a personal decision, although there are many influences on why we eat as we do. Taste, cost, convenience, availability, habit, peer pressure, emotional state, culture, and geographic location are some of the reasons we choose certain foods. Nutrition is one of the greatest determinants of our overall health, yet we usually don't think much about how the meal we are about to eat will affect our health. Using the results from your nutrition analysis lab in your Lab Booklet, answer the questions below to help you think more about your diet and understand why you make the choices you do.

1. How would you rate the quality of your diet (poor, fair, average, good), according to accepted dietary guidelines, the MyPyramid system and other recommendations for healthy eating?

2. Is your daily caloric intake too high, too low, or just about right for your activity level? Do you have concerns about your weight? What effect does your intake have on your present weight?

3. Which influences in your life or lifestyle have the most consequences on your food choices? If these result in poor choices, how can you modify these influences?

4. How often does your mood affect your diet? What emotions lead to unhealthy food choices?

5. Are there many "empty" calories in your diet, from items such as soda, candy, cookies and/or alcohol?

Which are the two largest sources? Why do you eat these foods?

6. Are you concerned about the amount of fast food in your diet? Why or why not?

7. Does your family history of disease suggest you should eat a certain way or avoid/modify certain foods?

Eating more healthfully doesn't just happen. It takes practice, patience and commitment to improve. What strategies can you develop to improve your eating? A couple of changes can make a big difference in your health, mood and energy levels.

CHAPTER

8 Making This Chapter Work for You

1. The classes of essential nutrients include which of the following?
   a. amino acids, antioxidants, fiber, and cholesterol
   b. proteins, calcium, calories, and folic acid
   c. carbohydrates, minerals, fat, and water
   d. iron, whole grains, fruits, and vegetables

2. Which type of fat is *not* considered a threat to heart health?
   a. omega–3 fatty acids
   b. trans fat
   c. triglycerides
   d. saturated fats

3. Antioxidants
   a. are nutrients important in the production of hemoglobin.
   b. are substances added to foods to make them more flavorful or physically appealing.
   c. are suspected triggers of food allergies.
   d. are substances that prevent the harmful effects of free radicals.

4. The MyPyramid System can be personalized to your age, gender, and activity level at www.MyPyramid.gov. Besides personalization, the MyPyramid System has these themes:
   a. variety, proportionality, moderation, and activity
   b. variety, bulimia, activity
   c. variety, moderation, activity, and food safety
   d. variety, moderation, activity, and correct food labeling

5. The MyPyramid System includes this recommendation:
   a. Make half your grains whole.
   b. Go lean with protein.
   c. Focus on fruits.
   d. All of the above.

6. The 2005 Dietary Guidelines for Americans include:
   a. Decrease intake of added sugars.
   b. Increase consumption of olive oil.
   c. Control calorie intake to manage body weight.
   d. Eat dessert no more than three days a week.

7. Food labels on packaged foods include all of the following *except*
   a. total weight of the package.
   b. total amount of nutrients contained in the food.
   c. the percent of nutrient Daily Values provided in the food.
   d. serving size.

8. Which of the following statements is true?
   a. The Chinese diet, which is high in fats and low in carbohydrates, leads to high incidence of obesity and heart disease.
   b. The French diet is considered to be healthful because the food is high in saturated fats.
   c. The Mediterranean diet is rich in fruits, vegetables, wine, and olive oil and may help prevent heart disease.
   d. African-American recipes often include okra or sweet potatoes, which are complete proteins.

9. Some vegetarians may
   a. include chicken and fish in their diets.
   b. avoid vitamin B_{12} supplements if they eat only plant foods.
   c. eat only legumes or nuts because these provide complete proteins.
   d. have high cholesterol levels because of the saturated fats in fruits and vegetables.

10. Common causes of foodborne infections include which of the following?
   a. the influenza virus
   b. *Salmonella* and *E. coli* bacteria
   c. additives
   d. irradiation

Answers to these questions can be found on page 376.

Critical Thinking

1. Which alternative or ethnic diet do you think has the best-tasting food? Which is the most healthy? Why?

2. Is it possible to meet nutritional requirements on a limited budget? Have you ever been in this situation? What would you recommend to someone who wanted to eat healthfully on $30 a week?

3. Consider the number of times a week you eat fast food. How much money would you have saved if you had eaten home-prepared meals? Which fast foods could you have selected that would have provided more nutritional value?

Media Menu

Health Now™

Don't forget to check out the wealth of resources on the HealthNow website at **http://healthnow.brookscole.com/itw** that will:

- Help you evaluate your knowledge of the material
- Allow you to take an exam-prep quiz
- Provide a Personalized Learning Plan targeting resources that address areas you should study
- Coach you through identifying target goals for behavior change and creating and monitoring your personal change plan throughout the semester.

INTERNET CONNECTIONS

U.S. Food and Nutrition Information Center

www.nal.usda.gov/fnic

This comprehensive governmental website features reports and scientific studies on a variety of nutrition information, including the 2005 USDA Dietary Guidelines, an updated Food Guide Pyramid, dietary supplements, dietary assessment, food composition searchable databases, educational brochures, historical food guides, and a topics A–Z section.

USDA Center for Nutrition Policy and Promotion

www.usda.gov/cnpp/

This interactive site, sponsored by the United States Center for Nutrition Policy and Promotion, features the Interactive Health Eating Index, an online dietary assessment that enables you to receive a personalized score on the overall quality of your diet, on a daily basis, based on the recommendations of the USDA Food Guide Pyramid. This tool provides you with information on total fat, cholesterol, sodium, and other nutrients. You can also download a series of brochures featuring dietary guidelines as well as healthy recipes.

Nutrient Analysis Tool

nat.crgq.com

This site, provided as a public service by the Food Science and Human Nutrition Department at the University of Illinois, features a free nutrient analysis interactive program that calculates the amount of calories, carbohydrates, protein, fat, vitamins, minerals, and fiber in the foods that make up your daily diet.

Cyberkitchen

www.nhlbi.nih.gov/chd/Tipsheets/cyberkit.htm

This interactive site helps you discover how much you are really eating with an activity on comparing standard serving sizes versus real serving sizes. You can also provide personal information regarding your age, gender, height, weight, and activity level, and the Cyberkitchen will provide you with a healthy diet plan to meet your weight management goals. It's fun and educational.

 InfoTrac College Edition Activities "Dark Chocolate May Help Hypertension, but chocolate's no 'health food'—it's the flavenoids," Tufts University Health & Nutrition Letter, October 25, 2005, v. 23m i. 8, p. 1.

1. Why do chocolate and cocoa seem to possess antioxidant properties?
2. Physiologically, how do the antioxidants found in chocolate promote vascular health?
3. How does chocolate affect blood pressure?

Conklin, Martha et al. "College students' use of point of selection nutrition information," *Topics in Clinical Nutrition,* April–June 2005 v20 i2 p97(12)

1. Which gender was more likely to use labels to make food choices? Why do you think this may occur?
2. What motivated women to select particular food items?
3. Which types of foods did men tend to select? What was their motive?

You can find additional readings related to personal health with InfoTrac College Edition, an online library of more than 900 journals and publications. Follow the instructions for accessing InfoTrac College Edition that were packaged with your textbook; then search for articles using a keyword search.

For additional links, resources, and suggested readings on the InfoTrac College Edition, visit our Health and Wellness Resource Center at **http://health.wadsworth.com.**

Key Terms

The terms listed are used on the page indicated. Definitions of the terms are in the Glossary at the end of this book.

amino acids 154
antioxidants 157
basal metabolic rate (BMR) 152
botulism 171
calories 152
carbohydrates 154
complementary proteins 167
complete proteins 154
complex carbohydrates 154
Daily Values (DVs) 169
dietary fiber 155
essential nutrients 152
folic acid 157
functional fiber 155
incomplete proteins 154
irradiation 172
lacto-vegetarians 166
listeria 171
macronutrients 152
micronutrients 152
minerals 158
nutrition 151
organic 172
osteoporosis 158
ovo-lacto-vegetarians 166
phytochemicals 159
proteins 154
saturated fats 155
simple carbohydrates 154
trans fat 156
unsaturated fats 155
vegans 166
vitamins 157

Taking Control of Your Weight

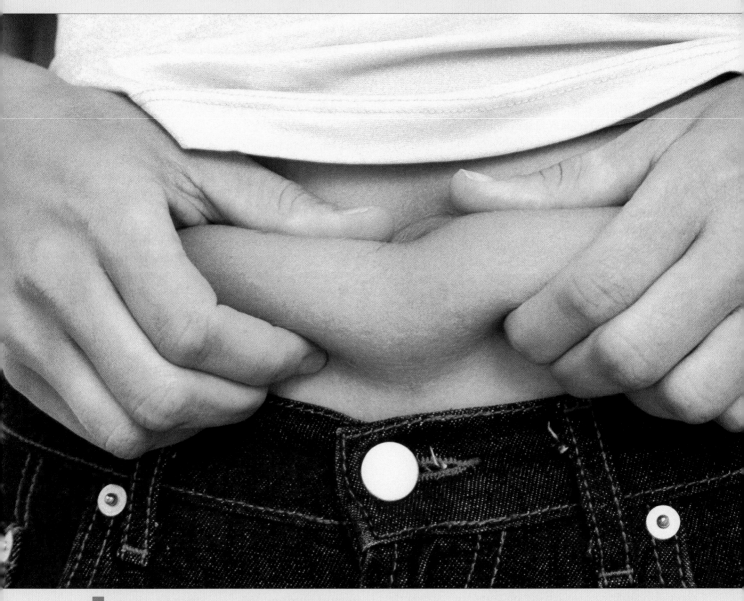

Deena's mother called it "baby fat." "You'll outgrow it soon enough," she said. Yet Deena's cheeks grew chubbier and her waist wider every year. "Wait for your growth spurt," her mother reassured her. But Deena remained one of the shortest girls in her class—and, she was convinced, the roundest.

Deena went on her first diet in high school. For three days she ate nothing but carrot sticks, cottage cheese, and apples. Then she scarfed down two double cheeseburgers with fries and a chocolate shake. Her other attempts at dieting didn't last much longer. By graduation she was grateful to hide under the flowing black robe as she walked on stage to get her diploma.

When Deena heard about the "freshman 15," the extra pounds many students acquire during their first year at college, she groaned at the prospect of putting on more weight. In her Personal Health and Wellness class, Deena set one primary goal: not to gain another pound. Rather than going on—and inevitably falling off—one diet after another, she developed a weight management plan that included healthy food choices and regular exercise. Armed with the information and tools provided in this chapter, Deena, for the first time in her life, took charge of her weight.

You can do the same. Excess weight weakens hearts; raises blood pressure; clogs arteries; strains backs and joints; increases the risk of diabetes, stroke, and certain cancers; and steals years of productive life. The earlier the weight gain, the greater the danger it poses. Obesity at age twenty can cut 20 years off a person's life.[1] According to preliminary data, the tide may be turning: The percentage of Americans who are obese does not seem to be increasing, although it remains at record levels.[2]

This chapter explains how we grew so big, tells what obesity is and why excess pounds are dangerous, describes current approaches to weight loss, discusses diets that work (and some that don't), offers practical guidelines for exercise and behavioral approaches to losing weight, and examines unhealthy eating patterns and eating disorders. Regardless of your current weight, you will find insights and skills you will need for healthy weight management throughout your life.

Peter Samuels GETTY

After studying the material in this chapter, you should be able to:

▌ **List** the factors besides genetics that have contributed to the global increase in overweight and obesity.

▌ **Define** overweight and obesity, and **describe** the three indicators of weight-related health risks.

▌ **Identify** the main health risks of excess weight.

▌ **Assess** various approaches to weight loss.

▌ **Design** a personal plan for sensible weight management.

▌ **Identify** and **describe** the symptoms and dangers associated with eating disorders.

Health ⊛ Now™

Don't forget to check out the wealth of resources on the HealthNow website at **http://healthnow.brookscole.com/itw** that will:

• Help you evaluate your knowledge of the material
• Allow you to take an exam-prep quiz
• Provide a Personalized Learning Plan targeting resources that address areas you should study
• Coach you through identifying target goals for behavior change and creating and monitoring your personal change plan throughout the semester.

✚ The Global Epidemic

For the first time in history, more than half of the people on the planet are overweight. Obesity, as headlines blare and health experts warn, is emerging as the number-one public health problem of the twenty-first century.

An estimated 1.1 billion people around the world—seven in ten of the Dutch and Spanish, two in three Americans and Canadians, and one in two Britons, Germans, and Italians—are overweight or obese. In Europe, excess weight ranks as the most common childhood disorder. Since 1980, obesity rates have tripled in parts of Eastern Europe, the Middle East, China, and the Pacific Islands.[3] In many poor countries, obesity is common among city dwellers, while people in rural areas remain underweight and malnourished.

The World Health Organization, in its first global diet, exercise, and health program to combat obesity, recommends that governments promote public knowledge about diet, exercise, and health; offer information that makes healthy choices easier for consumers to make; and require accurate, comprehensible food labels.[4] Although ultimately each individual decides what and how much to eat, policy makers agree that governments also must act to reverse the obesity epidemic.[5]

Exposure to a Western lifestyle seems to bring out susceptibility to excess weight. Obesity is much more common among the Pima Indians of Arizona compared to Pimas living in Mexico, who have maintained a more traditional lifestyle, with more physical activity and a diet lower in fat and richer in complex carbohydrates. Native Hawaiians who follow a more traditional diet and lifestyle also have lower rates of obesity and cardiovascular disease.[6]

Simply moving to America increases the risk of obesity. In a study of immigrants, the rate of obesity more than doubled within 15 years—from 8 percent among recent immigrants to 19 percent.[7]

Supersized Nation

Two-thirds of American adults, up from fewer than half 20 years ago, are overweight. About one in every three Americans is obese. Since the 1970s, the obesity rate has doubled for teens and tripled for children between the ages of 6 and 11.[8]

Although more men than women are overweight, more adult women (38 percent) are obese than men (28 percent). Non-Hispanic black women have the highest obesity rate (50 percent), compared with 40 percent of Hispanic women and 30 percent of white women (**Figure 9-1**).[9] In some Native American communities, up to 70 percent of all adults are dan-

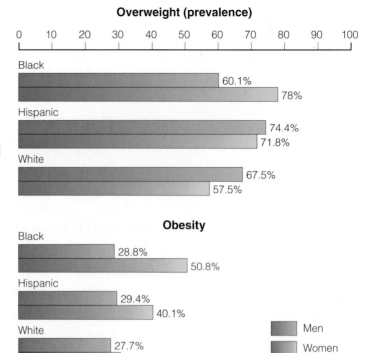

FIGURE 9-1 ❙ Weight Problems by Race/Ethnic Group and Gender

Source: American Obesity Association, "Obesity in Minority Populations," www.obesity.org.

gerously overweight. Differences in metabolic rates may be one factor.

Weight problems are starting earlier than ever. One in ten preschoolers and one in five grade schoolers are seriously overweight.[10] According to federal estimates, some 6 million American youngsters are so heavy that their health is in jeopardy. Another 5 million are on the threshold of this danger zone. Not only are more children overweight today, but they're 30 to 50 percent heavier than "fat" kids were a decade ago. The percentage of obese teenagers has tripled in the last 20 years.

Not all Americans are equally likely to be overweight or obese. As **Figure 9-2** shows, the southern states have the highest concentration of obese residents. Mississippi is home to the county with the highest percentage of people with a body mass index (BMI) between 30 and 40. (BMI is discussed in a later section—it is defined as the ratio between weight and height that correlates with percentage of body fat.)

States also vary in their efforts to control obesity. According to an ongoing evaluation program at the University of Baltimore, no states deserve an A overall. Only one state—California—earned an A in the report card. The researchers credited the state's legislative package targeted at the nutrition and diets of schoolchildren at risk of becoming obese for the high grade. Overall,

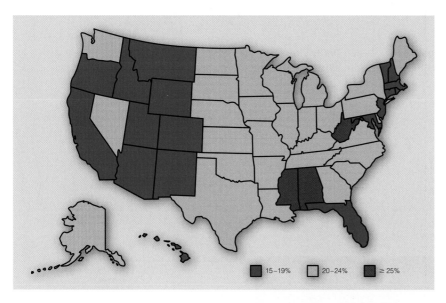

FIGURE 9-2 ▌ Obesity in the United States

This map shows the percentage of people in each state who are obese, that is, who have a body mass index between 30 and 40.

Source: Data from National Center for Chronic Disease Prevention and Health Promotion.

California earned a B for its anti-obesity work for all populations.

While most states made strides in this year's report card, several states continue to lag behind in taking corrective steps. The three states with the highest prevalence of obesity—Mississippi, West Virginia, and Michigan—have done little to correct the problem, although Mississippi did pass legislation specifying requirements for recess and physical education in schools and established a commission on obesity.

The report card indicates that it is costing the United States nearly $120 billion a year in medical care alone to deal with obesity. The report card's authors—Zoltan Acs, professor of economics and entrepreneurship, Kenneth Stanton, professor of finance, and Ann Cotten, director of the University of Baltimore's Schaefer Center—recommend that states use the same lessons learned from the tobacco wars and employ a mix of legislative efforts, private-sector influence, litigation, and common sense to combat obesity.[11]

Five states—Idaho, Nevada, South Dakota, Utah, and Wyoming—received an F on the report card for failing to take any action in combating obesity.

How Did We Get So Fat?

A variety of factors, ranging from behavior to environment to heredity, played a role in the increase in overweight and obesity. They include:

1. **More calories.** Bombarded by nonstop commercials for taste treats, tempted by foods in every form to munch and crunch, Americans are eating more—some 200 to 400 calories more a day than they did several decades ago. Many of these extra calories come from refined carbohydrates, which can raise levels of heart-damaging blood fats called triglycerides and increase the risk of diabetes as well as obesity.

2. **Bigger portions.** As Table 9-1 shows, the size of many popular restaurant and packaged foods has increased two to five times during the past 20 years.[12] Some foods, like chocolate bars, have grown more than ten times since they were first introduced. Popular 64-ounce sodas can pack a whopping 800 calories. According to studies of appetite and satiety, people presented with larger portions eat up to 30 percent more than they otherwise would.

3. **Fast Food.** Young adults who eat frequently at fast-food restaurants gain more weight and develop metabolic abnormalities that increase their risk of diabetes in early middle age. In a recent study, those who ate fast food at least twice a week gained an extra 10 pounds and had a two-fold greater increase in insulin resistance, a risk factor for diabetes. The men in the study visited fast food restaurants more often than the women, blacks did so more frequently than whites.[13]

4. **Physical inactivity.** As Americans eat more, they exercise less. Experts estimate that most adults expend 200 to 300 fewer calories than people did 25 years ago. The most dramatic drop in physical activity often occurs during the college years.[14]

5. **Passive entertainment.** Television is a culprit in an estimated 30 percent of new cases of obesity. TV viewing may increase weight in several ways: It takes up time that otherwise might be spent in physical activities. It increases food intake since people tend to eat more while watching TV. And compared with sewing, reading, driving, or other sedentary pursuits, television watching lowers metabolic rate so viewers burn fewer calories.[15] The combination of watching television (at least two and one-half hours a day) and eating fast food more than twice a week triples the risk of obesity, according to a 15-year study of more than 3,700 white and black young adults.[16]

6. **Modernization.** The growth of industry and technology has led to an abundance of food, less need for physical activity, urbanization, labor-saving devices, and a more sedentary lifestyle. Suburban sprawl directly contributes to obesity, according to a recent

TABLE 9-1 ▌ Supersized Portions

Food/Beverage	Original Size (year introduced)	Today (largest available)
Budweiser (bottle)	7 oz. (1976)	40 oz.
Nestle's Crunch	1.6 oz. (1938)	5 oz.
Soda (Coca Cola)	6.5 oz. (1916)	34 oz.
French fries (Burger King)	2.6 oz. (1954)	6.9 oz.
Hamburger (McDonald's) (beef only)	1.6 oz. (1955)	8 oz.

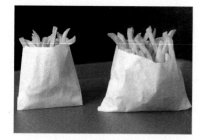 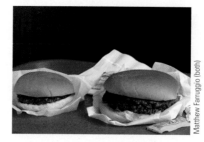

Matthew Farruggio (both)

Source: "Are Growing Portion Sizes Leading to Expanding Waistlines?" American Dietetic Association, www.eatright.org.

study. People who live in neighborhoods where they must drive to get anywhere are significantly more likely to be obese than those who can easily walk to their destinations. Each hour spent in a car was associated with a 6 percent increase in the likelihood of obesity and each half-mile walked per day reduced those odds by nearly 5 percent.[17]

7. **Socioeconomics.** The less money you make, the more likely you are to be overweight. One in four adults below the poverty level is obese, compared with one in six in households earning $67,000 or more. Minorities are at even greater risk. One in three poor African Americans is obese.[18]

8. **Prenatal factors.** A woman's weight before conception and weight gain during pregnancy influence her child's weight. A substantial number of children are prone to gaining weight because their mothers developed gestational diabetes during their pregnancies. Children born to obese women are more than twice as likely to be overweight by age four.[19]

9. **Childhood development.** Today's children don't necessarily eat more food than in the past, but they eat more high-fat, high-calorie foods and they exercise much, much less. On days when they eat fast food, youngsters consume an average of 187 more calories per day.[20] Fewer than half of grade schoolers participate in daily physical education classes. Many spend five hours or more a day in front of a computer or television screen.[21]

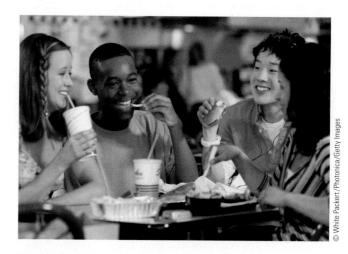

© White Packert/Photonica/Getty Images

▌ Round-the-clock snacking, fast-food restaurants around every corner, and hours in front of the TV have all contributed to the increase in obesity.

10. **Genetics.** Although scientists have identified genes involved in appetite and metabolism, they have not found a genetic cause for obesity. It may be that various genes contribute a small increase in risk or that rare abnormalities in many genes create a predisposition to weight gain and obesity.[22]

11. **Emotional influences.** Obese people are neither more nor less psychologically troubled than others. Psychological problems, such as irritability, depres-

sion, and anxiety, are more likely to be the result of obesity than the cause. As discussed later in this chapter, emotions do play a role in weight problems. Just as some people reach for a drink or a drug when they're upset, others cope by overeating, bingeing, or purging.

✚ Understanding Weight Problems

Weight problems don't develop overnight. Fat accumulates meal by meal, day by day, pound by pound. Ultimately all weight problems are the result of a prolonged energy imbalance—of consuming too many calories and burning too few in daily activities (**Figure 9-3**).

How many calories you need depends on your gender, age, body-frame size, weight, percentage of body fat, and your **basal metabolic rate (BMR)**—the number of calories needed to sustain your body at rest. Your activity level also affects your calorie requirements. Regardless of whether you consume fat, protein, or carbohydrates, if you take in more calories than required to maintain your size and don't work them off in some sort of physical activity, your body will convert the excess to fat.

The average American consumes about one million calories a year. Given that number, what difference does an extra 100-calorie soda or 300-calorie brownie make? A lot, because the extra calories that you don't burn every day accumulate, adding an average of 2 to 4 pounds to your weight every year.

Weight and the College Student

Obesity rates have increased most rapidly among 18- to 29-year-olds. According to the National College Health Risk Behavior Study, as many as 35 percent of college

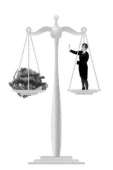

But . . .
Calories   > Calories = Weight gain
consumed   used

Calories   < Calories = Weight loss
consumed   used

No Weight Change:
Calories   = Calories
consumed   used

FIGURE 9-3 ▍ Energy Imbalance

Balancing the calories you eat with the calories you use through physical activity will help you maintain a healthy weight.

STRATEGIES for PREVENTION

Holding the Line on College Weight Gain

▍ **Plan meals.** Most campus cafeterias post the week's menus in advance. Plan which items you will eat before you see or smell high-fat dishes.

▍ **Don't linger.** If you use the cafeteria as a social gathering place, you may end up eating with two or three different groups of people. Set a time limit to eat—then leave.

▍ **Plan alternative behaviors.** People who eat when they are stressed or bored need substitute activities ready when they need them. Make a list of things you can do—shower, phone a friend, take a hike—when stress strikes.

▍ **Eat at "home."** If the dormitory has a small kitchen, cook some healthful dishes and invite friends to join you.

▍ **Take advantage of physical activity programs.** Many college students become less active during their years in college. Aim to maintain or increase the amount of exercise you did in high school. Join a biking club, take a salsa class, learn yoga.

students may be overweight or obese. In other studies, about one in five college students had an unhealthy weight as well as at least one risk factor for metabolic disorder, an important cause of cardiovascular disease (discussed in Chapter 10).[23] (See Student Snapshot: "Dangerous Weights.")

As many students discover, it's easy to gain weight on campuses, which are typically crammed with vending machines, fast-food counters, and cafeterias serving up hearty meals. But the infamous "freshman 15," the extra pounds acquired in the first year at college, seems to be a myth. Several studies have documented much lower weight gains, ranging from 2.45 to 7 pounds. In one study of changes in both weight and body fat, freshmen estimated that they had gained an average of 4.1 pounds. In fact, their weights fluctuated from a gain of 15 pounds to a loss of 15 pounds. Among the 60 percent of freshmen who did put on weight, the average gain was 4.6 pounds.[24]

Even international students may gain weight and body fat after arriving on American campuses. Ohio University researchers found that after 20 weeks, foreign students, who had incorporated foods high in fat, salt, and sugar into their diets, gained

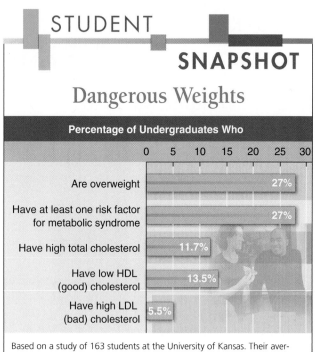

STUDENT SNAPSHOT

Dangerous Weights

Percentage of Undergraduates Who

Are overweight	27%
Have at least one risk factor for metabolic syndrome	27%
Have high total cholesterol	11.7%
Have low HDL (good) cholesterol	13.5%
Have high LDL (bad) cholesterol	5.5%

Based on a study of 163 students at the University of Kansas. Their average age was 22.2 years; 81 percent were white; 70 percent were female; 26 percent were smokers.
Source: Huang, Terry, et al. "Overweight and Components of the Metabolic Syndrome in College Students." *Diabetes Care,* Vol. 27, No. 12, December 2004, p. 3000.

about 3 pounds on average and their percentage of body fat rose by about 5 percent.

Is My Weight Healthy?

Rather than relying on a range of ideal weights for various heights, as they did in the past, medical experts use various methods to assess body composition and weight. The best indicators of weight-related health risks are Body Mass Index (BMI); waist circumference (WC); and waist-hip ratio (WHR).

If you're a young adult, even mild to moderate overweight poses a threat to your health because it puts you at risk for gaining even more weight—and for facing greater health risks. Obesity has been implicated as a culprit in rising rates of disability among younger Americans as well as a factor in chronic health problems.[25]

Body Composition

A combination of regular exercise and good nutrition is the best way to maintain a healthy body composition. Aerobic exercise helps by burning calories and increasing metabolic rate (the rate at which the body uses calories) for several hours after a workout. Strength training increases the proportion of lean body tissue by building muscle mass, which also increases the metabolic rate.

Most techniques for estimating body composition measure the relative amounts of fat and fat-free mass (bone, muscle, connective tissue, water, organs, and teeth) in the body. Some so-called field methods are used regularly by fitness professionals in gyms and training centers. Others are laboratory tools used primarily in clinical and research settings.

Knowing your specific body composition can provide useful information about body fat and health. Ideal body fat percentages for men range from 7 to 25 percent and for women from 16 to 35 percent. Methods of assessing body composition include anthropometric tests and body fat measurements.

Anthropometric Techniques

Body composition can be estimated by simply measuring the size and proportions of the human body and its various components, including height, body weight, circumferences, and waist-to-hip ratios. Easy and practical to use, anthropometric techniques are often employed in large epidemiological studies, and all provide some useful information about an individual's health and risk for various diseases. (See your Lab Booklet.)

Body Mass Index (BMI)

Body mass index (BMI), a ratio between weight and height, is a mathematical formula that correlates with body fat. You can determine your BMI from **Figure 9-4** on p. 185. (See your Lab Booklet on how to calculate your BMI.) A healthy BMI ranges from 18.5 to 24.9.

A BMI of 25 or greater defines **overweight** and marks the point at which excess weight increases the risk of disease. If your BMI is between 25 and 29.9 (23.4 for Asians), your weight is undermining the quality of your life. You suffer more aches and pains. You find it harder to perform everyday tasks. You run a greater risk of serious health problems.

A BMI of 30 or greater defines **obesity** and marks the point at which excess weight increases the risk of death. If your BMI is over 30, you face all the preceding dangers plus one more: dying. The risk of premature death increases even more if your BMI is over 40, a sign of severe or "morbid" obesity.

Doctors use BMI to determine whether a person is at risk for weight-related diseases like diabetes. However, using BMI as an assessment tool has limitations. Muscular individuals, including athletes and body builders, may be miscategorized as overweight or obese because they have greater lean muscle mass. BMI also does not reliably reflect body fat, an independent predictor of health risk, and is not useful for growing children, women who are pregnant or nursing, or the elderly. In addition, BMI, which was developed in Western nations, may not accurately indicate the risk of obesity-related diseases in Asian men and women.

If your BMI is high, you may be at increased risk of developing certain diseases, including hypertension, cardiovascular disease, adult-onset diabetes (type 2), sleep

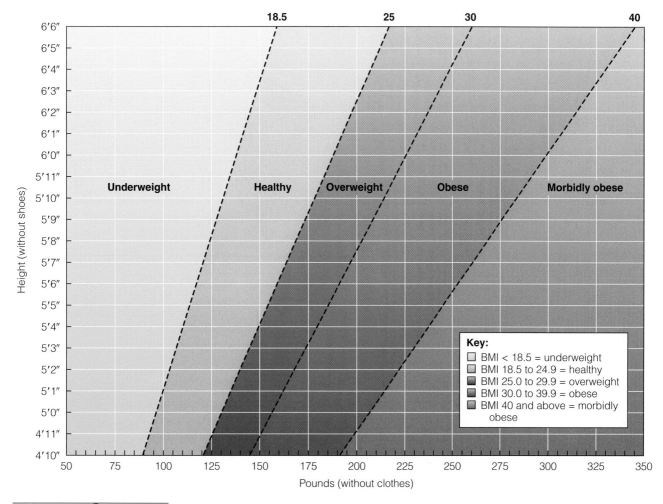

FIGURE 9-4 ▌ BMI Values Used to Assess Weight for Adults

apnea, and osteoarthritis. Although BMIs below 25 are considered healthy, individuals with BMIs between 22 and 24.9 are significantly more likely to develop a weight-related disease, such as high blood pressure, than leaner individuals with BMIs under 22.

Waist Circumference

Even if your scale shows that you haven't gained a lot of weight, your waist may widen—particularly if you've been under stress. Because of the physiological impact of stress hormones, fat accumulates around your midsection in times of tension and turmoil.

A widening waist or "apple" shape is a warning signal. In young women, a wider waist correlates with high levels of harmful blood fats, such as LDL cholesterol and triglycerides.[26] In both sexes, abdominal fat, unlike fat in the thighs or hips, increases the risk of high blood pressure, type 2 diabetes, high cholesterol, and metabolic syndrome (a perilous combination of over-weight, high blood pressure, and high levels of cholesterol and blood sugar, discussed in Chapter 10).[27]

To measure your waist circumference, place a tape measure around your bare abdomen just above your hip bone. Be sure that the tape is snug but does not compress your skin. Relax, exhale, and measure.

When is a waist too wide? Various studies have produced different results, but the general guideline is that a waist measuring more than 35 inches in a woman or more than 40 inches in a man signals greater health risks. These waist circumferences indicate "central" obesity, which is characterized by fat deposited deep within the central abdominal area of the body. Such "visceral" fat is more dangerous than "subcutaneous" fat just below the skin because it moves more readily into the bloodstream and directly raises levels of harmful cholesterol.

Body composition varies with race and ethnicity. Asians, for instance, may be more likely and African Americans less likely to accumulate visceral fat than Caucasians.[28]

Waist-to-Hip Ratio

Another way of determining your health risk is your **waist-to-hip ratio (WHR).** In addition to measuring your waist, measure your hips at the widest part. Divide your hip measurement into your waist measurement. For women, a ratio of 0.80 or less is considered safe; for men,

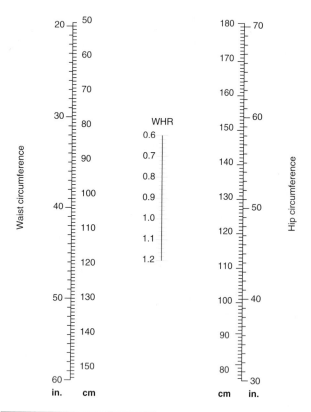

FIGURE 9-5 ❚ Determining Waist-to-Hip Ratio (WHR)

Use a straight edge to draw a line from your waist circumference (left) to your hip circumference (right). The point at which the line crosses the center column is your WHR.

Source: Data from Gray, G. A., and D. S. Gray. "Obesity: Part I: Pathenogenesis." *Western Journal of Medicine,* Vol. 149, 1988. In Christian, Janet, and Janet Greger, *Nutrition for Living,* 4th ed. Redwood City, CA: Benjamin Cummings, 1994.

the recommended ratio is 0.90 or less. For both men and women, a 1.0 or higher is considered "at risk" or in the danger zone for undesirable health consequences, such as heart disease and other ailments associated with being overweight. You can also use **Figure 9-5** to determine your WHR.

Men of all ages are more prone to develop the "apple" shape characteristic of central obesity; women in their reproductive years are more likely to accumulate fat around the hips and thighs and acquire a pear shape (**Figure 9-6**).

When men and women diet, men lose more visceral fat located around the abdominal area. This weight loss produces more cardiovascular benefits for men, including a decrease in triglycerides (fats circulating in the blood) and an increase in the "good" form of cholesterol, high-density lipoprotein (HDL).

Body Fat Measurements

You can check your body fat in various ways, including handheld body fat analyzers, stand-on body fat monitors, calipers, and sophisticated medical imaging devices.

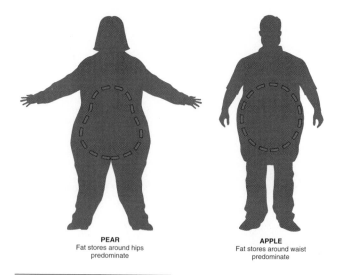

PEAR
Fat stores around hips predominate

APPLE
Fat stores around waist predominate

FIGURE 9-6 ❚ Pear-Shaped Versus Apple-Shaped Bodies

Skinfold Fat Measurements

Because of the relatively low cost and simplicity, the measurement of skinfolds is a popular method of estimating body composition. **Skinfold measurements** are taken with pressure calipers at designated body sites. The usual sites include the chest, abdomen, and thigh for men and the triceps, suprailium (hip), and thigh for women. The measurement is taken by pinching the skin with the thumb and forefinger, pulling it away from the body slightly, and placing the calipers on the fold. This technique measures the thickness of the two layers of skin and the underlying subcutaneous fat. Various equations are available to determine body fat percentage, including calculations that take into account age, gender, race, and other factors.

The skinfold method requires considerable technical skill and precision in selecting sites and calculating the measurements. Many types of calipers are available, ranging from research calipers that cost more than $200 to less expensive (but not necessarily less accurate) ones that sell for $10 to $50. Some research suggests that the same skinfold calipers should be used as were employed in formulating the specific equations for body fat percentages, because skinfold thicknesses can differ even among the highest-priced research calipers. Different technicians may also get somewhat different readings from the same person.

Skinfold measurements are not a good method for evaluating body composition in older men and women with loose connective tissue or obese individuals with large skinfolds. They are accurate for most athletes, however, so this approach has been recommended for specific uses, such as estimating minimal weights for competitors in weight-restrictive sports like wrestling.

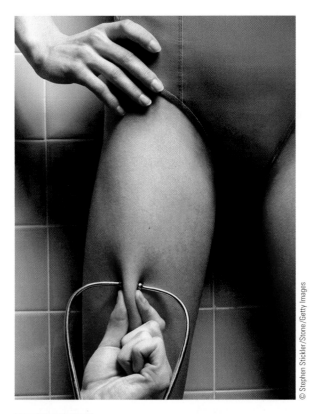

Accurate skinfold measurement can determine body fat percentage.

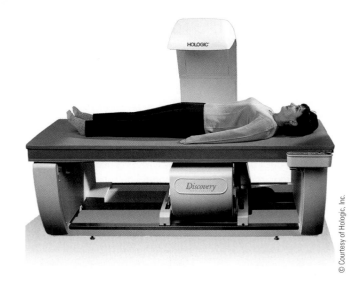

DXA directly measures body composition with the use of X rays.

Home Body Fat Analyzers

Handheld devices and stand-on monitors sold online and in specialty stores promise to make measuring your body fat percentage as easy as finding your weight. None has been extensively tested.

Laboratory Methods

Several approaches to body composition assessment are used primarily in clinical and research settings. Regardless of which test is used to assess body composition, each method is only as good as the measurement technique and the conversion formula that it employs. To limit errors, those conducting the test must meticulously follow the standard guidelines and protocols associated with each method. Additionally, the conversion formulas and prediction equations selected for use apply only to the populations (for example, men, women, athletes, or the elderly) on which they were based.

- **Hydrostatic (Underwater) Weighing.** Underwater weighing is a complex technique based on Archimedes' principle that a body immersed in a fluid is buoyed by a force equal to the weight of the displaced fluid. Because muscle has a higher density than water and fat has a lower density, fat people tend to displace less water than lean people.

  Although still considered the best body composition test by some researchers, **hydrostatic weighing** has many drawbacks. Individuals must exhale completely to force all air out of the lungs and remain completely still while submerged in a sitting position for five to ten seconds. This challenging exercise must be repeated several times, because at least three underwater weights are required to get an accurate reading. In addition, hydrostatic weighing is expensive and time-consuming.

- **Dual-Energy X-Ray Absorptiometry (DXA).** DXA uses X rays to quantify the skeletal and soft tissue components of body mass. Whereas other methods are based on variables indirectly related to body composition (such as water content of tissues), DXA provides a direct measurement of body composition. The test itself is simple and quick, usually requiring just 10 to 20 minutes, and the radiation dosage is low (800 to 2,000 times lower than a typical chest X ray).

  Although the accuracy and precision of DXA have been confirmed, this method has limitations. Variations in hydration, body thickness, fat distribution, and different technologies and software for dual-energy densitometers may limit its potential usefulness. Nevertheless, some researchers believe that DXA will supplant hydrostatic weighing as the gold standard for body composition assessment.

- **Bioelectrical Impedance Analysis (BIA).** This noninvasive method is based on the principle that electrical current applied to the body meets greater resistance with different types of tissue. Lean tissue, which contains large amounts of water and electrolytes, is a good electrical conductor; fat, which does not, is a poor conductor. In theory, the easier the electrical conduction, the greater an individual's lean body mass.

  In a BIA test, an individual is hooked up to a machine, and a weak electrical current is transmitted

STRATEGIES for CHANGE

Maintaining a Healthy Body Composition

- Keep track of what you eat. By choosing healthful foods and monitoring how many calories you consume, you can prevent weight gain.

- Spend half an hour a day on the move. Just 30 minutes of the exercise-equivalent of brisk walking can keep your body fat percentage from rising.

- Lose a little. If you are overweight, losing as little as 5 to 10 percent of your body weight can improve your body composition and your health.

- Work your muscles. Strength training can increase fat-free mass and reduce body fat.

through the body. Mathematical equations estimate the percent body fat based on the readings. Because it is difficult to obtain accurate skinfold measurements on older adults and obese individuals, BIA is the preferred field method for estimating body fat percentage in these men and women. It has also proved to be the most precise method for assessing the body composition of young female athletes and dancers.

- **The Bod Pod®.** This large, egg-shaped fiberglass chamber uses an approach based on air displacement plethysmography, that is, the calculation of the relationship between pressure and volume.

    Quicker, more convenient, and easier to administer than hydrostatic testing, the Bod Pod® has been reported to be a highly reliable method for determining percent body fat. It may prove especially useful for older adults, physically challenged individuals, and those afraid of being submerged underwater.

✚ Health Dangers of Excess Weight

The federal government has recognized obesity as a serious, potentially fatal disease. This designation cleared the way for insurance coverage for obesity treatments, rather than just for the medical problems it can cause. The effects of obesity on health are the equivalent of 20 years of aging.[29] They include increased risk of cardiovascular disease, diabetes, and cancer, as well as disability, rheumatoid arthritis, sleep apnea, gout, and liver disease (**Figure 9-7**). Total costs, both direct and indirect, amount to more than $117 billion a year.[30]

The Impact on the Body

The incidence of diabetes, gallstones, hypertension, heart disease, and colon cancer increases with the degree of overweight in both sexes. Those with BMIs of 35 or more are approximately 20 times more likely to develop diabetes. Individuals who are overweight but not obese, with BMIs between 25 and 29.9, are significantly more likely than leaner women to develop gallstones, high blood pressure, high cholesterol, and heart disease. Overweight men are also more likely to suffer strokes.

Health risks may vary in different races, ethnic groups, and at-risk populations.[31] Even relatively small amounts of excess fat—as little as 5 pounds —can add to the dangers in those already at risk for hypertension and diabetes. According to the National Heart, Lung, and Blood Institute, being overweight, even if not obese, increases the risk of heart failure. Obesity also causes alterations in various measures of immune function and increases the risk of kidney stones and disease.[32]

Major diseases linked to obesity include:

- **Type 2 diabetes.** More than 80 percent of people with type 2 diabetes are overweight. Although the reasons why are not known, being overweight may make cells less efficient at using sugar from the blood. This then puts stress on the cells that produce insulin (a hormone that carries sugar from the blood to cells) and makes them gradually fail. You can lower your risk for developing type 2 diabetes by losing weight and increasing the amount of physical activity you do. If you have type 2 diabetes, losing weight and becoming more physically active can help you control your blood sugar levels and may allow you to reduce the amount of diabetes medication you take.[33]

- **Heart disease and stroke.** People who are overweight are more likely to suffer from high blood pressure, high levels of triglycerides (blood fats) and harmful LDL cholesterol, and low levels of beneficial HDL cholesterol. In addition, people with more body fat have higher blood levels of substances that cause inflammation, which may raise heart disease risk. Losing 5 to 15 percent of your weight can lower your chances for developing heart disease or having a stroke.

    People who both smoke and are obese are at especially high risk of cardiovascular disease. Although some smokers have felt that they couldn't lose weight until they stopped smoking, researchers have found that weight loss among smokers is possible and beneficial, leading to a reduction in other risk factors, such as lower blood pressure and lower cholesterol.

- **Cancer.** According to a study of 900,000 people, the largest ever of its kind, excess weight may account for 14 percent of all cancer deaths in men and 20 percent of those in women. Losing weight, researchers estimate, could prevent as many as one of every six cancer deaths.[34]

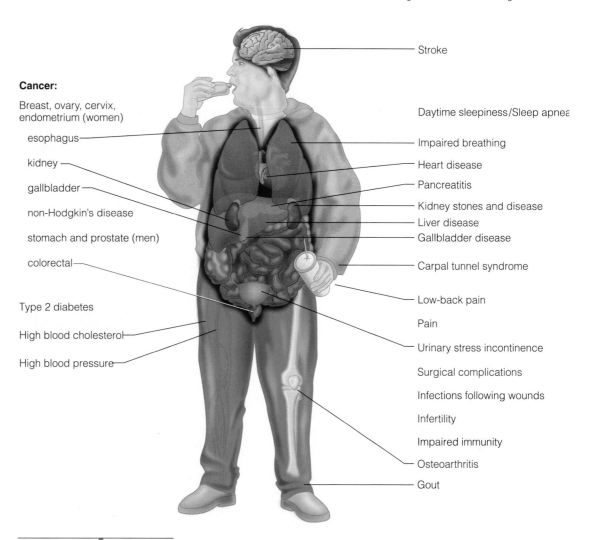

Stroke

Cancer:

Breast, ovary, cervix,
endometrium (women)

esophagus

kidney

gallbladder

non-Hodgkin's disease

stomach and prostate (men)

colorectal

Type 2 diabetes

High blood cholesterol

High blood pressure

Daytime sleepiness/Sleep apnea

Impaired breathing

Heart disease

Pancreatitis

Kidney stones and disease

Liver disease

Gallbladder disease

Carpal tunnel syndrome

Low-back pain

Pain

Urinary stress incontinence

Surgical complications

Infections following wounds

Infertility

Impaired immunity

Osteoarthritis

Gout

FIGURE 9-7 ▍ Health Dangers of Excess Weight

While earlier research had linked excess weight to cancers of the breast and uterus, colon and rectum, kidney, esophagus, and gallbladder, this study also linked weight to other cancers, including non-Hodgkin's lymphoma; multiple myeloma; and cancers of the pancreas and liver, the cervix and ovary (in women), and the stomach and prostate (in men). Those with BMIs over 40 had death rates from cancer that were 52 percent higher for men and 62 percent higher for women than those of normal-weight individuals.[35]

Body size and higher BMI are linked with increased risk of breast cancer in pre-menopausal women and in postmenopausal women not using hormone replacement therapy.[36]

Too much body fat can influence cancer in several ways: It increases the amount of estrogen in the blood, raising the risk of cancers of the female reproductive system. It raises the levels of insulin, which prompts the body to create a hormone that causes cells to multiply. Acid reflux, which can cause cancer of the esophagus, occurs more frequently in heavy men and women. Obesity also makes cancer harder to diagnose and treat.

Excess pounds affect people around the clock. Overweight and obese individuals sleep less than those with normal weights. Individuals with lower BMIs get an extra 16 minutes of rest a night or two hours a week. (See Chapter 7 for a discussion of sleep.) The lost sleep could add to the risk of medical problems.[37]

Life Expectancy

In the past, experts had estimated that obesity might claim more than 300,000 lives a year. However, the CDC recently reported that obesity is becoming less lethal than in the past, possibly as a result of improvements in public health and medical care. Based on BMI, extremely obese individuals are most likely to die. People who are overweight but not obese have a lower risk of death than those of normal weight.[38] The reasons are not clear, although rates of high blood pressure and high cholesterol in the obese have declined in recent decades, to a great extent because of breakthroughs in medications.[39] Since most deaths occur in old age, some researchers theorize that some extra weight might be beneficial in the elderly if it contributes to stronger bones and muscles. Decades of overweight and obesity may take a greater toll on wellness and possibly on lifespan.[40]

The Emotional Toll

In our calorie-conscious and thinness-obsessed society, obesity also affects quality of life, including sense of vitality and physical pain. Many see it as a psychological burden, a sign of failure, laziness, or inadequate willpower. Overweight men and women often blame themselves for becoming heavy and feel guilty and depressed as a result. In fact, the psychological problems once considered the cause of obesity may be its consequence.

A Canadian study found so many overweight and obese individuals (14 percent of the sample) at risk for depression that its authors suggested that all health professionals assess obese patients for depression.[41]

✚ A Practical Guide to Weight Loss

Readiness to change is key to successful weight loss. (See Self-Survey on p. 205.) However, individuals vary in their readiness to change their diets, increase their physical activity, and seek professional counseling. In one study, participants also varied in specific dietary changes. For instance, some were ready to eat more fruits and vegetables but not to reduce total calories.[42]

One indicator of readiness to change is willingness to talk with a health-care provider about diet or exercise.[43] Unfortunately, only about 40 percent of doctors report counseling patients about weight management.[44] When physicians do provide weight loss counseling, patients are more likely to understand the risks of obesity and the benefits of weight loss and move to a higher stage of readiness.[45]

Why Do I Overeat? 📭🔍

The answer lies not just in the belly, but in the brain. Both **hunger,** the physiological drive to consume food, and **appetite,** the psychological desire to eat, influence and control our desire for food. Scientists have discovered appetite receptors within the brain that specifically respond to hunger messengers carried by hormones produced in the digestive tract (**Figure 9–8**).

Appetite usually begins with the fear of the unpleasant sensation of hunger. We learn to avoid hunger by eating a certain amount of food at certain times of the day, just as dogs in the laboratory learn to avoid electric shocks by jumping at the sound of a warning bell. But appetite is easily led into temptation. In one famous experiment, psychologists bought bags of high-calorie goodies—peanut butter, marshmallows, chocolate-chip cookies, and salami—for their test rats. The animals ate so much on this "supermarket diet" that they gained

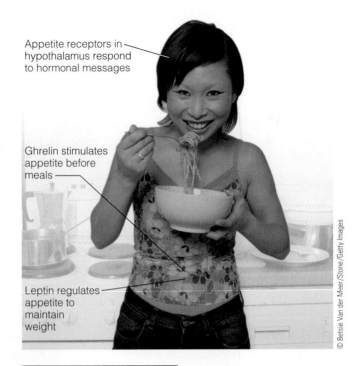

Appetite receptors in hypothalamus respond to hormonal messages

Ghrelin stimulates appetite before meals

Leptin regulates appetite to maintain weight

© Betsie Van der Meer/Stone/Getty Images

FIGURE 9-8 ▌ Hormones help regulate our appetite

more weight than any laboratory rats ever had before. The snack-food diet that fattened up these rats was particularly high in fats. Biologists speculate that creamy, buttery, or greasy foods may cause internal changes that increase appetite and, consequently, weight.

A hormone called leptin, produced by fat cells, sends signals to the brain that affect appetite. When leptin levels are normal, people eat just enough to maintain weight. When leptin is low, the brain responds as if fat stores had been depleted and slows down metabolism. This may be one reason why it is so difficult to lose weight by dieting alone.

Other hormones made in the stomach also influence how hungry we feel. One is ghrelin, a natural appetite stimulant. When given shots of ghrelin, people become very hungry and eat 30 percent more than they normally would. Ghrelin typically rises before meals and falls afterward. Dieters tend to have high levels of ghrelin, as if their bodies were trying to stimulate appetite so they regain lost fat.

We stop eating when we feel satisfied; this is called **satiety,** a feeling of fullness and relief from hunger. The neurotransmitter serotonin has been shown to produce feelings of satiety. In addition, several peptides, released from the digestive tract as we ingest food, may signal the brain to stop or restrict eating. However, it takes 20 minutes for the brain to register fullness.

Weight Loss Diets

Never before have so many had so much to lose. More than two-thirds of Americans—77 percent of women and 63 percent of men—are either dieting or struggling to

STRATEGIES for PREVENTION

Managing Your Weight

The 2005 Dietary Guidelines for Americans recommend the following steps for weight management:

▮ To maintain body weight in a healthy range, balance calories from foods and beverages with calories expended.

▮ To prevent gradual weight gain over time, make small decreases in food and beverage calories and increase physical activity.

Key Recommendations for Specific Population Groups

▮ **Those who need to lose weight.** Aim for a slow, steady weight loss by decreasing calorie intake while maintaining an adequate nutrient intake and increasing physical activity.

▮ **Overweight children.** Reduce the rate of body weight gain while allowing growth and development. Consult a health-care provider before placing a child on a weight-reduction diet.

▮ **Pregnant women.** Ensure appropriate weight gain as specified by a health-care provider.

▮ **Breastfeeding women.** Moderate weight reduction is safe and does not compromise weight gain of the nursing infant.

▮ **Overweight adults and overweight children with chronic diseases and/or on medication.** Consult a health-care provider about weight loss strategies prior to starting a weight-reduction program to ensure appropriate management of other health conditions.[46]

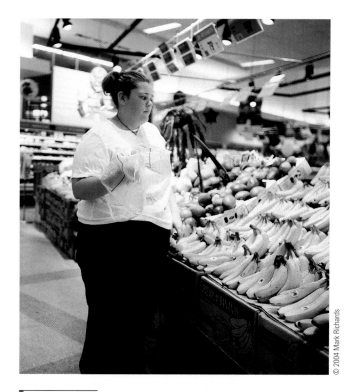

▮ Today's Goal: Have fruit instead of dessert at lunch.

maintain their weight. You've probably heard that 95 percent of people who lose weight gain it all back. That widely quoted statistic, based on a small study from 1959, is no longer true, if it ever was.[47] Diets can and do work. Tens of thousands of dieters have lost excess pounds and maintained lower, healthier weights. Although many regain some weight, most manage to keep off about two-thirds of the weight lost by dieting for at least a year.[48]

Which diet is best? That's a confusing and controversial question (**Table 9-2**). The heated debate over carbohydrates, fats, and calories continues to rage, but research is providing better understanding of what works and what doesn't, both in the short and long run.

You've seen the commercials and read the claims that a popular new diet can pare away pounds. Don't believe the hype. According to a review of commercial weight loss programs, there is little scientific evidence to back up any claims that popular diets help overweight individuals slim down. In almost any program, people lose weight because they are paying more attention to their food choices and limiting their calories.[49]

Diets do work—for a while. Low-calorie (1,000 to 1,200 calories daily) and very low-calorie diets produce similar results a year later. Physical activity alone leads to a weight loss of about 2 to 3 percent of initial weight and reduces abdominal fat. A combination of diet and physical activity, particularly along with behavioral therapy, produces greater reductions in weight and abdominal fat than either approach alone. "High-intensity" programs, which provide person-to-person contact more than once a month, are more effective than those with less frequent contact.[50]

In a year-long "battle of the bulge," researchers compared four popular diets: Atkins, Weight Watchers, The Zone, and Ornish. All produced similar results, including a weight loss of about 7 pounds and a lowering of heart disease risk factors—but only in those who stuck with the program. Nearly half of the dieters dropped out before the year was up because the diets were too hard to follow or weren't working. The Atkins and Ornish plans had the highest dropout rates.[51] In another study, Weight-Watchers dieters who regularly attended the program lost approximately 5 percent of their body weight in three to six months. Those on very low-calorie diets who finished the program lost up to 25 percent of their initial weight but were at high risk of regaining at least half of it back.[52]

Because of the high relapse rate, researchers are searching for ways to motivate dieters and sustain weight loss for five to ten years. In the meantime, the best

TABLE 9-2 ▮ Dueling Diets

Better ◀——————▶ Worse
◉ ◒ ○ ◓ ●

Diet	Price[1]	Overall score	Nutrition	Analytical results 6 months Weight loss	Dropout rate	1 year Weight loss	Dropout rate	Average daily calories	Nutritional content — Percentage of calories — Fat	Saturated fat	Carbohydrates	Protein	Grams of fiber/1,000 cal.	Fruits, veggies—daily servings
1 Weight Watchers	$10–13/week	◒	◉	○	◒	○	◒	1,450	24	7	56	20	20	11
2 Slim-Fast	$2–3/day for bars or drinks	◒	◉	◒	◒	◒	●	1,540	22	6	57	21	21	12
3 Zone (men's menu) (The Zone, Barry Sears, with Bill Lawren)[2]	$25.00	◒	◉	○	○	○	◓	1,660	27	7	42	30	21	17
4 Ornish (Eat More, Weigh Less, Dean Omnish)	$15.00	○	○	○	●	◒	●	1,520	6	1	77	16	31	17
5 Atkins Ongoing Weight Loss Dr. Atkins' New Diet Revolution, Robert C. Atkins[3]	$13.95	◓	●	◒	○	○	◓	1,520	60	20	11	29	12	6
6 Atkins Induction Dr. Atkins' New Diet Revolution, Robert C. Atkins[3]	$13.95	◓	●	◒	○	○	◓	1,640	61	19	8	31	8	6
Not Rated: Insufficient Study Data (diets listed in alphabetical order)														
7 eDiets	$12–32/month	—	◉	—	—	—	—	1,450	23	5	53	24	19	12
8 Jenny Craig	$6–7.65/week, $11–15/day (food)	—	◉	—	—	—	—	1,520	18	7	62	20	16	6
9 South Beach Phase One (The South Beach Diet, Arthur Agatston)	$24.95	—	◓	—	—	—	—	1,530	51	14	15	34	9	12
10 South Beach Phase Two (The South Beach Diet, Arthur Agatston)	$24.95	—	◒	—	—	—	—	1,340	39	9	38	22	19	13
11 Volumetrics (The Volumetrics Eating Plan, Barbara Rolls)	$25.95	—	◉	—	—	—	—	1,500	23	7	55	22	20	14

Source: © 2000–2004 Consumers Union of U.S., Inc. No reproduction, in whole or in part, without written permission.

[1] Except where noted, price is for the book. [2] Women's menu similar but about 1,300 calories. [3] Studies of Atkins used first the induction and then the ongoing diet plans, so our 6-month and 1-year results include both phases.

treatment of obesity is a "low-fad" approach, with an emphasis on healthy food choices and regular physical activity.[53]

No one approach suits everyone. Some people would rather restrict what they eat than work up a sweat. Others prefer to move their muscles and not worry about what they put in their mouths. Which approach works better? That depends on your goals.

To shed pounds, you have to cut back on how much you eat so you're consuming fewer calories than you

TABLE 9-3 ▮ Countdown to Weight Loss

The combination of walking and cutting calories results in greater weight loss than either alone.

If you walk (minutes)	& If you cut daily calories by	Days to Lose Weight				
		5 lb.	10 lb.	15 lb.	20 lb.	25 lb.
30	400	27	54	81	108	135
30	800	16	32	48	64	80
45	400	23	46	69	92	115
45	800	14	28	42	56	70
60	400	21	42	63	84	105
60	800	13	26	39	54	65

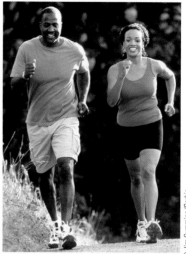

© Jim Cummins/Corbis

expend. If you eat less but don't exercise, you will lose pounds, but about one-quarter of the lost weight will come from muscle tissue rather than fat—and you're more likely to regain whatever you lose because, as you lose muscle, your metabolic rate slows down.

To improve your health and lower your risk of death and disease, exercise has proved more beneficial than diet alone. If you increase exercise without decreasing food intake, you will improve fitness, build lean muscle mass, and reduce body fat. Don't expect your scale to register a major change, but once you drop excess pounds, exercise will help keep them off.

Losing weight is not a question of "either/or" but of doing both. A combination of dietary change and moderate to high-level intensity of exercise leads to greater weight loss than either alone (**Table 9–3**). Putting psychology to work and adding behavioral changes can boost your chances of success, regardless of whether you focus more on diet or physical activity.

Low-Carbohydrate Diets

An estimated 17 million Americans have tried a low-carb diet in the last year. The diet popularized by the late Dr. Robert Atkins is high in protein and extremely low in carbohydrates. Followers of the Atkins diet eat unlimited amounts of meat, eggs, and cheese and cut back on bread, pasta, crackers, cakes, cookies, and other carbohydrates. Because they avoid many high-calorie foods and fill up on proteins, which take longer to digest, these dieters typically lose weight without feeling hungry.

Particularly in the initial stages, followers of the Atkins diet may consume 40 percent of their calories in fat, much of it saturated. For years professional groups such as the American Dietetic Association and the American Heart Association warned that low-carb, high-fat weight loss plans like the Atkins diet pose serious health dangers, primarily because the high fat content may increase the risk of heart disease, diabetes, stroke, and kidney and liver disease.

Several studies have challenged these assumptions, at least in the short term. In one six-month trial, participants were more likely to stick with an Atkins-style diet and lost more weight (26 pounds compared with 14 pounds) than volunteers on a low-fat, low-cholesterol diet. Triglyceride and HDL cholesterol levels improved considerably on the low-carb diet, but its followers reported more negative symptoms, such as constipation, headache, and muscle cramps. "Over six months the diet appears relatively safe, but we need to study the safety for longer durations," said the lead researcher, Dr. Will Yancy, who noted that potential long-term health risks include increases in harmful LDL cholesterol, bone loss, and kidney stones.[54]

In a year-long study, those on a low-carb diet lost more weight in the first six months, but at the end of the year their weight loss was comparable to the participants on a low-fat diet, whose weight declined slowly but steadily. As in the shorter study, the low-carb diet had a more beneficial effect on triglyceride and HDL levels than the low-fat diet.[55]

Diets such as Sugar Busters! and the Glucose Revolution distinguish between "correct" carbs (fruits, vegetables, and whole grains) and "harmful" ones (refined sugars and processed grains). Other popular diets call for specific proportions of nutrients. For instance, The Zone diet advocates meals and snacks that consist of 40 percent carbohydrate, 30 percent fat, and 30 percent protein. Dieters may lose weight because they're paying more attention to what they eat and making better food choices. However, approaches like this generally make smart eating more complicated than it has to be.[56]

Low-Fat Diets

Various diets reduce daily fat intake—some to 25 to 30 percent of calories; others, such as the Dean Ornish program, to less than 10 percent. The Ornish diet has proved effective in reversing atherosclerotic buildup. Low-fat diets also may enhance the immune response.

However, although experts support a decrease in trans and saturated fats for the sake of cardiovascular health, they have challenged the scientific evidence for reducing fat below 30 to 35 percent for the sake of preventing heart disease in healthy individuals. Epidemiological studies have not shown that dietary fat directly increases body fat. "Healthy" fats such as olive oil and fatty acids in fish oils may help control appetite and maintain long-term weight loss.

Low-Calorie Diets

Any diet that restricts calories will lead to weight loss. "There is no substitute for the simple formula that 'calories in must equal calories out' in order to control weight," said the FDA Deputy Commissioner when the agency's Obesity Working Group issued its report in 2004 and called for more focus on calories. The Department of Health and Human Services has launched a public education campaign, similar to earlier stop-smoking initiatives, that emphasizes the simple message, "Calories count."

Cutting back 500 to 1,000 calories a day typically leads to a loss of 1 to 2 pounds a week and an average weight loss of about 8 percent of body weight in six months. Expert groups, such as the American Society for Clinical Nutrition, the North American Association for the Study of Obesity, and the National Heart, Lung, and Blood Institute Obesity Education Initiative recommend going no lower than 1,000 to 1,200 calories a day for women and 1,200 to 1,600 calories for men.

Very low-calorie diets, which provide fewer than 800 calories a day, lead to rapid weight loss but pose serious, potentially deadly health risks. Whenever people cut back drastically on calories, they immediately lose several pounds because of a loss of fluid. As soon as they return to a more normal way of eating, they regain this weight.

On a very low-calorie diet, as much as 50 percent of the weight you lose may be muscle (so you'll actually look flabbier). Because your heart is a muscle, it may become so weak that it no longer can pump blood through your body. In addition, your blood pressure may plummet, causing dizziness, light-headedness, and fatigue. You may develop nausea and abdominal pain. You may lose hair. If you're a woman, your menstrual cycle may become irregular, or you may stop menstruating altogether. As you lose more water, you also lose essential vitamins, and your metabolism slows down. Even reaction time slows, and crash dieters may not be able to respond as quickly as usual.

Once you go off an extreme diet—as you inevitably must—your metabolism remains slow, even though you're no longer restricting your food intake. The human body appears to alter its energy use to compensate for weight loss. These metabolic changes may make it

STRATEGIES for CHANGE

Designing a Diet

There is no one perfect diet that will work for everyone who needs to lose weight. "Experiment with various methods for weight control," suggests Dr. Walter Willett of the Harvard School of Public Health. "Patients should focus on finding ways to eat that they can maintain indefinitely rather than seeking diets that promote rapid weight loss."[57] In other words, design an eating plan that you can stick with for the rest of your life.

Whether you decide to focus on carbohydrates, fat, or calories, the following strategies can help you get to and maintain a healthy weight:

▌ Avoid "bad" fats, including trans-fatty acids and partially hydrogenated fats.

▌ Consume "good" fats, such as omega-3 fatty acids every day.

▌ Eat fewer "bad" carbohydrates, such as sugar and white flour.

▌ Eat more "good" carbs, including fruits, vegetables, legumes, and unrefined grains like whole-wheat flour and brown rice.

▌ Have three or more daily servings of low-fat dairy products, which accelerate fat loss.

▌ Opt for quality over quantity. Eating a smaller amount of something delicious and nutritious can be far more satisfying than larger portions of junk foods.

▌ Exercise more. The key to balancing the equation between calories consumed and calories used is physical activity.

harder for people to maintain a reduced body weight after dieting.

Avoiding Diet Traps

Whatever your eating style, there are only two effective strategies for losing weight: eating less and exercising more. Unfortunately, most people search for easier alternatives that almost invariably turn into dietary dead ends or unexpected dangers. (See Savvy Consumer: "How to Spot a Dubious Diet.") Three common traps to avoid are diet pills, diet foods, and the yo-yo syndrome.

Diet Pills

In their search for a quick fix to weight problems, millions of people have tried often risky remedies. In the 1920s, some women swallowed patented weight loss

HOW TO SPOT A DUBIOUS DIET

The National Council Against Health Fraud cautions dieters to watch for these warnings of dangerous or fraudulent programs.

▌ Promises of very rapid weight loss.

▌ Claims that the diet can eliminate *cellulite* (a term used to describe dimply fatty tissue on the arms and legs).

▌ "Counselors" who are really salespersons pushing a product or program.

▌ No mention of any risks associated with the diet.

▌ Unproven gimmicks, such as body wraps, starch blockers, hormones, diuretics, or "unique" pills or potions.

▌ No maintenance program.

If you hear about a new diet that promises to melt away fat, don't try it until you get answers to the following questions:

▌ Does it include a wide variety of nutritious foods?

▌ Does it provide at least 1,200 calories a day?

▌ Is it designed to reduce your weight by one-half to two pounds per week?

▌ Does it emphasize moderate portions?

▌ Does it use foods that are easy to find and prepare?

▌ Can you follow it wherever you eat —at home, work, restaurants, or parties?

▌ Is its cost reasonable?

If the answer to any of these questions is no, don't try the diet; then ask yourself one more question: Is losing weight worth losing your well-being?

---

capsules that turned out to be tapeworm eggs. In the 1960s and 1970s, addictive amphetamines were common diet aids. In the 1990s, appetite suppressants known as fen-phen became popular. They were taken off the market after being linked to heart valve problems.

The Food and Drug Administration has warned users of the popular herb ephedra (also identified as ephedrine and ma huang and often combined with caffeine) about heart attacks, strokes, and even death. In a meta-analysis of studies conducted on ephedra products for weight loss, researchers concluded that use of high doses of ephedra or ephedra and caffeine for six months or less does promote weight loss—but also takes a toll on physical and mental well-being. Ephedra products are associated with two to three times the normal risk of psychiatric symptoms, upper gastrointestinal symptoms, and heart palpitations.

Diet Foods

According to the Calorie Control Council, 90 percent of Americans choose some foods labeled "light." But even though these foods keep growing in popularity, Americans' weight keeps rising. There are several reasons: Many people think choosing a food that's lower in calories, fat-free, or "light" gives them a license to eat as much as they want. What they don't realize is that many foods that are low in fat are still high in sugar and calories. Refined carbohydrates, rapidly absorbed into the bloodstream, raise blood glucose levels. As they fall, appetite increases.

Diet products, including diet sodas and low-fat foods, are a very big business. Many people rely on meal replacements, usually shakes or snack bars, to lose or keep off weight. If used appropriately—as actual replacements rather than supplements to regular meals and snacks—they can be a useful strategy for weight loss. Yet people who use these products often gain weight because they think that they can afford to add high-calorie treats to their diet.

What about the artificial sweeteners and fake fats that appear in many diet products? Nutritionists caution to use them in moderation and not to substitute them for

© Radhika Chalasani /Corbis

▌ The foods you choose at every meal can affect both your weight and your health.

basic foods, such as grains, fruits, and vegetables. Foods made with fat substitutes may have fewer grams of fat, but they don't necessarily have significantly fewer calories. Many people who consume reduced-fat, fat-free, or sugar-free sodas, cookies, chips, and other snacks often cut back on more nutritious foods, such as fruits and vegetables. They also tend to eat more of the low- or no-fat foods so that their daily calorie intake either stays the same or actually increases.

The Yo-Yo Syndrome

On-and-off-again dieting, especially by means of very low-calorie diets (under 800 calories a day), can be self-defeating and dangerous. Some studies have shown that weight cycling may make it more difficult to lose weight or keep it off (**Figure 9-9**). Repeated cycles of rapid weight loss followed by weight gain may even change food preferences. Chronic crash dieters often come to prefer foods that combine sugar and fat, such as cake frosting.

To avoid the yo-yo syndrome and overcome its negative effects: Exercise. Researchers at the University of Pennsylvania found that when overweight women who also exercised went off a very low-calorie diet, their metabolism did not stay slow but bounced back to the appropriate level for their new, lower body weight. The reason may be exercise's ability to preserve muscle tissue. The more muscle tissue you have, the higher your metabolic rate.

If you've been losing (and regaining) the same 5 or 10 pounds for years, try the following suggestions for long-term success:

▌ **Set a danger zone.** Once you've reached your desired weight, don't let your weight climb more than 3 or 4 pounds higher. Take into account normal fluctuations, but watch out for an upward trend. Once you hit your upper weight limit, take action immediately rather than waiting until you gain 10 pounds.

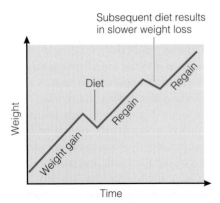

FIGURE 9-9 ▌ Weight-Cycling Effect of Repeated Dieting

Each round of dieting is typically followed by a rebound leading to a greater weight gain.

▌ **Be patient.** Think of weight loss as a road trip. If you're going across town, you expect to get there in 20 minutes. If your destination is 400 miles away, you know it'll take longer. Give yourself the time you need to lose weight safely and steadily.

▌ **Try, try again.** Dieters don't usually keep weight off on their first attempt. The people who eventually succeed don't give up. Through trial and error, they find a plan that works for them.

Physical Activity

Unplanned daily activity, such as fidgeting or pacing, can make a difference in preventing weight gain. Scientists use the acronym **NEAT**—for **nonexercise activity thermogenesis**—to describe such "nonvolitional" movement and have verified that it can be an effective way of burning calories. In a study of 10 lean and 10 mildly obese people—all self-confessed couch potatoes—the thinner ones sat an average of two hours less and moved and stood more often than the heavier individuals.[58] Small steps such as taking the stairs for a flight or two or parking farther away can make a difference.[59]

Although physical activity and exercise can prevent weight gain and improve health, usually it does not lead to significant weight loss. However, when combined with diet, exercise ensures that you lose fat rather than muscle and helps keep off excess pounds. Moderate exercise, such as 30 to 60 minutes of daily physical activity, has proved effective in reducing the risk of heart disease and other health threats. Although there are no definitive data, experts generally agree that more exercise—an estimated 60 to 90 minutes daily of moderately intense activity—is necessary to prevent weight gain. Recommending such higher levels of activity to overweight men and women does indeed lead to more exercise—and more lasting weight loss (**Table 9-4**).

Exercise has other benefits: It increases energy expenditure, builds up muscle tissue, burns off fat stores, and stimulates the immune system. Exercise also may reprogram metabolism so that more calories are burned during and after a workout.

An exercise program designed for both health benefits and weight loss should include both aerobic activity and resistance training. People who start and stick with an exercise program during or after a weight loss program are consistently more successful in keeping off most of the pounds they've shed.

✚ The Psychology of Losing Weight

Diets change what you eat. Exercise changes body composition, stamina, and strength. But changing your food-related thoughts and behaviors can be the key to lasting weight loss. If you think that you can shed pounds, if

TABLE 9-4 ▌ Calories/Hour Expended in Some Common Physical Activities

The second column shows the average number of calories a 154-pound individual will expend by engaging in the activity for 1 hour. The expenditure value encompasses both resting metabolic rate calories and activity expenditure.

Moderate Physical Activity	Approximate Calories/Hr for a 154-lb Person*
Hiking	370
Light gardening/yard work	330
Dancing	330
Golf (walking and carrying clubs)	330
Bicycling (< 10 mph)	290
Walking (3.5 mph)	280
Weight lifting (general light workout)	220
Stretching	180

Vigorous Physical Activity	Approximate Calories/Hr for a 154-lb Person*
Running/jogging (5 mph)	590
Bicycling (> 10 mph)	590
Swimming (slow freestyle laps)	510
Aerobics	480
Walking (4.5 mph)	460
Heavy yard work (chopping wood)	440
Weight lifting (vigorous effort)	440
Basketball (vigorous)	440

[a]Calories burned per hour will be higher for persons who weigh more than 154 lbs. (70 kg) and lower for persons who weigh less.

Source: Adapted from the *Dietary Guidelines for Americans 2005,* U.S. Department of Health and Human Services, U.S. Department of Agriculture, www.healthierus.gov/dietaryguidelines.

STRATEGIES for CHANGE

How to Boost Your Body Esteem

Whatever your weight or shape, here are some ways to improve your body image:

▌ Start walking with more bounce in your step.

▌ Focus on the parts of your body you like. Take pride in your powerful shoulders or large eyes.

▌ Treat yourself with the respect you'd like to receive from others. Don't put yourself down or joke about your weight.

▌ Work with hand weights. As you build your muscles, your sense of strength and self-confidence also will grow.

▌ Don't put off special plans, such as learning to kayak or signing up for an exchange program, until you reach a certain magical weight: Do what you want to do *now*.

▌ Pull your shoulders back, suck in your stomach, and stand up straight. You'll look and feel better.

you think that you can control what you put in your mouth, if you think that there is a form of exercise that you could enjoy, then you are on your way to reaching your weight loss goals.

Body Image

Influenced by the media, many Americans are paying more attention to their body images than ever before—and at a younger age. In a study of high school girls, those who regularly read women's health and fitness magazines, which may present unrealistic physical ideals, were more likely to go on low-calorie diets, take pills to suppress their appetites, use laxatives, or force themselves to vomit

after eating. In other research, girls who watched a lot of television and expressed concern about slimness and popularity were more dissatisfied with their bodies than girls involved in sports. Boys' body images also are influenced by media images depicting superstrong, highly muscular males.

African-American women often have more positive attitudes toward their bodies, feeling more satisfied with their weight and seeing themselves as more attractive. However, there are no significant differences between African-American women who diet and white women who diet in terms of self-esteem and body dissatisfaction.

Being overweight for a long period of time has a cumulative negative impact on body image. In a study of 266 college women, those who described themselves as "always overweight" ranked much lower in current body self-esteem than those with more recent weight problems.[60]

College students of different ethnic and racial backgrounds, including Asians, express as much —and sometimes more—concern about their body shape and weight as whites. Men and women are prone to different distortions in body image. Women tend to see themselves as overweight, whether or not they are; men perceive themselves as underweight, even when their weights are normal or above normal.

Behavioral Change

The most successful weight loss programs target the brain, rather than the belly, by focusing on the attitudes and behaviors that affect eating.

Who's in Charge?

As discussed in Chapter 2, if you see yourself as having control over your destiny, you have an internal locus of control. And your sense of self-efficacy is the belief in your ability to change and to reach a goal. Feeling in control and self-efficacy go hand in hand. The stronger your faith in yourself, the more energy and persistence you can put into making a change. The opposite is also true, especially for health behaviors.

How do you rate on locus of control and self-efficacy? Read the following statements, and jot down true or false.

1. I am overweight because I eat too much.
2. Weight problems run in my family.
3. Diet pills are my best hope for losing weight.
4. I would keep weight off if I exercised regularly.
5. I wouldn't overeat if I didn't have to cook for my family.
6. Some people are born thin and never have to diet.
7. I lose weight when I eat only diet shakes or prepared foods.
8. I could make time for exercise if I really wanted to.
9. My doctor will make sure I'm at a healthy weight.
10. I'm determined to lose weight, and I know I will.

"True" answers to numbers 1, 4, 8, and 10 indicate that you take responsibility for and see yourself in control of your weight. "True" answers to numbers 2, 3, 5, 6, 7, and 9 suggest that you credit or blame others for your weight. The more that you see external forces as in charge, the more difficult you will find it to make changes and lose weight permanently.[61]

Reach Out for Support— Real and Virtual

Behind most successful dieters is a friend, spouse, coach, mentor, colleague, support group, or online community. In various studies, dieters with supportive "buddies" were more likely to stick to their diet and workout program and lost more weight.

If you decide to diet with a roommate, friend, parent, spouse, or coworker, decide on a plan. You might walk or work out together, or check in with each other every evening when you're most prone to overeating. Another alternative is to join a weight loss group, either one that is part of a commercial program or a more informal group that meets on campus or at a church or community center. Support has proved one of the most critical factors in weight management for African-American women.[62]

Every month, an estimated five million Americans log on to commercial websites targeted to dieters. Online dieting is convenient, anonymous, and available around the clock. Some dieters post their weekly weights or before-and-after photos of the way (and weight) they were and how far they've come. Others find support in various blogs and chat groups, where they can commiserate, exchange tales of setbacks and successes, and encourage each other to stay the course. Simply reading diet blogs can help you feel less lonely in your quest.

Although e-dieting is popular, little is known about its usefulness. In a one-year study that compared two groups of women who used either a weight loss manual or eDiets.com, the manual users lost significantly more than those who used the Internet.[63] Other studies suggest that interactive online programs that provide diet and fitness advice are more effective than sites offering support alone.

✚ WELLNESS COACH

✚ Get a Grip on Emotional Eating

Occasionally all of us seek comfort at the tip of a spoon. However, many people use food as a way of coping with anger, frustration, stress, boredom, or fatigue. Whatever its motivation, emotional eating always involves eating for reasons other than physiological hunger. If you're not sure whether you do this, ask yourself the following questions:

▌ Do you eat when you're not hungry?
▌ Do you eat or continue eating even if the food doesn't taste good?
▌ Do you eat when you can't think of anything else to do?
▌ Do you eat when you're emotionally vulnerable— tired, frustrated, or worried?
▌ Do you eat after an argument or stressful situation to calm down?
▌ Do you eat as one of your favorite ways of enjoying yourself?
▌ Do you eat to reward yourself?
▌ Do you keep eating even after you're full?

If you answer yes to more than three of these, you're eating in response to what you feel, not what you need. Diets may work for you, but the extra weight will inevitably creep back unless you confront your hidden motives for overeating. Since neither emotions nor food ever go away, you have to learn to deal with both for as long as you live.

To get a grip on your emotional eating, try this three-step plan:

Step 1: Know Your Triggers

Whatever its specific motivation, emotional eating always involves eating for reasons other than physiological hunger. The key to getting it under control is awareness.

What are the feelings that set off an eating binge?

▌ **Anger?** Many women swallow their anger by eating because they're afraid of what might happen if they express it.
▌ **Guilt?** Some women eat because they feel they're always falling short as daughters, sisters, wives, or mothers.
▌ **Rebellion?** Eating may be the only way some women give themselves permission to take a break from being dutiful caregivers for others.
▌ **Deprivation?** At the end of a long day, a woman may justify turning to food as a well-deserved reward, maybe the first nice thing she's done for herself all day.

Did any of these possibilities hit home? If so, train yourself to take a step back and ask yourself a series of questions before you take a bite: Are you hungry? If not, how are you feeling? Stressed, tired, bored, anxious, sad, happy? Once you identify your true feeling, push deeper and ask why you feel this way. Try writing down your answers in your notebook. This is an even more effective way to help make sure that every bite you take is a conscious one.

Step 2: Put Your Body, Not Your Emotions, In Charge of What You Eat

To keep mind and body on an even keel, avoid getting so hungry and feeling so deprived that you become desperate and panicky. If you're facing an emotionally intense period—a corporate reorganization or a visit from an ornery relative—plan your meals and snacks in advance and try, as much as you can, to stick with your program. Rather than swearing off sweets forever, work indulgences into your weekly routine. If you plan to have a brownie for dessert on Friday night, you can look forward to it all week and not waste calories on a candy bar that won't taste as good.

Step 3: Focus on Your Feelings

Let yourself feel how you're feeling without eating. Breathe deeply for a minute or two. Focus on the places in your body that feel tense. Rate the intensity of the emotion on a scale from ten (life or death) to one (truly trivial). Ask yourself: What's the worst-case scenario of feeling this way? Is food going to make it better in any way? Will it make it worse?

When you're tempted to eat but aren't hungry, write down the circumstances and try to discern the underlying reasons. If you eat cookies at night, ask, "What does it get me?" "The answer might be that it relaxes you. Once you realize that the cookies are a means to an end, you can figure out something else you can do to get the same emotional benefits.

✚ Maintaining Weight Loss

Surveys of people who lost significant amounts of weight and kept it off for several years show that most did so on their own—without medication, meal substitutes, or membership in an organized weight loss group. When a National Institutes of Health panel reviewed 48 separate weight loss trials, they found that participants lost about 8 percent of their body weight on average and kept it off.

Rather than focusing on why dieters fail, the creators of the National Weight Control Registry study the habits and lifestyles of those who've maintained a weight loss of at least 30 pounds for at least a year. The nearly 4,000 people in the registry have averaged a weight loss of 66 pounds, which they've kept off for 5.5 years.[64]

No one diet or commercial weight loss program helped all these formerly fat individuals. Many, through years of trial and error, eventually came up with a permanent exercise and eating program that worked for them. Despite the immense variety, their customized approaches share certain characteristics:

▌ **Personal responsibility for change.** Weight loss winners develop an internal locus of control. Rather than blaming others for their weight problem or relying on a doctor or trainer to fix it, they believe that the keys to a healthy weight lie within themselves.
▌ **Exercise.** Registry members report an hour of moderate physical activity almost every day. Their favorite exercise? Three in four say walking, followed by cycling, weight lifting, aerobics, running, and stair climbing. On average, they burn about 2,545 calories per week through physical activity.
▌ **Monitoring.** About 44 percent of the registry members count calories, and almost all keep track of their food intake in some way, written or not.
▌ **Vigilance.** Rather than avoiding the scale or telling themselves their jeans shrunk in the wash, successful losers keep tabs on their weight and size. About a third check the scale every week. If the scale notches upward or their waistband starts to pinch, they take action.
▌ **Breakfast.** Your mother probably told you that breakfast is the most important meal of the day, and 40 years of breakfast-related studies, as well as the experience of registry members, have proved her right. A morning

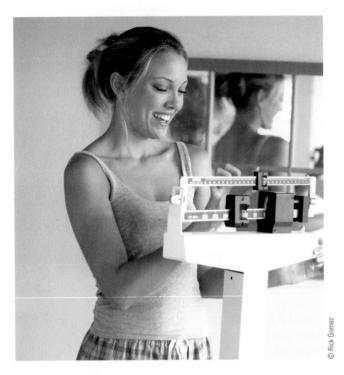

© Rick Gomez

▌ Vigilance helps keep weight off. If the number on the scale creeps upward, take action.

meal improves concentration and problem-solving ability, boosts energy levels, and helps control weight. Regular breakfast skippers are four times more likely to be obese than those who eat a morning meal.

✚ Treating Severe Obesity

The biggest Americans are getting bigger. The prevalence of severe or "morbid" obesity is increasing faster than obesity itself. The number of extremely obese adults—those at least 100 pounds overweight with BMIs over 40—has quadrupled in the last two decades from 1 in 200 to about 1 in every 50 men and women. The number with BMIs greater than 50 has jumped from 1 in 2,000 in the 1980s to 1 in 400.

Extreme obesity poses extreme danger to health and survival and undermines quality of life. White women report more impairment than men or African-American women, even when they have lower BMIs.[65] Severe obesity also has a profound effect on every aspect of an adolescent's life.

Drug Therapy

Obesity medications are recommended only for patients with BMIs equal to or greater than 30 or those with a BMI equal to or greater than 27 with risk factors (like high blood pressure) that increase their risk of disease. Researchers are experimenting with other medications, such as the epilepsy drug zonisamide, to enhance weight loss. Currently, only two weight loss drugs are FDA approved.

Xenical (orlistat) blocks fat absorption by the gut but also inhibits absorption of water and vitamins in some patients and may cause cramping and diarrhea. It produces a weight loss of 2 to 3 percent of initial weight beyond the weight lost by dieting over the course of a year.

Meridia (sibutramine) is in the same chemical class as amphetamines and works by suppressing appetite. It also may increase blood pressure, heart rate, or both. Other side effects include headache, insomnia, dry mouth, and constipation. Patients taking these drugs generally lose less than 10 percent of their body weight, and many regain weight after they stop treatment.

Obesity Surgery

Gastric or bariatric surgery is recommended only for individuals whose BMIs are higher than 40 or who have BMIs of 35 along with severe health complications. The most common operation uses bands or staples to section off a small portion of the stomach. A small outlet, about the size of a pencil eraser, is left at the bottom of the stomach pouch. Since the outlet is small, food stays in the pouch longer so people feel full for a longer time.

About 80 percent of patients lose some weight; 30 percent reach a normal BMI. The long-term weight loss success rate is 40 to 63 percent of excess body weight over a three-year period and 50 to 60 percent after five years.[66] Besides weight loss, bariatric surgery also eliminates or improves diabetes, high blood pressure, high cholesterol, and obstructive sleep apnea.[67] Possible complications include leaking of stomach juices into the abdomen, injury to the spleen, slippage or erosion of the band, breakdown of the staple line, and stretching of the stomach pouch with overeating. Up to 25 percent of patients may require reoperation within five years. Serious infection or death has been reported in fewer than 1 percent of patients.

✚ Unhealthy Eating Behavior

Unhealthy eating behavior takes many forms, ranging from not eating enough to eating too much too quickly. Its roots are complex. In addition to media and external pressures, family history can play a role. Researchers have linked specific genes to some cases of anorexia nervosa and binge eating, but most believe that a variety of factors, including stress and culture, combine to cause disordered eating.

About a third of female athletes in every sport show symptoms of disordered eating or eating disorders. Girls and adolescent females who participate regularly in sports are at risk for disordered eating, menstrual dysfunction, and decreased bone mineral density, according to the American Academy of Pediatrics. The combination of these three disorders is known as the *female athlete triad*.

Sooner or later many people don't eat the way they should. They may skip meals, thereby increasing the likelihood that they'll end up with more body fat, a higher weight, and a higher blood cholesterol level. They may live on diet foods but consume so much of them that they gain weight anyway. Some even engage in more extreme eating behavior: Dissatisfied with almost all aspects of their appearance, they continuously go on and off diets, eat compulsively, or binge on high-fat treats. Such behaviors can be warning signs of potentially serious eating disorders that should not be ignored.

Disordered Eating in College Students

College students—particularly women, including varsity athletes—are at risk for unhealthy eating behaviors. While some college students have full-blown eating disorders, many others develop "partial syndromes" and experience symptoms that are not severe or numerous enough for a diagnosis of anorexia nervosa or bulimia nervosa. Body dissatisfaction often precedes these problems, and researchers also have linked them to depression and alienation from a father.[68]

In a survey at a large, public, rural university in the mid-Atlantic states, 17 percent of the women were struggling with disordered eating. Younger women (ages 18 to 21) were more likely than older students to have an eating disorder. In this study, eating disorders did not discriminate, equally affecting women of different races (white, Asian, African American, Native American, and Hispanic), religions, athletic involvement, and living arrangements (on or off campus; with roommates, boyfriends, or family). Although the students viewed eating disorders as both mental and physical problems and felt that individual therapy would be most helpful, all said that they would first turn to a friend for help.

In another study of 1,620 students, almost 11 percent of the women and 4 percent of the men were at risk for eating disorders. About 17 percent of the women and 10 percent of the men said concerns about weight interfered with their academic work. Women in sororities were at slightly increased risk of an eating disorder compared with those in dormitories.

In a study of Australian male undergraduates, one in four men worried about shape and weight; one in five displayed attitudes and behaviors characteristic of disordered eating and eating disorders. None ever sought treatment, even if the students recognized they had a problem. The reason, the researchers theorized, may be that the young men hesitated to seek treatment for an illness stigmatized as a problem that affects only women. Some men exercised extremely intensively almost every day, even if ill or injured. None felt they had a problem with excessive exercise.[69]

The unique demands and stressors of the transition to college do not increase the likelihood of disordered eating for all freshmen. One study that followed more than 100 undergraduate women through their freshman year found that those who re-

ported the most body dissatisfaction and unhealthy eating patterns at the beginning of the first semester were most likely to experience more eating problems, such as losing control of their eating when feeling strong emotions. The strongest predictor that eating symptoms would get worse over the freshman year was not BMI or weight, but body dissatisfaction.

Extreme Dieting

About half of girls attempt to control their weight by dieting. In a year-long study of teenagers, both parents and the media had the most influence on the development of weight concerns and weight control practices, including dieting, among adolescents and preadolescents.

Extreme dieters go beyond cutting back on calories or increasing physical activity. They become preoccupied with what they eat and weigh. Although their weight never falls below 85 percent of normal, their weight loss is severe enough to cause uncomfortable physical consequences, such as weakness and sensitivity to cold. Technically, these dieters do not have anorexia nervosa (discussed later in the chapter), but they are at increased risk for it.

Extreme dieters may think they know a great deal about nutrition, yet many of their beliefs about food and weight are misconceptions or myths. For instance, they may eat only protein because they believe complex carbohydrates, including fruits and breads, are fattening.

Sometimes nutritional education alone can help change this eating pattern. However, many avid dieters who deny that they have a problem with food may need counseling (which they usually agree to only at their family's insistence) to correct dangerous eating behavior and prevent further complications.

Compulsive Overeating

People who eat compulsively cannot stop putting food in their mouths. They eat fast and they eat a lot. They eat even when they're full. They may eat around the clock rather than at set meal times, often in private because of embarrassment over how much they consume.

Some mental health professionals describe compulsive eating as a food addiction that is much more likely to develop in women. According to Overeaters Anonymous (OA), an international 12-step program, many women who eat compulsively view food as a source of comfort against feelings of inner emptiness, low self-esteem, and fear of abandonment.

The following behaviors may signal a potential problem with compulsive overeating:

▮ Turning to food when depressed or lonely, when feeling rejected, or as a reward
▮ A history of failed diets and anxiety when dieting
▮ Thinking about food throughout the day
▮ Eating quickly and without pleasure

▮ Continuing to eat even when you're no longer hungry
▮ Frequently talking about food, or refusing to talk about food
▮ Fear of not being able to stop eating once you start

Recovery from compulsive eating can be challenging because people with this problem cannot give up entirely the substance they abuse. Like everyone else, they must eat. However, they can learn new eating habits and ways of dealing with underlying emotional problems. An OA survey found that most of its members joined to lose weight but later felt the most important effect was their improved emotional, mental, and physical health. As one woman put it, "I came for vanity but stayed for sanity."

Binge Eating

Binge eating—the rapid consumption of an abnormally large amount of food in a relatively short time—often occurs in compulsive eaters. Individuals with a binge-eating disorder typically eat a larger than ordinary amount of food during a relatively brief period, feel a lack of control over eating, and binge at least twice a week for at least a six-month period. During most of these episodes, binge eaters experience at least three of the following:

▮ Eating much more rapidly than usual
▮ Eating until they feel uncomfortably full
▮ Eating large amounts of food when not feeling physically hungry
▮ Eating large amounts of food throughout the day with no planned mealtimes
▮ Eating alone because they are embarrassed by how much they eat and by their eating habits

Binge eaters may spend up to several hours eating and consume 2,000 or more calories worth of food in a single binge—more than many people eat in a day. After such binges, they usually do not induce vomiting, use laxatives, or rely on other means (such as exercise) to control weight. They simply get fatter. As their weight climbs, they become depressed, anxious, or troubled by other psychological symptoms to a much greater extent than others of comparable weight.

Probably the most common eating disorder, binge-eating strikes up to 4 million Americans according to the National Institutes of Health. Binge eaters are usually overweight or obese. An estimated 8 to 19 percent of obese patients in weight loss programs are binge eaters.

✚ Eating Disorders

According to the American Psychiatric Association, patients with **eating disorders** display a broad range of symptoms that occur along a continuum between those of anorexia nervosa and those of bulimia nervosa.

As many as 10 percent of teenage girls develop symptoms of or full-blown eating disorders. Among the factors that increase the risk are preoccupation with a thin body; social pressure; and childhood traits such as perfectionism and excessive cautiousness, which can reflect an obsessive-compulsive personality.

The best known eating disorders are anorexia nervosa, which affects fewer than 1 percent of adolescent women, and bulimia nervosa, which strikes 2 to 3 percent. Many more young women do not have the characteristic symptoms of these disorders but are preoccupied with their weight or experiment with unhealthy forms of dieting.

The American Psychiatric Association has developed practice guidelines for the treatment of patients with eating disorders, which include medical, psychological, and behavioral approaches.[70] One of the most scientifically supported is cognitive-behavioral therapy.

If you occasionally go on eating binges, use the behavioral technique called *habit reversal,* and replace your bingeing with a competing behavior. For example, every time you're tempted to binge, immediately do something—text-message a friend, play solitaire, check your e-mail—that keeps food out of your mouth.

If you binge twice a week or more for at least a six-month period, you may have binge-eating disorder, which can require professional help. Treatment usually consists of cognitive-behavioral therapy, either individually or in a group setting. As chronic binge eaters recog-

---

STRATEGIES for PREVENTION

Do You Have an Eating Disorder?

Physicians have developed a simple screening test for eating disorders, consisting of the following questions:

▮ Do you make yourself sick because you feel uncomfortably full?

▮ Do you worry you have lost control over how much you eat?

▮ Have you recently lost more than 14 pounds in a three-month period?

▮ Do you believe yourself to be fat when others say you are too thin?

▮ Would you say that food dominates your life?

Score one point for every "yes." A score of two or more is a likely indication of anorexia nervosa or bulimia nervosa.

Source: Miller, Karl. "Treatment Guideline for Eating Disorders." *American Family Physician,* Vol. 62, No. 1, July 1, 2000.

nize their unhealthy behavior and confront the underlying issues, they usually are able to stop bingeing and resume normal eating patterns.

Who Develops Eating Disorders?

Eating disorders affect an estimated 5 to 10 million women and 1 million men. Despite past evidence that eating disorders were primarily problems for white women, they are increasing among men and members of different ethnic and racial groups.

In the few studies of eating disorders in minority college students that have been completed, African-American female undergraduates had a slightly lower prevalence of eating disorder than whites. Asian Americans reported fewer symptoms of eating disorders but more body dissatisfaction, concerns about shape, and more intense efforts to lose weight.

In a survey of health-care professionals at the country's largest colleges and universities, 69 percent have professionals on staff who specialize in diagnosing and treating eating disorders. Of all the hurdles to helping students with eating disorders, 39 percent said denial is the biggest, while 24 percent felt it was unwillingness to seek treatment, and 20 percent blamed pressure from peers and the media to stay thin.

Eating disorders affect every aspect of college students' lives, including dating. Both men and women tend to avoid dating individuals with eating disorders, but men are far less accepting of obesity than women.

Male and female athletes are vulnerable to eating disorders, either because of the pressure to maintain ideal body weight or to achieve a weight that might enhance their performance. Many female athletes, particularly those participating in sports or activities that emphasize leanness (such as gymnastics, distance running, diving, figure skating, and classical ballet) have subclinical eating disorders that could undermine their nutritional status and energy levels. However, there is often little awareness or recognition of their disordered eating.

If someone you know has an eating disorder, let your friend know you're concerned and that you care. Don't criticize or make fun of his or her eating habits. Encourage your friend to talk about other problems and feelings, and suggest that he or she talk to the school counselor or someone at the mental health center, the family doctor, or another trusted adult. Offer to go along if you think that will make a difference.

Anorexia Nervosa

Although *anorexia* means "loss of appetite," most individuals with **anorexia nervosa** are, in fact, hungry all the time. For them, food is an enemy—a threat to their sense of self, identity, and autonomy. In the distorted mirror of their mind's eye, they see themselves as fat or flabby even at a normal or below-normal body weight. Some simply feel fat; others think that they are thin in some places and too fat in others, such as the abdomen, buttocks, or thighs.

The incidence of anorexia nervosa has increased in the last three decades in most developed countries. The peak ages for its onset are 14½ and 18 years. According to the American Psychiatric Association's Work Group on Eating Disorders, cases are increasing among males, minorities, women of all ages, and possibly preteens.

In the *restricting* type of anorexia, individuals lose weight by avoiding any fatty foods and by dieting, fasting, and exercising. Some start smoking as a way of controlling their weight. In the *binge-eating/purging* type, they engage in binge eating, purging (through self-induced vomiting, laxatives, diuretics, or enemas), or both. Obsessed with an intense fear of fatness, they may weigh themselves several times a day, measure various parts of their body, check mirrors to see if they look fat, and try on different items of clothing to see if they feel tight.

The medical consequences of anorexia nervosa are serious (**Figure 9-10**). Treatment of anorexia nervosa includes medical therapy (such as refeeding to overcome malnutrition) and cognitive-behavioral, psychodynamic, and family therapy. Antidepressant medication sometimes can help, particularly when there is a personal or family history of depression.

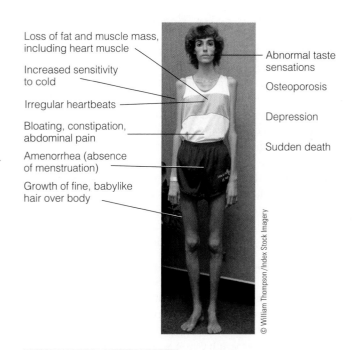

FIGURE 9-10 ▎ Medical Complications of Weight Loss from Anorexia Nervosa

Bulimia Nervosa

Individuals with **bulimia nervosa** go on repeated eating binges and rapidly consume large amounts of food, usually sweets, stopping only because of severe abdominal pain or sleep, or because they are interrupted. Those with *purging* bulimia induce vomiting or take large doses of laxatives to relieve guilt and control their weight. (**Figure 9–11** lists the medical complications of purging.) In *nonpurging* bulimia, individuals use other means, such as fasting or excessive exercise, to compensate for binges.

An estimated 1 to 3 percent of adolescent and young American women develop bulimia. Some experiment with bingeing and purging for a few months and then stop when they change their social or living situation. Others develop longer-term bulimia. Among males, this disorder is about one-tenth as common. The average age for developing bulimia is 18.

Most mental health professionals treat bulimia with a combination of nutritional counseling, psychodynamic or cognitive-behavioral therapy, individual or group psychotherapy, and medication. The drug most often prescribed is an antidepressant medication, such as fluoxetine (Prozac), which increases levels of the neurotransmitter serotonin. About 70 percent of those who complete treatment programs reduce their bingeing and purging, although flare-ups are common in times of stress.

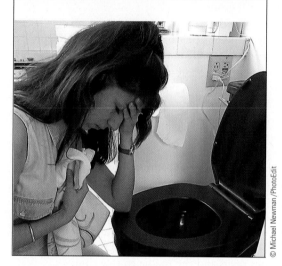

Abnormal levels of crucial chemicals
Inflammation of the salivary glands
Erosion of the esophagus and stomach
Severe abdominal pain
Erosion and decay of dental enamel, particularly of front teeth
Fatigue and weakness
Seizures

© Michael Newman/PhotoEdit

FIGURE 9-11 ▌ Medical Complications Related to Purging

MAKING HEALTHY CHOICES

To Manage Your Weight

No diet—high-protein, low-fat, or high-carbohydrate—can produce permanent weight loss. Successful weight management, the American Dietetic Association has concluded, "requires a lifelong commitment to healthful lifestyle behaviors emphasizing sustainable and enjoyable eating practices and daily physical activity."[71] Studies have shown that successful dieters are highly motivated, monitor their food intake, increase their activity, set realistic goals, and receive social support from others. Another key to long-term success is tailoring any weight loss program to an individual's gender, lifestyle, and cultural, racial, and ethnic values.

Here are some practical guidelines.

▌ **Be realistic.** Trying to shrink to an impossibly low weight dooms you to defeat. Start off slowly and make steady progress. If your weight creeps up 5 pounds, go back to the basics of your program. Take into account normal fluctuations, but watch out for an upward trend. If you let your weight continue to creep up, it may not stop until you have a serious weight problem—again.

▌ **Recognize that there are no quick fixes.** Ultimately, quick-loss diets are very damaging physically and psychologically because when you stop dieting and put the pounds back on, you feel like a failure.

▌ **Note your progress.** Make a graph, with your initial weight as the base, to indicate your progress. View plateaus or occasional gains as temporary setbacks rather than disasters.

▌ **Adopt the 90 percent rule.** If you practice good eating habits 90 percent of the time, a few indiscretions won't make a difference. In effect, you should allow for occasional cheating so that you don't have to feel guilty about it.

▌ **Look for joy and meaning beyond your food life.** Make your personal goals and your relationships your priorities, and treat food as the fuel that allows you to bring your best to both.

▌ **Try, try again.** Remember, dieters usually don't keep weight off on their first attempt. The people who eventually succeed try various methods until they find the plan that works for them.

SELF-SURVEY

Are You Ready to Lose Weight?

As discussed in Chapter 2, people change the way they behave stage by stage and step by step. The same is true for changing behaviors related to weight. If you need to lose excess pounds, knowing your stage of readiness for change is a crucial first step. Here is a guide to identifying where you are right now.

If you are still in the *precontemplation* stage, you don't think of yourself as having a weight problem, even though others may. If you can't fit into some of your clothes, you blame the dry cleaners. Or you look around and think, "I'm no bigger than anyone else in this class." Unconsciously, you may feel helpless to do anything about your weight. So you deny or dismiss its importance.

In the *contemplation* stage, you would prefer not to have to change, but you can't avoid reality. Your coach or doctor may comment on your weight. You wince at the vacation photos of you in a swimsuit. You look in the mirror, try to suck in your stomach, and say, "I've got to do something about my weight."

In the *preparation* stage, you're gearing up by taking small but necessary steps. You may buy athletic shoes or check out several diet books from the library. Maybe you experiment with some minor changes, such as having fruit instead of cookies for an afternoon snack. Internally, you are getting accustomed to the idea of change.

In the *action* stage of change, you are deliberately working to lose weight. You no longer snack all evening long. You stick to a specific diet and track calories, carbs, or points. You hop on a treadmill or stationary bike for 30 minutes a day. Your resolve is strong, and you know you're on your way to a thinner, healthier you.

In the *maintenance* stage, you strengthen, enhance, and extend the changes you've made. Whether or not you have lost all the weight you want, you've made significant progress. As you continue to watch what you eat and to be physically active, you lock in healthy new habits.

Where are you right now? Read each of the following statements and decide which best applies to you.

1. I never think about my weight. **Precontemplation Stage**
2. I'm trying to zip up a pair of jeans and wondering when was the last time they fit. **Contemplation Stage**
3. I'm downloading a food diary to keep track of what I eat. **Preparation Stage**
4. I have been following a diet for three weeks and have started working out. **Action Stage**
5. I have been sticking to a diet and engaging in regular physical activity for at least six months. **Maintenance Stage**

ACTION PLAN

Your Action Plan for Losing Weight

Here is a guide to strategies most likely to help you at your particular stage of readiness to change:

Precontemplation (Not Active and Not Thinking about Becoming Active)

▌ **Set a small, reasonable goal** that does not involve working up a sweat, such as standing rather than sitting when blow-drying your hair or doing squats while brushing your teeth.

▌ **Start paying attention** to what, when, where, and why you eat. Take note of the times you eat or continue eating even though you're not hungry.

▌ **List what you see** as the cons of physical activity. For example, do you fear it will take up too much time? Write down three activities you could do if you woke up half an hour earlier.

Contemplation (Not Active But Thinking about Becoming Active)

▌ **Think back to activities** you found enjoyable in the past. Did you ever try inline skating? Play softball? Row? Ask friends if they can put you in touch with others with the same interest.

▌ **Start drinking more water.** Get used to the idea of ending every meal with water to wash away the taste of what you've eaten and signal that you've stopped putting food in your mouth.

▌ **Determine the types of activity** you can realistically fit into your daily schedule. If you have classes and work most of the day, sign up for an evening body-sculpting or spinning class.

▌ **Find an image of the slimmer body** you'd like to have—from a magazine advertisement, for example—and post it where you can see it often.

Preparation (Active But Not at Recommended Levels)

▌ **Record everything you put in your mouth.** List calories and carbs next to each entry. Also describe how you feel as you eat.

▌ **Set specific daily and weekly action-oriented goals.** Your daily goal might begin with 10 or 15 minutes of activity and increase by 5 minutes every week or two. Your weekly goal might be to try a new activity, such as kick-boxing or a dance class.

▌ **Document your progress.** You could use a monthly calendar to keep track of the number of days you've exercised as well as the length of each workout. Or you can keep a more detailed record, noting the types of exercise you do every day, the intensity you work at, the duration of each workout, and so forth.

Action and Maintenance (Active at Recommended Levels for Less than Six Months)

▌ **Find new comfort foods.** Good options include air-popped popcorn, chocolate fruit sundaes (fresh fruit with a spoonful of rich syrup), hot chocolate (with skim milk), and fudgsicles (creamy but low in calories).

▌ **Avoid boredom.** Think through ways to vary your exercise routine. Take different routes on your walks. Invite different friends to join you. Alternate working with free weights with resistance machines at the gym.

▌ **Develop new athletic and sports skills.** Try snowshoeing, kayaking, rock climbing, hiphop dancing. Don't expect instant expertise. It usually takes four to six weeks to feel competent and get in the swing of a new activity.

Don't expect to progress through these stages just once. Most people "recycle" several times before a change becomes permanent. Whether you're moving forward or have temporarily fallen back, remember that change is a journey that happens step by step, meal by meal, day by day, stage by stage.

SETTING GOALS

Setting Personal Weight Loss Goals

You may wish that you didn't have such a big appetite, that you didn't enjoy food so much, or that you had more time to exercise. But you're more likely to slim down if you stop wishing and take concrete steps toward what you want. As you launch your weight loss program, set goals that are both at reach and reachable. As you progress, add or modify your goals so they continue to inspire rather than overwhelm you.

Here are suggestions for creating goals worth going for.

▌ **Create an image of your goal.** Maybe you see yourself dazzling old friends or buttoning the pants that fit just last year. Describe and define your goal in your mind. Then put it in words, and commit it to paper. Set aside a page or section of your Wellness Journal to record, amend, modify, refine, expand, and

extend your goals—and check off each one as your reach it.

▌ **Aim for five.** Anticipate the sense of accomplishment you'll feel as you hit each five-pound marker. Each small win can add up to a big boost in motivation. Even if you want to shed more pounds, this difference alone will lower your health risks and boost your self-confidence.

▌ **Identify your resources.** Do you have what you need—knowledge, skills, time—to succeed? For instance, if you're committing yourself to a daily walk, make sure you have good shoes. Decide if you'll go alone or ask a friend to join you. Clear thirty minutes of your day so you'll be sure to hit the trail or the treadmill.

▌ **Systematically analyze barriers.** Think through, in very concrete and specific terms, what is likely to get in your way. For each obstacle, list solutions. If your dorm overflows with junk food, study at the library. If seeing other people eat rich, fatty foods makes you crave them, eat meals with a friend who's also counting calories.

▌ **Set goals that go beyond pounds.** Thinking only in terms of pounds can be both limiting and frustrating. Set goals that focus on changing behavior, and make them as specific as possible, for example:

Today's goal	I will take a 15-minute walk at lunch time, and I'll have low-fat milk instead of a milk shake with my lunch.
This week's goal	At least three evenings this week, I'll have fruit for dessert or no dessert at all.
This month's goal	I'm going to get off the bus one stop sooner and walk the rest of the way to and from work. If the weather's bad, I'll walk up one flight before taking the elevator up to my office or apartment. By the end of the month, I'll get off two stops away and walk two or three flights before getting on the elevator.

Source: Helmering, Doris Wild, and Dianne Hales. *Think Thin, Be Thin.* New York: Broadway Books, 2005.

Your Personal Weight Loss Goal:

Is It S.M.A.R.T.?
    Specific? _____
    Measurable? _____
    Achievable? _____
    Rewarding? _____
    Time Defined? _____
Strategies for Success:
    1. _____
    2. _____
    3. _____

Potential Obstacles:
  1. _____
  2. _____
  3. _____

Ways Around Them:
  1. _____
  2. _____
  3. _____

Daily Report

The Week that Was:

What Went Right?
What Could I Do Better?

WELLNESS JOURNAL

Using Food Diaries to Write Off Weight

Food Diaries

A food diary (see figure) can serve different purposes at different points in a weight loss program. In studies of dieters, keeping a diary helped people lose weight because it forced them to be accountable for their food choices.

▎ **If you are thinking about or starting a diet:** Use your food diary as a research tool. Without changing your usual routine or judging yourself, record in your notebook when, where, why, and how much you eat. After a week, analyze the data. Look for patterns and problems. Are you skipping breakfast? Do you snack all day long on weekends? The answers can provide valuable information as you launch your weight loss program.

▎ **If you're on a diet:** Use your food diary as a periodic reality check that provides a snapshot of your food intake. For three days (including one weekend day), tally your daily total in calories, carbs, points, or fat grams. Are they higher than your diet allows? Highlight every "diet-right" choice you've made. Circle every diet stumble or no-no. Don't criticize yourself for less than perfect compliance. Just use the new information to fine-tune your weight loss strategies.

▎ **If you hit a plateau:** Use your food diary to figure out why. For a week, conscientiously record every morsel that you eat—down to each lick of icing or cookie dough. If your diary reveals that you're a food sneak thief, catch yourself before you take a bite. Use sticky notes to remind yourself to write down every thing you put in your mouth. Simply knowing you have to do so can discourage you from sneaking a treat.

▎ **If you overeat:** Use your food diary to overcome "overboard" eating when you just can't stop stuffing yourself. Each time you overeat, write an O for "overboard." If you go overboard three times in a day, you'll have three Os. If you cross over the line five times, put down five Os. Recording overeating will help you become more conscious of just how much you're putting in your mouth.

Food/Drink	Amount	Time	Place	Activity	Mood	By Myself?
orange juice	small glass	7:30 a.m.	dorm	studying for chem. test	tired	yes
bagel with cream cheese	1	same				
doughnuts	2	10:10 a.m.	rec center	break between classes	nervous about test	no
turkey sandwich	1	noon	cafeteria	lunch—talking with friends	good	no
chips	small bag	2:00 p.m.	Main Quad	walking	thinking about weekend	yes
iced tea	large	4:00 p.m.	Internet cafe	checking e-mail	okay	yes
brownie	$1^1/2$	4:20 p.m.	same	surfing Internet	bored	yes

▎ Food diary

A food diary provides a realistic picture of what you're eating.

Making This Chapter Work for You

1. Which of the following statements is true?
   a. Obesity is a problem only in industrialized countries.
   b. Obesity is a problem that starts in middle age.
   c. The southern states have the highest percentage of people who are obese.
   d. If you were heavy as a child, you will always be obese.

2. If you are a healthy weight,
   a. you are always hungry.
   b. your BMI is between 18.5 and 24.9.
   c. your waist measurement is 25 to 28 inches.
   d. your waist-to-hip ratio is greater than 1.0.

3. The health dangers of excess weight include all of the following *except*
   a. increased risk of type 2 diabetes, heart disease, and cancer.
   b. increased risk of impaired immunity.
   c. increased risk of auto accidents.
   d. increased risk of dying prematurely.

4. If you have gone online to check out weight-reduction support groups in your area, which stage of readiness for weight behavior change are you in?
   a. precontemplation stage
   b. contemplation stage
   c. preparation stage
   d. action stage

5. Which of the following statements is *incorrect?*
   a. I can lose weight successfully on a low-carbohydrate diet.
   b. I can lose weight successfully on a low-fat diet.
   c. I can lose weight successfully on a low-calorie diet.
   d. I can lose weight successfully by working out once a week.

6. Successful weight management strategies include which of the following?
   a. Learn to distinguish between actual and emotional hunger.
   b. Ask friends for recommendations for methods that helped them to lose weight quickly.
   c. Practice good eating habits 50 percent of the time so that you can balance your cravings with healthy food.
   d. Look at celebrity photos and pick one for a model.

7. Which of the following statements is true?
   a. Very low-calorie diets increase metabolism, which helps burn calories more quickly.
   b. An individual eating low-calorie or fat-free foods can increase the serving sizes.

   c. Low-carbohydrate diets have been shown safe over the short term, but long-term studies have not been completed.
   d. Yo-yo dieting works best for long-term weight loss.

8. Which of the following eating behaviors may be a warning sign of a serious eating disorder?
   a. vegetarianism
   b. compulsive food washing
   c. binge eating
   d. weight gain during the first year of college

9. Individuals with anorexia nervosa
   a. believe they are overweight even if they are extremely thin.
   b. typically feel full all the time, which limits their food intake.
   c. usually look overweight, even though their body mass index is normal.
   d. have a reduced risk for heart-related abnormalities.

10. Bulimia nervosa is
    a. characterized by excessive sleeping followed by periods of insomnia.
    b. found primarily in older women who are concerned with the aging process.
    c. associated with the use of laxatives or excessive exercise to control weight.
    d. does not have serious health consequences.

Answers to these questions can be found on page 376.

Critical Thinking

1. In a poll conducted by *Time*/ABC, 87 percent of respondents said that individual Americans bore a "great deal of responsibility" for the nation's obesity problem because of their choice of diet and lack of exercise, while 64 percent identified fast-food restaurants and schools that allow high-calorie snacks and sweets. Where do you think the responsibility lies? Why?

2. Do you think you have a weight problem? If so, what makes you think so? Is your perception based on your actual BMI measurement or on how you believe you look? If you found out that your BMI was within the ideal range, would that change your opinion about your body? Why or why not?

3. Suppose one of your roommates appears to have symptoms of an eating disorder. You have told him or her of your concerns, but your roommate has denied having a problem and brushed off your fears. What can you do to help this individual? Should you contact his or her parent? Why or why not?

Media Menu

Health🏃Now™

Don't forget to check out the wealth of resources on the HealthNow website at **http://healthnow.brookscole.com/itw** that will:

- Help you evaluate your knowledge of the material
- Allow you to take an exam-prep quiz
- Provide a Personalized Learning Plan targeting resources that address areas you should study
- Coach you through identifying target goals for behavior change and creating and monitoring your personal change plan throughout the semester.

INTERNET CONNECTIONS

American Obesity Association

www.obesity.org

The American Obesity Association is the leading organization for advocacy and education on the nation's obesity epidemic. This comprehensive website features statistics on overweight and obesity in the United States, research articles, consumer protection links, prevention topics, library resources, fact sheets on a variety of weight management topics, and more.

Weight Control Information Network

http://win.niddk.nih.gov/index.htm

This government-sponsored website features a variety of publications in English and Spanish on nutrition, physical activity, and weight control for the general public and for health care professionals. In addition, there are links for research, a newsletter, statistical data, and a bibliography of journal articles on various aspects of weight management and obesity.

Body Composition Laboratory

www.bcm.edu/bodycomplab/

The Body Composition Laboratory at the Children's Nutrition Research Center in Houston, Texas, sponsors this informative website, which explains the techniques for and applications of body composition measurements in all populations, ranging from low-birth-weight infants to adults. Learn how high-precision instruments are used to measure total body levels of body water, minerals, protein, and fat.

Something Fishy, A Website on Eating Disorders

www.something-fishy.org

This very comprehensive and popular site features the latest news on eating disorders as well as links regarding signs to watch for, "Recovery Reach-out," treatment finders, doctors and patients, cultural issues, and a support chat.

 InfoTrac College Edition Activities Jancin, Bruce. "Maintain young adult weight to limit CV risks," *Family Practice News,* Feb 15, 2005 v35 i4 p10(1)

1. What can young adults do to prevent the development of cardiovascular disease and metabolic syndromes as they age?

2. Why is weight stabilization a more realistic goal than weight loss?

3. What single step do researchers suggest to hold the line on weight gain?

You can find additional readings related to personal health with InfoTrac College Edition, an online library of more than 900 journals and publications. Follow the instructions for accessing InfoTrac College Edition that were packaged with your textbook; then search for articles using a keyword search.

For additional links, resources, and suggested readings on the InfoTrac College Edition, visit our Health and Wellness Resource Center at **http://health .wadsworth.com.**

Key Terms

The terms listed are used on the page indicated. Definitions of the terms are in the Glossary at the end of the book.

anorexia nervosa 203
appetite 190
basal metabolic rate (BMR) 183
binge eating 202
body mass index (BMI) 184
bulimia nervosa 204
dual-energy X-ray absorptiometry (DXA) 187

eating disorders 202
hunger 190
hydrostatic weighing 187
NEAT (nonexercise activity thermogenesis) 196
obesity 184
overweight 184
satiety 190
skinfold measurement 186
waist-to-hip ratio (WHR) 185

Keeping Your Heart Healthy

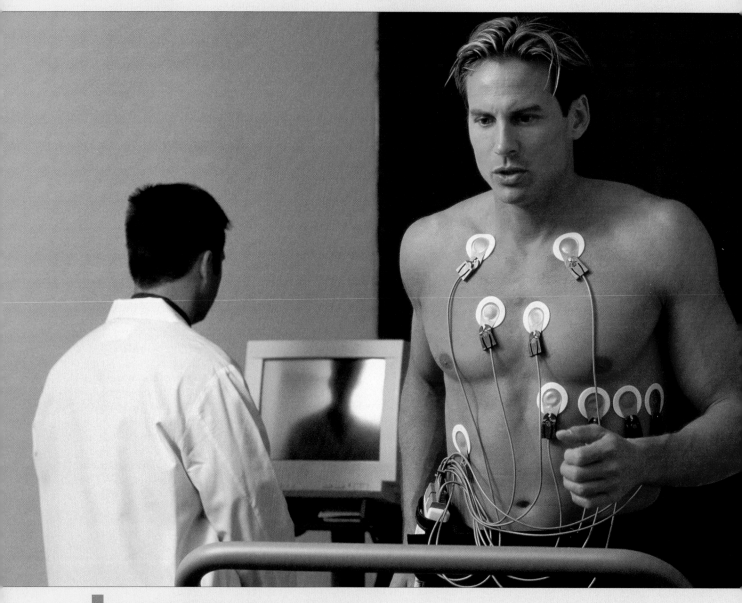

Jamal never forgot the terror he felt when his Dad had his first heart attack. Only ten, he couldn't understand why this towering giant of a man had fallen to the ground, his face twisted in pain, his fist pressed against his chest. His father seemed different when he came home from the hospital, as if something had gone out of him. But his face would still light up with an impish grin, especially when he'd sneak a cigarette and wink at Jamal so he wouldn't tell his mother. The second heart attack came four years later. This time Jamal's Dad didn't come home.

Jamal promised his mother that he'd take better care of his heart. He wouldn't smoke; he'd watch his blood pressure and weight; he'd keep tabs on his diet; he'd exercise regularly. Jamal didn't forget these promises as time passed. But like many college students, he felt invincible. He was shocked when a sports physical revealed that his blood pressure was high and his levels of the most dangerous type of cholesterol were elevated. But he also felt lucky: "I got my wake-up call," he explains. "And I'm not going to ignore it."

As Jamal realizes, it's never too soon, or too late, to start being heart smart. Death rates from cardiovascular disease have dropped by 60 percent since 1950, one of the major U.S. health achievements of the twentieth century. The medical advances described in this chapter have contributed to this decline, but much of the credit goes to lifestyle changes, such as quitting smoking and making dietary changes that lower blood pressure and cholesterol levels.

Yet we still have a long way to go to keep the hearts of all Americans healthy. One of every two men and one of every three women in the United States will develop some form of cardiovascular illness. Each year an estimated one million Americans suffer a heart attack; nearly half of them die.

This chapter provides the information you need about risk factors, silent dangers such as high blood pressure and cholesterol, and medical advances that can improve your chances to have a healthier heart and a longer life.

Steve Craft

After studying the material in this chapter, you should be able to:

▌ **Name** three changes you can make to keep your heart healthy.

▌ **Identify** the risk factors for cardiovascular disease that you can control and those that you cannot control.

▌ **Define** hypertension, and **discuss** why it is dangerous and ways to prevent it.

▌ **Describe** the types of cholesterol that compose your lipoprotein profile and the effects of each on heart health.

▌ **Identify** three strategies for lowering LDL cholesterol and C-reactive protein.

▌ **Explain** what happens during a myocardial infarction (MI) and what can be done to prevent and treat such attacks.

▌ **Define** stroke and transient ischemic attacks (TIAs), and **list** five risk factors for them.

Health⊛Now™

Don't forget to check out the wealth of resources on the HealthNow website at **http://healthnow.brookscole.com/itw** that will:

- Help you evaluate your knowledge of the material
- Allow you to take an exam-prep quiz
- Provide a Personalized Learning Plan targeting resources that address areas you should study
- Coach you through identifying target goals for behavior change and creating and monitoring your personal change plan throughout the semester.

✚ Preventing Heart Problems

For the first time ever, the number of deaths from heart disease for Americans under age 85 has dropped lower than those caused by cancer.[1] This decline reflects the success of new treatments that can save damaged hearts, but it is also a testimony to the power of prevention.

As years of research have confirmed, heart disease does not have to happen. However, avoiding or delaying it must start early. Some of the risk factors for heart disease discussed in this chapter begin in childhood with too much time in front of the television, too many fatty foods, and too many extra pounds. Other behaviors that endanger a heart's health begin in adolescence and young adulthood, including tobacco use, high-fat diets, sedentary lifestyles, and high stress. The choices that you make in your college years can affect your heart's health for decades to come.

As research shows, young women with a low-risk profile for heart disease—that is, those who don't smoke, who exercise 30 minutes or more a day, who have BMIs under 25, who consume alcohol only moderately (one drink a day), and who eat healthfully—have a much lower risk of heart disease and fatal heart attacks throughout life. In the Nurses Health Study, only 3 percent of the more than 84,000 female participants were low risk, but their odds of having heart problems were 83 percent lower than the other women. These women also were less likely to die of any cause over a 31-year period.[2]

Simply holding the line on weight can make a difference. In a 15-year study that followed over 5,000 men and women initially aged 18 to 30, those who maintained their starting weight showed no significant change in risk factors for heart disease as they reached middle age. However, only about one in five of the study participants managed to avoid gaining weight with the passing years.[3]

Why Should I Worry About Heart Disease? ✚◉

Many people, including college students and other young adults, are unaware of habits and conditions that put their hearts at risk. In a survey of almost 1,500 undergraduates, the majority viewed heart disease as mainly a problem for white men and underestimated the risks for women and ethnic groups. (See Student Snapshot: "How Heart-Smart Are College Students?") Students rated their own knowledge of heart disease as lower than that of sexually transmitted infections and psychological disorders. Most—88 percent—

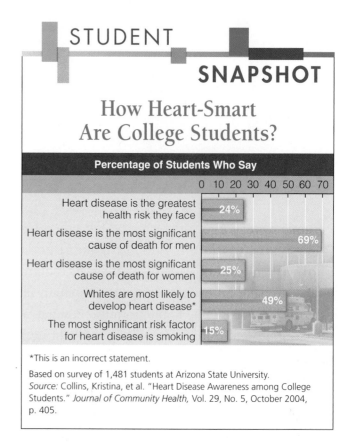

STUDENT SNAPSHOT

How Heart-Smart Are College Students?

Percentage of Students Who Say

	0 10 20 30 40 50 60 70
Heart disease is the greatest health risk they face	24%
Heart disease is the most significant cause of death for men	69%
Heart disease is the most significant cause of death for women	25%
Whites are most likely to develop heart disease*	49%
The most sighnificant risk factor for heart disease is smoking	15%

*This is an incorrect statement.

Based on survey of 1,481 students at Arizona State University.
Source: Collins, Kristina, et al. "Heart Disease Awareness among College Students." *Journal of Community Health,* Vol. 29, No. 5, October 2004, p. 405.

said a doctor had never discussed heart disease with them.[4] Yet heart disease is the third leading cause of death among adults aged 25 to 44.

In another study of undergraduates enrolled in physical activity classes at a large university, 68 percent rated their risk of heart disease as lower or much lower than that of their peers, reflecting what researchers called "a clear optimistic bias." The undergraduates who exercised regularly rated their risk as lower than those who did not. Men and women did not realize that diabetes, family history, and other risk, factors increase their likelihood of heart disease.[5]

Even college students who indicate that they're aware of cardiovascular risks often behave in ways that do not reflect their knowledge. In one study of 226 students at a New Jersey college, half or more ate a high-fat diet or reported moderate to severe stress. Many did not exercise frequently; some already had high cholesterol or high blood pressure.[6]

Young athletes face special risks. Each year seemingly healthy teens or young adults die suddenly on playing fields and courts. The culprit in one of every three cases of sudden cardiac death in young athletes is a silent condition called hypertrophic cardiomyopathy (HCM), an excessive thickness of the heart muscle. Because of HCM, the heart is more prone to dangerous heart irregularities.

Making Heart-Healthy Changes

Chances are that you don't have any noticeable symptoms of heart disease: no pain, no swelling, no breathlessness when you walk or climb stairs. But that doesn't mean that you're home safe. Depending on your age, family history, blood pressure, cholesterol levels, and other risk factors, your heart's health may be in jeopardy.

Yes, advances in treatment can help if you eventually develop heart disease. But change in lifestyle can do even more: They can prevent or reverse heart-related symptoms. In one recent study, a 12-week program of therapeutic life changes, sometimes called TLC, helped lower blood pressure, cholesterol, blood sugar, and weight without medications.[7]

If you don't feel any need to make changes, you are in the precontemplation stage of behavioral change (see Chapter 2 for a complete discussion). Read this entire chapter with an open mind, and think of family members or friends who have heart disease or who are clearly at risk because they smoke or are overweight. What effect have their habits had on their health? Make a list of the benefits heart-healthy habits might have for you.

If you do want to make some heart-healthy changes, begin by assessing your cardiovascular health and knowledge by completing Lab 10.1 in your Lab Booklet. Once you have a good sense of the current state of your heart's health, set goals for yourself. Write them down in your Wellness Journal, and develop a step-by-step Action Plan.

Changes You Can Make Today

▌ **Eat a good breakfast: whole-grain cereal, juice, yogurt, and so on.**
▌ **Take a walk after lunch.**
▌ **Skip dessert at dinner.**
▌ **Eat one more serving of vegetables.**
▌ **Eat one more piece of fruit.**
▌ **Drink one more glass of water.**
▌ **Take the stairs for one or two flights** rather than riding the elevator in your dorm or classroom building.
▌ **Get seven to eight hours of sleep tonight.**

Changes You Can Make This Week

▌ Block out time for exercise on your calendar. Try for at least 30 minutes of physical activity most days.

▌ If you haven't had your lipoproteins checked within the last year, schedule a test.
▌ If you don't know your blood pressure, find out what it is. If you know it, compare your reading with those in Table 10-1 (page 222) to determine if it is too high.
▌ Make a list of stress-reducing activities (see Wellness Coach, p. 127). Select two or three to do each week.
▌ Get in touch with an old friend and enjoy catching up on each other's lives.
▌ If you meet the weekly goals in your Action Plan, reward yourself by renting a special DVD or going to a concert or sports event on campus.

Changes You Can Make This Term

▌ Keep a log in your Wellness Journal of everything you do. Every few weeks, review this log and revise your Action Plan. Allow for interruptions or slowdowns due to a cold, a holiday break, or a pulled muscle.
▌ Look for new ways to meet your goals. For example, try new and different foods each week, or join a volleyball team.
▌ Be patient. Don't get discouraged if change seems harder and slower than you thought it would be.
▌ If you slip up and smoke again or blow your diet, don't give up. Analyze what triggered your relapse. Was it the smell of smoke at the party Saturday night? Did you try to console yourself for a poor grade with a carton of chocolate ice cream? Think of how you might handle similar situations differ-

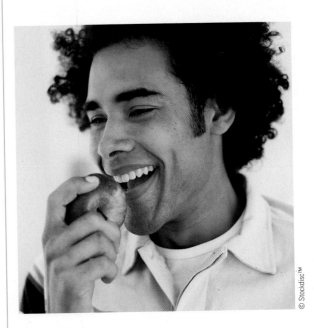

▌ You can do something today to prevent heart disease in your future: Eat some fruit.

ently in the future, such as staying away from smokers at parties or listening to music to lift your mood rather than turning to food.

❚ Develop and use a support system of friends and family members. Identify individuals you can talk to, work out with, or call.

Getting Physical

Physical activity prevents or reduces many of the risk factors for heart disease discussed later in this chapter by:

❚ **Reducing body weight.**
❚ **Reducing blood pressure.**
❚ **Reducing harmful low-density-lipoprotein** (LDL) and total cholesterol.
❚ **Increasing beneficial high-density lipoprotein** (HDL) cholesterol.
❚ **Increasing insulin sensitivity** (and lowering the risk of diabetes).[8]
❚ Lowering C-reactive protein, a marker of inflammation.

Sometimes exercise alone can lower an individual's risk of heart problems; in other cases exercise enhances the benefits of other treatments, such as cholesterol-lowering medications.

To maintain cardiovascular fitness, many medical groups, including the American Heart Association, American College of Sports Medicine, and the CDC, recommend 30 to 60 minutes or more of moderate-

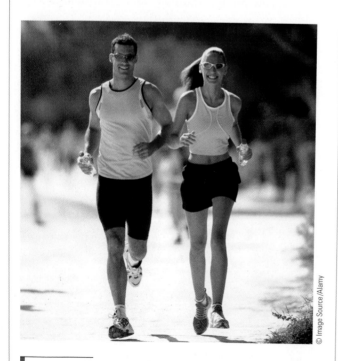
Regular physical activity can lower your risk of developing cardiovascular disease.

© Image Source/Alamy

intensity physical activity such as brisk walking on most, if not all, days of the week. Simply meeting this recommendation for activity would reduce heart disease by 30 to 40 percent.[9] The greatest cardiovascular gains occur in people who go from being sedentary to engaging in low-intensity to moderate activities, such as gardening, walking, and housecleaning. Their blood pressure falls; they lose weight; their hearts function more efficiently.

The greater the exercise "dose," the more benefits it yields. In studies that compared individuals of different fitness levels, the least fit were at much greater risk of dying. In men, more rigorous exercise, such as jogging, produces greater protection against heart disease and boosts longevity.[10] (See Chapter 4 on cardiorespiratory exercise.)

Choosing Heart-Healthy Foods

A balanced, low-fat diet is the best recipe for a healthy heart. Fruits and vegetables, in particular, are associated with a reduced risk of cardiovascular disease, including lower blood pressure.

The American Heart Association (AHA) also recommends including cholesterol-lowering foods, such as oats, barley, soy protein, and nuts, in your daily diet. A diet rich in bran, one of the major components of whole grains, lowers the risk of heart disease. In a study of 43,000 men, those who ate the most oatmeal, brown rice, and other whole grain products had the lowest rates of heart disease.[11]

Another dietary heart-helper is fish. Eating fish two times a week, as the AHA recommends, can reduce blood pressure, decrease levels of the blood fats known as triglycerides, and increase HDL ("good") cholesterol levels. The more fish you eat, the slower your heart beats. This may protect against the fast irregular heart beats that can lead to sudden death.[12]

Federal researchers have concluded that the evidence is insufficient to recommend for or against the use of supplements of vitamins A, C, or E; multivitamins with folic acid; or antioxidant combinations for the prevention of cardiovascular disease. They also advise against the use of beta-carotene supplements.[13]

✚ Risk Factors for Cardiovascular Disease

Heart disease, contrary to a common misperception, generally does not strike "out of the blue." According to research, 80 to 90 percent of those who develop heart disease and 95 percent of those who suffer a fatal heart attack have at least one major risk factor. Recognition of the risk factors for heart disease has helped prevent many heart-related problems and saved countless lives.

Approximately 25 percent of adults have multiple risk factors, some form of heart disease, or type 2 diabetes. These high-risk men and women should work with their physicians on specific strategies to protect their hearts. Roughly 40 percent of adults with one or more elevated risk factors are at intermediate risk. They should undergo regular testing by a physician.[14]

Risk Factors You Can Control

The choices you make and the habits you follow can have a significant impact on whether or not your heart remains healthy. You can choose to avoid the following potential risks for the sake of your heart's health.

Physical Inactivity

As discussed in Chapter 3, about one-quarter of U.S. adults are sedentary and another third are not active enough to reach a healthy level of fitness. (See the Self-Survey to assess your own level of activity.) The risk for heart disease is 1.5 to 2.4 times higher for people who are inactive compared with those who engage in regular physical activity.[15]

Women who report higher levels of physical fitness have less risk of cardiovascular disease, regardless of their body mass index (BMI), waist circumference, or waist-hip ratio (see Chapter 9). This suggests that fitness may be more important than overweight or obesity per se for women's cardiovascular risk.[16] A minimum of 30 minutes a day of moderate activity at least five days a week can lift a woman from the "low-fitness category" and lessen her risk of heart disease.[17]

In men, more rigorous exercise produced greater protection against heart disease.[18] Those who ran for an hour or more per week reduced their risk of heart disease by 42 percent, compared with an 18 percent reduction for those who walked briskly for a half-hour per day or more. With walking, pace, not duration, was linked with lower danger of heart disease.

Tobacco

Smoking may be the single most significant risk factor for cardiovascular disease—and quitting may do more to reduce the risk of mortality among heart disease patients who smoke than any other intervention or treatment. Each year smoking causes more than 250,000 deaths from cardiovascular disease—far more than it causes from cancer and lung disease. Smokers who have heart attacks are more likely to die from them than are nonsmokers. Smoking is the major risk factor for *peripheral vascular disease,* in which the vessels that carry blood to the leg and arm muscles become hardened and clogged.

Cigar smoking causes a moderate, but significant increase in an individual's risk for coronary artery disease,

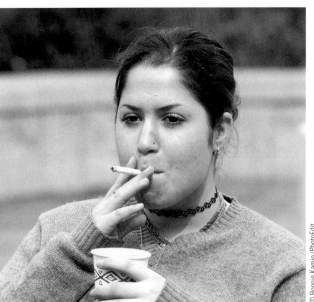

▌ Quitting smoking is the best thing you can do for your heart—regardless of your age.

as well as for cancers of the upper digestive tract and chronic obstructive pulmonary disease.

Both active and passive smoking accelerate the process by which arteries become clogged and increase the risk of heart attacks and strokes.[19] Overall, nonsmokers exposed to environmental tobacco smoke are at a 25 percent higher relative risk of developing coronary heart disease than non-smokers not exposed to environmental tobacco smoke.

In various studies, quitting has reduced the risk of heart disease and subsequent death among patients with heart disease by as much as 50 percent. After 18 years without cigarettes, the risk of dying among ex-smokers is no greater than that of never-smokers.[20]

Obesity

Obesity has emerged as an increasingly common and dangerous risk factor for cardiovascular disease, increasing the risk for hypertension, diabetes, coronary artery disease, and congestive heart failure in both men and women. BMI and measurement of waist circumference, discussed in Chapter 9, are good indicators of increased risk.

According to the National Heart, Lung, and Blood Institute (NHLBI), losing weight at any age can help reduce the risk of heart problems. For women, obesity is as great a cause of death and disability from heart disease as smoking and heavy drinking. Even mild-to-moderately obese women are more likely to suffer chest pain or a heart attack than thinner women. Weight loss significantly reduces high blood pressure, another risk factor for heart disease. (See Chapter 9 for a discussion of obesity.)

High Blood Pressure (Hypertension)

Blood pressure is a result of the contractions of the heart muscle, which pumps blood through your body, and the resistance of the walls of the vessels through which the blood flows. Each time your heart beats, your blood pressure goes up and down within a certain range. It's highest when the heart contracts; this is called **systolic blood pressure.** It's lowest between contractions; this is called **diastolic blood pressure.** A blood pressure reading consists of the systolic measurement "over" the diastolic measurement, recorded in millimeters of mercury (mm Hg) by a sphygmomanometer (**Figure 10-1**).

High blood pressure, or **hypertension,** occurs when the artery walls become constricted so that the force exerted as the blood flows through them is greater than it should be. Physicians see blood pressure as a continuum: The higher the reading, the greater the risk of stroke and heart disease. New guidelines have lowered the levels considered dangerous and identified *prehypertension* as a potential threat to the heart's health. (See the discussion of high blood pressure later in this chapter.)

Blood Fats (Lipids)

Cholesterol is a fatty substance found in certain foods and also manufactured by the body. The measurement of cholesterol in the blood is one of the most reliable indicators of the formation of plaque, the sludgelike substance that builds up on the inner walls of arteries. You can lower blood cholesterol levels by cutting back on high-fat foods and exercising more, thereby reducing the risk of a heart attack. According to the NHLBI, for every 1 percent drop in blood cholesterol, studies show a 2 percent decrease in the likelihood of a heart attack.

Lipoproteins are compounds in the blood that are made up of proteins and fat. The different types are classified by their size or density. The heaviest are *high-density lipoproteins,* or HDLs, which have the highest proportion of protein. These "good guys," as some cardiologists refer to them, pick up excess cholesterol in the blood and carry it back to the liver for removal from the body. An HDL level of 40 mg/dL or lower substantially increases the risk of heart disease. (Cholesterol levels are measured in milligrams of cholesterol per deciliter of blood—mg/dL.) The average HDL for men is about 45 mg/dL; for women, it is about 55 mg/dL.

Low-density lipoproteins, or LDLs, and very low-density lipoproteins (VLDLs) carry more cholesterol than HDLs and deposit it on the walls of arteries—they're the "bad guys." The higher your LDL cholesterol, the greater your risk for heart disease. If you are at high risk of heart disease, any level of LDL higher than 100 mg/dL may increase your danger. (See "Your Lipoprotein Profile" later in this chapter.)

Triglycerides are fats that flow through the blood after meals and have been linked to increased risk of coronary artery disease, especially in women. Triglyceride levels tend to be highest in those whose diets are high in calories, sugar, alcohol, and refined starches. High levels of these fats may increase the risk of obesity, and cutting back on these foods can reduce high triglyceride levels.

Metabolic Syndrome

Metabolic syndrome, once called Syndrome X or insulin-resistant syndrome, is emerging as a major risk factor for heart disease.[21] This condition is not a disease, but a cluster of disorders of your body's metabolism—including high blood pressure, high insulin levels, excess body weight, and abnormal cholesterol levels—that make you more likely to develop diabetes, heart disease, or stroke. Each of these conditions is by itself a risk factor for other diseases. In combination, they dramatically boost your chances of developing potentially life-threatening illnesses.

This dangerous syndrome has become so widespread that health officials describe it as an epidemic that affects one in three Americans. As

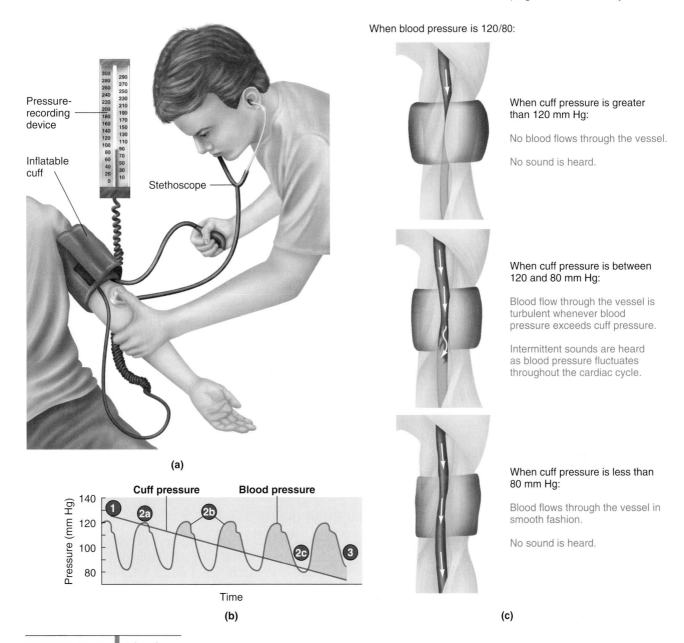

Pressure-recording device

Inflatable cuff

Stethoscope

(a)

When blood pressure is 120/80:

When cuff pressure is greater than 120 mm Hg:

No blood flows through the vessel.

No sound is heard.

When cuff pressure is between 120 and 80 mm Hg:

Blood flow through the vessel is turbulent whenever blood pressure exceeds cuff pressure.

Intermittent sounds are heard as blood pressure fluctuates throughout the cardiac cycle.

When cuff pressure is less than 80 mm Hg:

Blood flows through the vessel in smooth fashion.

No sound is heard.

Cuff pressure   Blood pressure

Pressure (mm Hg)

Time

(b)   **(c)**

FIGURE 10-1 ▌ Blood Pressure

Three steps in measuring blood pressure: (1) Increasing cuff pressure until no blood flows through (① in graph). (2) Releasing the cuff slowly so blood starts to flow through (②ⓐ, ②ⓑ, ②ⓒ)—your systolic pressure is at ②ⓐ. (3) As release of the cuff pressure continues, your diastolic pressure is the point when no sound is heard (③ on graph).

Figure 10-2 shows, it is especially common in Hispanic men and women. College-age men and women who maintain their weight as they get older are much less likely to develop metabolic syndrome.[22] However, about one in four undergraduates already has one risk factor for metabolic syndrome.[23]

According to the National Institutes of Health, three or more of the following symptoms indicate metabolic syndrome:

▮ **Waist measurement of 40 inches or more** in men and 35 inches or more in women.
▮ **Levels of triglycerides of 150 mg/dL** or more.
▮ **Levels of high-density lipoprotein**—"good" cholesterol—of less than 40 mg/dL in men or 50 mg/dL in women.
▮ **Blood pressure of 130 mmHg** systole over 85 mmHg diastole (130/85) or higher.
▮ **Fasting blood sugar of 110 mg/dL** or higher.

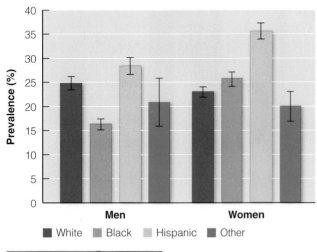

FIGURE 10-2 ❙ Prevalence of the Metabolic Syndrome

Source: Deen, Darwin. "Metabolic Syndrome: What Is It and What Can I Do about It?" *American Family Physician,* Vol. 69, No. 12, June 2004, p. 2887.

Men with three factors of metabolic syndrome are nearly twice as likely to have a heart attack or stroke and more than three times more likely to develop heart disease than those with none. Men with four or five characteristics of the syndrome have nearly four times the risk of heart attack or stroke and more than 24 times the risk of diabetes.[24]

Diabetes Mellitus

Diabetes mellitus, a disorder of the endocrine system discussed in Chapter 11, increases the likelihood of hypertension and atherosclerosis, thereby increasing the risk of heart attack and stroke. A physician can detect diabetes and prescribe a diet, exercise program, and if necessary, medication to keep it in check. Even before developing diabetes, individuals at high risk for this disease —those who are overweight, have a family history of the disease, have mildly elevated blood pressure and blood sugar levels, and above-ideal levels of harmful blood fats —may already be at increased risk of heart disease. Up to one-half of diabetics also have hypertension, another risk factor.

Psychosocial Factors

How you respond to everyday sources of stress can affect your heart as well as your overall health. While you may not be able to control the sources of stress, you can change how you habitually respond to it.

Researchers classify psychological risk factors for heart disease into three categories: chronic, episodic, and acute. Chronic factors, such as Type A behavior, play an important role in the buildup of artery-clogging plaque.

Episodic factors, such as depression, can last from several weeks to two years and may lead to the creation of "unstable" plaque (discussed later in this chapter), which is more likely to break off and block a blood vessel within the heart. Short-term or acute psychological risk factors, such as an angry outburst, can directly trigger a heart attack in people with underlying heart disease.

These factors may act alone or combine and exert different effects at different ages and stages of life. They may influence behaviors such as smoking, diet, alcohol consumption, and physical activity, as well as directly cause changes in physiology.

Depression and heart disease often occur together. People with heart disease are more likely to be depressed, and some seemingly healthy people with depression are at greater risk of heart problems. Depressed women younger than age 60 are twice as likely to suffer a heart attack than those who do not suffer from depression. After a heart attack, depression is common in both men and women, but physicians are less likely to recognize and treat depression in African-American patients.[25] Patients who suffer heart attacks and develop clinical depression have higher rates of complications and an increased risk of dying.

Job stress also can be hard on the heart, particularly for employees who have little control over their work. A lack of social support also seems to increase risk, possibly because intimate, caring relationships may buffer the effect of other stressors in life.

Drug Use

Illegal Drugs. Illegal drugs pose many dangers—one of the most serious is their potentially deadly impact on the cardiovascular system. Cocaine, ecstasy, and amphetamines can cause a sudden rise in blood pressure, heart rate, and contractions of the left ventricle (the pumping chamber) of the heart, which can increase the risk of a heart attack.

The hallucinogens lysergic acid diethylamide (LSD) and psilocybin (psychoactive mushrooms) also have the potential for triggering irregular heartbeats and heart attacks, although less serious cardiac complications, such as a temporary rise in blood pressure, are more common. Morphine and heroin, which account for almost half of drug-related deaths, can lower blood pressure and affect the heart rate. Inhalants can produce fatal heartbeat irregularities. Marijuana, the most widely used illegal drug among young adults, can affect blood pressure and heart rate, but it is not known whether it can trigger a heart attack.

Prescription Painkillers. Legal prescription drugs also can endanger the heart. Vioxx, a popular painkiller, was removed from the market in 2004 because of increased risks of heart attack and strokes in patients taking it for more than 18 months. The Food and Drug Administration (FDA) estimates that Vioxx may have contributed to as many as 80,000 to 140,000 cases of serious heart disease, many of them fatal.[26] Similar drugs in the category known as COX-2 inhibitors, used primarily to relieve arthritis pain, may also increase the risk of heart problems.[27]

Risk Factors You Can't Control

Heredity

Anyone whose parents, siblings, or other close relatives suffered heart attacks before age 50 is at increased risk of developing heart disease. Certain risk factors, such as abnormally high blood levels of lipids, can be passed down from generation to generation. Although you can't rewrite your family history, individuals with an inherited vulnerability to cardiovascular disease can lower the danger by changing the risk factors within their control. Your heart's health depends to a great extent on your behavior, including the decisions you make about the foods you eat or the decision not to smoke. As an added preventive step, cardiologists may prescribe a small daily dose of aspirin to individuals with a history of coronary artery disease who are at risk of forming clots that could block blood supplies to the heart, brain, and other organs. (Note: Daily aspirin is not advised for individuals who are not at risk because of their age or health history.)

Race and Ethnicity

African Americans are twice as likely to develop high blood pressure as whites. African Americans also suffer strokes at an earlier age and of greater severity. Poverty may be an unrecognized risk factor for members of this minority group, who are less likely to receive medical treatments or undergo corrective surgery. Family history, lifestyle, diet, and stress may also play a role, starting early in life. However, researchers have found no single explanation for why African-American youngsters, like their parents, tend to have higher blood pressure than white children.

Black women are twice as likely as white women to suffer heart attacks and to die from heart disease, according to a four-year study of 2,700 women nationwide.[28] Common risk factors—high blood pressure, diabetes, and high cholesterol—account for this increased jeopardy. In addition, black women are less likely to receive common medications, such as aspirin and cholesterol-lowering drugs, to lower their risk.

Age

Almost four out of five people who die of a heart attack are over age 65. Heart disease accounts for more than 40 percent of deaths among people between 65 and 74

and almost 60 percent at age 85 and above. However, the risk factors that are likely to cause heart disease later in life, including high blood pressure and high levels of "bad" cholesterol, may begin to develop in childhood. Nevertheless, although cardiovascular function declines with age, heart disease is not an inevitable consequence of aging. Many 80- and 90-year-olds have strong, healthy hearts.

Gender

Many people still think of heart disease as a "guy problem." However, in every year since 1984, heart disease has claimed the lives of more females than males. Cardiovascular diseases are the number-one killer of women as well as men.

For the U.S. population as a whole, as many women as men eventually die of heart disease. Yet most women are far more afraid of breast cancer (the cause of 1 in 27 female deaths) than heart disease (which is responsible for almost 1 in 2 female deaths).

Each gender also faces some unique heart-related issues, including male pattern baldness and menopause. **Male pattern baldness** (the loss of hair at the vertex, or top, of the head) is associated with increased risk of heart attack in men under age 55. The speed at which men lose their hair also may be an indicator of risk. Men with male pattern baldness who lose their hair quickly may metabolize male sex hormones differently than others, thereby increasing the likelihood of heart disease. Although it's premature to say that baldness is definitely bad news for the heart, health experts advise bald men to follow basic guidelines, such as not smoking and controlling their cholesterol levels, to lower any possible risk.

A woman's risk increases sharply after menopause. Researchers long believed that postmenopausal hormone therapy (HT) protected women from heart disease. However, recent studies have shown this not to be true. A major long-term study, the Women's Health Initiative, has shown that women on certain types of HT actually have an increased risk of heart attack and stroke.

Bacterial Infection

Certain bacteria may indeed put the heart at risk. *Streptococcus sanguis,* the bacterium found in dental plaque, has been implicated in the buildup of atherosclerotic plaque. Individuals with periodontal disease are at increased risk of heart disease and stroke. Regular brushing, flossing, and dental visits can reduce this danger.

Another common bacterium, *Chlamydia pneumoniae,* long linked to respiratory infections, also may threaten the heart. Individuals with high levels of antibodies to this bacteria are more likely to suffer a heart-related problem. Researchers have reported that antibiotics, taken to treat common infections, may protect against first-time heart attacks. A national clinical trial to determine whether antibiotics can reduce the risk of heart attack and stroke is underway.

High Blood Pressure (Hypertension)

Blood pressure refers to the force of blood against the walls of arteries. When blood pressure remains elevated over time—a condition called hypertension—it forces the heart to pump harder than is healthy. Because the heart must force blood into arteries that are offering increased resistance to blood flow, the left side of the heart becomes enlarged. If untreated, high blood pressure can cause a variety of cardiovascular complications, including heart attack and stroke—two of the three leading causes of death among U.S. adults—as well as kidney failure and blindness (**Figure 10-3**).

The World Health Organization estimates that hypertension causes one in every eight deaths globally, making it the third leading killer in the world. In the United States, high blood pressure is responsible for about a third of cardiovascular problems like heart attack or stroke and a quarter of all premature deaths.

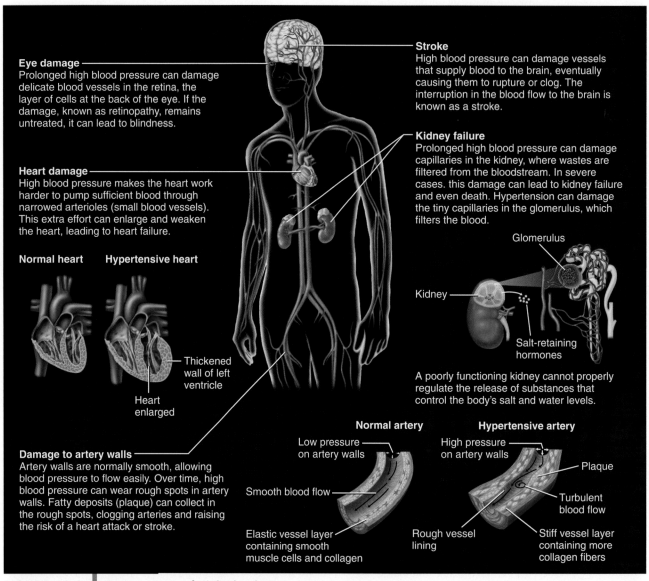

Eye damage
Prolonged high blood pressure can damage delicate blood vessels in the retina, the layer of cells at the back of the eye. If the damage, known as retinopathy, remains untreated, it can lead to blindness.

Heart damage
High blood pressure makes the heart work harder to pump sufficient blood through narrowed arterioles (small blood vessels). This extra effort can enlarge and weaken the heart, leading to heart failure.

Normal heart   Hypertensive heart

Thickened wall of left ventricle

Heart enlarged

Damage to artery walls
Artery walls are normally smooth, allowing blood pressure to flow easily. Over time, high blood pressure can wear rough spots in artery walls. Fatty deposits (plaque) can collect in the rough spots, clogging arteries and raising the risk of a heart attack or stroke.

Stroke
High blood pressure can damage vessels that supply blood to the brain, eventually causing them to rupture or clog. The interruption in the blood flow to the brain is known as a stroke.

Kidney failure
Prolonged high blood pressure can damage capillaries in the kidney, where wastes are filtered from the bloodstream. In severe cases. this damage can lead to kidney failure and even death. Hypertension can damage the tiny capillaries in the glomerulus, which filters the blood.

Glomerulus

Kidney

Salt-retaining hormones

A poorly functioning kidney cannot properly regulate the release of substances that control the body's salt and water levels.

Normal artery   Hypertensive artery

Low pressure on artery walls   High pressure on artery walls

Plaque

Smooth blood flow

Turbulent blood flow

Elastic vessel layer containing smooth muscle cells and collagen

Rough vessel lining

Stiff vessel layer containing more collagen fibers

FIGURE 10-3 ▮ Consequences of High Blood Pressure
If left untreated, elevated blood pressure can damage blood vessels in several areas of the body and lead to serious health problems.

About a third of adults age 18 and older in the United States—some 65 million men and women—have high blood pressure.[29] In the last decade, hypertension grew by about 8 percent, with a 30 percent jump in the total number of adults with high blood pressure. Blood pressure has also increased among children and adolescents over the last decade, with the highest rates among black and Mexican-American children. The primary culprit is the increase in obesity in the young.[30] No one knows why African Americans are more vulnerable, although some speculate that overweight or dietary factors may contribute.

Family history also plays a role. "If you study healthy college students with normal blood pressures, those who have one parent with hypertension will have blood pressure that's little higher than average," notes Rose Marie Robertson, M.D., of the American Heart Association. "If two parents have high blood pressure, their levels will be a little higher, and they're destined to go higher still. If your parents have high blood pressure, have yours checked regularly."[31]

Men and women are equally likely to develop hypertension, but in women, blood pressure tends to rise around the time of menopause. Half of all women over age 45 have hypertension. For individuals who smoke, are overweight, don't exercise, or have high cholesterol levels, hypertension multiplies the risk of heart disease and stroke. At ultrahigh risk are people with diabetes or kidney disease.

In its most recent report, the Joint National Committee on Prevention, Detection, Evaluation, and Treatment of High Blood Pressure identified the following key messages:[32]

▮ Beginning at 115/75 mm HG, cardiovascular disease risk doubles for each increment of 20/10 mm Hg.

▮ In those older than age 50, a systolic blood pressure greater than 140 mm Hg is a more important risk factor for cardiovascular disease than diastolic blood pressure. The risk of cardiovascular disease, beginning at 115/75 doubles with each increment of 20/10 mm Hg.

▮ Men and women with normal blood pressure at age 55 have a 90 percent lifetime risk of developing hypertension.

In a young person even mild hypertension can cause organs such as the heart, brain, and kidneys to start to deteriorate. By age 50 or 60, the damage may be irreversible.

Different races suffer different consequences of high blood pressure. An African American with the same elevated blood pressure reading as a Caucasian faces a greater risk of stroke, heart disease, and kidney problems.

Preventing Hypertension

Prevention pays off when it comes to high blood pressure. The most effective preventive measures involve lifestyle changes. Losing weight is the best approach for individuals with high normal values. Exercise may be effective in lowering mildly elevated blood pressure. High intake of folate, a B vitamin discussed in Chapter 8, can significantly reduce the risk of hypertension. In a study of women under age 35, those who consumed the most folate had one third of the risk of developing high blood pressure as those consuming very little.[33] Among the approaches that have not proved effective are dietary supplements, such as calcium, magnesium, potassium, and fish oil.

The National Heart, Lung, and Blood Institute has developed what is known as the DASH diet. Following DASH, which stands for Dietary Approaches to Stop Hypertension, has proved as effective as drug therapy in lowering blood pressure. An additional benefit: The DASH diet also lowers harmful blood fats, including cholesterol and low-density lipoprotein, and the amino acid homocysteine (one of the new suspects in heart disease risk).

Restriction of sodium intake also helps. Most Americans consume more salt than they need. The 2005 *Dietary Guidelines for Americans* recommend limiting sodium to 2,300 milligrams a day—about a teaspoonful—including salt used at the table and in cooking. Diets of less than 1,500 milligrams of sodium produce greater benefits and help blood pressure medicines work better.

The lower the amount of sodium in the diet, the lower the blood pressure for both those with and those without hypertension and for both genders and all racial and ethnic groups. However, reducing dietary sodium has an even greater effect on blood pressure in blacks than whites, in women than men, and in individuals with hypertension.

What Is a Healthy Blood Pressure?

The answer to this question has changed. The past standard for normal—120/80 millimeters of mercury (mm Hg)—is no longer considered low enough to prevent serious health consequences. Guidelines released in 2003 (Table 10-1) categorize a reading of 120/80 as **prehypertension,** a condition that is likely to worsen in time. A healthy reading is 115/75 mm Hg. Once blood pressure rises above this threshold, the risk of cardiovascular disease increases.

In healthy adults, blood pressure screening should begin at age 21, with repeat evaluations at least every two years, or more often depending on your current health, medical history, and risk factors for cardiovascular disease.

To get an accurate blood pressure reading, you should visit the doctor's office at least twice and have your blood

TABLE 10-1 ▌ What Your Blood Pressure Means

Top Number (systolic)		Bottom Number (diastolic)	Your Group	What to Do
Below 120	and	Below 80	Normal blood pressure	Maintain a healthy lifestyle
120–139	or	80–89	Prehypertension	Adopt a healthy lifestyle
140–159	or	90–99	Stage 1 hypertension	Adopt a healthy lifestyle; take medication
160 or more	or	100 or more	Stage 2 hypertension	Adopt a healthy lifestyle; take more than one medication

Numbers are expressed in millimeters of mercury (mm Hg).

Source: Seventh Report of the Joint National Committee on Prevention, Detection, Evaluation and Treatment of High Blood Pressure, 2003.

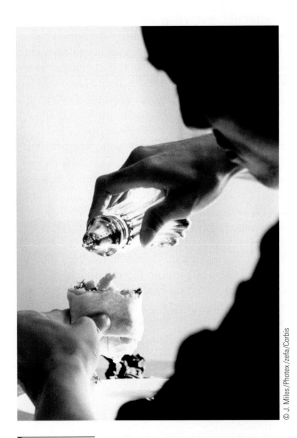

© J. Miles /Photex /zefa/Corbis

▌ Reducing your salt intake can help lower your blood pressure.

pressure taken two or more times while you're seated. The average of those measurements determines how your blood pressure is classified.

The new guidelines classify hypertension into two categories:

▌ **Stage 1.** This consists of a systolic pressure ranging from 140 to 159 or a diastolic pressure ranging from 90 to 99.

▌ **Stage 2.** The most severe form of hypertension occurs with a systolic pressure of 160 or higher or a diastolic reading of 100 or higher.

Only one of the numbers—the top or bottom—needs to be high to meet these criteria. In people over age 50, systolic pressure is more important than diastolic. If it rises to 140 mm Hg or higher, doctors advise treatment regardless of the diastolic pressure.

Controlling High Blood Pressure

Lifestyle changes are a first-line weapon in the fight against high blood pressure. Rather than making a single change, a combination of behavioral changes, including losing weight, eating heart-healthy foods, reducing sodium, and exercising more, yields the best results. For uncomplicated hypertension, the recommended treatment is a thiazide diuretic, either alone or combined with other antihypertensive medications.

Making healthy lifestyle modifications can help reduce Stage 1 hypertension, but most people also require a medication. Those with Stage 2 hypertension typically need at least two types of high blood pressure medications (antihypertensives) to reduce blood pressure to a safer level. The goal for most people with hypertension is to reduce blood pressure to below 140/90 mm Hg.

Only about one-third of people with hypertension have it effectively controlled—below 140/90 mm Hg. Yet the higher your blood pressure, the higher your risk of heart attack, heart failure, stroke, and kidney disease.

Reducing systolic blood pressure 12 mm Hg for 10 years can prevent one death in every 11 people treated for hypertension. In those with existing cardiovascular disease or organ damage, such as kidney disease, that reduction has an even bigger benefit, preventing one death in every nine people treated.

✚ Your Lipoprotein Profile

Medical science has changed the way it views and targets the blood fats that endanger the healthy heart. In the past, the focus was primarily on total cholesterol in the blood. The higher this number was, the greater the risk

SAVVY

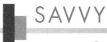

CONSUMER

WHAT YOU NEED TO KNOW ABOUT
TESTING CHOLESTEROL

❚ Go to your primary health-care provider to get a lipoprotein profile. Although cholesterol tests at shopping malls or health fairs can help identify people at risk, the analyzers are often not certified technicians, and the readings may be inaccurate. In addition, without a health expert to counsel them, some people may be unnecessarily frightened by a high reading—or falsely reassured by a low one.

❚ Ask about accuracy. Even at first-rate laboratories, cholesterol readings are often inaccurate. Find out if the lab is using the National Institutes of Health standards, and ask about the lab's margin of error (which should be less than 5 percent).

❚ Fast beforehand. Cholesterol tests are most accurate after a 9- to 14-hour fast. Schedule the test before breakfast if you can. Women may not want to get tested at the end of their menstrual cycles, when minor elevations in cholesterol levels occur because of lower estrogen levels. Cholesterol levels can also rise 5 to 10 percent during periods of stress. Reschedule the test if you come down with an intestinal flu because the viral infection could interfere with the absorption of food and thus with cholesterol levels. Let your doctor know if you're taking any drugs. Common medications, including birth control pills and hypertension drugs, can affect cholesterol levels.

❚ Sit down before allowing blood to be drawn or your finger to be pricked; fluids pool differently in the body when you're standing than when you're sitting. Don't let a technician squeeze blood from your finger, which forces fluid from cells, diluting the blood sample and possibly leading to a falsely low reading.

❚ Get real numbers. Don't settle for "normal" or "high" because laboratories can inaccurately label results. Find out exactly what your reading is. Find out your HDL/LDL ratio, and HDL and LDL levels.

---

of heart disease. The NHLBI's National Cholesterol Education Program has recommended more comprehensive testing, called a *lipoprotein profile,* for all individuals age 20 or older. (See Savvy Consumer: "What You Need to Know About Testing Cholesterol.")

This blood test, which should be performed after a 9- to 12-hour fast and repeated at least once every five years, provides readings of:

❚ **Total cholesterol.**
❚ **LDL (bad) cholesterol,** the main culprit in the buildup of plaque within the arteries.
❚ **HDL (good, or Healthy) cholesterol,** which helps prevent cholesterol buildup.
❚ **Triglycerides,** the blood fats released into the bloodstream after a meal.

What Is a Healthy Cholesterol Reading?

The updated guidelines of the National Cholesterol Education Program (NCEP) focus on the greatest threat to your heart's health: LDL cholesterol. However, the degree of danger of a higher reading depends not just on the number itself but on whether or not you have other risk factors for heart disease. These include age (over 45 in men, over 55 in women), smoking, high blood pressure, high blood sugar, diabetes, abdominal obesity ("belly" fat), and a family history of heart disease. The new guidelines set lower target goals for LDL cholesterol, particularly for those at greatest risk of a heart attack or death from cardiovascular disease[34] (**Table 10–2**).

HDL, good cholesterol, also is important, particularly in women. Federal guidelines define an HDL reading of less than 40 mg/dL as a major risk factor for developing heart disease. HDL levels of 60 mg/dL or more are protective and lower the risk of heart disease.

A lipoprotein profile also measures triglycerides, the free-floating molecules that transport fats in the bloodstream. Ideally this should be below 150 mg/dL. Individuals with readings of 150 to 199 mg/dL, considered borderline, as well as those with higher readings, may benefit from weight control, physical activity, and, if necessary, medication.

TABLE 10-2 ▮ New Targets for Lowering LDL

Risk Category	LDL Goal
Low Risk (1 or 0 risk factors for heart disease)	Less than 160 mg/dL
Moderate Risk (2 or more risk factors that create a 10 percent or lower risk of a heart attack in the next 10 years)	Less than 130 mg/dL
Moderately High Risk (2 or more risk factors that create a 10 to 20 percent chance of a heart attack in next 10 years)	Less than 130 mg/dL
High Risk (heart disease or diabetes, diseased blood vessels, 2 or more risk factors)	Less than 100 mg/dL
Very High Risk (heart disease and multiple, severe, or poorly controlled risk factors, espe- cially smoking, or a history of heart attack or angina)	Less than 70 mg/dL

Source: Based on the National Cholesterol Education Program Adult Treatment Panel III Guidelines, www.circulationaha.org.

Lowering Cholesterol

Lifestyle changes can lower harmful LDL levels by 5 to 10 percent. However, a greater reduction of 30 to 40 percent requires either the kind of intensive lifestyle changes promoted by Dr. Dean Ornish, including an extremely low-fat diet, or the addition of cholesterol-lowering medication. All medications, including the ones used to lower LDL, cost money and sometimes cause side effects. However, if you are at high risk of having a heart attack, their benefits far outweigh the costs and risks of medication.

The most widely used cholesterol-lowering medications are statins, currently used by an estimated 11 million Americans. Because of the new LDL targets, the number of people on statins—better known by brand names such as Lipitor and Pravachol—could rise to about 50 million.

Statins work in the liver to block production of cholesterol. When the liver can't make cholesterol, it draws LDL cholesterol from the blood to use as raw material. This means that less LDL is available to trigger or promote the artery-clogging process known as atherosclerosis. Statins also appear to stabilize cholesterol-filled deposits in artery walls and to cool down inflammation.

All of these actions can help prevent a heart attack or other forms of cardiovascular trouble. Long-term therapy with statins reduces the risk for death, heart attack, and stroke among people with heart disease, even when LDL levels are not elevated.

Raising HDL—which can be done with lifestyle changes, vitamins such as niacin (B_3), or a combination of both—can both stop and reverse the progression of cardiovascular plaque. Other medications, called fibrates, can help lower triglycerides, the main fat-carrying particles in the blood.

✚ C-Reactive Protein (CRP)

C-reactive protein is a marker of inflammation in the blood vessels, which may make atherosclerotic plaque more likely to rupture. As several studies have shown, the higher the concentrations of CRP in the blood, the greater the risk for heart disease and sudden death.[35] Among those who have had a heart attack, lowering CRP with statin medications, which also reduce harmful cholesterol levels, helps open clogged arteries.[36] Based on these findings, researchers are urging doctors and their patients to reduce both "bad" cholesterol and CRP.

A simple and inexpensive blood test called hs-CRP (for high-sensitivity CRP) that measures very low levels of CRP can detect inflammation within blood vessels and indicate increased danger of heart disease.

The CDC and American Heart Association have not endorsed CRP testing as a standard screening tool for the general public but recommend it for those at intermediate risk of developing coronary heart disease in the next 10 years. The test can help a cardiologist decide on further evaluations and the need for more aggressive therapy to prevent cardiovascular disease. The test may be especially useful in evaluating heart disease risk in women.

Testing for CRP usually requires two blood tests two weeks apart. C-reactive protein is measured in milligrams per liter (mg/L) of blood, and **Table 10-3** shows the risk associated with level of CRP.

✚ Aspirin and the Heart

Daily aspirin is recommended as a preventive step for people at high risk of cardiovascular disease because it reduces the stickiness of platelets (cells that cause blood clotting). This lowers the risk of blood clots, which can block a blood vessel and trigger a heart attack or stroke. Several research studies, such as the Hypertension Optimal Treatment study, have demonstrated an association

TABLE 10-3 ▮ C-Reactive Protein (CRP) Levels and Cardiovascular Risk

CRP (milligrams per liter)	Level of cardiovascular risk
Less than 0.5 mg/L	Lowest
Less than 1 mg/L	Low
1–3 mg/L	Moderate
Greater than 3 mg/L	High (risk doubles)

Lowering LDL and C-Reactive Protein

▍ Stop smoking.

▍ Eat a diet rich in fruit and vegetables.

▍ Increase your daily servings of whole grains and bran-containing foods.

▍ Cut back on high-fat foods.

▍ Exercise regularly for at least 30 minutes each day.

▍ Aim for a healthy weight by thinking long-term and making gradual changes.

▍ Know your numbers, including blood pressure and lipoprotein levels, and follow your doctor's advice on whether you would benefit from medication.

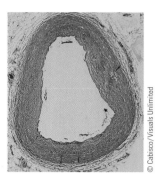 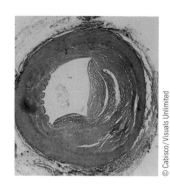

FIGURE 10-4 ▍ Plaque in the arteries

Left: A healthy coronary artery. Right: An artery partially blocked by the buildup of atherosclerotic plaque.

between aspirin use and reductions in heart attacks and strokes. Aspirin lowers the risk of death from any cause, not just heart disease. Its protective effects are strongest in the elderly and those with heart disease. People who regularly take other painkillers, such as ibuprofen, may not benefit from aspirin.

Aspirin has different effects in men and women. In men, daily low-dose aspirin significantly lowers the risk of heart attack but has little effect on preventing stoke. In women ages 45 to 64, aspirin therapy does little, if anything, to ward off a first heart attack, but it may reduce the risk of stroke.[37] Doctors no longer recommend daily aspirin for all healthy women under age 65, but they may advise it for those at risk of stroke.

Aspirin can produce side effects, including gastro-intestinal bleeding, allergic reactions, and peptic ulcers. However, the very low doses recommended for heart disease prevention generally do not cause serious problems. They are not advised for people taking anticlotting medication, who have stomach ulcers, or who have kidney or liver disease. Some individuals are aspirin-resistant and do not benefit from its protective effects.

✚ Crises of the Heart

Coronary Artery Disease

The general term for any impairment of blood flow through the blood vessels, often referred to as "hardening of the arteries," is **arteriosclerosis.** The most common

form is **atherosclerosis,** a disease of the lining of the arteries in which **plaque**—deposits of fat, fibrin (a clotting material), cholesterol, other cell parts, and calcium—narrows the artery channels as shown in **Figure 10-3** on page 220 and the photos above.

Atherosclerosis

Atherosclerosis, or atherosclerotic vascular disease (ASVD), is the most common form of cardiovascular disease. While it may begin in childhood, atherosclerosis worsens with the continued buildup of plaque on the arterial lining. The arteries lose their ability to expand and contract. Blood moves with increasing difficulty through the narrowed channels, making it easier for a clot (thrombus) to form, perhaps blocking the channel and depriving vital organs of blood. When such a blockage is in a coronary artery, the result is coronary thrombosis, one form of heart attack. When the clot occurs in the brain, the result is cerebral thrombosis, one form of stroke (discussed later in this chapter).

Unstable Plaque

Extra cholesterol deposited on an artery wall creates a "bump" covered by a hard scar. This plaque narrows the space in the arteries, and the heart may not receive an adequate supply of oxygen-carrying blood, which may lead to chest pain (angina) or a heart attack.

Cardiologists long believed that the most dangerous plaques were the largest ones, which were most likely to cause total blockage of the coronary arteries. However, small plaques are now thought to be very unstable and more likely to burst or rupture, spewing cholesterol into the bloodstream. This triggers blood clotting, which blocks the artery, stops blood flow, and leads to a heart attack.

Lowering cholesterol can make plaque more stable and less prone to rupture. A possible early warning of unstable plaque is an elevated level of C-reactive protein (see page 224).

Unclogging the Arteries

For years, heart specialists said that, once clogged, arteries couldn't be unclogged. However, research has now shown that it is possible to reverse the buildup of plaque inside the arteries by means of cholesterol-lowering drugs and a low-fat diet. A strict program of dietary and lifestyle change without any medication, developed by Dean Ornish, M.D., of the University of California, San Francisco, also has proved effective in reversing coronary artery disease. The following are the key elements of this approach:

- **A very low-fat, vegetarian diet,** including nonfat dairy products and egg whites, keeping fat intake to below 8 percent of total calories consumed. Ornish's recommended diet allows no meat, poultry, fish, butter, cheese, ice cream, or any form of oil.
- **Moderate exercise,** consisting of an hour of aerobic activity three times a week. Walking is recommended because more rigorous exercise might be dangerous for heart patients, who may develop increased risk of blood clots, irregular heartbeats, or coronary artery spasms during exertion.
- **Stress counseling.** Ornish's patients learn how the body's stress response can cause a rapid heartbeat and narrowing of the arteries, and how stress reduction can reduce cholesterol levels.
- **An hour a day of yoga,** meditation, breathing, and progressive relaxation. Some patients use visualization, for instance, imagining their arteries being cleared by a tunneling machine.

Angina Pectoris

A temporary drop in the supply of oxygen to the heart tissue causes feelings of pain or discomfort in the chest known as **angina pectoris.** Some people suffer angina only when the demands on their hearts increase, such as during exercise or when under stress. Many people have angina for years and yet never suffer a heart attack; in some, the angina even disappears. However, angina should be considered a warning of danger if it becomes more severe or more frequent, occurs with less activity or exertion, begins to waken a person from a sound sleep at night, persists for more than ten to fifteen minutes, or causes unusual perspiration.

Coronary Artery Spasms

Sometimes the arteries tighten suddenly or go into a spasm, cutting off or reducing blood flow. Spasms can produce heart attacks, as well as angina, and can be fatal. Several factors may trigger spasms in the heart, including the following:

- **Clumping of platelets.** When *platelets* (a type of blood cell) clump together, they produce a substance called thromboxane A-2, which causes the narrowing of a blood vessel.
- **Smoking.** When some angina victims stop smoking, their chest pain declines or disappears.
- **Stress.** No one knows exactly how stress may lead to spasms, but many heart specialists believe that it's a culprit.
- **Increased calcium flow.** Calcium regularly flows into smooth muscle cells; too much calcium, however, may lead to a spasm. (This calcium flow is not regulated by the amount of calcium in your diet.)

Heart Attack (Myocardial Infarction)

Each year, about 1.1 million Americans suffer a heart attack. About 460,000 are fatal. Half of the deaths occur within an hour of the start of symptoms and before the person reaches the hospital. The medical name for a heart attack, or coronary, is **myocardial infarction (MI).** The *myocardium* is the cardiac muscle layer of the wall of the heart. It receives its blood supply, and thus its oxygen and other nutrients, from the coronary arteries. If an artery is blocked by a clot or plaque, or by a spasm, the myocardial cells do not get sufficient oxygen, and the portion of the myocardium deprived of its blood supply begins to die (**Figure 10-5**). Although such an attack may seem sudden, usually it has been building up for years, particularly if the person has ignored risk factors and early warning signs.

How Do I Know It's a Heart Attack?

Individuals should seek immediate medical care if they experience the following symptoms:

- **A tight ache, heavy, squeezing pain,** or discomfort in the center of the chest, which may last for 30 minutes or more and is not relieved by rest.
- **Chest pain** that radiates to the shoulder, arm, neck, back, or jaw.
- **Anxiety.**
- **Sweating or cold, clammy skin.**
- **Nausea and vomiting.**
- **Shortness of breath.**
- **Dizziness, fainting, or loss of consciousness.**

If you're with someone who's exhibiting the classic signs of heart attack, and if they last for two minutes or more, act at once. Expect the person to deny the possibility of anything as serious as a heart attack, but insist on taking prompt action.

Time is of the essence when a heart attack occurs. If you develop symptoms or if you're with someone who does, call the emergency system (911 in most places) immediately. The sooner emergency personnel get to someone having a heart attack and administer cardiac life support, the greater the odds of survival. Yet, according to the American Heart Association, most patients wait

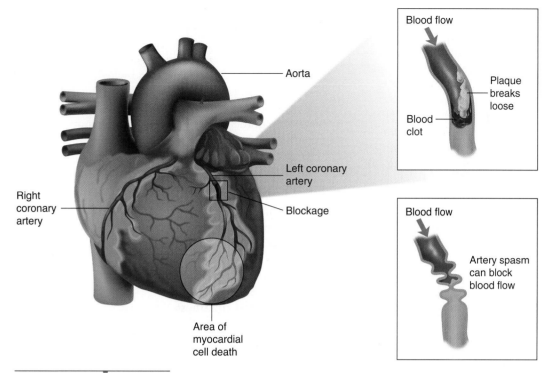

FIGURE 10-5 ▌ Heart Attack

If blood flow within a coronary artery is blocked, the lack of blood supply causes cells in that area of the heart to die. This blockage is most often caused by plaque breaking loose, and a blood clot forms and blocks the artery. A coronary artery spasm can also stop the flow of blood.

three hours after the initial symptoms begin before seeking help. By that time, half of the affected heart muscle may already be lost.

Individuals trained in **cardiopulmonary resuscitation (CPR),** a combination of mouth-to-mouth breathing and chest compression, should use this technique only after calling or having someone else call for help. CPR is most effective when started within minutes of a cardiac arrest and when trained medical personnel arrive within 8 to 12 minutes. CPR should be performed only by individuals trained in this technique. If performed incorrectly, CPR may be ineffective or harmful.[38]

Treatments That Save Hearts

State-of-the-art treatments for heart attacks include clot-dissolving drugs, early administration of medications to thin the blood, intravenous nitroglycerin, and in some cases, a beta-blocker (which blocks many of the effects of adrenaline in the body, particularly its stimulating impact on the heart).

Clot-dissolving drugs called thrombolytic agents are the treatment of choice for acute myocardial infarction in most clinical settings. Administered through a *catheter* (flexible tube) threaded through the arteries to the site of the blockage (the more effective method of delivery) or injected intravenously (the faster, cheaper method of delivery), these agents can save lives and dissolve clots but don't remove the underlying atherosclerotic plaque.

Two clot-thinning drugs may be better than one for treating heart attacks. One drug, called a thrombolytic, dissolves blood clots. The second drug, a platelet receptor blocker, keeps platelets from clumping and forming the blood clots that can obstruct blood flow and thereby trigger a heart attack or stroke.

Emergency balloon **angioplasty** has shown greater effectiveness than clot-dissolving medication in restoring blood flow in arteries immediately after an attack. With this approach, arteries are less likely to close down again and patients have shorter hospital stays and fewer hospital readmissions. Angioplasty patients also are less likely to die of the heart attack or to experience repeat attacks.

Women who have heart attacks are less likely than men to survive over both the short and the long term. A woman's risk of dying within a month of a heart attack is up to 75 percent higher than a man's, in part because women typically take an hour longer to get to the hospital than men. Women also have more complications than men during hospitalization and a higher death rate. Men are more likely to receive therapy with aspirin, beta-blockers, or angiotensin-converting enzyme inhibitors and to undergo angioplasty or bypass surgery.

✚ Stroke

When the blood supply to a portion of the brain is blocked, a cerebrovascular incident, or **stroke,** occurs. Someone in the United States suffers a stroke every 53 seconds; more than a quarter are under age 65. An estimated 20 percent of stroke victims die within three months; 50 to 60 percent are disabled. About half of those who have a stroke are partially paralyzed on one side of their body; between a quarter and a half are partially or completely dependent on others for daily living; a third become depressed; a fifth cannot walk.

Strokes rank third, after heart disease and cancer, as a cause of death in this country. Worldwide, stroke is second only to heart disease as a cause of death. After decades of steady decline, the number of strokes per year has begun to rise. The main reasons seem to be that more people in the United States are living longer, advanced medical care is allowing more people to survive heart disease, and doctors are better able to diagnose and detect strokes. Yet 80 percent of strokes are preventable, and key risk factors can be modified through either lifestyle changes or drugs. The most important steps are treating hypertension, not smoking, lowering cholesterol, and exercise.

Strokes continue to occur 40 percent more often in the Southeast (the so-called Stroke Belt) than in other regions of the United States. However, stroke rates have fallen in Mississippi and Alabama while they've increased in Oregon, Washington, and Arkansas. The decline in deaths among stroke victims has been greatest in white men and smallest among black men.

What Causes a Stroke? 📠

There are two types of stroke: *ischemic stroke,* which is the result of a blockage that disrupts blood flow to the brain, and *hemorrhagic stroke,* which occurs when blood vessels rupture. One of the most common causes of ischemic stroke is the blockage of a brain artery by a thrombus, or blood clot—a *cerebral thrombosis.* Clots generally form around deposits sticking out from the arterial wall. Sometimes a wandering blood clot (embolus), carried in the bloodstream, becomes wedged in one of the cerebral arteries. This is called a *cerebral embolism,* and it can completely plug up a cerebral artery.

In hemorrhagic stroke, a diseased artery in the brain floods the surrounding tissue with blood. The cells nourished by the artery are deprived of blood and can't function, and the blood from the artery forms a clot that may interfere with brain function. This is most likely to occur if the patient suffers from a combination of hypertension and atherosclerosis. Hemorrhage (bleeding) may also be caused by a head injury or by the bursting of an aneurysm, a blood-filled pouch that balloons out from a weak spot in the wall of an artery.

Brain tissue, like heart muscle, begins to die if deprived of oxygen, which may then cause difficulty speaking and walking and loss of memory. These effects may be slight or severe, temporary or permanent, depending on how widespread the damage and whether other areas of the brain can take over the function of the damaged area. About 30 percent of stroke survivors develop dementia, a disorder that robs a person of memory and other intellectual abilities.

The following symptoms should alert you to the possibility that you or someone with you has suffered a stroke:

▌ **Sudden weakness or loss of strength.**
▌ **Numbness of face, arm, or leg.**
▌ **Loss of speech, or difficulty speaking** or understanding speech.
▌ **Dimness or loss of vision,** particularly double vision in one eye.
▌ **Unexplained dizziness.**
▌ **Change in personality.**
▌ **Change in pattern of headaches.**

Risk Factors for Strokes

People who've experienced **transient ischemic attacks (TIAs),** "little strokes" that cause minimal damage, are at the highest risk for stroke. Other risk factors, like those for heart disease, include some that can't be changed (such as gender and race) and some that can be controlled:

▌ **Gender.** Men have a greater risk of stroke than women. However, women are at increased risk at times of marked hormonal changes, particularly pregnancy and childbirth. Past studies have shown an association between oral contraceptive use and stroke, particularly in women over age 35 who smoke. The newer low-dose oral contraceptives have not shown an increased stroke risk among women ages 18 to 44. A woman's stroke risk may increase markedly at menopause.
▌ **Race.** The incidence of strokes is two to three times greater in blacks than whites in the same communities. Hispanics also are more likely to develop hemorrhagic strokes than whites.
▌ **Age.** A person's risk of stroke more than doubles every decade after age 55.
▌ **Hypertension.** Detection and treatment of high blood pressure are the best means of stroke prevention.
▌ **High red blood cell count.** A moderate to marked increase in the number of a person's red blood cells increases the risk of stroke.
▌ **Heart disease.** Heart problems can interfere with the flow of blood to the brain; clots that form in the heart can travel to the brain, where they may clog an artery.
▌ **Blood fats.** Although the standard advice from cardiologists is to lower harmful LDL levels, what may be

more important to lower stroke risk is a drop in the levels of protective HDL.

▌ **Diabetes mellitus.** Diabetics have a higher incidence of stroke than nondiabetics.

▌ **Estrogen therapy.** In 2004, the Women's Health Initiative—a series of clinical trials of hormone therapy for postmenopausal women —halted its study of estrogen-only therapy because of an increase in the risk of stroke. Women on estrogen experienced 12 more strokes per 10,000 persons, compared to women not taking hormones.[39]

▌ **A diet high in fat and sodium.** Individuals consuming the largest amounts of fatty foods and sodium are at much greater risk then those eating low-fat, low-salt diets.[40]

MAKING HEALTHY CHOICES

To Protect Your Heart

Heart disease is not inevitable. We can keep our hearts healthy for as long as we live, but the process of doing so must start early and continue throughout life.

▌ **Don't smoke.** There's no bigger favor you can do your heart—and lungs!

▌ **Watch your weight.** Even relatively modest gains can have a big effect on your risk of heart disease.

▌ **Cut down on saturated fats and cholesterol.** This can help prevent high blood cholesterol levels, obesity, and heart disease.

▌ **Get moving.** Engage in regular physical activity. A little is better than none; more is even better.

▌ **Lower your stress levels.** If too much stress is a problem in your life, try the relaxation techniques described in Chapter 7.

▌ **Know your family history.** Inheriting a predisposition to high blood pressure or heart disease means that your heart needs extra preventive care.

▌ **Get your blood pressure checked regularly.** Knowing your numbers can alert you to a potential problem long before you develop any symptoms.

▌ **Tame your temper.** Hostility can be hazardous to the heart. Look for other ways of releasing anger and frustration.

▌ **Get a lipoprotein profile.** You can't know if your heart is in danger unless you know your cholesterol and lipoprotein levels. Get a blood test at your next physical, and discuss the results with your physician.

▌ **Take appropriate medications.** Those with high cholesterol or high blood pressure should seek their physicians' advice.

SELF-SURVEY

What Do You Know About Heart Disease?

Checkmark the following statements either True or False to test your knowledge about Heart Disease.

True	False	
1. ___	___	A major risk factor for heart disease is lack of regular physical activity.
2. ___	___	Smoking is directly related to about 20% of deaths from cardiovascular disease.
3. ___	___	For best heart health, it is recommended to cut out all fat from the diet.
4. ___	___	Women have less chance of dying from heart disease than do men.
5. ___	___	Obesity increases the chances of getting heart disease.
6. ___	___	Because heredity can't be changed, there is nothing you can do about it.
7. ___	___	Signs of heart disease can be seen in teenagers.
8. ___	___	Chest pain, shortness of breath, cold sweat and nausea are heart attack symptoms.
9. ___	___	The major cause of high blood pressure is a high stress lifestyle.
10. ___	___	Cardiovascular disease is the leading cause of death in the United States.

Answers

1. **True.** Inactive people are almost twice as likely to develop heart disease. Fortunately, it doesn't take a lot of time to incorporate physical activity into your life. As little as 20 minutes a day can help you reap the benefits associated with physical activity. Regular activity helps reduce stress, control weight, improve HDL cholesterol and blood pressure readings, and increase one's insulin sensitivity, which lowers the risk for diabetes.

2. **True.** Nicotine is abrasive to the inner lining of the arteries and makes it easier for cholesterol and other fatty deposits to collect plaque and obstruct blood flow, forcing the heart to work harder pumping blood through a narrower artery. Nicotine also increases heart rate and blood pressure, which forces the heart to increase overall work output. Carbon monoxide, a

by-product of tobacco smoke, decreases the ability of the blood to carry adequate oxygen to the heart, decreasing the amount of oxygen available to the heart muscle and making the heart work harder to get the oxygen it needs for proper functioning.

3. **False.** Reducing the amount of saturated fat in the diet is a good idea, because this will help reduce cholesterol levels and make the blood less susceptible to clotting. But cutting out all fat is unhealthy. Fat is needed as a source of essential fatty acids, which help to metabolize fat in the body. Adequate fat also is needed to assist with digestion and absorption of fat-soluble vitamins, which are critical to overall health. Dietary fat should be consumed in moderation from a variety of sources: Vegetable oils, nuts, seeds, dairy and other animal products, including meat and poultry.

4. **False.** Even though heart disease is the primary killer of men and women, in each year since 1984 more women than men have died from heart disease. Clinical symptoms in women don't appear until about ten years later than men. Women suffer from the same risk factors as men and should take similar proactive steps early in life toward the prevention of heart disease.

5. **True.** The more body fat there is, the harder the heart works to pump blood through all the additional blood vessels needed to feed the extra tissue. Over time, this can result in a tremendous strain placed on the heart. In addition, other risk factors such as diabetes, high blood pressure, physical inactivity and high cholesterol levels are often seen in an obese person. The more risk factors you have, the higher your chances for developing heart disease.

6. **False.** Family history helps you to be more aware of your *potential* risk for certain diseases and conditions. Although your risk may be greater, it does not guarantee you will end up with a disease. Knowing what may "run in the family" can help you be more careful in your lifestyle and initiate healthy behaviors at an earlier age to help reduce and offset the inherited risks you may have.

7. **True.** Autopsy observations of teens that have died have shown early stages of atherosclerosis (a buildup of plaque in the arteries). Although heart disease is normally a chronic, long-term event, it has its beginnings in childhood. Excess consumption of high saturated fat foods and low levels of physical activity are related to the early development of heart disease. It is never too early to start improving your lifestyle and take a proactive approach to avoiding heart disease.

8. **True.** Other symptoms are a pain in the neck, jaw or back, tingling in the extremities, lightheadedness and drifting in and out of consciousness. The most critical time for successful treatment following a

heart attack is within the two hours after it occurs. Once you recognize symptoms, don't waste time— call 911 for help. Get the victim to a hospital right away, but don't drive him or her yourself. Emergency medical services can transport the victim to a hospital faster, provide lifesaving treatment, if necessary, along the way and get the person into the care of hospital personnel much more quickly.

9. **False.** Blood pressure can rise due to stressful events but this is only a temporary increase. Blood pressure readings should be taken and averaged over time to get an accurate evaluation. High blood pressure is known as the "silent killer" because it is not detectable unless a blood pressure reading is taken. If your family history includes high blood pressure it is a good idea to monitor it on a frequent basis.

10. **True.** Over 1,000,000 people die annually from cardiovascular disease, making it by far the number one cause of death in the United States. The major cardiovascular diseases include atherosclerosis, heart attack, stroke, hypertension and congestive heart failure.

ACTION PLAN

Your Action Plan for Lowering Heart Disease Risk

1. **Maintain a healthy weight**
   ▌ Check with your health care provider to see if you need to lose weight.
   ▌ If you do, lose weight slowly using a healthy eating plan and engaging in physical activity.

2. **Be physically active**
   ▌ Engage in physical activity for a minimum of 30 minutes on most days of the week.
   ▌ Combine every day chores with moderate-level sporting activities, such as walking to achieve your physical activity goals.

3. **Follow a healthy eating plan**
   ▌ Set up a healthy eating plan with foods low in saturated fat, total fat, and cholesterol, and high in fruits, vegetables, and low fat dairy foods.
   ▌ Write down everything that you eat and drink in a food diary. Note areas that are successful or need improvement.
   ▌ If you are trying to lose weight, choose an eating plan that is lower in calories.

4. **Reduce sodium in your diet**
   ▌ Choose foods that are low in salt and other forms of sodium.
   ▌ Use spices, garlic, and onions to add flavor to your meals without adding more sodium.

5. **Drink alcohol only in moderation**
   - ▌ In addition to raising blood pressure, too much alcohol can add unneeded calories to your diet.
   - ▌ If you drink alcoholic beverages, have only a moderate amount—one drink a day for women, two drinks a day for men.
6. **Take prescribed drugs as directed**
   - ▌ If you need drugs to help lower your blood pressure or cholesterol, you still must follow the lifestyle changes mentioned above.
   - ▌ Use notes and other reminders to help you remember to take your drugs.

SETTING GOALS

Setting Heart-Healthy Goals

Your Heart-Healthy Goal:

Is It S.M.A.R.T.?
Specific? _____
Measurable? _____
Achievable? _____

Rewarding? _____
Time Defined? _____

Strategies for Success
1. _____
2. _____
3. _____

Potential Obstacles
1. _____
2. _____
3. _____

Ways Around Them
1. _____
2. _____
3. _____

Daily Report

The Week that Was:

What Went Right?
What Could I Do Better?

WELLNESS JOURNAL

Notes on Negativity

As discussed in this chapter, negative emotions, particularly anger, hostility, and cynicism, are hazardous to your heart's health. One highly effective way of tuning into your emotional life and gaining insight is by keeping an emotional journal. If you often react negatively, make note of intense negative emotions you experience in the course of the day. Record what triggered them, where you were, what you were doing, who you were with, what you were feeling before and after. After a week or two, you should see patterns emerge. Once you recognize what sets you off, you can develop a plan to turn negatives into more positive experiences.

	Event	Setting	Feelings	Trigger	Aftermath
1					
2					
3					
4					
5					
6					

CHAPTER 10

Making This Chapter Work for You

1. You can help maintain a healthy heart by doing all the following except
   a. getting regular moderate levels of exercise every day.
   b. stopping smoking and avoiding regular exposure to secondhand smoke.
   c. eating a diet high in levels of free radicals.
   d. controlling your blood pressure.

2. You can control all of these risk factors for heart disease *except*
   a. male pattern baldness
   b. diabetes mellitus
   c. sedentary lifestyle
   d. blood fat cells

3. You can also control all of these risk factors *except*
   a. tobacco use
   b. illegal drug use
   c. family history
   d. job stress

4. Which of the following statements about blood pressure is true?
   a. blood pressure increases when the heart relaxes.
   b. systolic blood pressure is the pressure of the blood entering the atrium of the heart.
   c. high blood pressure is usually the cause of sudden cardiac death in young athletes.
   d. blood pressure decreases during diastole.

5. Hypertension
   a. is diagnosed when blood pressure is consistently lower than 130/85 mm Hg.
   b. may be treated with dietary changes, which include eating low-fat foods and avoiding sodium.
   c. can cause fatty deposits to collect on the artery walls.
   d. usually does not respond to medication, especially in severe cases.

6. Your lipoprotein profile
   a. provides a breakdown of the different types and levels of blood fats circulating in your body.
   b. is best obtained at a health fair where the results are uniformly accurate.
   c. will give a total cholesterol level, which is the amount of triglycerides and LDL cholesterol levels added together.
   d. should be evaluated after eating a full meal.

7. Having a high level of this blood element is a good thing:
   a. LDL cholesterol
   b. HDL cholesterol
   c. C-reactive protein
   d. triglyceride

8. Cholesterol-lowering medications—the statins—
   a. work directly in the heart.
   b. have no side effects.
   c. block production of cholesterol in the liver.
   d. increase the amount of LDL in the blood.

9. A heart attack
   a. occurs when the myocardium receives an excessive amount of blood from the coronary arteries.
   b. is typically suffered by individuals who have irregular episodes of atherosclerosis.
   c. can be treated successfully up to four hours after the event.
   d. occurs when the myocardial cells are deprived of oxygen-carrying blood, causing them to die.

10. Which of the following statements about stroke is true?
    a. A stroke occurs when the blood supply to the aorta is blocked.
    b. Ischemic stroke is usually caused by a blood clot in the brain.
    c. Little strokes, also called transient ischemic attacks, can cause permanent blindness and paralysis of one side of the body.
    d. Risk factors for stroke include gender and occupation.

Answers to these questions can be found on page 376.

Critical Thinking

1. "White coat syndrome" occurs when patients have high blood pressure in the doctor's office but nowhere else. What can you do to ensure that you and members of your family get accurate blood pressure readings?

2. Have you had a lipoprotein profile lately? Do you think it's necessary for you to obtain one? If your reading was/is borderline or high, what lifestyle changes can you make to help control your cholesterol level?

3. The costs for a heart transplant are over $100,000. The annual price tag for a year's worth of cyclosporine, the drug that prevents rejection and must be taken for the rest of a transplant recipient's life, is about $5,000. The total medical bill can come to hundreds of thousands of dollars—enough to fund programs to improve the nutrition of poor pregnant women, to treat alcoholism, or to provide regular preventive care. Does treatment of any single individual justify such huge costs? Should our society try to balance the costs versus the benefits of such heroic measures as heart transplants? How would you go about making such decisions?

Media Menu

Health ⊗ Now ™

Don't forget to check out the wealth of resources on the HealthNow website at **http://healthnow.brookscole.com/itw** that will:
- Help you evaluate your knowledge of the material
- Allow you to take an exam-prep quiz
- Provide a Personalized Learning Plan targeting resources that address areas you should study
- Coach you through identifying target goals for behavior change and creating and monitoring your personal change plan throughout the semester.

INTERNET CONNECTIONS

National Cholesterol Education Program

www.nhlbi.nih.gov/chd/

This comprehensive site features interactive sessions on planning a low-cholesterol diet and lots more. It provides helpful information for those with heart disease, as well as information to prevent heart disease. You can also hear radio messages from the Heart Beat Radio Network. This site is highly recommended.

Create a Diet to Lower Your Cholesterol

www.nhlbisupport.com/chd1/create.htm

This interactive site will provide personalized guidelines on how to eat healthy and decrease your risk of heart disease, based on your height, weight, gender, and activity level.

HeartSite.com

www.heartsite.com

This site, developed by two prominent cardiologists at the Medical College of Georgia, features many color diagrams to illustrate what you need to know about cardiac disease, including diagnostic tests, procedures, and treatment. The site also features a multimedia presentation on heart disease and heart failure with slides and accompanying audio.

The Heart: An Online Exploration

www.fi.edu/biosci/heart.html

This interesting site, developed by the Franklin Institute of Science, provides an interactive multimedia tour of the heart, as well as statistics, resources, links, and information on how to monitor your heart's health by becoming aware of your vital signs.

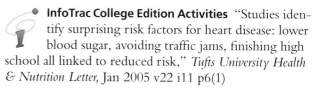 **InfoTrac College Edition Activities** "Studies identify surprising risk factors for heart disease: lower blood sugar, avoiding traffic jams, finishing high school all linked to reduced risk," *Tufts University Health & Nutrition Letter,* Jan 2005 v22 i11 p6(1)

1. How might lowering your blood sugar affect your risk of heart disease?

2. How does traffic gridlock threaten the heart?

3. How can education reduce the danger of heart disease?

You can find additional readings related to personal health with InfoTrac College Edition, an online library of more than 900 journals and publications. Follow the instructions for accessing InfoTrac College Edition that were packaged with your textbook; then search for articles using a keyword search.

For additional links, resources, and suggested readings on the InfoTrac College Edition, visit our Health and Wellness Resource Center at **http://health .wadsworth.com.**

Key Terms

The terms listed are used on the page indicated. Definitions of the terms are in the Glossary at the end of the book.

angina pectoris 226	**male pattern baldness** 219
angioplasty 227	**metabolic syndrome** 216
arteriosclerosis 225	**myocardial**
atherosclerosis 225	**infarction (MI)** 226
cardiopulmonary	**plaque** 225
resuscitation 227	**prehypertension** 221
cholesterol 216	**stroke** 228
diabetes mellitus 218	**systolic blood pressure** 216
disastolic blood	**transient ischemic**
pressure 216	**attack (TIA)** 228
hypertension 216	**triglycerides** 216
lipoproteins 216	

Preventing Cancer and Other Illnesses

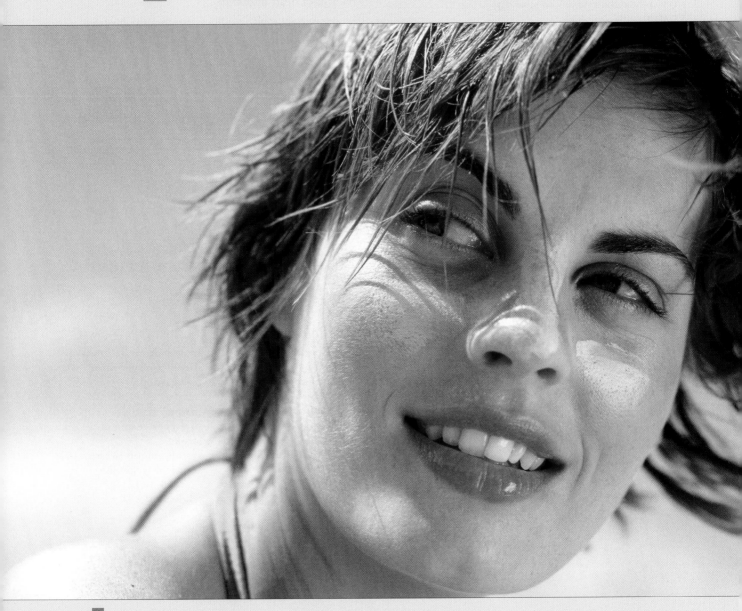

eline knows that she inherited her mother's brown eyes and buoyant sense of humor. She wonders whether she's also inherited "the bad gene"—the cancer-causing one that killed her grandmother and great-grandmother. Celine's mother was 42 years old when she learned that she, too, had cancer. She died two years later, leaving behind eight sisters. Within the next decade, six had developed breast or ovarian cancer.

Unlike most college students, Celine never thinks of cancer as something that affects only people much older than she. Three of her five sisters have tested positive for what is called "the breast cancer gene." Celine is struggling to decide whether she too will undergo testing.

An estimated 10 percent of cancers are hereditary, but no one is immune from the threat of cancer or other serious diseases.

Cancer has overtaken heart disease as the number-one killer of Americans under age 85. Yet many of the almost 500,000 deaths caused by cancer each year could be prevented. A third of cancers are related to smoking; another third, to obesity, poor diet, and lack of exercise.[1] Many of the other serious illnesses discussed in this chapter, including infectious diseases and diabetes mellitus, also can be prevented by lifestyle changes and appropriate immunizations.

This chapter is a lesson in self-defense against the illnesses that can threaten your well-being and your survival. The information that it provides can help you boost your defenses, recognize and avoid health threats, protect yourself, and realize when to seek medical help.

After studying the material in this chapter, you should be able to:

▮ **List** the risk factors for cancer, and **describe** practical ways to reduce the risk.

▮ **Discuss** the major forms of cancer and **explain** their risk factors and prevention.

▮ **Name** the agents of infection that spread disease.

▮ **Describe** how your body protects itself from infectious disease.

▮ **List** and **describe** some common infectious diseases.

▮ **Name** the risk factors for diabetes mellitus.

Health✪Now™

Don't forget to check out the wealth of resources on the HealthNow website at **http://healthnow.brookscole.com/itw** that will:

• Help you evaluate your knowledge of the material

• Allow you to take an exam-prep quiz

• Provide a Personalized Learning Plan targeting resources that address areas you should study

• Coach you through identifying target goals for behavior change and creating and monitoring your personal change plan throughout the semester.

✚ Understanding Cancer

The uncontrolled growth and spread of abnormal cells causes cancer. Normal cells follow the code of instructions embedded in DNA (the body's genetic material); cancer cells do not. Think of the DNA within the nucleus of a cell as a computer program that controls the cell's functioning, including its ability to grow and reproduce itself. If this program or its operation is altered, the cell goes out of control. The nucleus no longer regulates growth. The abnormal cell divides to create other abnormal cells, which again divide, eventually forming **neoplasms** (new formations), or tumors.

Tumors can be either *benign* (slightly abnormal, not considered life-threatening) or *malignant* (cancerous). The only way to determine whether a tumor is benign is by microscopic examination of its cells. Cancer cells have larger nuclei than the cells in benign tumors, they vary more in shape and size, and they divide more often.

At one time cancer was thought to be a single disease that attacked different parts of the body. Now scientists believe that cancer comes in countless forms, each with a genetically determined molecular "fingerprint" that indicates how deadly it is. With this understanding, doctors can identify how aggressively a tumor should be treated.

Without treatment, cancer cells continue to grow, crowding out and replacing healthy cells. This process is called **infiltration**, or invasion. Cancer cells may also **metastasize**, or spread to other parts of the body via the bloodstream or lymphatic system (**Figure 11-1**). For many cancers, as many as 60 percent of patients may have metastases (which may be too small to be felt or seen without a microscope) at the time of diagnosis.

✚ Who Is at Risk for 📠 Developing Cancer?

According to the American Cancer Society, 1.37 million individuals are diagnosed with cancer each year; about 570,280 die of it. Cancer death rates have decreased in men by about 1 percent per year since 1992. The five-year survival rate for all cancer is 64 percent, up from 50 percent three decades ago.[2]

Since the occurrence of cancer increases over time, most cases affect adults who are middle-aged or older (**Table 11-1**). In the United States, men have a one in two lifetime risk of developing cancer; for women, the risk is one in three (**Figure 11-2**).

The term **relative risk** compares the risk of developing cancer in people with a certain exposure or trait to the risk in those who do not have this exposure or trait. Smokers, for instance, have a ten-times-greater relative risk of developing lung cancer than nonsmokers. Most relative risks are smaller. For example, women who have a first-degree (mother, sister, or daughter) family history of breast cancer have about a twofold increased risk of developing breast cancer compared with women who do not have a family history

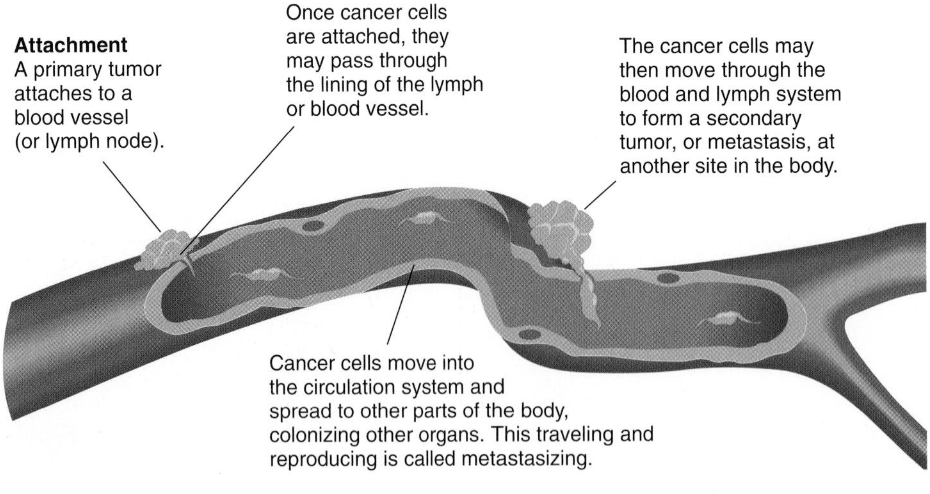

Attachment
A primary tumor attaches to a blood vessel (or lymph node).

Once cancer cells are attached, they may pass through the lining of the lymph or blood vessel.

The cancer cells may then move through the blood and lymph system to form a secondary tumor, or metastasis, at another site in the body.

Cancer cells move into the circulation system and spread to other parts of the body, colonizing other organs. This traveling and reproducing is called metastasizing.

FIGURE 11-1 ▮ Metastasis, or Spread of Cancer

Cancer cells can travel through the blood vessels to spread to other organs, or through the lymphatic system to form secondary tumors.

TABLE 11-1 ▌ Age and the Risk of Cancer (All Sites)

	Men	Women
Birth to age 39	1 in 64	1 in 51
Ages 40 to 59	1 in 12	1 in 11
Ages 60 to 79	1 in 3	1 in 4
Birth to death	1 in 2	1 in 3

Source: Cancer Facts & Figures—2005. Atlanta, GA: American Cancer Society, 2005.

of the disease. This means that they are about twice as likely to develop breast cancer.

Heredity

Maybe curly hair or dimples run in your family. Vulnerability to certain illnesses, including asthma, diabetes, can-

cer, and heart disease, may do so too. You can't change your genes, but you can change unhealthy behaviors, such as smoking or poor eating habits. In many cases, such changes can greatly reduce your risk for the diseases that run in your family. Everyone's family history is different. You can use the Wellness Journal Lab on page 258 to learn more about your relatives and your risks.

An estimated 13 to 14 million Americans may be at risk of a hereditary cancer. In hereditary cancers, such as retinoblastoma (an eye cancer that strikes young children) or certain colon cancers, a specific cancer-causing gene is passed down from generation to generation. The odds of any child with one affected parent inheriting this gene and developing the cancer are fifty/fifty.

Other people are born with genes that make them susceptible to having certain cells grow and divide uncontrollably, which may contribute to cancer development. The most well known are mutations of the BRCA gene, linked with increased risk of breast, colon, and ovarian

Estimated New Cases*		Estimated Deaths	
Male	**Female**	**Male**	**Female**
Prostate 232,090 (33%)	Breast 211,240 (32%)	Lung and bronchus 90,490 (31%)	Lung and bronchus 73,020 (27%)
Lung and bronchus 93,010 (13%)	Lung and bronchus 79,560 (12%)	Prostate 30,350 (10%)	Breast 40,410 (15%)
Colon and rectum 71,820 (10%)	Colon and rectum 73,470 (11%)	Colon and rectum 28,540 (10%)	Colon and rectum 27,750 (10%)
Urinary bladder 47,010 (7%)	Uterine corpus 40,880 (6%)	Pancreas 15,820 (5%)	Ovary 16,210 (6%)
Melanoma of the skin 33,580 (5%)	Non-Hodgkin's lymphoma 27,320 (4%)	Leukemia 12,540 (4%)	Pancreas 15,980 (6%)
Non-Hodgkin's lymphoma 29,070 (4%)	Melanoma of the skin 26,000 (4%)	Esophagus 10,530 (4%)	Leukemia 10,030 (4%)
Kidney and renal pelvis 22,490 (3%)	Ovary 22,220 (3%)	Liver 10,330 (3%)	Non-Hodgkin's lymphoma 9,020 (3%)
Leukemia 19,640 (3%)	Thyroid 19,190 (3%)	Non-Hodgkin's lymphoma 10,150 (3%)	Uterine corpus 7,310 (3%)
Oral cavity 19,100 (3%)	Urinary bladder 16,200 (2%)	Urinary bladder 8,970 (3%)	Multiple myeloma 5,640 (2%)
Pancreas 16,100 (2%)	Pancreas 16,080 (2%)	Kidney and renal pelvis 8,020 (3%)	Brain and nervous system 5,480 (2%)
All sites 710,040 (100%)	All sites 662,870 (100%)	All sites 295,280 (100%)	All sites 275,000 (100%)
All sites 699,560	All sites 668,470	All sites 290,890	All sites 272,810

FIGURE 11-2 ▌ Sex Differences in Cancer Rates and Deaths

*Excludes basal and squamous cell skin cancers and in situ carcinoma except urinary bladder. Percentages may not total 100% due to rounding.

Source: ©2005, American Cancer Society, Inc., Surveillance Research

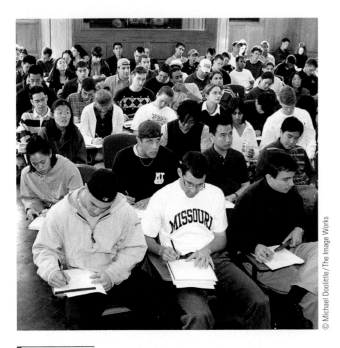

By age 39, 1 in 64 men and 1 in 51 women will have cancer. Look at your risk factors and lifestyle–what do you think are your odds?

cancer. Researchers recently recognized an even more common inherited cancer susceptibility gene, known as TGFRB1*6A, carried by nearly one in eight people, that increases cancer risk by 26 percent.[3]

Genetic tests can identify some individuals who are born with an increased susceptibility to cancer. By spotting a mutated gene in an individual, doctors can sometimes detect cancer years earlier through increased cancer screening. The most likely sites for inherited cancers to develop are the breast, brain, blood, muscles, bones, and adrenal glands. The telltale signs of inherited cancers include:

▌ **Early development.** Genetic forms of certain diseases strike earlier than noninherited cancers. For example, the average age of women diagnosed with breast cancer is 62. But if breast cancer is inherited, the average age at diagnosis is 44, an 18-year difference.

▌ **Family history.** Anyone with a close relative (mother, father, sibling, child) with cancer has about three times the usual chance of getting the same type of cancer.

▌ **Multiple targets.** The same type of hereditary cancer often strikes more than once—in both breasts or both kidneys, for instance, or in two separate parts of the same organ.

▌ **Unusual gender pattern.** Genes may be responsible for cancers that generally don't strike a certain gender —for example, breast cancer in a man.

▌ **Cancer family syndrome.** Some families, with unusually large numbers of relatives affected by cancer, seem clearly cancer-prone. For instance, in Lynch syndrome (a form of colon cancer), more than 20 percent of the family members in at least two generations de-

velop cancer of both the colon and the endometrium (lining of the uterus).

Racial and Ethnic Groups

More cases of cancer occur in black Americans than in any other racial or ethnic group.[4] Blacks are 30 percent more likely to die of cancer than whites. African-American women have the highest incidence of colorectal and lung cancers of any ethnic group, while black men have the highest rates of prostate, colorectal, and lung cancer. African Americans also have higher rates of incidence and deaths from other cancers, including those of the mouth, throat, esophagus, stomach, pancreas, and larynx.

Cancer rates also vary in other racial and ethnic groups. Hispanics have six times lower risk of developing melanoma than Caucasians, yet tend to have a worse prognosis than Caucasians when they do develop this skin cancer. The incidence of female breast cancer is highest among white women and lowest among Native American women. Cervical cancer is most common in Hispanic women.

Obesity

Long recognized as threats to cardiovascular health, overweight and obesity may play a role in an estimated 90,000 cancer deaths each year. According to American Cancer Society researchers who examined the relationship between body mass index (BMI) and risk of dying from cancer, 14 percent of cancer deaths in men and 20 percent of cancer deaths in women may stem from excess weight.

The higher an individual's BMI, the greater the likelihood of dying of cancer. A woman with a BMI of 25 to 30 faces a 30 percent higher risk of breast cancer, while the risk is 63 percent higher for women with BMIs in the 30 to 35 range and 70 percent higher for those with a BMI between 35 and 40. The heaviest men had a 52 percent higher death rate from all cancers, while the heaviest women had a 62 percent higher death rate.[5]

An unhealthy body weight increases the risk of many types of cancer, including breast (in postmenopausal women), colon and rectum, kidney, cervix, ovary, uterus, esophagus, gallbladder, stomach (in men), liver, pancreas, prostate, non-Hodgkin's lymphoma, and multiple myeloma.

Infectious Agents

Worldwide, an estimated 17 percent of cancers can be attributed to infection. In economically developing countries, infections cause or contribute to 26 percent of cancers. In developed countries, they play a role in 7 percent of new cases of cancer.[6]

Among the cancers that have been linked with infectious agents are human papilloma virus (HPV) with cervical cancer and *Helicobacter pylori* with stomach cancer.

Viruses have been implicated in certain leukemias (cancers of the blood system) and lymphomas (cancers of the lymphatic system), cancers of the nose and pharynx, liver cancer, and cervical cancer. Human immune deficiency virus (HIV) can lead to certain lymphomas and leukemias and to a type of cancer called Kaposi's sarcoma.

Generally, the presence of a bacterium or a virus, per se, is not enough to cause cancer. A predisposing environment and other cofactors—most still unknown—are needed for cancer development and growth.

WELLNESS COACH

Lowering Your Cancer Risk

Environmental factors may cause between 80 and 90 percent of cancers. At least in theory, these cancers can be prevented by avoiding cancer-causing substances (such as tobacco and sunlight) or using substances that protect against cancer-causing factors (such as antioxidants and vitamin D). How do you start protecting yourself? Simple changes in lifestyle—smart eating, losing excess weight, not smoking, protecting yourself from the sun, exercising regularly—are essential.

Stay Smoke-Free

Cigarette smoking is the single most devastating and preventable cause of cancer deaths in the United States. If you don't smoke, don't start—and limit the time you spend around smokers. If you smoke, read Chapter 13 for advice on quitting. Your life could depend on it.

People who smoke two or more packs of cigarettes a day are 15 to 25 times more likely to die of cancer than nonsmokers. Cigarettes cause most cases of lung cancer and increase the risk of cancer of the mouth, pharynx, larynx, esophagus, pancreas, and bladder. Pipes, cigars, and smokeless tobacco also increase the danger of cancers of the mouth and throat.

Environmental tobacco smoke can increase the risk of cancer even among those who've never smoked. For example, exposure to others' tobacco smoke for as little as three hours a day can increase the risk of developing cancer. (See the discussion of environmental tobacco smoke in Chapter 13.)

Eat Smart

The links between diet and cancer are complex, and medical advice is constantly evolving. According to recent studies, cutting down on high-fat foods, particularly in middle age, does little to reduce the risk of breast and colon cancer.[7] In large epidemiological studies, increasing fruits and vegetables did not significantly lower rates of breast cancer.[8] However, there is evidence linking red meat consumption and colon cancer.[9]

The best approach is to follow the guidelines designed for overall well-being. The same foods that keep your heart healthy, your blood pressure low, your bones strong, and your weight under control are most likely to help you reduce your risk of cancer and other major illnesses.

Pay attention to food processing and preparation. Whenever possible, select foods close to their natural state, grown locally and without pesticides. Avoid cured, pickled, or smoked meats. When cooking, try not to fry or barbecue often; these cooking methods can produce mutagens that induce cancer in animals. The process of smoking or charcoal-grilling releases carcinogenic tar that may increase the risk of cancer of the stomach and esophagus.

Maintain a Healthy Weight

Obesity, as discussed in Chapter 9, causes one in six cancer deaths. Excess weight may account for 14 to 20 percent of all cancers, including cancer of the breast, uterus, cervix, ovary, stomach, prostate, colon and rectum, kidney, esophagus, pancreas, liver, and gallbladder as well as non-Hodgkin's lymphoma and multiple myeloma.

Women who gain more than 20 pounds from age 18 to midlife double their risk of breast cancer compared to those whose weight remains stable. Too much body fat increases cancer risk in several ways: It raises the amount of estrogen in a woman's blood, which may contribute to cancers of the female reproductive system. It also raises levels of insulin, which prompts the body to create a hormone that causes cells to multiply. Obesity also makes various types of cancer harder to diagnose and treat.

Limit Exposure to Environmental Risks

Although it may not be possible to avoid all possible **carcinogens** (cancer-causing chemicals), you can take steps to minimize your danger. Many chemicals used in industry, including nickel, chromate, asbestos, and vinyl chloride, are carcinogens; employees as well as people living near a factory that creates smoke, dust, or gases are at risk. If your job involves their use, follow safety precautions at work. If you are concerned about possible hazards in your community, check with local environmental protection officials.

Women and men who frequently dye their hair, particularly with very dark shades of permanent coloring, may be at increased risk for leukemia (cancer of blood-forming cells), non-Hodgkin's lymphoma (cancer of the lymph system), multiple myeloma (cancer of the bone marrow), and, in women, ovarian cancer. Lighter shades and less permanent tints do not seem to

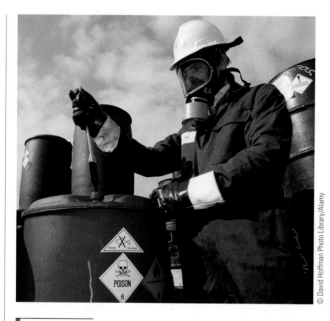

© David Hoffman Photo Library/Alamy

■ Follow workplace safety precautions to avoid unnecessary exposure to carcinogens.

be a danger. (Chapter 15 discusses pesticides and other environmental threats.)

Be Vigilant

Proven methods of cancer prevention and early detection could save more than 60,000 lives a year. Screening examinations, conducted regularly by a health-care professional, can lead to early diagnosis of cancers of the breast, colon, rectum, cervix, prostate, testicles, and oral cavity and can improve the odds of successful treatment. Self-examinations for cancers of the breast, testicles, and skin may also result in detection of tumors at earlier stages. The five-year relative survival rate for all these cancers is about 81 percent. If all Americans participated in regular cancer screenings, this rate could increase to more than 95 percent. (See Your Action Plan for the latest guidelines on cancer screenings.)

✚ Common Types of Cancer

Cancer refers to a group of more than a hundred diseases characterized by abnormal cell growth. Although all cancers have similar characteristics, each is distinct. Some cancers are relatively simple to cure, whereas others are more threatening and mysterious. The earlier any cancer is found, the easier it is to treat and the better the patient's chances of survival.

Cancers are classified according to the type of cell and the organ in which they originate, such as the following:

■ **Carcinoma,** the most common kind, which starts in the epithelium, the layers of cells that cover the body's surface or line internal organs and glands.

■ **Sarcoma,** which forms in the supporting, or connective, tissues of the body: bones, muscles, blood vessels.
■ **Leukemia,** which begins in the blood-forming tissues: bone marrow, lymph nodes, and the spleen.
■ **Lymphoma,** which arises in the cells of the lymph system, the network that filters out impurities.

Skin Cancer

Skin cancer is diagnosed in more than 1.5 million Americans every year.[10] One of every five Americans can expect to develop skin cancer in their lifetimes. Once scientists thought exposure to the B range of ultraviolet light (UVB), the wavelength of light responsible for sunburn, posed the greatest danger. However, longer-wavelength UVA, which penetrates deeper into the skin, also plays a major role in skin cancers. An estimated 80 percent of total lifetime sun exposure occurs during childhood, so sun protection is especially important in youngsters. Tanning salons and sunlamps also increase the risk of skin cancer because they produce ultraviolet radiation. A half-hour dose of radiation from a sunlamp can be equivalent to the amount you'd get from an entire day in the sun.

Young adults spend the most time in the sun and also frequent tanning salons. Even when they perceive the seriousness of skin cancer, college students—particularly women—describe suntanned skin as attractive, healthy, and athletic-looking and view the benefits of getting a suntan as outweighing the risks of skin cancer of premature aging.[11] A third of students do not use sunscreen while sunbathing: half do not use it for incidental exposure.[12] (See Student Snapshot).

The most common skin cancers are *basal-cell* (involving the base of the epidermis, the top level of the skin)

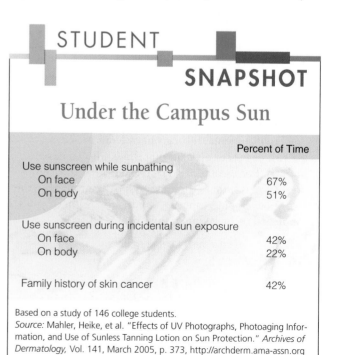

STUDENT SNAPSHOT

Under the Campus Sun

	Percent of Time
Use sunscreen while sunbathing	
On face	67%
On body	51%
Use sunscreen during incidental sun exposure	
On face	42%
On body	22%
Family history of skin cancer	42%

Based on a study of 146 college students.
Source: Mahler, Heike, et al. "Effects of UV Photographs, Photoaging Information, and Use of Sunless Tanning Lotion on Sun Protection." *Archives of Dermatology,* Vol. 141, March 2005, p. 373, http://archderm.ama-assn.org

and *squamous-cell* (involving cells in the epidermis). Every year more than 5 million Americans develop skin lesions known as actinic keratoses (AKs), rough red or brown scaly patches that develop in the upper layer of the skin, usually on the face, lower lip, bald scalp, neck, and back of the hands and forearms. Forty percent of squamous cell carcinomas, the second leading cause of skin cancer deaths, begin as AKs. Treatments include surgical removal, cryosurgery (freezing the skin), electrodesiccation (heat generated by an electric current), topical chemotherapy, and removal with lasers, chemical peels, or dermabrasion.

Smoking and exposure to certain hydrocarbons in asphalt, coal tar, and pitch may increase the risk of squamous-cell skin cancer. Other risk factors include occupational exposure to carcinogens and inherited skin disorders, such as xeroderma pigmentosum and familial atypical multiple-mole melanoma.

Malignant *melanoma,* the deadliest type of skin cancer, causes 1 to 2 percent of all cancer deaths. During the 1930s, the lifetime risk of melanoma was about 1 in 1,500. Today it is 1 in 75. This increase in risk is due mostly to overexposure to UV radiation. The use of a tanning bed ten times or more a year doubles the risk for individuals over age 30.

Both the amount and the intensity of lifetime sun exposure play key roles in determining risk for melanoma. People living in areas where the sun's ultraviolet rays reach the earth with extra intensity, such as tropical or high-altitude regions, are at increased risk. Although melanoma occurs more often among people over 40, it is increasing in younger people, particularly those who had severe sunburns in childhood. The rate of increase in melanoma also has risen more in men (4.6 percent a year) than for women (3.2 percent). Men are more likely than women to be diagnosed with melanoma after age 40.

Individuals with any of the following characteristics are at increased risk:

▌ **Fair skin,** light eyes, or fair hair.
▌ **A tendency to develop freckles** and to burn instead of tan.
▌ **A history of childhood sunburn** or intermittent, intense sun exposure.
▌ **A personal or family history** of melanoma.
▌ **A large number of nevi,** or moles (200 or more, or 50 or more if under age 20), or dysplastic (atypical) moles.

Detection

The most common predictor for melanoma is a change in an existing mole or development of a new and changing pigmented mole. The most important early indicators are change in color, an increase in diameter, and changes in the borders of a mole (**Figure 11-3**). An increase in height signals a corresponding growth in depth under the skin. Itching in a new or long-standing mole also should not be ignored.

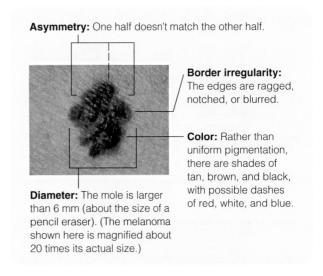

Asymmetry: One half doesn't match the other half.

Border irregularity: The edges are ragged, notched, or blurred.

Color: Rather than uniform pigmentation, there are shades of tan, brown, and black, with possible dashes of red, white, and blue.

Diameter: The mole is larger than 6 mm (about the size of a pencil eraser). (The melanoma shown here is magnified about 20 times its actual size.)

FIGURE 11-3 ▌ **ABCD: The Warning Signs of Melanoma**

An estimated 95 percent of cases of melanoma arise from an existing mole. A normal mole is usually round or oval, less than 6 millimeters (about 1/4 inch) in diameter, and evenly colored (black, brown, or tan). Seek prompt evaluation of any moles that change in ways shown in the photo.

Source: American Academy of Dermatology. All rights reserved.

Treatment

If caught early, melanoma is highly curable, usually with surgery alone. Once it has spread, chemotherapy with a single drug or a combination can temporarily shrink tumors in some people. However, the five-year survival rate for metastatic melanoma is 14 percent.

Breast Cancer

Every 3 minutes a woman in the United States learns that she has breast cancer. Every 12 minutes a woman dies of breast cancer. Many women misjudge their own likelihood of developing breast cancer, either overestimating or underestimating their susceptibility. In a national poll, one in every ten surveyed considered herself at no risk at all. This is never the case. "Every woman is at risk for breast cancer simply because she's female," says Leslie Ford, M.D., associate director for early detection at the National Cancer Institute (NCI).[13]

However, not all women's risks are equal. NCI has developed a computerized Breast Cancer Risk Assessment Tool, based on data from more than 280,000 women, that allows a woman to sit down with her doctor and discuss her own odds of developing breast cancer within the next five years and over her entire lifetime.

The most common risk factors include the following:

▌ **Age.** As shown in **Figure 11-4**, at 25, a woman's chance of developing breast cancer is 1 in 19,608; by age 45, it has increased to 1 in 93; by 65, it is 1 in 17. By age 90 to 95, 1 in 8 women will have developed breast

By age 25	1 in 19,608
By age 30	1 in 2,525
By age 35	1 in 622
By age 40	1 in 217
By age 45	1 in 93
By age 50	1 in 50
By age 55	1 in 33
By age 60	1 in 24
By age 65	1 in 17
By age 70	1 in 14
By age 75	1 in 11
By age 80	1 in 10
By age 85	1 in 9
Ever	1 in 8

FIGURE 11-4 A Woman's Risk of Developing Breast Cancer

Source: Surveillance Program, National Cancer Institute.

cancer. The mean age at which women are diagnosed is 63.

- **Family history.** The overwhelming majority of breast cancers—90 to 95 percent—are not due to strong genetic factors. However, having a first-degree relative —mother, sister, or daughter—with breast cancer does increase risk, and if the relative developed breast cancer before menopause, the cancer is more likely to be hereditary. Genetic testing, controversial but sometimes recommended for women in cancer-prone families, can identify these defects. However, it's not yet clear how many women with a defective gene actually will develop breast cancer; estimates range from 50 to 80 percent, or higher in families with many affected members.

- **Long menstrual history.** Women who had their first period before age 12 are at greater risk than women who began menstruating later. The reason is that the more menstrual cycles a woman has, the longer her exposure to estrogen, a hormone known to increase breast cancer danger. For similar reasons, childless women, who menstruate continuously for several decades, are also at greater risk.

- **Age at birth of first child.** An early pregnancy— in a woman's teens or twenties—changes the actual maturation of breast cells and decreases risk. But if a woman has her first child in her forties, precancerous cells may actually flourish with the high hormone levels of the pregnancy.

- **Breast biopsies.** Even if laboratory analysis finds no precancerous abnormalities, women who require such tests are more likely to develop breast cancer. Fibrocystic breast disease, a term often used for "lumpy" breasts, is not a risk factor.

- **Race.** Breast cancer rates are lower in Hispanic and Asian populations than in whites, but higher in African-American women up to age

50. In postmenopausal African-American women, rates are lower. Nonetheless, African-American women are still more likely to die of breast cancer than whites. Scientists don't know if that's because they don't have equal access to care, if they don't get optimal care, or if the disease itself is more aggressive in black women.

- **Occupation.** Based on two decades of following more than a million women, Swedish researchers have developed a list of jobs linked with a high risk of breast cancer. These include pharmacists, certain types of teachers, systems analysts and programmers, telephone operators, telegraph and radio operators, metal platers and coaters, and beauticians.

- **Alcohol.** Women's risk of breast cancer increases with the amount of alcohol they drink. Those who take two or more drinks per day are 40 percent more likely to develop breast cancer than women who don't drink at all. For a nondrinking woman, the lifetime risk of breast cancer by age 80 is 1 in 11. For heavy drinkers it's about 1 in 7, regardless of race, education, family history, use of hormone therapy, or other risk factors.[14]

- **Hormone therapy.** After years of debate over postmenopausal hormone therapy (HT), several studies confirmed an increased risk with a combination of estrogen and progestin, particularly in women who use combination HT for five years or longer.[15] Women taking combination HT are more likely to have abnormal mammograms requiring further testing and to be diagnosed at a more advanced stage of breast cancer. Researchers theorize that estrogen and progestin may stimulate breast cancer growth and hinder cancer diagnosis by increasing breast density. Women using only estrogen did not have an elevated rate of breast cancer.

- **Obesity.** Excess weight, particularly after menopause, increases the risk of getting breast cancer. Overweight women, both pre- and postmenopausal, with breast cancer are more likely to die of their disease.

Detection

Doctors long advised women to perform monthly breast self-exams (BSE) after their periods (**Figure 11-5**). In its newest guidelines, the American Cancer Society now describes BSE as "an option" for women starting in their twenties and urges all women to report any breast changes promptly.[16] It recommends a breast exam by a trained practitioner every three years for women in their twenties and thirties and every year for women 40 and over and a yearly mammogram for all women, starting at age 40.[17]

The best tool for early detection is the diagnostic X-ray exam called **mammography.** Overall, screening mammograms could reduce breast cancer deaths by 25 percent. Mammograms can detect a tumor two to three years before it can be detected by manual exam.

Feeling

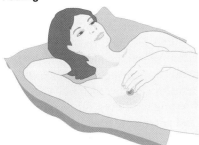

1. Lie flat on your back. Place a pillow or towel under one shoulder, and raise that arm over your head. With the opposite hand, you'll feel with the pads, not the fingertips, of the three middle fingers, for lumps or any change in the texture of the breast or skin.

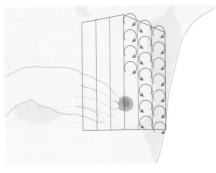

2. The area you'll examine is from your collarbone to your bra line and from your breastbone to the center of your armpit. Imagine the area divided into vertical strips. Using small circular motions (the size of a dime), move your fingers up and down the strips. Apply light, medium, and deep pressure to examine each spot. Repeat this same process for your other breast.

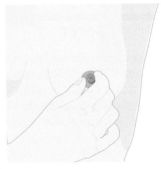

3. Gently squeeze the nipple of each breast between your thumb and index finger. Any discharge, clear or bloody, should be reported to your doctor immediately.

FIGURE 11-5 ▍ Breast Self-Exam

The best time to examine your breasts is after your menstrual period every month.

According to a recent report, annual mammography for women in their forties is more cost-effective than Pap smear tests for cervical cancer and installation of airbags and seat belts in vehicles.

Treatment

Breast cancer can be treated with surgery, radiation, and drugs (chemotherapy and hormonal therapy). Doctors may use one of these options or a combination, depending on the type and location of the cancer and whether the disease has spread.

Most women undergo some type of surgery. **Lumpectomy** or breast-conserving surgery removes only the cancerous tissue and a surrounding margin of normal tissue. A modified radical **mastectomy** includes the entire breast and some of the underarm lymph nodes. Radical mastectomy, in which the breast, lymph nodes, and chest wall muscles under the breast are removed, is rarely performed today because modified radical mastectomy has proved just as effective. Removing underarm lymph nodes is important to determine if the cancer has spread, but a technique called sentinel node biopsy allows physicians to pinpoint the first lymph node into which a tumor drains (the sentinel node) and remove only the nodes most likely to contain cancer cells.

Radiation therapy is treatment with high-energy rays or particles to destroy cancer. In almost all cases, lumpectomy is followed by six to seven weeks of radiation. Chemotherapy is used to reach cancer cells that may have spread beyond the breast—in many cases even if no cancer is detected in the lymph nodes after surgery.

The use of drugs such as tamoxifen and aromatase inhibitors, in addition to standard chemotherapy, can significantly lower the risk of recurrence. A biological therapy—a monoclonal antibody that zeros in an cancer cells like a miniature guided missile—also has shown promise against some aggressive breast tumors. The drug Herceptin targets a defective growth-promoting gene (HER-2/neu) found in about 30 percent of women with breast cancer. The combination of Herceptin and standard chemotherapy has significantly improved survival rates in women with this gene.

Cervical Cancer

An estimated 16,370 cases of invasive cervical cancer are diagnosed in the United States every year, with about 3,710 annual deaths from this disease. The highest incidence rate occurs among Vietnamese women; Alaskan Native, Korean, and Hispanic women also have higher rates than the national average. The mortality rate for African-American women is more than twice that of whites, largely because of a high number of deaths among older black women.

The primary risk factor for cervical cancer is infection with certain types of the human papilloma virus (HPV), discussed in Chapter 14. HPV occurs in more than 99.7 percent of cervical cancer cases. However, not every HPV infection becomes cervical cancer, and while HPV infection is very common, cervical cancer is not. Other risk factors for cervical cancer include early age of first intercourse, multiple sex partners, genital herpes, and smoking or significant exposure to passive smoke.

The standard screening test for cervical cancer is the Pap smear. New, more precise forms of Pap testing and new screening tests for HPV may help detect cases of cervical cancer at earlier stages.

Ovarian Cancer

Ovarian cancer is the leading cause of death from from gynecological cancers. Risk factors include a family history of ovarian cancer; personal history of breast cancer; obesity; infertility (because the abnormality that interferes with conception may also play a role in cancer development); and low levels of transferase, an enzyme involved in the metabolism of dairy foods. Often women develop no obvious symptoms until the advanced stages, although they may experience painless swelling of the abdomen, irregular bleeding, lower abdominal pain, digestive and urinary abnormalities, fatigue, backache, bloating, and weight gain.

Colon and Rectal Cancer

Colon and rectal, or colorectal, cancer is the third most common cancer and accounts for 10 percent of cancer deaths. Most cases occur after age 50. Both age and gender influence the risk of colon cancer. Older individuals and men are more likely to develop polyps (nonmalignant growths that may turn cancerous at some point) and tumors in the colon than young people and women.

Risk factors include age (over 50), personal or family history of colon and rectal cancer, polyps in the colon or rectum, ulcerative colitis, smoking, alcohol consumption, high-fat or low-fiber diet, and inadequate intake of fruits and vegetables. Nonsteroidal anti-inflammatory drugs, such as aspirin and ibuprofen, and regular exercise may reduce the risk.

New guidelines recommend screening for colon cancer beginning at age 50, earlier for those at higher risk based on personal, family, or medical history.[18]

Early signs of colorectal cancer are bleeding from the rectum, blood in the stool, or a change in bowel habits. Treatment may involve surgery, radiation therapy, and/or chemotherapy.

Prostate Cancer

After skin cancer, prostate cancer is the most common form of cancer in American men. The risk of prostate cancer is 1 in 6; the risk of death to due metastatic prostate cancer is 1 in 30.[19] More than a quarter of men diagnosed with cancer have prostate cancer. The disease strikes African-American men more often than white; Asian and American Indian men are affected less often.

The risk of prostate cancer increases with age, family history, exposure to the heavy metal cadmium, high number of sexual partners, and history of frequent sexually transmitted diseases. An inherited predisposition may account for 5 to 10 percent of cases. A purported link between vasectomy and prostate cancer has been disproved.[20]

The development of a simple annual screening test that measures levels of a protein called prostate-specific antigen (PSA) in the blood has revolutionized the diagnosis of prostate cancer. PSA testing is recommended for men at high risk (African Americans and men with close relatives with prostate cancer) starting at age 45 and for all men at age 50. It remains controversial, however. Some claim that PSA testing saves lives; others, that it leads to unnecessary and potentially harmful treatments.

Treatment may include hormones, chemotherapy, and radiation. About 60,000 men undergo radical prostate surgery in the United States every year.[21] The five-year survival rate has increased from 67 percent to 99 percent over the past 20 years.[22]

Testicular Cancer

In the last 20 years, the incidence of testicular cancer has risen 51 percent in the United States—from 3.61 to 5.44 per 100,000. It is not clear why testicular cancer is on the rise, although researchers speculate that changing environmental or socioeconomic risk factors could have a role. Testicular cancer occurs mostly among young men between the ages of 18 and 35, who are not normally at risk of cancer. At highest risk are men with an undescended testicle (a condition that is almost always corrected in childhood to prevent this danger). To detect possibly cancerous growths, men should perform monthly testicular self-exams, as shown in **Figure 11-6**.

Although college-age men are among those at highest risk of testicular cancer, three in four do not know how to perform a testicular self-examination.

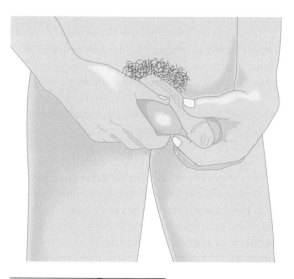

FIGURE 11-6 ▍ **Testicular Self-Exam**

The best time to examine your testicles is after a hot bath or shower, when the scrotum is most relaxed. Place your index and middle fingers under each testicle and the thumb on top, and roll the testicle between the thumb and fingers. If you feel a small, hard, usually painless lump or swelling, or anything unusual, consult a urologist.

Often the first sign of this cancer is a slight enlargement of one testicle. There also may be a change in the way it feels when touched. Sometimes men with testicular cancer report a dull ache in the lower abdomen or groin, along with a sense of heaviness or sluggishness. Lumps on the testicles also may indicate cancer.

A man who notices any abnormality should consult a physician. If a lump is indeed present, a surgical biopsy is necessary to find out if it is cancerous. If the biopsy is positive, a series of tests generally is needed to determine whether the disease has spread.

Treatment for testicular cancer generally involves surgical removal of the diseased testis, sometimes along with radiation therapy, chemotherapy, and the removal of nearby lymph nodes. The remaining testicle is capable of maintaining a man's sexual potency and fertility. Only in rare cases is removal of both testicles necessary. Testosterone injections following such surgery can maintain potency. The chance for a cure is very high if testicular cancer is spotted early.

✚ Understanding Infection

We live in a sea of microbes. Most of them don't threaten our health or survival; some, such as the bacteria that inhabit our intestines, are actually beneficial. Yet in the course of history, disease-causing microorganisms have claimed millions of lives. The twentieth century brought the conquest of infectious killers such as cholera and scarlet fever. Although modern science has won many victories against the agents of infection, infectious illnesses remain a serious health threat.

Infection is a complex process, triggered by various **pathogens** (disease-causing organisms) and countered by the body's own defenders. Physicians explain infection in terms of a **host** (either a person or a population) that contacts one or more agents in an environment. A **vector**—a biological or physical vehicle that carries the agent to the host—provides the means of transmission.

Agents of Infection

The types of microbes that can cause infection are viruses, bacteria, fungi, protozoa, and helminths (parasitic worms).

Viruses

The tiniest pathogens—**viruses**—are also the toughest; they consist of a bit of nucleic acid (DNA or RNA, but never both) within a protein coat. Unable to reproduce on its own, a virus takes over a body cell's reproductive machinery and instructs it to produce new viral particles, which are then released to enter other cells.

The problem in fighting viruses is that it's difficult to find drugs that harm the virus and not the cell it has commandeered. **Antibiotics** (drugs that inhibit or kill bacteria) have no effect on viruses. **Antiviral drugs** don't completely eradicate a viral infection, although they can decrease its severity and duration. Because viruses multiply very quickly, antiviral drugs are most effective when taken before an infection develops or in its early stages.

Bacteria

Simple one-celled organisms, **bacteria** are the most plentiful microorganisms as well as the most pathogenic. Most kinds of bacteria don't cause disease; some, like certain strains of *Escherichia coli* that aid in digestion, play important roles within our bodies. Even friendly bacteria, however, can get out of hand and cause acne, urinary tract infections, vaginal infections, and other problems.

Because bacteria are sufficiently different from the cells that make up our bodies, antibiotics can kill them without harming our cells. Antibiotics work only against specific types of bacteria. If your doctor thinks you have a bacterial infection, tests of your blood, pus, sputum, urine, or stool can identify the particular bacterial strain.

Fungi

Single-celled or multicelled organisms, **fungi** consist of threadlike fibers and reproductive spores. Fungi lack chlorophyll and must obtain their food from organic material, which may include human tissue. Fungi release enzymes that digest cells and are most likely to attack hair-covered areas of the body, including the scalp, beard, groin, and external ear canals. They also cause athlete's foot. Treatment consists of antifungal drugs.

Protozoa

These single-celled, microscopic animals release enzymes and toxins that destroy cells or interfere with their function. Diseases caused by **protozoa** are not a major health problem in this country, primarily because of public health measures.

The most common disease caused by protozoa in the United States is *giardiasis,* an intestinal infection caused by microorganisms in human and animal feces. It has become a threat at day-care centers, as well as among campers and hikers who drink contaminated water. Symptoms include nausea, lack of appetite, gas, diarrhea, fatigue, abdominal cramps, and bloating. Many people recover in a month or two without treatment. However, in some cases the microbe causes recurring attacks over many years. Giardiasis can be life-threatening in small children and the elderly, who are especially prone to severe dehydration from diarrhea. Treatment usually consists of antibiotics.

Helminths (Parasitic Worms)

Small parasitic worms that attack specific tissues or organs and compete with the host for nutrients are called **helminths.** One major worldwide health problem is *schistosomiasis,* a disease caused by a parasitic worm, the fluke, that burrows through the skin and enters the circulatory system. Infection with another helminth, the tapeworm, may be contracted from eating undercooked beef, pork, or fish containing larval forms of the tapeworm. Helminthic diseases are treated with appropriate medications.

How Do You Catch an Infection?

The major vectors, or means of transmission, for infectious disease are animals and insects, people, food, and water.

Animals and Insects

Disease can be transmitted by house pets, livestock, birds, and wild animals. Insects also spread a variety of diseases. The housefly may spread dysentery, diarrhea, typhoid fever, or trachoma (an eye disease rare in the United States but common in other parts of the world). Other insects, including mosquitoes, ticks, mites, fleas, and lice, can transmit such diseases as malaria, yellow fever, encephalitis, dengue fever (a growing threat in Mexico), and Lyme disease.

New threats in the United States include West Nile virus (WNV), which can be spread to humans by mosquitoes that bite infected birds, and monkeypox virus, carried by various animals, including prairie dogs.

People

The people you're closest to can transmit pathogens through the air, through touch, or through sexual contact. To avoid infection, stay out of range of anyone who's coughing, sniffling, or sneezing, and don't share food or dishes. Carefully wash your dishes, utensils, and hands, and abstain from sex or make self-protective decisions about sexual partners.

Food

Every year foodborne illnesses strike millions of Americans, sometimes with fatal consequences. Bacteria account for two-thirds of foodborne infections, and thousands of suspected cases of infection with *Escherichia coli* bacteria in undercooked or inadequately washed food have been reported.

Every year as many as 4 million Americans have a bout with *Salmonella* bacteria, which have been found in about a third of all poultry sold in the United States. These infections can be serious enough to require hospitalization and can lead to arthritis, neurological problems, and even deaths. Consumers can greatly reduce the number of salmonella infections by proper handling, cooking, and refrigeration of poultry.

Water

Waterborne diseases, such as typhoid fever and cholera, are still widespread in less developed areas of the world. They have been rare in the United States, although outbreaks caused by inadequate water purification have occurred.

How Your Body Protects Itself

Various parts of your body safeguard you against infectious diseases by providing **immunity,** or protection, from these health threats. Your skin, when unbroken, keeps out most potential invaders. Your tears, sweat, skin oils, saliva, and mucus contain chemicals that can kill bacteria. Cilia, the tiny hairs lining your respiratory passages, move mucus, which traps inhaled bacteria, viruses, dust, and other foreign matter, to the back of the throat, where it is swallowed; the digestive system then destroys the invaders.

When these protective mechanisms can't keep you infection-free, your body's immune system, which is on constant alert for foreign substances that might threaten the body, swings into action. The immune system includes structures of the lymphatic system—the spleen, thymus gland, lymph nodes, and lymph vessels—that help filter impurities from the body (**Figure 11-7**). More than a dozen different types of white blood cells (lymphocytes) are concentrated in the organs of the lymphatic system or patrol the entire body by way of the blood and lymph vessels. Attacked by pathogens, the body musters its forces and fights. Sometimes the invasion is handled like a minor border skirmish; other times a full-scale battle is waged throughout the body. Together, the immune cells work like an internal police force.

The **lymph nodes,** or glands, are small tissue masses in which some protective cells are stored. If pathogens invade your body, many of them are carried to the lymph nodes to be destroyed. This is why your lymph nodes often feel swollen when you have a cold or the flu.

If the microbes establish a foothold, the blood supply to the area increases, bringing oxygen and nutrients to the fighting cells. Tissue fluids, as well as antibacterial and antitoxic proteins, accumulate. You may develop redness, swelling, local warmth, and pain—the signs of **inflammation.** As more tissue is destroyed, a cavity, or **abscess,** forms and fills with fluid, battling cells, and dead white blood cells (pus). If the invaders aren't killed or inactivated, the pathogens are able to spread into the bloodstream and cause what is known as **systemic disease.**

Some people have an **immune deficiency**—either inborn or acquired. A very few children are born without an effective immune system; their lives can be endangered by any infection. Although still experimental, therapy to implant a missing or healthy gene may offer new hope for a normal life.

Immunity and Stress

Whenever we confront a crisis, large or small, our bodies produce powerful hormones that provide extra energy. However, this stress response dampens immunity, reducing the number of some key immune cells and the responsiveness of others.

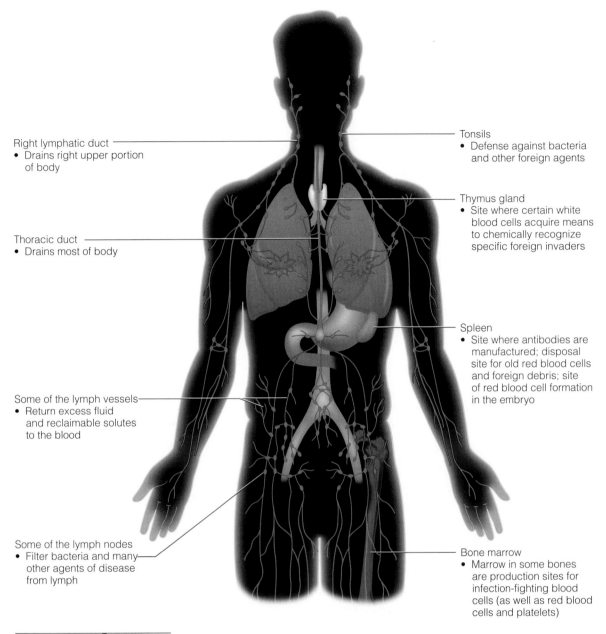

Right lymphatic duct
- Drains right upper portion of body

Thoracic duct
- Drains most of body

Some of the lymph vessels
- Return excess fluid and reclaimable solutes to the blood

Some of the lymph nodes
- Filter bacteria and many other agents of disease from lymph

Tonsils
- Defense against bacteria and other foreign agents

Thymus gland
- Site where certain white blood cells acquire means to chemically recognize specific foreign invaders

Spleen
- Site where antibodies are manufactured; disposal site for old red blood cells and foreign debris; site of red blood cell formation in the embryo

Bone marrow
- Marrow in some bones are production sites for infection-fighting blood cells (as well as red blood cells and platelets)

FIGURE 11-7 ▌ The Human Lymphatic System and Its Functions
The lymphatic system helps filter impurities from the body.

Stress affects the body's immune system in different ways, depending on two factors: the controllability or uncontrollability of the stressor and the mental effort required to cope with the stress. An uncontrollable stressor that lasts longer than 15 minutes may interfere with cytokine interleukin-6, which plays an essential role in activating the immune defenses. Uncontrollable stressors also produce high levels of the hormone cortisol, which suppresses immune system functioning. The mental efforts required to cope with high-level stressors produce only brief immune changes that appear to have little consequence for health. However, stress has been shown to slow pro-inflammatory cytokine production, which is essential for wound healing.

✚ Immunization: The Key to Prevention

One of the great success stories of modern medicine has been the development of vaccines that provide protection against many infectious diseases. Immunization has reduced cases of measles, mumps, tetanus, whooping cough, and other life-threatening illnesses by more than 95 percent.

Although many people think that vaccines are only for children, they remain an important part of protection throughout life. **Table 11-2** shows the recommended immunizations for adults. If you're uncertain about your

TABLE 11-2 ▌ Recommendations for Adult Immunization

Vaccine	Recommended for	Schedule
Tetanus, diphtheria	All adolescents and adults	Booster dose every 10 years
Hepatitis B	Adults at risk, including: • Patients receiving dialysis • Health-care workers and public safety workers who are exposed to blood • Students in schools of medicine, dentistry, nursing, laboratory technology, and other allied health professions • Injection-drug users • Persons with more than one sex partner in previous 6 months • People with recently diagnosed STIs • All clients in STI clinics • Men who have sex with men • Household contacts and sex partners of persons with chronic hepatitis B infection • Clients and staff of institutions for the developmentally disabled • Inmates of correctional facilities • Certain international travelers	Three doses over 6 months
Hepatitis A	• People with clotting-factor disorders or chronic liver disease • Men who have sex with men • Injection-drug users • People traveling to or working in countries that have high or intermediate endemicity of hepatitis A	Two doses over 6 months
Measles, mumps, rubella	One dose for adults: • Born during or after 1957 who do not have documentation for more than one dose of earlier vaccine • Women whose rubella vaccination history is unreliable Two doses for adults: • Recently exposed to measles • Previously vaccinated with killed measles vaccine • Vaccinated with unknown vaccine during 1963–1967 • Who are students in postsecondary educational institutions • Working in health-care facilities • Planning to travel internationally	One or two doses over 4 weeks
Varicella (chickenpox)	Adults lacking a reliable history of varicella infection who might be at high risk, including: • Health-care workers and family contacts of people with compromised immune systems • Teachers of young children, day-care employees • Residents and staff in institutional settings such as correctional institutions • College students • Military personnel • Adults living in households with children • Nonpregnant women of childbearing age	Two doses within 8 weeks
Meningococcal disease	• Travels to countries where the disease is hyperendemic or epidemic • College freshmen, especially those living in dormitories, should make an educated decision	One dose
Influenza	• Adults with chronic illness (e.g., asthma, diabetes) or other risk factors • Women who will be pregnant during flu season • Health-care workers • Employees of long-term-care and assisted-living facilities • Residents of nursing homes • Adults living or working with at-risk people • All adults older than 65 • Anyone who wishes to be vaccinated	One dose annually
Pneumococcal disease (includes bacterial pneumonia and ear infection)	• All adults older than 65 • Adults with chronic illness or other risk factors	One-time dose

Source: Centers for Disease Control and Prevention (CDC), Washington, DC, www.cdc.gov.

past immunizations, check with family members or your doctor. If you can't find answers, a blood test can show whether you carry antibodies to specific illnesses, such as the following.

- **Tetanus and diphtheria.** Most children complete their initial series of diphtheria and tetanus vaccinations at 4 to 6 years of age and receive their first booster dose during adolescence.
- **Hepatitis B.** The hepatitis B virus is easily transmitted by simple contact with a toothbrush or hand towel and primarily infects teenagers and young adults.
- **Measles, mumps, and rubella.** A blood test for antibodies is recommended for those who did not receive two doses of the vaccine. A second dose has been required since 1989, after several serious measles outbreaks. About 95 percent of people develop immunity after one dose of the vaccine; about 99 percent after two doses of the vaccine.

  CDC officials estimate that 5 to 15 percent of college students are susceptible to measles because they were vaccinated at 12 months of age rather than the currently recommended 15 months, or did not receive a second dose of the vaccine between ages 4 and 12. Others were given immune globulin, which was intended to lower the risk of reaction but which also reduced the vaccine's effectiveness. Many colleges require students to submit proof of measles immunization before allowing them to enroll.

- **Varicella** (chickenpox). An antibody test is recommended for those who have not had chickenpox or been vaccinated against it. Adults are ten times more likely than children to be hospitalized with the severe consequences of chickenpox, including pneumonia and encephalitis (inflammation of the brain).
- **Meningitis.** College students living in dormitories are at increased risk of infection with the meningococcus bacterium, which causes meningitis, an inflammation of the lining of the brain and spinal cord. Vaccination is discussed on page 252.

Infectious Diseases

Although infections can be unavoidable at times, the more you know about their causes, the more you can do to protect yourself.

Who Is at Highest Risk of Infectious Diseases?

Like human bullies, the viruses responsible for the most common infectious illnesses tend to pick on those least capable of fighting back. Among the most vulnerable are the following groups:

- **Children and their families.** Youngsters get up to a dozen colds annually; adults average two a year. When

---

STRATEGIES
for PREVENTION

Protecting Yourself from Infection

- **Wash your hands frequently** with hot water and soap. In a public restroom, use a paper towel to turn off the faucet after you wash your hands, and avoid touching the door-knob. Wash objects used by someone with a cold.
- **Don't share food, drinks, silverware, glasses,** and other objects that may carry infectious microbes.
- **Spend as little time as possible in crowds** during cold and flu season, especially in closed places, such as elevators and airplanes. When out, keep your distance from sneezers and coughers.
- **Don't touch your eyes, mouth, and nose** after being with someone who has cold symptoms.
- **Use tissues** rather than cloth handkerchiefs, which may harbor viruses for hours or days.
- **Avoid irritating air pollutants** whenever possible.

---

a flu epidemic hits a community, about 40 percent of school-age boys and girls get sick, compared with only 5 to 10 percent of adults. But parents get up to six times as many colds as other adults.

- **The elderly.** Statistically, fewer older men and women are likely to catch a cold or flu, yet when they do, they face greater danger than the rest of the population. People over 65 who get the flu have a one in ten chance of being hospitalized for pneumonia or other respiratory problems, and a one in fifty chance of dying from the disease.
- **The chronically ill.** Lifelong diseases, such as diabetes, kidney disease, or sickle-cell anemia, decrease an individual's ability to fend off infections. Individuals taking medications that suppress the immune system, such as steroids, are more vulnerable to infections, as are those with medical conditions that impair immunity, such as infection with HIV.
- **Smokers and those with respiratory problems.** Smokers are a high-risk group for respiratory infections and serious complications, such as pneumonia. Chronic breathing disorders, such as asthma and emphysema, also greatly increase the risk of respiratory infections.
- **Those who live or work in close contact with someone sick.** Health-care workers who treat high-risk patients, nursing home residents, and others living

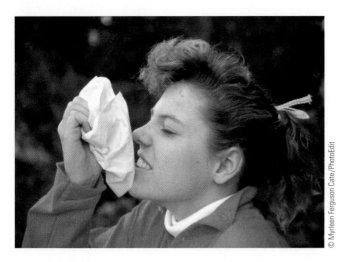

© Myrleen Ferguson Cate/PhotoEdit

▮ Colds spread by direct or indirect contact with an infected person. Wash your hands frequently to protect yourself.

in close quarters—such as students in dormitories—face greater odds of catching others' colds and flus.

▮ **Residents or workers in poorly ventilated buildings.** Building technology has helped spread certain airborne illnesses, such as tuberculosis, via recirculated air. Indoor air quality can be closely linked with disease transmission in winter, when people spend a great deal of time in tightly sealed rooms.

Common Cold

There are more than 200 distinct cold viruses. Although in a single season you may develop a temporary immunity to one or two, you may then be hit by a third. Americans come down with 1 billion colds annually.

Every year, about 25 million cold-sufferers in the United States visit their family doctors with uncomplicated upper respiratory infections. The common cold results in about 20 million days of absence from work and 22 million days of absence from school.

Colds can strike in any season, but different cold viruses are more common at different times of year. *Rhinoviruses* cause most spring, summer, and early fall colds and tend to cause more symptoms above the neck (stuffy nose, headache, runny eyes). *Adenoviruses, parainfluenza viruses, coronaviruses, influenza viruses,* and others that strike in the winter are more likely to get into the bronchi and trachea (the breathing passages) and cause more fever and bronchitis.

Cold viruses spread by coughs, sneezes, and touch. Cold-sufferers who sneeze and then touch a doorknob or countertop leave a trail of highly contagious viruses behind them. The best preventive tactics are frequent hand-washing, replacing toothbrushes regularly, exercising regularly, and avoiding stress overload. High levels of stress increase the risk of becoming infected by respiratory viruses and developing cold symptoms. People who feel

unable to deal with everyday stresses have an exaggerated immune reaction that may intensify cold or flu symptoms once they've contracted a virus. Those with a positive emotional outlook are less vulnerable.[23]

Until scientists develop truly effective treatments, experts advise against taking aspirin and acetaminophen (Tylenol), which may suppress the antibodies the body produces to fight cold viruses and increase symptoms such as nasal stuffiness. A better alternative for achiness is ibuprofen (brand names include Motrin, Advil, and Nuprin), which doesn't seem to affect immune response. Children, teenagers, and young adults should never take aspirin for a cold or flu because of the danger of Reye's syndrome, a potentially deadly disorder that can cause convulsions, coma, swelling of the brain, and kidney damage.

The main drawback of antihistamines, the most widely used cold remedy, is drowsiness, which can impair a person's ability to safely drive or operate machinery. Another common ingredient, pseudoephedrine, opens and drains sinus passages without drowsiness but can speed up heart rate and cause complications for individuals with high blood pressure, diabetes, heart disease, or thyroid disorders. Nasal sprays clear a stuffy nose, but they invariably cause a rebound effect.

In general, doctors recommend treating specific symptoms—headache, cough, chest congestion, sore throat—rather than taking a multisymptom medication. For a cough, the ingredient to look for in any suppressant is dextromethorphan, which turns down the brain's cough reflex. In expectorants, the only medicine the FDA has deemed effective is guaifenesin, which helps liquefy secretions so you can bring up mucus from the chest. Unless you're coughing up green or foul yellow mucus (signs of a secondary bacterial infection), antibiotics won't help. They have no effect against viruses and may make your body more resistant to such medications when you develop a bacterial infection in the future.

Many Americans try alternative remedies for colds. Vitamin C and extracts of the plant *Echinacea* are widely used to prevent the common cold, but there is no conclusive evidence that they help. In a carefully controlled study of college students, echinacea tablets proved no more effective than placebos in reducing the duration or severity of a cold.[24] Zinc lozenges, another popular alternative treatment in recent years, have not proved to be clearly beneficial.

Although colds and sore throats—a frequent cold symptom—are caused by viruses, many people seek treatment with antibiotics, which are effective only against bacteria. An estimated 5 to 17 percent of sore throats in adults are caused by bacteria (*Group A streptococci*). The inappropriate use of antibiotics contributes to the growing problem of bacteria becoming resistant to the antibiotics that previously were able to kill them.

Your own immune system can do something modern science cannot: cure a cold. All it needs is time, rest, and plenty of fluids. Usually cold symptoms last for one to two weeks, although chest colds (bronchitis) may last two or three weeks. Warmth is important because the aptly named "cold" viruses replicate at lower temperatures. Hot soups and drinks (particularly those with a touch of something pungent, like lemon or ginger) raise body temperature and help clear the nose. Tea may enhance the immune system.[25] Even more important is getting off your feet. Taking it easy reduces demands on the body, which helps speed recovery.

Influenza

Although similar to a cold, **influenza**—or the flu— causes more severe symptoms that last longer. Every year 10 to 20 percent of Americans develop influenza, more than 200,000 are hospitalized, and 36,000 die.[26]

Flu viruses, transmitted by coughs, sneezes, laughs, and even normal conversation, are extraordinarily contagious, particularly in the first three days of the disease. The usual incubation period is two days, but symptoms can hit hard and fast. Two varieties of viruses—influenza A and influenza B—cause most flus. In recent years, the deadliest flu epidemics have been caused by various forms of influenza A viruses.

Flu shots now are advised for almost everyone (Table 11-2), including college students living in dormitories, who are at higher risk of influenza than those in nondormitory settings.[27] In a recent study, researchers tried to identify the specific aspects of dormitory life that increase the risk of flu symptoms. As summarized in **Figure 11-8** students living in "triples," with three beds to a room; those sleeping in the same room with a roommate in a double; and those with uncarpeted floors had higher rates of flu symptoms, such as fever, sore throat, and fatigue.[28]

In older individuals, flu shots may offer significant protection against strokes and heart disease. The only individuals who should steer clear are those allergic to eggs, since the inactivated flu viruses are grown in chick embryos.

A new alternative to flu shots is FluMist, an intranasal spray containing a live, attenuated influenza virus vaccine. The aerosol vaccine significantly reduces flu severity, days lost from work, health-care visits, and the use of over-the-counter medication. The spray represents a particular advantage for children since more than 30 percent of youngsters get the flu, but most don't receive a flu shot.

For those who don't get vaccinated this year, antiviral drugs, such as Relenza (zanamivir) and Tamiflu (oseltamivir), are the next best line of defense. These agents act against both influenza A and influenza B viruses and cause few side effects. In research trials, they shortened the duration of flu by up to two days and decreased the likelihood of complications such as bronchitis, sinusitis, and ear infections. However, to be effective, treatment with either medication must begin within 36 to 48 hours of the first

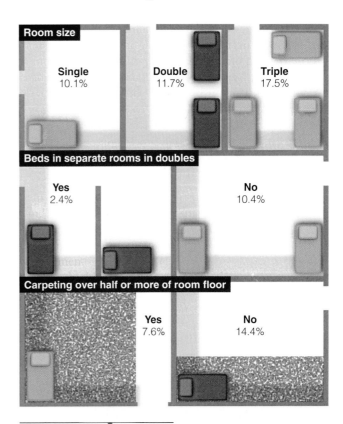

FIGURE 11-8 ∎ Rate of Flu in College Dorms

In a survey of 540 undergraduates, the rate of flu was highest for students living three to a room and lowest for those living alone. Students living in uncarpeted rooms had a higher flu rate than those living in carpeted rooms.

Source: Tsuang, Wayne, et al. "Influenza-like Symptoms in the College Dormitory Environment." *Journal of Environmental Health,* Vol. 66, No. 8, April 2004, p. 39.

flu symptom. Although approved only for use as a treatment, antiviral drugs also can prevent flu from spreading through a family, workplace, or school.

Meningitis

Meningitis, or invasive meningococcal disease, attacks the membranes around the brain and spinal cord and can result in hearing loss, kidney failure, and permanent brain damage. An estimated 2,400 to 3,000 cases occur every year; approximately 10 percent are fatal. One of the most common types is caused by the bacterium *Neisseria meningitidis,* which is spread through coughing; kissing; sharing drinks, eating utensils, or cigarettes; or prolonged exposure to infected individuals. Viral meningitis is typically less severe.

Most common in the first year of life, the incidence of bacterial meningitis rises in young people between ages 15 and 24.[29] College students are generally not at greater risk, except freshmen living in dormitories. In an analysis of data from 50 state health departments and 231 college health centers, CDC researchers found that the risk of meningitis is three times greater for freshmen in dorms than for other college students.[30]

Early symptoms of meningitis include rash, fever, severe headache, nausea, vomiting, and lethargy. A tell-tale symptom in many, but not all, cases is stiffness of the neck when bending forward. Meningitis progresses rapidly, often in as little time as 12 hours. If untreated, it can lead to permanent hearing loss, brain damage, seizures, or death. If it is caught early and treated with antibiotics, however, it is usually curable. Fatality rates are five times higher among 15- to 24-year-olds. As many as one in five survivors may suffer permanent complications, including hearing loss and neurological damage.[31]

Should I Be Vaccinated Against Meningitis?

The Advisory Committee on Immunization Practices of the CDC and the American Academy of Pediatrics have recommended that all college freshmen be informed that vaccination is effective against 70 percent of the bacterial meningitis strains found on campuses and could prevent 80 percent or more of cases among undergraduates. Immunization is recommended primarily for freshmen living in dormitories. The risk among college freshmen living in dormitories is 4.6 per 100,000, higher than among all dorm residents (2.2/100,000), freshmen in general (0.6/100,000), and all young adults between ages 18 and 23 (1.4/100,000).[32] Social behaviors common among college students—such as active or passive smoking, sharing beverage containers, excessive alcohol use, and patronizing bars and night-clubs—can increase their risk of exposure.[33]

Peak incidence for bacterial meningitis is November to March. The CDC is expected to consider new recommendations for college freshmen because a new, more effective vaccine has been developed.

At most schools, the cost of vaccination ranges from $50 to $75. Research into the success of meningococcal vaccination programs on college campuses has shown that women are more likely than men to be vaccinated and that vaccination rates for all nonwhite ethnic groups are somewhat lower than rates for whites. Students majoring in science-oriented fields have higher vaccination rates than those majoring in the humanities. More younger students living on campus than older ones get vaccinations, possibly because of greater parental influence or because they see themselves as being at higher risk.

The current vaccine protects against the most common strains of the *N. meningitidis* bacterium but does not provide complete protection and remains effective for only about three years. More effective vaccines that confer long-lasting immunity and could be administered with other routine infant immunizations have been developed. Some have been introduced in the United Kingdom and other European countries.

Hepatitis

An estimated 500,000 Americans contract hepatitis each year. At least five different viruses, referred to as **hepatitis** A, B, C, Delta, and E, can cause this inflammation of the liver. Newly identified viruses also may be responsible for some cases of what is called "non-A, non-B" hepatitis.

All forms of hepatitis target the liver, the body's largest internal organ. Symptoms include headaches, fever, fatigue, stiff or aching joints, nausea, vomiting, and diarrhea. The liver becomes enlarged and tender to the touch; sometimes the yellowish tinge of jaundice develops. Treatment consists of rest, a high-protein diet, and the avoidance of alcohol and drugs that may stress the liver. Alpha interferon, a protein that boosts immunity and prevents viruses from replicating, may be used for some forms.

Most people begin to feel better after two or three weeks of rest, although fatigue and other symptoms can linger. As many as 10 percent of those infected with hepatitis B and up to two-thirds of those with hepatitis C become carriers of the virus for several years or even life. Some have persistent inflammation of the liver, which may cause mild or severe symptoms and increase the risk of liver cancer.

Hepatitis A

Hepatitis A, a less serious form, is generally transmitted by poor sanitation, primarily fecal contamination of food or water, and is less common in industrialized nations than in developing countries. Among those at highest risk in the United States are children and staff at day-care centers, residents of institutions for the developmentally disabled, sanitation workers, and workers who handle primates such as monkeys. Gamma globulin can provide short-term immunity; vaccines against hepatitis A have been approved by the FDA. The CDC has recommended routine immunization against hepatitis A in 11 western states with high rates.

Hepatitis B

Hepatitis B, a potentially fatal disease transmitted through the blood and other bodily fluids, infects an estimated 350,000 people around the world each year. Once spread mainly by contaminated tattoo needles, needles shared by drug users, or transfusions of contaminated blood, hepatitis B is now transmitted mostly through sexual contact. It can lead to chronic liver infection, cirrhosis, and liver cancer.

Hepatitis B is a particular threat to young people; 75 percent of new cases are diagnosed in those between ages 15 to 39. They usually contract hepatitis B through high-risk behaviors such as multiple sex partners and use of injected drugs. Individuals who have tattoos or body piercings also may be at risk if procedures are not done under regulated conditions. At highest risk are male homosexuals, heterosexuals with multiple sex partners, health-care workers with frequent contact with blood, injection drug users, and infants born to infected mothers. Vaccination can prevent hepatitis B and is recommended for all children and teens, and adults at high risk.

Hepatitis C

Hepatitis C virus (HCV) is four times as widespread as HIV, infecting about 2 percent of Americans. A simple blood test can show if you are infected with HCV. However, few of the estimated 3 to 4 million carriers in the United States realize they are infected. Eighty percent of those infected with HCV have no symptoms.[34]

The risk factors for HCV infection are blood transfusion or organ transplant before 1992, exposure to infected blood, injection-drug use, tattoos, or body piercing. If you choose to have a body piercing, avoid piercing guns, and make certain that the piercing equipment has been sterilized.[35] (See Savvy Consumer: "Before You Get a Tattoo or Piercing.") Hepatitis C virus is not spread by hugging, kissing, or sharing food utensils. There is controversy over whether HCV also can be transmitted sexually.

About three-quarters of those infected with HCV develop chronic or long-term hepatitis. About one-quarter develop progressive, irreversible liver damage, with scar tissue (cirrhosis) gradually replacing healthy liver tissue.

The most common treatment for hepatitis C is a combination of interferon, which stops the virus from making copies of itself; and ribavirin, an antiviral medication. If the liver no longer functions adequately, a patient may require liver transplantation.

Mononucleosis

You can get **mononucleosis** through kissing—or any other form of close contact. "Mono" is a viral disease that targets people 15 to 24 years old. Its symptoms include a sore throat, headache, fever, nausea, and prolonged weakness. The spleen is swollen and the lymph nodes are enlarged. You may also develop jaundice or a skin rash similar to rubella.

The major symptoms usually disappear within two to three weeks, but weakness, fatigue, and often depression may linger for at least two more weeks. The greatest danger is from physical activity that might rupture the spleen, resulting in internal bleeding. The liver may also become inflamed. A blood test can determine whether you have mono. However, there's no specific treatment other than rest.

Insect- and Animal-Borne Infections

Common insects and animals, including ticks and mosquitoes, can transmit dangerous infections. Lyme disease is the most widespread in the United States, while West Nile virus continues to spread.

Lyme Disease

Lyme disease, a bacterial infection, is spread by ticks carrying a particular bacterium—the spirochete *Borrelia burgdorferi*. An infected person may have various symptoms, including joint inflammation, heart arrhythmias, blinding headaches, and memory lapses. The disease can also cause miscarriages and birth defects. Lyme disease is by far the most commonly reported vector-borne infectious disease in the United States. The vast majority of all reported cases have occurred in just ten

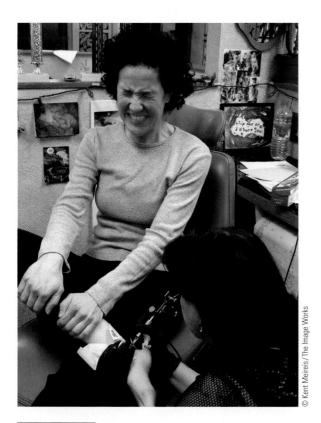

Getting a tattoo or a piercing can pose health risks, including bacterial infection and hepatitis.

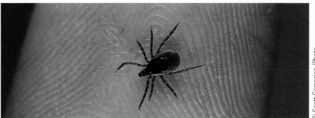

Ticks are responsible for the spread of Lyme disease. If you spot a tick, remove it as soon as possible with tweezers or small forceps. Put it in a plastic bag or sealed bottle and save it. If you develop a rash or other symptoms, take it with you to the doctor.

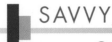

SAVVY CONSUMER

BEFORE YOU GET A TATTOO OR PIERCING

Body art—tattoos and piercings—may seem harmless, but health officials warn of hidden risks, including hepatitis B and C infection and transmission of HIV. In a survey of undergraduates at a university in New York, 51 percent reported body piercings, and 23 percent had gotten tattoos. Almost one in five of those with piercings reported medical complications. Bacterial infection was the most common, followed by bleeding and injury or tearing at the site.

With no state or federal regulations of "body artists," unsafe tattooing and piercing practices can put consumers in danger. In one survey of "skin-penetration operators," only half said that they followed governmental guidelines for infection control. Many were not knowledgeable about standard infection control principles and practices.

Epidemiologists have identified tattooing as a strong, independent risk factor for testing positive for hepatitis C virus (HCV), but not with development of acute hepatitis. In other words, individuals with tattoos may acquire HCV but may not develop symptoms themselves. This does not mean that they will never become symptomatic or that they cannot transmit HCV to others.

Even so-called temporary tattooing with henna is not without risk. Dermatologists have reported an increasing number of skin reactions. The culprit is an ingredient in many henna preparations (as well as many other dyes) called paraphenylenediamine (PPD). Allergic reactions to henna itself can occur but are much rarer. Piercings of the tongue, lips, or cheeks present different dangers, including recessed gums; loose, chipped, or fractured teeth; pain; infec-

tion; inflammation; nerve damage; and tooth loss.

You may think you're safe if you go to a licensed tattoo or piercing salon. However, there are no formal schools, no certification requirements, and no diplomas for these practitioners. In many states it is possible to get a license without the benefit of any kind of training. Your best assurance of quality is making sure that basic safety principles are followed:

- **Ask to see certification that the autoclave, a high-temperature pressure cooker used for medical instruments, has been sterilized.** Ask to see the autoclave itself. Is it clean? More importantly, are the shop personnel happy to show it to you, or do they seem to have something to hide? Autoclaves need to be regularly tested to ensure that they are working properly. Ask to see the results of their latest spore test. Check the date. The results should be no more than two months old.

- **Make sure the artist is wearing standard medical latex gloves.** Check the fit. If the gloves are too big or too small, the artist runs the risk of either poking a hole in the gloves or tearing them. All it takes is a pinhole to run the risk of cross-contamination.

- **Find out if the artist is vaccinated for hepatitis B.** As this infection has spread, vaccination has become essential for a tattoo artist's own safety as well as that of clients. If artists claim to be vaccinated, never just take their word for it. Can they show you proof, such as a doctor's record, that they were vaccinated? If

they tell you they don't remember if they've been vaccinated, they're probably lying. Most people vividly remember the vaccinations.

- **Make sure the artist uses only new sterile needles.** The needles should not be removed from the autoclave bag, the sort of pouch you see in dentists' offices, until you are ready for your tattoo. Ask to see the sterile confirmation logo on the bag itself. Usually the name of the company that made the bag will be visible on the front of the bag only when the equipment has been properly autoclaved. To determine if the needles are new and not just sterilized after previous use, check the color. They should be bright silver, not stained with ink or brownish looking.

- **Ask how the artist disposes of used needles.** They should be placed in a sharps container, a plastic container, usually red, with a biohazard symbol on the outside, and removed in a timely manner.

- **Always ask to see photos of the artist's finished work.** Examine the designs up close to check precision and skill. If you have the time, watch the artist work on another client before you go ahead with your tattoo.

- **If you require prophylactic antibiotics for dental cleanings or other procedures, do not get a tattoo.** Consumers with rheumatic heart disease and other conditions that increase their risk of infections have died as a result of bacterial infection contracted from a tattoo.

states; including New York, New Jersey, Connecticut, Pennsylvania, and Wisconsin.

The FDA has licensed a vaccine to prevent Lyme disease in individuals 15 to 70 years old. LYMErix, like most vaccines, stimulates the immune system to produce

antibodies, in this case against the bacterium that causes Lyme disease. But the vaccine, administered in three doses over a one-year period, is not 100 percent effective and should not be considered a substitute for protective clothing and tick repellent.

The primary culprit in most cases of Lyme disease is the deer tick, although other ticks, including the western black-legged tick, the dog tick, and the lone star tick, also may transmit the bacterium that causes Lyme disease.

West Nile Virus

West Nile virus (WNV) is transmitted by a mosquito that feeds on an infected bird and then bites a human. The first cases in the United States occurred in 1999. Experts now see WNV as a seasonal epidemic that flares up in the summer and continues into the fall. WNV also can be spread through blood transfusions, organ transplants, breast-feeding, and from mother to fetus during pregnancy.

WNV interferes with normal central nervous system functioning and causes inflammation of brain tissue. The risk of catching WNV is low. Relatively few mosquitoes carry WNV, and less than 1 percent of people who are bitten by mosquitoes experience any symptoms. There is no specific treatment for WNV infection. People with more severe cases usually require hospitalization.

✚ Diabetes Mellitus

About 100 million people around the world, including nearly 16 million people in the United States, have **diabetes mellitus,** a disease in which the body doesn't produce or respond properly to insulin, a hormone essential for daily life. In those who have diabetes, the pancreas, which produces insulin (the hormone that regulates carbohydrate and fat metabolism) doesn't function as it should. When the pancreas either stops producing insulin (type 1 or *insulin-dependent diabetes*) or doesn't produce sufficient insulin to meet the body's needs (type 2 or *non-insulin-dependent diabetes*), almost every body system can be damaged.

Who Is at Risk for Developing Diabetes?

One in three Americans with diabetes is not aware of having an illness that increases the risk of blindness, kidney failure, cardiovascular disease, and premature death. The incidence of this potential killer, which jumped about a third in the last decade, is growing so fast that Dr. Allen Spiegel, director of the National Institute of Diabetes and Digestive and Kidney Diseases (NIDDK), describes it as "a definite epidemic."[36] There has been a particularly dramatic rise in type 2 diabetes in children and adolescents, especially among minority populations.

Uncontrolled glucose levels slowly damage blood vessels throughout the body, thus individuals who become diabetic early in life may face devastating complications even before they reach middle age. "Diabetes is already the number one cause of blindness, nontraumatic amputations, and kidney failure, and diabetes increases by two or three times the risk of heart attack or stroke," says Dr. Robert Sherwin of Yale University, president of the American Diabetes Association, who estimates that the disease may affect 22 million Americans within the next two decades.[37]

Lifestyle factors, especially a lack of physical activity, greatly increase the risk for type 2 diabetes. Both obesity, as measured by BMI, and physical inactivity are independent risk factors for diabetes, but in women the impact of obesity is greater than fitness. Women who drink more than one sugar-sweetened beverage a day also are more likely to gain weight; those with a high consumption are at higher risk of type 2 diabetes.[38]

Television watching, more than other sedentary activities such as sewing, reading, writing, and driving, is strongly associated with weight and obesity, a risk factor for diabetes in both children and adults. In a ten-year study of 1,058 individuals with type 2 diabetes, watching television for 2 to 10 hours a week increased the risk of diabetes 66 percent; 21 to 40 hours per week more than doubled the risk; more than 40 hours a week nearly tripled the risk.

To identify individuals with this disease as early as possible, the American Diabetes Association now recommends screening every three years for all men and women beginning at age 45. Those at highest risk include relatives of diabetics, obese persons, older persons, and mothers of large babies (an indication of maternal prediabetes). A child of two parents with type 2 diabetes faces an 80 percent likelihood of also becoming diabetic.

The early signs of diabetes are frequent urination, excessive thirst, a craving for sweets and starches, and weakness. Diagnosis is based on tests of the sugar level

---

STRATEGIES for PREVENTION

Lowering Your Risk of Diabetes

▌ Eat a diet rich in complex carbohydrates (bread and other starches) and high-fiber foods, and low in sodium and fat.

▌ Eat fruits and vegetables that are rich in antioxidants, substances that prevent oxygen damage to cells.

▌ Keep your weight down. Weight loss for those who are overweight can sometimes decrease or eliminate the need for insulin or oral drugs. For individuals at high risk of developing type 2 diabetes, losing just half the pounds needed to reach their ideal weight can prevent the onset of the disease.

▌ Exercise regularly. Regular, vigorous aerobic activity reduces the risk of type 2 diabetes in men and women.

in the blood. Researchers are working to develop a test that would help identify telltale antibodies in the blood; this could indicate whether pancreas cells were being destroyed years before the first signs of diabetes.

Dangers of Diabetes

Before the development of insulin injections, diabetes was a fatal illness. Today diabetics can have normal life spans. However, both types of diabetes can lead to devastating complications, including increased risk of heart attack or stroke, blindness, and loss of circulation to the extremities. Diabetes is the most common cause of kidney failure.

Diabetic women who become pregnant face higher risks of miscarriage and babies with serious birth defects; however, precise control of blood sugar levels before conception and in early pregnancy can lower the likelihood of these problems. The development of diabetes during pregnancy, called *gestational diabetes,* may pose potentially serious health threats to mother and child years later. Women who develop gestational diabetes are more than three times as likely to develop type 2 diabetes if they have a second pregnancy; their infants may be at increased risk of cardiovascular disease later in life.

Diabetes and Ethnic Minorities

Several minority groups, especially African Americans, Native Americans, and Hispanics, are at high risk of developing diabetes. One in every ten African Americans and Hispanics has this disease. The members of some Native American tribes are 300 percent more likely to develop diabetes than the general population. For many, obesity and unhealthy food choices increase the risk. Researchers now believe that the interaction of environmental factors and genes varies among different racial and ethnic groups.

Treatment

The goal for diabetics is to keep blood sugar levels as stable as possible to prevent complications, such as kidney damage. Home glucose monitoring allows diabetics to check their blood sugar levels as many times a day as necessary and to adjust their diet or insulin doses as appropriate.

An estimated 6 to 7 million Americans use insulin or insulin analogues. Newer insulin therapies help patients with diabetes maintain better control of blood sugar levels around the clock. Types of insulin differ in how long they take to start working after injection (onset), when they work hardest (peak), and how long they last in the body (duration). Individuals with diabetes may use different types in various combinations, depending on time of day and timing of meals.

Those with type 1 diabetes require daily doses of insulin via injections, an insulin infusion pump, or oral medication. Those with type 2 diabetes can control their disease through a well-balanced diet, exercise, and weight management. However, insulin therapy may be needed to keep blood glucose levels near normal or normal, thereby reducing the risk of damage to the eyes, nerves, and kidneys.

▌MAKING HEALTHY CHOICES

To Prevent Serious Illnesses

You may not be able to control every risk factor in your life or environment, but you can protect yourself from the obvious ones.

▌ **Don't smoke.** There's no bigger favor you can do for yourself and those who live and work near you. Smoking decreases the levels of some immune cells and increases susceptibility to respiratory infections.

▌ **Eat a balanced diet** to be sure you get essential vitamins and minerals. Severe deficiencies in vitamins B_6, B_{12}, and folic acid impair immunity. Keep up your iron and zinc intake. Iron influences the number and vigor of certain immune cells, whereas zinc is crucial for cell repair. Too little vitamin C may also increase susceptibility to infectious diseases.

▌ **Avoid fatty foods.** A low-fat diet can increase the activity of immune cells that hunt down and knock out cells infected with viruses.

▌ **Watch your weight.** Overweight and obesity are associated with increased risk for cancers at several sites: breast (among postmenopausal women), colon, endometrium, adenocarcinoma of the esophagus, and kidney.

▌ **Get enough sleep.** Without adequate rest, your immune system cannot maintain and renew itself.

▌ **Exercise regularly.** Aerobic exercise stimulates the production of an immune-system booster called interleukin-2.

▌ **Avoid excessive exposure to ultraviolet light.** If you spend a lot of time outside, you can protect your skin by using sunscreen and wearing long-sleeve shirts and a hat. Also, wear sunglasses to protect your eyes. Don't purposely put yourself at risk by binge-sunbathing or by using sunlamps.

▌ **Avoid obvious cancer risks.** Besides ultraviolet light, other environmental factors that have been linked with cancer include tobacco, asbestos, and radiation.

■ **Control your alcohol intake.** Heavy drinking interferes with normal immune responses and lowers the number of defender cells. The risk of cancers of the mouth, pharynx, larynx, esophagus, liver, and breast increases substantially with intake of more than 2 drinks per day for men or one drink for women.

■ **Be alert to changes in your body.** You know your body's rhythms and appearance better than anyone else, and only you will know if certain things aren't right. Changes in bowel habits, skin changes, unusual lumps or discharges—anything out of the ordinary—may be clues that require further medical investigation.

SELF-SURVEY

Are You at Risk of Cancer?

Answer the following questions:

1. Do you protect your skin from overexposure to the sun? _____
2. Do you abstain from smoking or using tobacco in any form? _____
3. If you're over 40 or if family members have had colon cancer, do you get routine digital rectal exams? _____
4. Do you eat a balanced diet that includes the recommended Daily Value for vitamins A, B, and C? _____
5. If you're a woman, do you have regular Pap tests and pelvic exams? _____
6. If you're a man over 40, do you get regular prostate exams? _____
7. If you have burn scars or a history of chronic skin infections, do you get regular checkups? _____
8. Do you avoid smoked, salted, pickled, and high-nitrite foods? _____
9. If your job exposes you to asbestos, radiation, cadmium, or other environmental hazards, do you get regular checkups? _____
10. Do you limit your consumption of alcohol? _____
11. Do you avoid using tanning salons or home sunlamps? _____
12. If you're a woman, do you examine your breasts every month for lumps? _____
13. Do you eat plenty of vegetables and other sources of fiber? _____
14. If you're a man, do you perform regular testicular self-exams? _____
15. Do you wear protective sunglasses in sunlight? _____
16. Do you follow a low-fat diet? _____
17. Do you know the cancer warning signs? _____

Scoring:

If you answered no to any of the questions, your risk for developing various kinds of cancer may be increased.

ACTION PLAN

Your Action Plan for Early Detection of Cancer

Site	Recommendation
Breast	■ Yearly mammograms are recommended starting at age 40. The age at which screening should be stopped should be individualized by considering the potential risks and benefits of screening in the context of overall health status and longevity.

Breast

■ Clinical breast exam should be part of a periodic health exam, about every 3 years for women in their twenties and thirties, and every year for women 40 and older.

■ Women should know how their breasts normally feel and report any breast change promptly to their health-care providers. Breast self-exam is an option for women starting in their twenties.

■ Women at increased risk (e.g., family history, genetic tendency, past breast cancer) should talk with their doctors about the benefits and limitations of starting mammography screening earlier, having additional tests (i.e., breast ultrasound and MRI), or having more frequent exams.

Colon & rectum Beginning at age 50, men and women should begin screening with one of the following examination schedules:

■ A fecal occult blood test (FOBT) or fecal immunochemical test (FIT) every year

■ A flexible sigmoidoscopy (FSIG) every 5 years

■ Annual FOBT or FIT and flexible sigmoidoscopy every 5 years★

■ A double-contrast barium enema every 5 years

■ A colonoscopy every 10 years

★*Combined testing is preferred over either annual FOBT or FIT, or FSIG every 5 years, alone. People who are at moderate or high risk for colorectal cancer should talk with a doctor about a different testing schedule.*

Prostate The prostate-specific antigen (PSA) test and the digital rectal examination should be offered annually, beginning at age 50, to men who have a life expectancy of at least 10 years. Men at high risk (African-American men and men with a strong family history of one or more first-degree relatives diagnosed with prostate cancer at an early age) should begin testing at age 45. For both men at average risk and high risk, information should be provided about what is known and what is uncertain about the benefits and limitations of early detection and treatment of prostate cancer so that they can make an informed decision about testing.

Uterus **Cervix:** Screening should begin approximately 3 years after a woman begins having vaginal intercourse, but no later than 21 years of age. Screening should be done every year with regular Pap tests or every 2 years using liquid-based tests. At or after age 30, women who have had three normal test results in a row may get screened every 2 to 3 years. Alternatively, cervical cancer screening with HPV DNA (to detect human papilloma virus) testing and conventional or liquid-based cytology could be performed every 3 years. However, doctors may suggest a woman get screened more often if she has certain risk factors, such as HIV infection or a weak immune system. Women 70 years and older who have had three or more consecutive normal Pap tests in the last 10 years may choose to stop cervical cancer screening. Screening after total hysterectomy (with removal of the cervix) is not necessary unless the surgery was done as a treatment for cervical cancer.

Endometrium: The American Cancer Society recommends that at the time of menopause all women should be informed about the risks and symptoms of endometrial cancer and strongly encouraged to report any unexpected bleeding or spotting to their physicians. Annual screening for endometrial cancer with endometrial biopsy beginning at age 35 should be offered to women with or at risk for hereditary nonpolyposis colon cancer (HNPCC).

Cancer-related checkup For individuals undergoing periodic health examinations, a cancer-related checkup should include health counseling and, depending on a person's age and gender, might include examinations for cancers of the thyroid, oral cavity, skin, lymph nodes, tests, and ovaries, as well as for some nonmalignant diseases.

Source: ©2005, American Cancer Society, Inc.

SETTING GOALS

Your Personal Cancer Prevention Goal:

Is It S.M.A.R.T.?
Specific? _____
Measurable? _____
Achievable? _____
Rewarding? _____
Time Defined? _____

Strategies for Success
1. _____
2. _____
3. _____

Potential Obstacles
1. _____
2. _____
3. _____

Ways Around Them
1. _____
2. _____
3. _____

Daily Report

The Week that Was:

What Went Right?
What Could I Do Better?

WELLNESS JOURNAL 1

The Surgeon General's Family History Initiative: How to Create Your Family Health Portrait

The Surgeon General has launched a national initiative to encourage all American families to learn more about their family health histories. Knowing your family's medical history can save your life. With a copy of your family health history, you and a health care professional can individualize your care to prevent and screen for conditions for which you may be at higher risk. Family events, such as Thanksgiving or family reunions, offer a great chance to gather the information for "My Family Health Portrait."

Whom Should I Talk With?

To get the most accurate health history information, it is important to talk directly with your relatives. Explain to them that their health information can help improve prevention and screening of diseases for all family members.

Start by asking your relatives about any health conditions they have had—including history of chronic illnesses, such as heart disease; pregnancy complications, such as miscarriage; and any developmental disabilities. Get as much specific information as possible.

It is most useful if you can list the formal name of any medical condition that has affected you or your relatives.

You can get help finding information about health conditions that have affected you or your family members—living or deceased—by asking relatives or health-care professionals for information, or by getting copies of medical records.

If you are planning to have children, you and your partner should each create a family health portrait and show it to your health-care professional.

Knowing your family health history is a powerful guide to understanding risk for disease. However, keep in mind that a family history of a particular illness may increase risk, but it almost never *guarantees* that other family members will develop the illness.

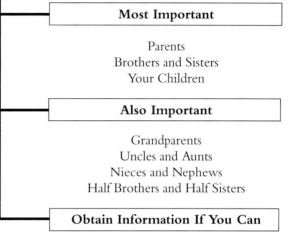

Most Important

Parents
Brothers and Sisters
Your Children

Also Important

Grandparents
Uncles and Aunts
Nieces and Nephews
Half Brothers and Half Sisters

Obtain Information If You Can

Cousins
Great-Uncles and Great-Aunts

How Do I Fill Out The Form?

The "My Family Health Portrait" form will help you collect and organize your family information. No form can reflect every version of the American family, so use this chart as a starting point and adapt it to your family's needs.

First, write each of your relatives' names in the designated boxes and circle whether they are male (M) or female (F). On the next line, write the name of any health conditions they have had. If you know the age at which they were diagnosed with a condition, write that in parentheses after the condition. For example: "diabetes (diagnosed—age 37)."

If family members have died, write "deceased" and the age at which they died. For example: "heart attack (deceased—age 63)."

For twins, write "twin" on the first line for both individuals. If the twins are identical, write "identical twin" on the first line for both.

If your family includes half brothers or half sisters, write "half brother" or "half sister" on the first line and note "different father" or "different mother" on the next line.

Some conditions are more common in people with a shared background or ancestry. It is important to record the ancestry of your relatives and be as specific as possible. For example, if you know that your grandmother is Hispanic and her family comes from Mexico, write "Mexican" underneath her name. Likewise, if your family is from Africa, Asia, Europe, or South America, note the country they came from, if possible.

Once you complete "My Family Health Portrait," take it to your health-care professional so that he or she can better individualize your health care. Be sure to make a copy for your records and update it as circumstances change or you learn more about your family's health history.

Congratulations on taking this step toward a longer, healthier life! "My Family Health Portrait" can be an effective way to improve your health—today and in the future.

My Family Health Portrait

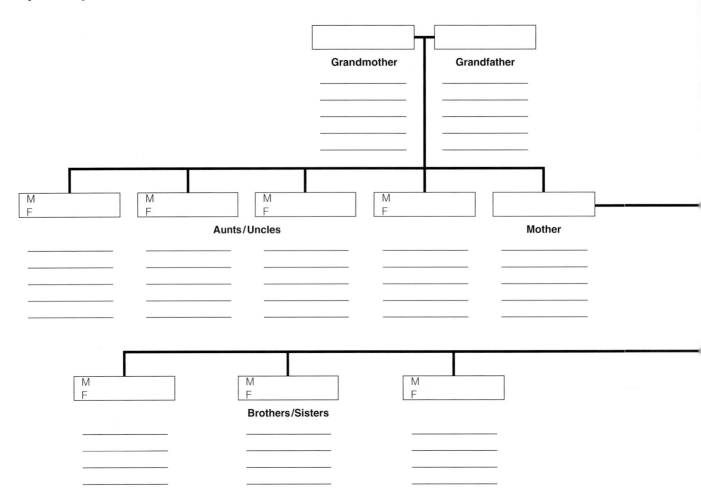

Grandmother   Grandfather

M
F

M
F

M
F

M
F

M
F

Aunts/Uncles   **Mother**

M
F

M
F

M
F

Brothers/Sisters

━━━ Cut out and add to chart as needed ━━━

M
F

M
F

M
F

Name: _____

Date: _____

Grandmother   Grandfather

_____   _____
_____   _____
_____   _____
_____   _____
_____   _____

Father   M   M   M   M
                     F   F   F   F
                              Aunts/Uncles

_____ _____ _____ _____ _____
_____ _____ _____ _____ _____
_____ _____ _____ _____ _____
_____ _____ _____ _____ _____
_____ _____ _____ _____ _____
_____ _____ _____ _____ _____

M   M
F   F
You   Spouse/Partner

_____   _____
_____   _____
_____   _____
_____   _____

M   M   M   M   M
F   F   F   F   F
              Your Children

_____ _____ _____ _____ _____
_____ _____ _____ _____ _____
_____ _____ _____ _____ _____
_____ _____ _____ _____ _____
_____ _____ _____ _____ _____

WELLNESS JOURNAL 2

What's the Risk?

After completing the Surgeon General's "Your Family Health Portrait" it is a good idea to assess the results of your research. Summarize your findings below and determine what steps you need to take in order to lower your potential risk(s).

Relative	Conditions/ Diseases(s)?	Your Risk of Getting It?	What are the recommended prevention tactics?	Do you need to have more info?
Father				
Mother				
Uncles				
Aunts				
Brothers				
Sisters				
Paternal Grandfather				
Paternal Grandmother				
Maternal Grandfather				
Maternal Grandmother				

Are there lifestyle habits you might need to change or initiate as a result of your assessment? Explain.

Making This Chapter Work for You

1. Which of the following statements about cancer is *true?*
   a. When cancer cells spread to another part of the body, the process is called infiltration.
   b. Cancer occurs when abnormal cells grow and spread uncontrollably until they form an ectoplasm.
   c. Those cancers that have been shown to be triggered by viruses are contagious.
   d. Every cancer has a genetically determined "fingerprint" that indicates how deadly it is.

2. You can protect yourself from certain types of cancer by:
   a. eating a diet rich in antioxidants.
   b. avoiding people who have had cancer.
   c. wearing sunscreen with an SPF of less than 15.
   d. using condoms during sexual intercourse.

3. Which of the following statements about skin cancer is *true?*
   a. Individuals with a large number of moles are at decreased risk for melanoma.
   b. The most serious type of skin cancer is squamous cell carcinoma.
   c. The safest way to get a tan and avoid skin cancer is to use tanning salons and sunlamps instead of sunbathing in direct sunlight.
   d. Individuals with a history of childhood sunburn are at increased risk for melanoma.

4. A woman's risk of developing breast cancer increase if:
   a. she is African American under the age of 50.
   b. she had her first child when in her teens or twenties.
   c. her husband's mother had breast cancer.
   d. she began menstruating when she was 15 or 16.

5. Prostate cancer:
   a. occurs mostly among men between the ages of 18 and 35.
   b. is usually more aggressive in white men.
   c. has a low survival rate.
   d. can be detected through a screening test that measures the levels of prostate-specific antigen in the blood.

6. To lower your cancer risk,
   a. minimize your exposure to carcinogens.
   b. don't smoke.
   c. perform monthly self-exams on your breasts or testicles.
   d. all of the above.

7. Which of these body tissues is *not* part of the body's immune system?
   a. thymus gland
   b. lymph nodes
   c. skin
   d. spleen

8. Which of the following statements about the common cold and influenza is *true?*
   a. Influenza is just a more severe form of the common cold.
   b. Aspirin should be avoided by children and young adults who have a cold or influenza.
   c. The flu vaccine is also effective against most of the viruses that cause the common cold.
   d. Antibiotics are appropriate treatments for colds but not for influenza.

9. Which of the following statements about specific infectious diseases is *false?*
   a. You can get mononucleosis by kissing an infected person.
   b. West Nile virus is transmitted by mosquitoes.
   c. Hepatitis A is usually transmitted through contaminated needles, transfusions, and sexual contact.
   d. College freshmen are at higher risk for contracting meningitis than the general population of young people between the ages of 18 and 23.

10. Which of the following statements about diabetes mellitus is *false?*
    a. The two types of diabetes are insulin-dependent and non-insulin-dependent.
    b. The incidence of diabetes has decreased in the last decade, especially among African Americans, Native Americans, and Latinos.
    c. Individuals with diabetes must measure the levels of glucose in their blood to ensure that it does not rise to unsafe levels.
    d. Untreated or uncontrolled diabetes can lead to coma and eventual death.

Answers to these questions can be found on page 376.

Critical Thinking

1. Do you have family members who have had cancer? Were these individuals at risk for cancer because of specific environmental factors, such as long-term exposure to tobacco smoke? If no particular cause was identified, what other factors could have triggered their diseases? Are you concerned that you might have inherited a genetic predisposition to any

particular type of cancer because of your family history?

2. A friend of yours, Karen, discovered a small lump in her breast during a routine self-examination. When she mentions it, you ask if she has seen a doctor. She tells you that she hasn't had time to schedule an appointment; besides, she says she's not sure it's really the kind of lump one has to worry about. It's clear to you that Karen is in denial and procrastinating about seeing a doctor. What advice would you give her?

3. Because of advances in antirejection treatment, organ transplants have proved highly successful in helping many people who otherwise might have died. Even elderly patients have clearly benefited from donated kidneys and livers. However, because the demand for organs to transplant greatly exceeds the supply, health experts have debated setting priorities. Should a 30-year-old be placed higher on the waiting list for a particular organ than a 70-year-old? Should a nurse who needs a liver because she contracted hepatitis on the job get priority over an alcoholic whose liver has been destroyed by cirrhosis? Who, if anyone, should make such decisions? Would a lottery be a fair way to determine who receives an available organ?

Media Menu

Health ⊗ Now™

Don't forget to check out the wealth of resources on the HealthNow website at **http://healthnow.brookscole.com/itw** that will:
- Help you evaluate your knowledge of the material
- Allow you to take an exam-prep quiz
- Provide a Personalized Learning Plan targeting resources that address areas you should study
- Coach you through identifying target goals for behavior change and creating and monitoring your personal change plan throughout the semester.

INTERNET CONNECTIONS

Cancer Prevention

www.cancer.org/docroot/PED/ped_0.asp
This site from the American Cancer Society features information on prevention, emphasizing nutrition and environmental toxins.

National Cancer Institute

www.nci.nih.gov
This government site, from the National Institutes of Health, provides statistics, frequently asked questions, as well as information on research and support resources. It includes links to web pages with information about specific cancers.

Cancer Prevention and Control

www.cdc.gov/cancer/index.htm
This site, sponsored by the Centers for Disease Control and Prevention (CDC), features current information on cancer of the breast, cervix, prostate, skin, and colon. The site also provides monthly spotlights on specific cancers, as well as links to the National Comprehensive Cancer Control Program and the National Program of Cancer Registries.

Women's Cancer Network: Cancer Risk Assessment Survey

www.wcn.org
Sponsored by Health Net, this site features a detailed personal breast cancer risk analysis; information about screening through self-exams, clinical exams, and mammograms; and teaching aids and resources.

 InfoTrac College Edition Activities Liebman, Bonnie. "Antioxidants: still hazy after all these years," *Nutrition Action Healthletter,* Nov 2005 v32 i9 p1(6).

1. How has scientific opinion of the value of antioxidants in preventing major diseases such as cancer changed in recent years?

2. Should you believe the health claims of products, such as teas and dietary supplements, that contain antioxidants?

3. What is the best advice for consumers until scientists sort out the possible benefits of antioxidants?

You can find additional readings related to personal health with InfoTrac College Edition, an online library of more than 900 journals and publications. Follow the instructions for accessing InfoTrac College Edition that were packaged with your textbook; then search for articles using a keyword search.

For additional links, resources, and suggested readings on the InfoTrac College Edition, visit our Health and Wellness Resource Center at **http://health .wadsworth.com.**

Key Terms

The terms listed are used on the page indicated. Definitions of the terms are in the Glossary at the end of the book.

abscess 246
antibiotics 245
antiviral drugs 245
bacteria 245
carcinogen 239
diabetes mellitus 255

fungi 245
helminth 245
hepatitis 252
host 245
immune deficiency 246
immunity 246

Taking Care of Yourself

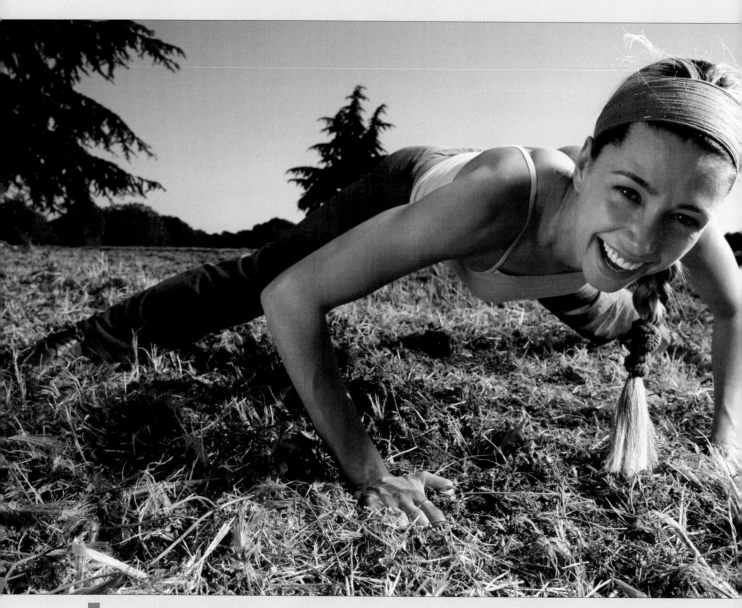

Long after she immigrated to the United States from India, Tapu's grandmother refused to go to Western doctors. She preferred practitioners who used the herbs and techniques she had relied on in her homeland. Tapu's father, an American-trained physician, would argue with his mother-in-law about what he considered her old-fashioned views. As a doctor's son, Tapu grew up believing in the superiority of Western medicine.

In his sophomore year at college, Tapu found out that he needed oral surgery. To his surprise, the oral surgeon suggested an alternative method of controlling post-operative pain: acupuncture. "My dad's never going to approve," he said. "And he's the one who's still paying my medical bills." The doctor referred Tapu—and his father—to recent studies conducted by National Institute of Health researchers on acupuncture's efficacy in relieving post-surgical pain. After doing more research online, Tapu agreed to try acupuncture following his operation.

Like Tapu, millions of Americans are turning to complementary and alternative medicine (CAM), a term that includes a broad range of healing philosophies, approaches, and therapies not traditionally taught in medical schools or provided in hospitals. But consumers are learning that they have to be just as savvy—and skeptical—about these therapies and practitioners as they are with any other form of health care.

Because there are so many health-care choices, you face a greater responsibility for your personal well-being. Whether you are monitoring your blood pressure, taking medication, or deciding whether to try an alternative therapy, you need to gather information, ask questions, weigh advantages and disadvantages, and take charge of your health. The reason: No one cares more about your health than you do, and no one will do more to promote your well-being than you.

After studying the material in this chapter, you should be able to:

▌ **Discuss** strategies for self-care, as well as how to get the best possible health care.

▌ **Identify** strategies for maintaining good oral health.

▌ **Describe** some problems involving use of over-the-counter medications and prescription drugs.

▌ **Describe** the different types of complementary and alternative therapies and **explain** what research has shown about their effectiveness.

▌ **Name** four long-term strategies for staying healthy longer.

Health❨❩Now™

Don't forget to check out the wealth of resources on the HealthNow website at **http://healthnow.brookscole.com/itw** that will:

• Help you evaluate your knowledge of the material

• Allow you to take an exam-prep quiz

• Provide a Personalized Learning Plan targeting resources that address areas you should study

• Coach you through identifying target goals for behavior change and creating and monitoring your personal change plan throughout the semester.

✚ Safeguarding Health and Wellness

It's up to you. By learning how to maintain your wellness, evaluate health information, and spot early signs of a problem, you're more likely to get the best possible care—and to keep down your medical bills. Self-care means head-to-toe maintenance, including good oral care, informed and prudent use of over-the-counter and prescription medications, and appropriate screening tests.

Chances are that you've tried—or will try—alternative therapies. Many use a "whole-person" approach that addresses all the dimensions of wellness, not just the physical. But you need to be just as savvy a consumer when considering a complementary or alternative treatment as you would with a more mainstream one. You also need to continue "wellness practices" throughout your life so you can function at your best for as long as possible. But your future begins with the healthy choices you make today and every day.

WELLNESS COACH

✚ Making Smart Health-Care Decisions

Although you may not realize it, you make crucial decisions that affect your wellness every day. You choose what you eat, whether you exercise, if you smoke or drink, when to fasten your seat belt. You decide when to see health professionals, what to tell them, and whether to follow their advice.

The responsibility for making smart choices about your health lies with you. Never before has so much information about health been available in so many forms and formats to so many people. However, not all of it is accurate, objective, or helpful. In order to base your decisions on a solid scientific basis, you have to develop and apply your critical-thinking skills.

The following sections can help.

How Can I Find Good 🔳 Advice Online?

An estimated 85 million Americans—three in four Internet users—are "e-health" consumers who seek information or support, communicate with health-care providers, or buy medical products online.[1] "They use the Internet as an adjunct to physicians, who remain their primary source of health advice," says Mark

STUDENT SNAPSHOT

Going Online for Health Information

	Percentage
Students who have used the Internet to get health information for themselves	74%
Did so in the past day or week	15%
Did so in the last month	32%
Said that online information improved the way they took care of their health	37%
Searched for information on fitness/exercise	50%
Searched for information on diet/nutrition	47%

Based on a survey of 743 undergraduates at two southeastern universities. *Source:* Escoffery, Cam, et al. "Internet Use for Health Information among College Students." *Journal of American College Health*, Vol. 53, No. 4, January–February 2004, p. 183.

Bard, president of Manhattan Research, a health-care marketing firm.[2] As noted in Student Snapshot: "Going Online for Health Information," about three in four college students have used the Internet to get health information.[3]

According to Manhattan Research, 57 percent of doctors suggest specific sites to patients. The American College of Physicians Foundation has launched an Information Rx campaign that refers patients to a website (www.medlineplus.gov) operated by the National Library of Medicine. Table 12-1 lists some doctor-endorsed websites.

About one in four doctors uses e-mail with patients. That number is expected to grow as more physicians realize that e-mail is an efficient, effective way of communicating with patients. Contrary to assumptions, e-health consumers aren't likely to seek more health care than others. In a Stanford University study, more than 90 percent of respondents said their use of e-mail and the Internet had no effect on how often they called or visited a doctor.[4] However, the new digital age is changing the way patients use health services, with increasing numbers going online to make appointments, refill prescriptions, or view electronic medical records.[5]

If you go to other websites for medical information, here are some guidelines for evaluating them:

❚ **Check the creator.** Websites are produced by health agencies, health support groups, school health

TABLE 12-1 ▌ Doctor-Recommended Websites

National Library of Medicine: MedlinePlus   **www.medlineplus.gov**
MedlinePlus contains links to information on hundreds of health conditions and issues. The site also includes a medical dictionary, an encyclopedia with pictures and diagrams, and links to physician directories.

FDA Center for Drug Evaluation and Research   **www.fda.gov**
Click on Drugs@FDA for information on approved prescription drugs and some over-the-counter medications.

WebMD   **www.webmd.com**
WebMD is full of information to help you manage your health. The site's quizzes and calculators are a fun way to test your medical knowledge. Get diet tips, information on drugs and herbs, and check out special sections on men's and women's health.

MayoClinic   **www.mayoclinic.com**
The renowned Mayo Clinic offers a one-stop health resource website. Use the site's Health Decision Guides to make decisions about prevention and treatment. Learn more about complementary and alternative medicine, sports medicine, and senior health in the Healthy Living Centers.

Centers for Disease Control   **www.cdc.gov**
Stay up to date on the latest public health news and get the CDC's recommendations on travelers' health, vaccines and immunizations, and protecting your health in case of a disaster.

Medscape   **www.medscape.com**
Medscape delivers news and research specifically tailored to your medical interests. The site requires free registration.

---

programs, health-product advertisers, health educators, and health-education organizations. Read site headers and footers carefully to distinguish biased commercial advertisements from unbiased sites created by scientists and health agencies.

- **If you are looking for the most recent research,** check the date the page was created and last updated as well as the links. Several nonworking links signal that the site isn't carefully maintained or/updated.
- **Check the references.** As with other health-education materials, web documents should provide the reader with references. Unreferenced suggestions may be scientifically unsound and possibly unsafe.
- **Consider the author.** Is he or she recognized in the field of health education or otherwise qualified to publish a health-information web document? Does the author list his or her occupation, experience, and education?
- **Look for possible bias.** Websites may be attempting to provide health information to consumers, but they also may be attempting to sell a product. Many sites are merely disguised advertisements.

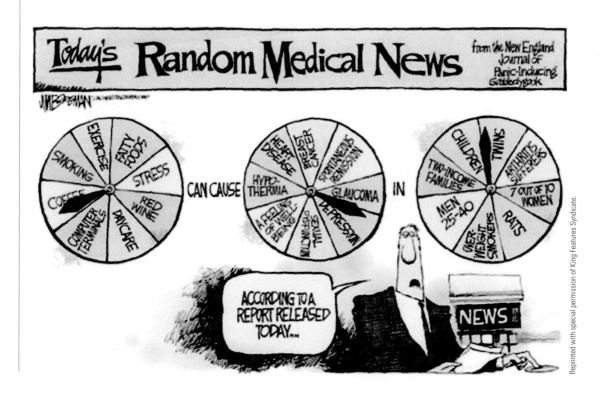

Evaluating Health News

Cure! Breakthrough! Medical miracle! These words make headlines. Remember that although medical breakthroughs and cures do occur, most scientific progress is made one small step at a time. Rather than putting your faith in the most recent report or the hottest trend, try to gather as much background information and as many opinions as you can. Weigh them carefully—ideally with a trusted physician—and make the decision that seems best for you.

When reading a newspaper or magazine story or listening to a radio or television report about a medical advance, look for answers to the following questions:

▮ **Who are the scientists involved?** Are they recognized, legitimate health professionals? What are their credentials? Are they affiliated with respected medical or scientific institutions? Be wary of individuals whose degrees or affiliations are from institutions you've never heard of, and be sure that the person's educational background is in a discipline related to the area of research reported.

▮ **Where did the scientists report their findings?** The best research is published in peer-reviewed professional journals, such as the *New England Journal of Medicine*. Research developments also may be reported at meetings of professional societies.

▮ **Is the information based on personal observations?** Does the report include testimonials from cured patients or satisfied customers? If the answer to either question is yes, be wary.

▮ **Does the article, report, or advertisement include words like *amazing, secret,* or *quick?*** Does it claim to be something the public has never seen or been offered before? Such sensationalized language is often a tip-off to a dubious treatment.

▮ **Is someone trying to sell you something?** Manufacturers who cite studies to sell a product have been known to embellish the truth.

▮ Self-Care

Most people do treat themselves. You probably prescribe aspirin for a headache, chicken soup or orange juice for a cold, or a weekend trip to unwind from stress. At the very least, you should know what your **vital signs** are and how they compare against normal readings (**Table 12-2**).

Once a thermometer was the only self-testing equipment found in most American homes. Now hundreds of home tests are available to help consumers monitor everything from fertility to blood pressure to cholesterol levels (**Table 12-3**). More convenient and less expensive than a visit to a clinic or doctor's office, the new tests are generally as accurate as those administered by a professional.

Self-care also can mean getting involved in the self-help movement, which has grown into a major national trend. An estimated 20 million people participate in self-help support groups. Many others join virtual support communities online.

TABLE 12-2 ▮ Take Your Own Vital Signs

Vital Sign	Normal Values
Temperature	The upper limit of the normal oral temperature for people 40 years old or younger is 98.9°F in the morning or 99.9°F later in the day. • Women's temperatures are slightly higher than men's. • African Americans' temperatures are slightly higher than white Americans. Measure your temperature with a mercury or digital thermometer.
Blood pressure 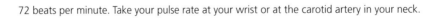	Below 120 (systolic) and below 80 (diastolic). You can measure your own blood pressure if you want to invest in blood pressure equipment. Check your local drugstore to purchase a blood pressure cuff or digital blood pressure monitor.
Pulse	72 beats per minute. Take your pulse rate at your wrist or at the carotid artery in your neck.
Respiration rate	15–20 breaths per minute.

TABLE 12-3 ▌ Home Health Tests: A Consumer's Guide

Type of Test	What It Does
Pregnancy	Determines if a woman is pregnant by detecting the presence of human chorionic gonadotropin in urine. Considered 99 percent accurate.
Fertility	Measures levels of luteinizing hormone (LH), which rise 24 to 36 hours before a woman conceives. Can help women increase their odds of conceiving.
Blood pressure	Measures blood pressure by means of an automatically inflating armband or a cuff for the finger or wrist; helps people taking hypertension medication or suffering from high blood pressure monitor their condition.
Cholesterol	Checks cholesterol in blood from a finger prick; good for anyone concerned about cholesterol.
Colon cancer	Screening test to detect hidden blood in stool; recommended for anyone over 40 or concerned about colorectal disease.
Urinary tract infection	Diagnoses infection by screening for certain white blood cells in urine; advised for women who get frequent UTIs and whose doctors will prescribe antibiotics without a visit.
HIV infection	Detects antibodies to HIV in a blood sample sent anonymously to a lab. Controversial because no face-to-face counseling is available for those who test positive.

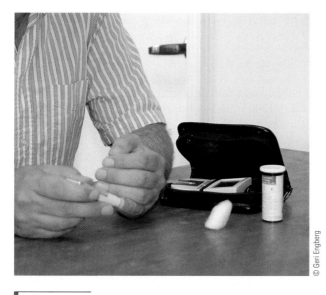

Home health tests can be more convenient and less expensive than a trip to a clinic or doctor's office.

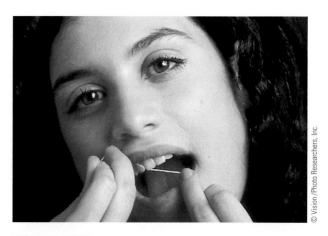

Flossing every day helps prevent gum disease and other health problems. Using a gentle sawing motion, work the floss down to your gum line. Move the floss up and down to scrape the sides of each tooth. Clean between all your teeth, using a fresh section of floss for each tooth.

✚ Oral Health

Oral health involves more than healthy teeth—it refers to the entire mouth, including all the structures that allow us to talk, bite, chew, taste, swallow, smile, scream, or scowl. Oral health is a critical part of overall health. Research has revealed links between chronic oral infection and heart and lung diseases, stroke, low birthweight, premature births, and diabetes.

Thanks to fluoridated water and toothpaste, and improved dental care, Americans' oral health is better than in the past. However, without good self-care, you probably will lose some teeth to decay and gum disease. The best way to prevent such problems is through proper and regular brushing and flossing.

Gum, or periodontal **disease** is an inflammation that attacks the gum and bone that hold your teeth in place. The culprit is **plaque,** the sticky film of bacteria that forms on teeth. More than 300 species of bacteria live under the gum line, and about half a dozen have been linked to serious gum problems. The early stage of gum disease is called **gingivitis.** If untreated, it develops into a more serious form known as **periodontitis,** in which plaque moves down the tooth to the roots, which then become infected. In advanced periodontitis, the infection destroys the bone and fibers that hold teeth in place.

STRATEGIES
for PREVENTION

Taking Care of Your Mouth

▌ Brush your teeth every morning and every night. Oral bacteria reach their highest count during sleep because fluids in the mouth accumulate. Nighttime cleaning reduces the bacterial population; morning cleaning lets you reduce the buildup.

▌ Use a toothpaste that has the American Dental Association (ADA) seal of acceptance and a toothbrush with soft, rounded bristles. Replace your toothbrush every three months.

▌ Hold the brush at a 45-degree angle from your gums. Pay particular attention to the space between your teeth and gums, especially on the inside, toward your tongue. Brush for two to five minutes. Don't brush too vigorously. If you scrub as hard as you can, you may damage your teeth and gums. Abrasion—a problem for more than half of American adults—erodes tooth surfaces, weakens teeth, and increases sensitivity to hot and cold foods.

▌ Because brushing can't reach plaque and food trapped between teeth, daily flossing is essential. Using waxed or unwaxed floss, start behind the upper and lower molars at one side of your mouth and work toward the other side.

▌ See your dentist twice a year for routine cleaning and examination. Your dentist should take a complete medical history from you and update it every six months, examine your mouth for signs of cancer, and thoroughly outline all treatment options.

▌ Make sure that everyone who works on the inside of your mouth wears a mask and rubber gloves to reduce the risk of disease transmission (that is, bacterial and viral infections, such as hepatitis, herpes, and HIV).

Symptoms of gum disease include bleeding during brushing or flossing, redness and puffiness of gums, tenderness or pain, persistent bad breath or a bad taste in the mouth, receding gums, shifted or loosened teeth, and changes in the way your teeth fit together when you bite. New treatments, which offer an alternative to traditional gum surgery, include a single antibiotic injection or the implant of a small antibiotic chip in the periodontal pockets to promote healing.

Taking care of your mouth isn't important only for dental health: It may affect how long you live. Gingivitis and periodontitis trigger an inflammatory response that causes the arteries to swell, which leads to a constriction of blood flow that can increase the incidence of cardio-vascular disease. Periodontal disease also leads to a higher white blood cell count, an indicator that the immune system is under increased stress. The good news: You can prevent these problems by flossing daily and brushing your teeth and your tongue (to get rid of bacteria that can cause gum disease and bad breath).

✚ Medications

Many of the medications and pharmaceutical products available in this country do indeed relieve symptoms and help cure various illnesses. However, as many as half of all patients take the wrong medications, in the wrong doses, at the wrong times, or in the wrong ways. Every year these inadvertent errors lead to an estimated 125,000 deaths and more than $8.5 billion in hospital costs.[6] Because drugs are powerful and increasingly marketed directly to consumers, it's important to know how to evaluate and use them appropriately.

What Should I Know About Buying Over-the-Counter Drugs?

More than half a million health products—remedies for everything from bad breath to bunions—are readily available without a doctor's prescription. This doesn't mean that they're necessarily safe or effective. Indeed, many widely used **over-the-counter (OTC) drugs** pose unsuspected hazards.

Among the most potentially dangerous is aspirin, the "wonder drug" in practically everyone's home pharmacy. When taken by someone who's been drinking (often to prevent or relieve hangover symptoms), for instance, aspirin increases blood-alcohol concentrations. (Chapter 13 defines blood-alcohol concentration.) Along with other nonsteroidal anti-inflammatory drugs, such as ibuprofen (brand names include Motrin, Advil, and Nuprin), aspirin can damage the lining of the stomach and lead to ulcers in those who take large daily doses for arthritis or other problems. Kidney problems also have been traced to some pain relievers, including acetaminophen (Tylenol).

Some health products that aren't even considered true drugs also can cause problems. Many Americans take food supplements, even though the Food and Drug Administration (FDA) has never approved their use for any medical disorder.

A growing number of drugs that once were available only with a doctor's prescription can now be bought over the counter. These include Gyne-Lotrimin and Monistat, which combat vaginal yeast infections, and famotidine (sold as Pepcid AC) and cimetidine (sold as Tagamet), which offer an alternative to antacids for people suffering from heartburn and acid indigestion.

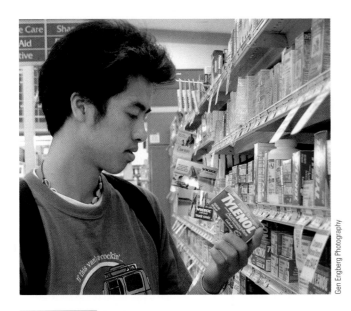

▌ OTC drugs. Practically all of these packages have warnings on the back. Read them before you use the drug.

Gen Engberg Photography

For consumers, the advantages of this greater availability include lower prices and fewer visits to the doctor. The disadvantages, however, are the risks of misdiagnosing a problem and misusing or overusing medications.

Like other drugs, OTC medications can be used improperly, often simply because of a lack of education about proper use. Among those most often misused are the following:

▌ **Nasal sprays.** Nasal sprays relieve congestion by shrinking blood vessels in the nose. If they are used too often or for too many days in a row, the blood vessels widen instead of contracting, and the surrounding tissues become swollen, causing more congestion. To make the vessels shrink again, many people use more spray more often. The result can be permanent damage to nasal membranes, bleeding, infection, and partial or complete loss of smell.

▌ **Laxatives.** Believing that they must have one bowel movement a day (a common misconception), many people rely on laxatives. Brands that contain phenolphthalein irritate the lining of the intestines and cause muscles to contract or tighten, often making constipation worse rather than better. Bulk laxatives are less dangerous, but regular use is not advised. A high-fiber diet and more exercise are safer and more effective remedies for constipation.

▌ **Eye drops.** Eye drops make the blood vessels of the eye contract. However, as in the case of nasal sprays, with overuse (several times a day for several weeks), the blood vessels expand, making the eye look redder than before.

▌ **Sleep aids.** Although OTC sleeping pills are widely used, there has been little research on their use and possible risks.

▌ **Cough syrup.** Chugging cough syrup (also called "roboing" after the OTC medication Robitussin) is a growing problem, in part because young people think of dextromethorphan (DXM), a common ingredient in cough medicine, as a "poor man's version" of the popular drug ecstasy.

Prescription Drugs

Medications are a big business in this country. However, the latest, most expensive drugs aren't necessarily the best. Each year the FDA approves about 20 new drugs, yet no more than 4 are rated as truly meaningful advances. The others often are no better or worse than what's already on the market. Some, such as the painkiller Vioxx, which has been taken off the market can cause deadly side effects. (For tips on using prescription drugs, see Savvy Consumer: "Getting the Most Out of Medications.")

College students, like other consumers, often take medicines, particularly nonprescription pain pills, without discussing them with their physicians. Both doctors and patients make mistakes when it comes to prescription drugs. The most frequent mistakes doctors make are over- or under-dosing, omitting information from prescriptions, ordering the wrong dosage form (a pill instead of a liquid, for example), and not recognizing a patient's allergy to a drug.

Nonadherence

Many prescribed medications aren't taken the way they should be; millions simply aren't taken at all. As many as 70 percent of adults have trouble understanding dosage information and 30 percent can't read standard labels, according to the FDA, which has called for larger, clearer

STRATEGIES

for PREVENTION

When You Get a Prescription

Before you leave with a prescription, be sure to ask the following questions:

▌ What is the name of the drug?

▌ What's it supposed to do?

▌ How and when do I take it? For how long?

▌ What foods, drinks, other medications, or activities should I avoid while taking this drug?

▌ Are there any side effects? What do I do if they occur?

▌ What written information is available on this drug?

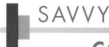

GETTING THE MOST OUT OF MEDICATIONS

"Home medication errors are a major public health problem," says Judy Smetzer, vice president of the Institute for Safe Medication Practices (ISMP). "Mistakes occur among people of all ages, both genders, and every race, occupation, level of education, and personality type." Their number-one cause: not understanding directions. Here are some common-sense precautions that can ensure that your medications help rather than harm:

■ **Keep a record of all your medicines,** listing both their brand and generic (chemical) names and the reason you are taking them, and update it regularly. If you manage medicines for others—children, spouses, elderly parents—do the same for them. Give a copy of this list to every physician and every pharmacy providing healthcare services.

■ **Inform your doctors** of any over-the-counter drugs, vitamins, and herbal products you use regularly.

■ **Keep the patient insert** that comes with your prescription. To avoid confusion, keep each medicine in its original bottle.

■ **Keep medicines high** (out of children's reach) **and dry.** The worst place is a bathroom medicine chest, where heat and humidity can break down medications so they're less effective.

■ **Always turn on the light when you take your medication.** Familiarize yourself with the imprint on each tablet or capsule so you can recognize each pill.

■ **Don't crush or chew a medicine** without checking with your doctor or pharmacist first. Some medications are designed for gradual release rather than all at once and could be harmful if absorbed too quickly.

■ **Don't use a kitchen spoon to dispense liquid medications.** Household teaspoons can hold between three and seven milligrams; a prescription "teaspoon" means five milligrams. Either measure the dose in the cup or dropper that came with the medicine or ask the pharmacist for a measuring device.

■ **Never take someone else's medications.** Even if several family members are taking the same medicine, each may be taking different strengths or doses.

■ **Don't take medicine with grapefruit juice,** which can interact with more than 200 medications, including cholesterol-lowering statins, sleeping pills, and antianxiety agents.

■ **When travelling, don't try to save space** by putting different drugs in the same bottle. Check with your doctor or pharmacist if you're changing time zones. Timing can be crucial with some medications, such as those used to treat diabetes.

■ **Keep your medications in your carry-on luggage** rather than checked baggage. Don't leave medicines in a car for prolonged periods. Temperature extremes, along with moisture, light, and oxygen, can affect the potency of many medications.

---

drug labeling. The dangers of nonadherence (not properly taking prescription drugs) include recurrent infections, serious medical complications, and emergency hospital treatment. The drugs most likely to be taken incorrectly are those that treat problems with no obvious symptoms (such as high blood pressure), require complex dosage schedules, treat psychiatric disorders, or have unpleasant side effects.

Side Effects

Most medications, taken correctly, cause only minor complications. However, no drug is entirely without side effects for all individuals taking it. Serious complications that may occur include heart failure, heart attack, seizures, kidney and liver failure, severe blood disorders, birth defects, blindness, memory problems, and allergic reactions.

Allergic reactions to drugs are common. The drugs that most often provoke allergic responses are penicillin and other antibiotics (drugs used to treat infection).

Allergic reactions range from mild rashes or hives to anaphylaxis—a life-threatening constriction of the airways and sudden drop of blood pressure. This extreme response, which is rare, requires immediate treatment with an injection of epinephrine (adrenaline) to open the airways and blood vessels.

Both over-the-counter and prescription drugs—can cause changes in the way people think, feel, and behave. Unfortunately, neither patients nor their physicians usually connect such symptoms with medications. Doctors may not even mention potential mental and emotional problems because they don't want to scare patients away from what otherwise may be a very effective treatment. What you don't know about a drug's effects on your mind *can* hurt you.

Among the medications most likely to cause psychiatric side effects are drugs for high blood pressure, heart disease, asthma, epilepsy, arthritis, Parkinson's disease, anxiety, insomnia, and depression. Some drugs—such as the powerful hormones called *corticosteroids,* used for asthma, autoimmune diseases, and cancer—can cause different psychiatric symptoms, depending on dosage and other factors.

Any medication that slows down bodily systems, as many high blood pressure and cardiac drugs do, can cause depressive symptoms. Estrogen in birth control pills can cause mood changes. As many as 15 percent of women using oral contraceptives have reported feeling depressed or moody. For many people, switching to another medication quickly lifts a drug-induced depression.

All drugs that stimulate or speed up the central nervous system can cause agitation and anxiety—including the almost 200 allergy, cold, and congestion remedies containing pseudoephedrine hydrochloride (Sudafed). Other common culprits in inducing anxiety are caffeine and theophylline, a chemical relative of caffeine found in many medications for asthma and other respiratory problems. These drugs act like mild amphetamines in the body, making people feel hyper and restless.

Drug Interactions

OTC and prescription drugs can interact in a variety of ways. For example, mixing some cold medications with tranquilizers can cause drowsiness and coordination problems, thus making driving dangerous. Moreover, what you eat or drink can impair or completely wipe out the effectiveness of drugs or lead to unexpected effects on the body. For instance, aspirin takes five to ten times as long to be absorbed when taken with food or shortly after a meal than when taken on an empty stomach.

To avoid potentially dangerous interactions, check the label(s) for any instructions on how or when to take a medication, such as "with a meal." If the directions say that you should take a drug on an empty stomach, take it at least one hour before eating or two or three hours after eating.

Whenever you take a drug, be especially careful of your intake of alcohol, which can change the rate of metabolism and the effects of many different drugs.

✚ Getting the Best Health Care

Once patients simply put their faith in physicians and assumed that they knew best and would make the correct medical decisions. Today health care has become far more complex and impersonal. Increasingly, doctors as well as consumer advocates insist that patients need to take responsibility for their own care. Rather than assuming that health care providers will do whatever is necessary and appropriate, you must take the initiative to ensure that you get quality care.

How Should I Choose My Primary Care Physician?

Why does a healthy young adult need a doctor? Answer: To stay healthy as long as possible. At some point in early adulthood, you should establish a relationship with a physician who will do basic screening tests (**Table 12-4**), record your family history, and help you prevent problems down the road.

The primary care physicians who are playing increasingly important roles in American health care include family practitioners, general internists, and pediatricians. Obstetrician-gynecologists serve as the primary providers of health care for more than half of all women. If you're a woman and your gynecologist is the only physician you see, make sure that he or she performs other tests, such as measuring your blood pressure, in addition to a pelvic and breast exam. If you develop other symptoms or health concerns, ask for an appropriate referral.

At college health centers, clinics, and some health-care organizations, consumers may be assigned to a primary physician or restricted to certain doctors. Even if your choices are limited, don't suspend your critical judg-

---

STRATEGIES *for* CHANGE

How to Talk with Your Doctor

■ Prepare in advance. Write down your questions, organize them in a logical fashion, and select the top ten queries you want answered. Make a copy of all your questions to review and leave with your doctor. (See Wellness Journal Lab.)

■ Ask about a "question hour." Many health-care practitioners set aside a specific time of day for patients with call-in questions. Find out if your college health center offers this service. Does a nurse field all calls? Can you get specific advice?

■ Go online. Many doctors' offices answer queries by e-mail. Ask your doctor if you can e-mail follow-up questions or progress reports on how you're feeling.

■ Interrupt the interrupter. If you're having difficulty explaining what's wrong, say so. If your doctor tries to put words in your mouth, say, "Please just listen so I can tell you the whole story without getting sidetracked."

TABLE 12-4 ▌ Screening Tests and Recommendations

Anemia	Beginning in adolescence, all nonpregnant women should be screened every 5–10 years until menopause.
Clinical breast exam/ mammography	Women ages 20–39 should receive a clinical breast exam every 3 years. Women age 40 and older should receive an annual clinical breast exam and mammography.
Cervical cancer screening (Pap smear)	Three years after first sexual intercourse or by age 21, whichever comes first, until age 30 women should receive an annual Pap smear. After age 30, the screening rate may decrease. See "Your Action Plan for Early Detection of Cancer" in Chapter 11.
Cholesterol and lipids	Adults over age 20 should have a lipoprotein panel test every 5 years.
Colorectal cancer screening	Adults age 50 and older should receive an annual fecal occult blood test and sigmoidoscopy every 5 years or colonoscopy every 10 years.
Type 2 diabetes	Beginning at age 45, adults should have a fasting plasma glucose test every 3 years.
Hypertension screening	Adults age 18 and older should have an annual blood pressure (BP) check. If the BP is less than 130/85, then it should be checked every 2 years. If the BP is between 130–139/85–89, then it should be checked annually. After age 60, BP should be checked annually.
Osteoporosis	Women age 65 and older should have a baseline bone mineral density test. To reduce the risk of fractures, women should increase dietary calcium and vitamin D, perform weight bearing exercise, stop smoking, and moderate alcohol intake.
Prostate cancer screening	Men age 50 and older should discuss potential benefits and known harms of screening with prostate-specific antigen (PSA) test and digital rectal exam.
Skin cancer screening	Between the ages of 20–39, adults should receive a skin exam every 3 years. After age 40, adults should receive an annual skin exam.
Visual exam	Adults age 18–40 years should have a complete visual examination every 2–3 years; ages 41–60, every 2 years; and ages 61 and older, every year.

ment. If your assigned physician does not listen to your concerns or is not providing adequate care, you can—and should—request another physician. Your rapport with your primary physician and the feelings of mutual trust and respect that develop between you can have as much of an impact on your well-being as your doctor's technical expertise.

One key to making the health-care system work for you lies in choosing a good physician. After seeing your primary care physician, ask yourself the following questions to evaluate the quality of care you are getting.

▌ Did your physician take a comprehensive history? Was the physical examination thorough?

▌ Did your physician explain what he or she was doing during the exam?

▌ Did he or she spend enough time with you?

▌ Did you feel free to ask questions? Did your physician give you straight answers? Did he or she reassure you when you were worried?

▌ Does your physician seem willing to admit that he or she doesn't know the answers to some questions?

▌ Does your physician hesitate to refer you to a specialist even when you have a complex problem that warrants such care?

Look back at your answers. If they make you feel uneasy, have a talk with your physician. Or find a physician or a health plan that provides better service.

Health Care and the College Student

All of the more than 14 million men and women enrolled in institutions of higher learning need some health-care services, regardless of their age or general health. The Preventive Services Task Force of the U.S. Public Health Service recommends that all adolescents and young adults have periodic screenings for high blood pressure, obesity, and problem alcohol consumption and that they receive regular counseling concerning the use of drugs, tobacco, and alcohol; sexually transmitted infections; effective contraception; a healthy diet; exercise; oral health; and prevention of motor vehicle injuries and other accidents.

✚ Complementary and Alternative Medicine

The medical research community uses the term **complementary and alternative medicine (CAM)** to apply to all health-care approaches, practices, and treatments not widely taught in medical schools and not generally used in hospitals.[7] CAM includes many healing philosophies, approaches, and therapies, including preventive techniques designed to delay or prevent serious health problems before they start and **holistic** methods that focus on the whole person and the physical, mental, emotional, and spiritual aspects of well-being. Some approaches are based on the same physiological principles as traditional Western methods; others, such as acupuncture, are based on different healing systems.

According to a recent nationwide government survey of more than 31,000 adults aged 18 and over, 50 percent have used CAM at some time and 46 percent have tried some form of complementary and alternative medicine in the last year. When CAM includes megavitamins and prayer specifically for health, the number reporting they ever used some form of CAM rises to 75 percent; 62 percent did so in the past year.[8]

CAM use varies among different groups. Those most likely to use CAM include women; people with higher education; those hospitalized within the past year; and former smokers (compared to current smokers or those who never smoked). African-American adults are more likely than white or Asian-American adults to use CAM practices, including megavitamin therapy and prayer (**Figure 12-1**).

Some states have mandated health insurance coverage for CAM therapies, which also are becoming more common in Canada and Europe. Many medical schools now include training in CAM in their curricula. **Integrative medicine,** which combines selected elements of both conventional and alternative medicine in a comprehensive approach to diagnosis and treatment, has gained greater acceptance within the medical community.

Why People Use CAM Therapies

Rather than turning to CAM as an alternative to conventional treatments, consumers combine the two approaches. About half (55 percent of those surveyed) use CAM because they believe that it could help them when combined with conventional medical care, 50 percent thought CAM would be interesting to try. Almost one in three (28 percent) used CAM because they believed conventional medical treatments would not help their health problem. About a quarter used CAM because a conventional medical professional suggested it; 13 percent turned to CAM because they felt that conventional medicine was too expensive.

Consumers turn to CAM most often for chronic or recurring pain—of the back, neck, or joints—and for colds, anxiety, or depression. Most use CAM as a form of self-care; only about 12 percent seek care from a licensed CAM practitioner, suggesting that most people who use CAM do so without consulting a practitioner. According to the survey, the ten most commonly used CAM therapies are:

- **Prayer** for own health (used by 43 percent)
- **Prayer by others** for the respondent's health (24 percent)
- **Natural products,** such as herbs, other botanicals, and enzymes (19 percent)
- **Deep-breathing** exercises (12 percent)
- **Participation in prayer** group for own health (10 percent)
- **Meditation** (8 percent)
- **Chiropractic care** (8 percent)
- **Yoga** (5 percent)
- **Massage** (5 percent)
- **Diet-based therapies,** such as Atkins, Pritikin, Ornish, and Zone diets (4 percent)

Individuals with a psychiatric disorder are significantly more likely to use a CAM therapy than the general population. Those with severe depression or anxiety disorders use CAM most often. Most patients who use CAM for mental health problems also use conventional therapies. The most popular CAM therapies in mental health care are relaxation techniques and "spiritual healing." The efficacy and safety of most CAM therapies used to self-treat or treat mental health problems are not yet established.

An estimated 10 to 50 percent of cancer patients try alternative treatments, many without their physicians' knowledge. These include dietary changes, antioxidant vitamins, soy, herbs, and other natural products, acupuncture, massage, exercise, and psychologic and mind-

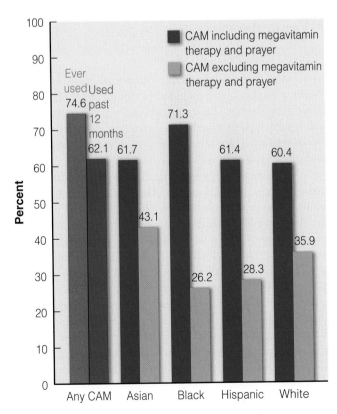

FIGURE 12-1 | CAM Use by U.S. Adults and by Race/Ethnicity

Source: NCCAM, http://nccam.nih.gov.

body interventions. Based on the best evidence available, cancer specialists have ranked these approaches on a continuum ranging from "recommend" to "discourage."

A reduction in dietary fat was deemed acceptable, but the use of antioxidant vitamins A, C, and E may cause more harm than benefit because of the risks of cancer progression and effects on blood clotting. Doctors discourage the use of soy supplements in women with breast cancer but accept their use by men with prostate cancer. The efficacy of shark cartilage remains unclear. Acupuncture was deemed acceptable to help control chemotherapy-related nausea and vomiting among cancer patients. Massage has not demonstrated any positive effect on cancer progression or pain relief. Psychologic and mind-body therapies such as individual and group therapy, relaxation, imagery, hypnosis, and meditation can relieve distress and pain as well as some of the physical symptoms of disease and side effects of conventional therapy.

What Should I Know Before I Try CAM?

You should never decide on any treatment—traditional or CAM—without fully evaluating it. Here are some key questions to ask:

▌ **Is it safe?** Be particularly wary of unregulated products.
▌ **Is it effective?** Check the website of the National Center for CAM: http://nccam.nih.gov.
▌ **Will it interact with other medicines or conventional treatments?** Many widely used alternative remedies can interact with prescription medications in dangerous ways.
▌ **Is the practitioner qualified?** Find out if your state licenses practitioners who provide acupuncture, chiropractic services, naturopathy, herbal medicine, homeopathy, and other treatments.
▌ **What has been the experience of others?** Talk to people who have used CAM for a similar problem, both recently and in the past.
▌ **Can you talk openly and easily with the practitioner?** You should feel comfortable asking questions and confident in the answers you receive. And the practitioner's office should put you at ease.
▌ **What are the costs?** Many CAM services are not covered by HMOs or health insurers.

Types of CAM

The National Center for Complementary and Alternative Medicine (NCCAM) has classified CAM therapies into five categories (**Figure 12-2**).

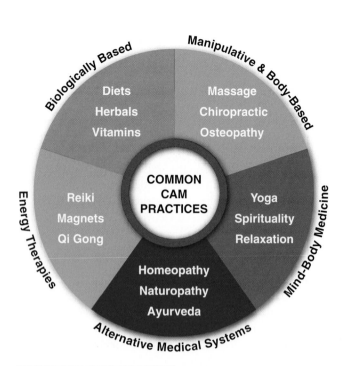

FIGURE 12-2 ▌ The Five Categories of CAM

Source: NCCAM, http://nccam.nih.gov.

▌ **Alternative medical systems**
▌ **Mind-body medicine**
▌ **Biologically based therapies**
▌ **Manipulative and body-based methods**
▌ **Energy therapies**

Alternative Medical Systems

Systems of theory and practice other than traditional Western medicine are included in this group. They include acupuncture, Eastern medicine, t'ai chi, external and internal qi, Ayurvedic medicine, naturopathy, and unconventional Western systems, such as homeopathy and orthomolecular medicine.

Acupuncture is an ancient Chinese form of medicine, based on the philosophy that a cycle of energy circulating through the body controls health. Pain and disease are the result of a disturbance in the energy flow, which can be corrected by inserting long, thin needles at specific points along longitudinal lines, or *meridians,* throughout the body. Each point controls a different corresponding part of the body. Once inserted, the needles are rotated gently back and forth or charged with a small electric current for a short time. Western scientists aren't sure exactly how acupuncture works, but some believe that the needles alter the functioning of the nervous system.

A National Institute of Health (NIH) consensus development panel that evaluated current research into acupuncture concluded that there is "clear evidence" that acupuncture can control nausea and vomiting in patients after surgery or while undergoing chemotherapy and

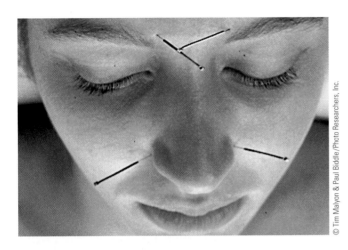

▌ The ancient Chinese practice of acupuncture produces healing through the insertion and manipulation of needles at specific points throughout the body.

relieve postoperative dental pain. The panel said that acupuncture is "probably" also effective in the control of nausea in early pregnancy and that there were "reasonable" studies showing satisfactory treatment of addiction to illicit drugs and alcohol (but not to tobacco), stroke rehabilitation, headache, menstrual cramps, tennis elbow, general muscle pain, low-back pain, carpal tunnel syndrome, and asthma. Ongoing studies are evaluating its efficacy for chronic headaches and migraines.

Considered alternative here, **Ayurveda** is a traditional form of medical treatment in India, where it has evolved over thousands of years. Its basic premise is that illness stems from incorrect mental attitudes, diet, and posture. Practitioners use a discipline of exercise, meditation, herbal medication, and proper nutrition to cope with such stress-induced conditions as hypertension, the desire to smoke, and obesity.

Homeopathy is based on three fundamental principles: like cures like; treatment must always be individualized; and less is more—the idea that increasing dilution (and lowering the dosage) can increase efficacy. By administering doses of animal, vegetable, or mineral substances to a large number of healthy people to see if they all develop the same symptoms, homeopaths determine which substances may be given, in small quantities, to alleviate the symptoms. Some of these substances are the same as those used in conventional medicine: nitroglycerin for certain heart conditions, for example, although the dose is minuscule.

Naturopathy emphasizes natural remedies, such as sun, water, heat, and air, as the best treatments for disease. Therapies might include dietary changes (such as more vegetables and no salt or stimulants), steam baths, and exercise. Some naturopathic physicians (who are not M.Ds) work closely with medical doctors in helping patients.

Mind-Body Medicine

Mind-body medicine uses techniques designed to enhance the mind's capacity to affect bodily function and symptoms. Some techniques that were considered alternative in the past have become mainstream (for example, patient support groups and cognitive-behavioral therapy). Other mind-body approaches are still considered CAM, including meditation, prayer (see Chapter 7), mental healing, and therapies that use creative outlets such as art, music, or dance.

Biofeedback uses machines that measure temperature or skin responses and then relay this information to the subject. In this way, people can learn to control usually involuntary functions, such as circulation to the hands and feet, tension in the jaws, and heartbeat rates. Biofeedback has been used to treat dozens of ailments, including asthma, epilepsy, pain, and Reynaud's disease (a condition in which the fingers become painful and white when exposed to cold). Many health insurers now cover biofeedback treatments.

Creative **visualization,** or imaging, helps patients, including some diagnosed as terminally ill with cancer, heal. On the premise that positive and negative beliefs and attitudes have a great deal to do with whether people get well or die of disease, patients imagine themselves getting well—they "see," for instance, immune-system cells marching to conquer cancer cells. Other patients use visualization in different ways—for example, to create a clear idea of what they want to achieve, whether the goal is weight loss or relaxation.

Biologically Based Therapies

Biologically based CAM therapies use substances such as herbs, foods, and vitamins. They include botanical medicine or phytotherapy, the use of individual herbs or combinations; special diet therapies, such as macrobiotics, Ornish, McDougall, and high fiber; Mediterranean orthomolecular medicine (use of nutritional and food supplements for preventive or therapeutic purposes); and use of other products (such as shark cartilage) and procedures applied in an unconventional manner.

Herbal medicine has become an estimated $4 billion-a-year industry, yet questions about the safety and effectiveness of herbal supplements persist. Although more than 1,500 different preparations are on the U.S. market, just a few single-herb preparations account for about half the sales in the United States: echinacea, garlic, ginkgo, ginseng, kava, St. John's wort, and valerian. Unlike medications, herbal products are exempt from the FDA's regulatory scrutiny. The ingredients and the potency of active ingredients can vary from batch to batch.

Rigorous research studies are producing the first scientific evidence on the safety and efficacy of herbal sup-

TABLE 12-5 ▮ Evidence-Based Evaluations of Herbal Supplements

Herb	Evidence
Saw Palmetto	Reduces an enlarged prostate, but the effect is small compared with prescription medication
Ginseng	No demonstrated benefits or proven effect on energy
Echinacea	No proven benefits as a cold remedy; can trigger an allergic reaction
Kava	May reduce anxiety but can cause liver damage
Gingko biloba	No improvement in memory or thinking in the healthy elderly but a small benefit for patients with dementia
Garlic	Lowers cholesterol when taken in higher doses than you would get with food; much less effective than cholesterol-lowering medications
Black Cohosh	Currently under study as a treatment for hot flashes; long-term effects unknown

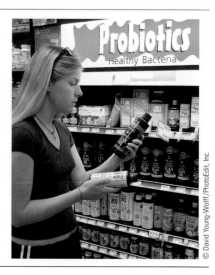

© David Young-Wolff/PhotoEdit, Inc.

plements.[9] Their benefits, if any, have proved modest (Table 12-5). Ginkgo biloba, for instance, temporarily boosts memory, but no more so than eating a candy bar.[10] Other agents, such as saw palmetto or garlic, produce slight benefits, but far less than available medications.

Most of the herbs tested have proved generally safe, although side effects such as headaches and nausea can occur. However, some herbs can cause serious, even fatal dangers. Echinacea, widely used as a cold remedy, may cause liver damage if taken in combination with anabolic steroids.

Several widely used herbs, including ginger, garlic, and ginkgo, are dangerous if taken prior to surgery—yet it's been estimated that more than 70 percent of patients fail to disclose their use of herbal medicine before an operation. Herbs such as ginseng and goldenseal can cause unexpected rises in blood pressure and heart rate during an operation, while St. John's wort and kava may interact with and prolong anesthesia medications. All herbal supplements should be discontinued for periods of several days or longer prior to surgery.

The most dangerous herbal products, sold as ephedra, ma huang, sinica, and sida cordifolia, contain ephedrine, which stimulates the heart to beat faster and increases blood pressure. Ephedra has been linked with dozens of deaths and more than 1,000 adverse reactions. In 2004, the FDA prohibited the sale of dietary supplements containing ephedra.[11] The FDA has issued warnings on other potentially dangerous herbs, including chaparral, comfrey, yohimbe, lobelia, germander, willow bark, jin bu huan, and products containing magnolia or stephania.[12]

Manipulative and Body-Based Methods

CAM therapies based on manipulation and/or movement of the body are divided into three subcategories:

▮ **Chiropractic medicine**
▮ **Massage and body work** (including osteopathic manipulation, Swedish massage, Alexander technique, reflexology, Pilates, acupressure, and rolfing)
▮ **Unconventional physical therapies** (including colonics, hydrotherapy, and light and color therapies)

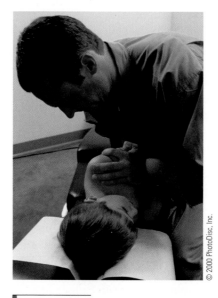

© 2000 PhotoDisc, Inc.

▮ People often turn to chiropractors for pain relief following an injury.

Chiropractic is a treatment method based on the theory that many human diseases are caused by misalignment of the bones (subluxation). Chiropractors are licensed in all 50 states, but chiropractic is considered a mainstream therapy by some and a form of CAM by others. Significant research in the last ten years has demonstrated its efficacy for acute lower-back pain. NIH is funding research on other potential benefits, including headaches, asthma, middle ear inflammation, menstrual cramps, and arthritis.

Chiropractors, who emphasize wellness and healing without drugs or surgery, may use X rays and magnetic resonance imaging (MRI) as well as orthopedic, neurological, and manual examinations in making diagnoses. However, chiropractic treatment consists solely of the manipulation of misaligned bones that may be putting pressure on nerve tissue and affecting other parts of the body. Many HMOs offer chiropractic services, which are the most widely used alternative treatment among managed care patients.

Massage therapy is the manipulation of body tissues to promote wellness and reduce pain and stress. Techniques include stroking and kneading, as in Swedish massage, and applying pressure to specific areas, as used in Shiatsu and acupuncture. It has been shown helpful in relieving pain and muscle soreness, controlling asthma, relieving constipation, and lowering stress and anxiety.

In *acupressure,* the therapist uses his or her finger and thumb to stimulate certain points, relieve pain, and relax muscles. **Reflexology** is based on the theory that massaging certain points on the foot or hand relieves stress or pain in corresponding parts of the body.

Massage appears to be an effective way to treat back pain according to a new, in-depth review of evidence from dozens of studies of alternative treatments. Spinal manipulation (commonly done by chiropractors and osteopaths) has small clinical benefits for back pain—about the same as conventional medical treatments such as over-the-counter pain relievers and various types of physical therapy.[13]

Energy Therapies

Various approaches focus on energy fields believed to exist in and around the body. Some use external energy sources, such as electromagnetic fields. Magnets are marketed to relieve pain but there is little scientific evidence of their efficacy. Others, such as therapeutic touch, use a therapist's healing energy to repair imbalances in an individual's biofield.

Aging Well

Too young to worry about getting old? Think again. Whether you're in your teens, twenties, thirties, or older, now is the time to start taking the steps that will add healthy, active, productive years to your life.

Aging—the characteristic pattern of normal life changes that occurs as humans, plants, and animals grow older—remains inevitable. However, at any age, at any stage of life, at any level of fitness, you can do a great deal to influence the impact that the passage of time has on you. More and more Americans are extending not just their lifespan but also their *health span*—their years of health and vitality. You can do the same.

How Long Can I Expect to Live?

The answer depends on you. Statistically, you're likely to live longer than your parents or grandparents. Life expectancy has been increasing steadily over the last century, reaching an all-time high in the United States of 77.4 years.[14] (As **Table 12-6** indicates, the United States is not in the top five countries.) A child born in the United States in 2020 should expect to live 79.25 years; one born in 2050, 82.91 years.

Women's lifespans average 5 to 10 percent longer than men's. No one knows exactly why. But the gender gap in longevity narrows over time. At birth a baby boy has a life expectancy about five years shorter than a girl's. By age 65, a man can expect to live an additional 15.1 years, just 3.8 years less than a woman. By age 85, the difference in projected life expectancies is down to 1.2 years.

Staying Healthy Longer

If you want to feel young when you're older, the time to start taking care of yourself is now—whether you're 19, 29, 49, or 69. The healthier you become now, the longer you're likely to stay healthy in the future.

Genes, as studies of identical twins have revealed, influence only about 30 percent of the rate and ways in which we age. "The rest is up to us," says Michael Roizen,

TABLE 12-6 | Life Expectancies Around the World (in years)

Top 5		Bottom 5	
Japan	81.6	Zambia	32.4
Sweden	80.1	Botswana	39.7
Hong Kong	79.9	Afghanistan	43.1
Iceland	79.8	Ethiopia	45.5
Canada	79.3	Laos	54.5

M.D., author of *You: The Owner's Manual,* who notes that it's possible to turn back the biological clock. "With relatively simple changes, someone whose chronological age is 69 can have a physiological age of 45. And the most amazing thing is that it's never too late to live younger— until one foot is six feet under." [15]

Keep Your Arteries Young

"You are as young—or as old—as your arteries," says Roizen. Problems like high blood pressure, high cholesterol, and buildup of atherosclerotic plaque increase the likelihood of stroke, heart disease, kidney problems, even memory impairment. If your arteries are healthy, you're much more likely to have a healthy heart and a healthy brain. People with "young" arteries tend to retain a higher level of cognitive functioning.

Premature aging of the arteries is largely self-inflicted; common culprits are a high-fat diet, lack of exercise, obesity, and a high-stress lifestyle. At any age, the un-exercised body—though free of the symptoms of illness —will rust out long before it could ever wear out. Inactivity can make anyone old before his or her time. Just as inactivity accelerates aging, activity slows it down. The effects of ongoing activity are so profound that gerontologists sometimes refer to exercise as "the closest thing to an antiaging pill." Exercise can reverse many of the changes that occur with age, including increases in body fat and decreases in muscle strength. The bottom line: What you *don't* do may matter more than what you do do. [16]

Exercise slows many changes associated with advancing age, such as loss of lean muscle tissue, increase in body fat, and decreased work capacity. It lowers the risk of heart disease and stroke in the elderly—and greatly improves general health. Male and female runners over age 50 have much lower rates of disability and much lower health-care expenses than less active seniors. Even less intense activities, such as gardening, dancing, and brisk walking, can delay chronic physical disability and cognitive decline.

Avoid Illness

In studies of centenarians, most have had no serious chronic illnesses. Among the most important strategies: not smoking, avoiding weight gain in middle age, and recognizing and treating conditions like elevated cholesterol and high blood pressure.

Also important is keeping up with immunizations against diseases, such as influenza and pneumococcal pneumonia, that take a greater toll on the elderly. For women at risk of osteoporosis, new options, including "designer estrogens" like raloxifene, can preserve their bones' health. A healthy diet, chockful of fruits and vegetables, also can contribute to a healthy old age, in part because they contain antioxidants that may ward off many age-related problems.

Maintain Your Zest for Living

Age may indeed be a matter of attitude. The healthiest seniors are "engaged" in life, resilient, optimistic, productive, and socially involved. While they are not immune to life's slings and arrows, successful agers bounce back after a setback and have a "can-do" attitude about the challenges they face. They also tend to be lifelong learners who may take up entirely new hobbies late in life— pursuits that stimulate production of more connections between neurons and may slow aging within the brain.

Just as with muscles, the best advice to keep your brain healthy as you age is "use it or lose it." Some memory losses among healthy older people are normal—but reversible with training in simple methods, such as word associations, that improve recall.

Stay Strong

For years, experts assumed that older meant weaker. Landmark research with frail nursing home residents in their eighties and nineties showed this isn't so. After just

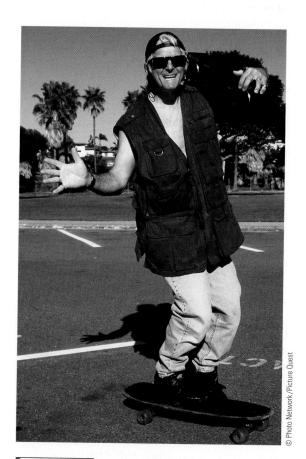

▌ Age is just a matter of attitude.

eight to ten weeks of strength training, even the oldest seniors increased muscle and bone, speeded up their metabolic rate, improved sleep and mobility, boosted their spirits, and gained in self-confidence. Other studies have found that exercise programs can increase lung capacity, double leg strength, and decrease the risk of disability and premature death.

The Challenges of Age

No matter how well we eat, exercise, and take care of ourselves, some physical changes are inevitable as we age. Aging brains and bodies also become vulnerable to diseases like Alzheimer's and osteoporosis.

Alzheimer's Disease

About 15 percent of older Americans lose previous mental capabilities, a brain disorder called **dementia.** Sixty percent of these—a total of 4 million men and women over age 65—suffer from the type of dementia called **Alzheimer's disease,** a progressive deterioration of brain cells and mental capacity.

The percentage of people with Alzheimer's doubles for every five-year age group beyond 65. By age 85, nearly half of men and women have Alzheimer's. A person with the disease typically lives eight years after the onset of symptoms, but some live as long as 20 years. Some 13.2 million older Americans will develop Alzheimer's disease by 2050, up from 4.5 million today. The greatest increase will be among people age 85 and older.

Women are more likely to develop Alzheimer's than men, and women with Alzheimer's perform significantly worse than men in various visual, spatial, and memory tests. Initiating hormone therapy after age 60 increases the risk of Alzheimer's disease, but earlier use may reduce a woman's risk of this devastating illness.[17]

African Americans have higher rates of Alzheimer's disease than Africans living in Africa, according to the first study to find differences in the incidence of this illness in an industrial and a non-industrial country.

The early signs of dementia—insomnia, irritability, increased sensitivity to alcohol and other drugs, and decreased energy and tolerance of frustration—are usually subtle and insidious. Diagnosis requires a comprehensive assessment of an individual's medical history, physical health, and mental status, often involving brain scans and a variety of other tests.[18]

Even though medical science cannot restore a brain that is in the process of being destroyed by an organic brain disease like Alzheimer's, medications can control difficult behavioral symptoms and enhance or partially restore cognitive ability. Often physicians find other medical or psychiatric problems, such as depression, in these patients; recognizing and treating these conditions can have a dramatic impact.

The FDA has approved several prescription drugs for people with mild to moderate Alzheimer's, including Cognex, Aricept, Exelon, and Reminyl. They all increase the level of the brain chemical acetylcholine. Researchers are studying other medications that might delay Alzheimer's or stop its progression.

Osteoporosis

Another age-related disease is **osteoporosis,** a condition in which losses in bone density become so severe that a bone will break after even slight trauma or injury. A chronic disease, osteoporosis is silent for years or decades before a fracture occurs.

Women, who have smaller skeletons, are more vulnerable than men; in extreme cases, their spines may become so fragile that just bending causes severe pain. But although commonly seen as an illness of women, osteoporosis occurs frequently in men. One in every two women and one in four men over 50 will have an osteoporosis-related fracture in their lifetime (**Figure 12-3**).[19] An estimated 44 million men and women aged 50 and older currently have osteoporosis or low bone mass.[20]

Osteoporosis doesn't begin in old age. The bone weakness that increases the risk of osteoporosis may actu-

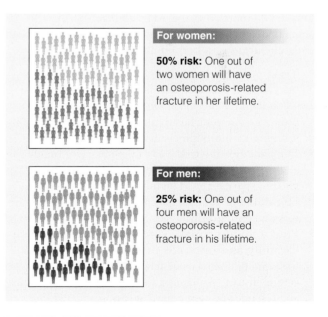

For women:

50% risk: One out of two women will have an osteoporosis-related fracture in her lifetime.

For men:

25% risk: One out of four men will have an osteoporosis-related fracture in his lifetime.

FIGURE 12-3 ▎ Bone Fracture Risk in Women and Men

STRATEGIES for PREVENTION

Lowering Your Risk of Osteoporosis

Regardless of your age and gender, you can prevent future bone problems by taking some protective steps now. The most important guidelines are as follows:

- Get adequate calcium. See Chapter 8.

- Exercise regularly. Both aerobic exercise and weight training can help preserve bone density.

- Limit alcohol. More than two alcoholic beverages a day impairs intestinal calcium absorption.

- Don't smoke. Smokers tend to be thin (a risk factor for osteoporosis) and enter menopause earlier, thus extending the period of jeopardy from estrogen loss.

- Let the sunshine in (but don't forget your sunscreen). Vitamin D, a vitamin produced in the skin in reaction to sunlight, boosts calcium absorption.

ally begin before birth. Infants undernourished in the womb are small when born, remain smaller than their age peers at age 1, have low bone mass at 25, and an increased risk of fractures in late adulthood.[21]

The ideal time to start preventing osteoporosis is adolescence and young adulthood. You can strengthen your bones and reduce your risk of osteoporosis by increasing your calcium intake and physical activity.

Various factors can increase a woman's risk of developing osteoporosis, including a family history (a mother, grandmother, or sister with osteoporosis, fractures, height loss, or humped shoulders); petite body structure; white or Asian background; menopause before age 40; smoking; heavy alcohol consumption; loss of ovarian function through chemotherapy, radiation, or hysterectomy; low calcium intake; and a sedentary lifestyle.

MAKING HEALTHY CHOICES

To Live Long and Well

You can do more to safeguard and enhance your well-being than any health-care provider. Here are some recommendations to keep in mind:

- **Trust your instincts.** You know your body better than anyone else. If something is bothering you, it deserves medical attention. Don't let your health-care provider—or your health plan administrator—dismiss it without a thorough evaluation.

- **Do your homework.** Go to the library or online and find authoritative articles that describe what you're experiencing. The more you know about possible causes of your symptoms, the more likely you are to be taken seriously.

- **Find a good primary care physician who listens carefully and responds to your concerns.** Look for a family doctor or general internist who takes a careful history, performs a thorough exam, and listens and responds to your concerns.

- **See your doctor regularly.** If you're in your twenties or thirties, you may not need an annual exam, but it's important to get checkups at least every two or three years so you and your doctor can get to know

each other and develop a trusting, mutually respectful relationship.

- **Get a second opinion.** If you are uncertain of whether to undergo treatment or which therapy is best, see another physician and listen carefully for any doubts or hesitation about what you're considering.

- **Seek support.** Patient support and advocacy groups can offer emotional support, information on many common problems, and referral to knowledgeable physicians.

- **If your doctor cannot or will not respond to your concerns, get another one.** Regardless of your health coverage, you have the right to replace a physician who is not meeting your health-care needs.

- **Speak up.** If you don't understand, ask. If you feel that you're not being taken seriously or being treated with respect, say so. Sometimes the only difference between being a patient or becoming a victim is making sure your needs and rights are not forgotten or overlooked.

- **Bring your own advocate.** If you become intimidated or anxious talking to physicians, ask a friend to accompany you, to ask questions on your behalf, and to take notes.

SELF-SURVEY

Are You a Savvy Health-Care Consumer?

1. You want a second opinion, but your doctor dismisses your request for other physicians' names as unnecessary. Do you:
   a. Assume that he or she is right and you would merely be wasting time.
   b. Suspect that your physician has something to hide and immediately switch doctors.
   c. Contact your health plan and request a second opinion.

2. As soon as you enter your doctor's office, you get tongue-tied. When you try to find the words to describe what's wrong, your physician keeps interrupting. When giving advice, your doctor uses such technical language that you can't understand what it means. Do you:
   a. Prepare better for your next appointment.
   b. Pretend that you understand what your doctor is talking about.
   c. Decide you'd be better off with someone who specializes in complementary/alternative therapies and seems less intimidating.

3. You feel like you're running on empty, tired all the time, worn to the bone. A friend suggests some herbal supplements that promise to boost energy and restore vitality. Do you:
   a. Immediately start taking them.
   b. Say that you think herbs are for cooking.
   c. Find out as much as you can about the herbal compounds and ask your doctor if they're safe and effective.

4. Your hometown physician's office won't give you a copy of your medical records to take with you to college. Do you:
   a. Hope you won't need them and head off without your records.
   b. Threaten to sue.
   c. Politely ask the office administrator to tell you the particular law or statute that bars you from your records.

5. Your doctor has been treating you for an infection for three weeks, and you don't seem to be getting any better. Do you:
   a. Talk to your doctor, by phone or in person, and say, "This doesn't seem to be working. Is there anything else we can try?"
   b. Stop taking the antibiotic.
   c. Try an herbal remedy that your roommate recommends.

6. Your doctor suggests a cutting-edge treatment for your condition, but your health plan or HMO refuses to pay for it. Do you:
   a. Try to get a loan to cover the costs.
   b. Settle for whatever treatment options are covered.
   c. Challenge your health plan.

7. You call for an appointment with your doctor and are told nothing is available for four months. Do you:
   a. Take whatever time you can get whenever you can get it.
   b. Explain your condition to the nurse or receptionist, detailing any symptoms and pain you're experiencing.
   c. Give up and decide you don't need to see a doctor at all.

8. Even though you've been doing sit-ups faithfully, your waist still looks flabby. When you see an ad for waist-whittling liposuction, do you:
   a. Call for an appointment.
   b. Talk to a health-care professional about a total fitness program that may help you lose excess pounds.
   c. Carefully research the risks and costs of the procedure.

9. You have a condition that you do not want anyone to know about, including your health insurer and any potential employer. Do you:
   a. Use a false name.
   b. Give your physician a written request for confidentiality about this condition.
   c. Seek help outside the health-care system.

10. Your doctor suggests a biopsy of a funny-looking mole that's sprouted on your nose. Rather than using a laboratory that specializes in skin analysis, your HMO requires that all samples be sent to a general lab, where results may not be as precise. Do you:
    a. Ask your doctor to request that a specialty pathologist at the general lab perform the analysis.
    b. Hope that in your case, the general lab will do a good enough job.
    c. Threaten to change HMOs.

Answers:

1: c; 2: a; 3: c; 4: c; 5: a; 6: c; 7: b; 8: b and c; 9: b; 10: a

ACTION PLAN

Your Action Plan for Protecting Yourself from Medical Mistakes and Misdeeds

Just as physicians practice "defensive" medicine to protect themselves from legal liability, today's patients should take preventive steps to defend themselves from potentially harmful health services.

The Whats, Whys, and Hows of Medical Testing

▮ Before undergoing any test, find out why you need it. Get a specific answer, not a "just in case" or "for your peace of mind." If you've had the test before, could the earlier results be used? Would a follow-up exam be just as helpful?

▮ Get some practical information as well: Should you do specific things before the test (such as not eat for a specified period)? How long will the test take? What will the test feel like? Will you need help getting home afterward?

▮ Check out the risks. Any invasive test—one that penetrates the body with a needle, tube, or viewing instrument—involves some risk of infection, bleeding, or tissue damage. Tests involving radiation also present risks, and some people develop allergic reactions to the materials used in testing.

▮ Get information on the laboratory that will be evaluating the test. Ask how often *false positives* or *false negatives* occur. (False positives are abnormal results indicating that you have a particular condition when you really don't; false negatives indicate that you don't have a particular condition when you really do.) Find out about civil or criminal *negligence* suits filed against the laboratory on charges such as failing to diagnose cervical cancer because of incorrect reading of Pap smears.

▮ You'll also want to know what happens when the test indicates a problem: Will the test be repeated? Will a different test be performed? Will treatment begin immediately? Could any medications you're taking (including nonprescription drugs, like aspirin) affect the testing procedures or results?

▮ If you have a test, don't assume that no news is good news. Check back to get the results.

SETTING GOALS

Setting Self-Care Goals

Your Personal Self-Care Goal:

Is It S.M.A.R.T.?
  Specific? _____
  Measurable? _____
  Achievable? _____
  Rewarding? _____
  Time Defined? _____

Strategies for Success
  1. _____
  2. _____
  3. _____

Potential Obstacles
  1. _____
  2. _____
  3. _____

Ways Around Them
  1. _____
  2. _____
  3. _____

Daily Report

The Week that Was:

What Went Right?
What Could I Do Better?

WELLNESS JOURNAL

Things to Tell Your Doctor

Many people feel flustered or anxious during a medical exam and forget to bring up questions they would like answered or ask for information the doctor should have. In your Wellness Journal, start jotting down notes that you can use to make the most of your next visit to the doctor.

    Here are some topics to get you started:

▮ **Any changes you've noticed**. Is there something you once did but no longer can, such as climb the stairs without breathing hard or use your computer without feeling pain in your wrist? Lab tests or a physical examination won't reveal such symptoms. If you don't tell your doctor about them, you may be missing out on treatments that could help.

▮ **Any fears you have.** If your mother had breast cancer or your father had a heart attack at a young age, you may be afraid that the same will happen to you. Your doctor needs to know what you're afraid of and why in order to provide the information and care you need to stay well.

▪ **Over-the-counter pills and supplements.** Patients often forget to tell doctors about nonprescription medications or deliberately conceal their use of herbal medications. Yet both can have dangerous interactions with conventional medications.

▪ **Medications prescribed by other doctors.** Your family doctor may have prescribed allergy or asthma medications that you've been taking for years. Bring a list or the pill bottles themselves to the physician who is providing your current care. Also let your doctor know about medications you were supposed to take but don't—maybe because of side effects, maybe because you don't like taking pills. Your physician needs to know the whole story.

▪ **If you smoke or drink heavily.** You may be embarrassed because you know your doctor won't approve, but your use of tobacco or alcohol can affect your health and your medical treatments.

▪ **If you've been depressed or under stress.** Many people still don't like to admit they're depressed or overwhelmed. But talking about your feelings can be the first step to feeling better.

▪ **If you're sexually active.** Your sexual health—and your partner's—depends on your use of birth control and safe sex practices. Your doctor can help with both. You also can discuss sexual problems, such as erectile dysfunction, with your physician.

CHAPTER

12 Making This Chapter Work for You

1. Which of the following statements about health information on the Internet is *true*?
   a. Chat rooms are the most reliable source of accurate medical information.
   b. Physicians who have websites must adhere to a strict set of standards set by the American Medical Association.
   c. Government-sponsored sites such as that of the Centers for Disease Control and Prevention are excellent sources of accurate health-care information.
   d. The Internet is a safe and cost-effective source of prescription drugs.

2. Self-care includes all of these *except*
   a. taking a home health test for colon cancer
   b. brushing and flossing every day
   c. filling a prescription
   d. searching online for an article on back pain

3. Periodontal disease
   a. results from poor eating habits.
   b. can lead to cardiovascular problems.
   c. in its early stage can be prevented by brushing alone.
   d. is caused by a variety of bacteria and viruses.

4. To help ensure that an over-the-counter or prescription drug is safe and effective,
   a. take smaller doses than indicated in the instructions.
   b. test your response to the drug by borrowing a similar medication from a friend.
   c. ask your doctor or pharmacist about possible interactions with other medications.
   d. buy all of your medications online.

5. People use complementary and alternative therapies
   a. to spend less money on health care.
   b. to take an active role in their own treatment.
   c. to show their disdain for the medical establishment.
   d. to take more prescription drugs.

6. Examples of complementary and alternative therapies include all of the following *except*
   a. psychiatry
   b. acupuncture
   c. chiropractic
   d. homeopathy

7. Herbal remedies that appear to have positive health effects include
   a. Ayurveda for controlling asthma.
   b. acidophilus for improving memory.
   c. aloe vera for diabetes.
   d. garlic for lowering cholesterol.

8. Which statement is *false?*
   a. Acupuncture has been shown to control nausea in patients after surgery.
   b. Reflexologists massage points on the foot or hand to relieve stress or pain in corresponding parts of the body.
   c. People can learn to control involuntary functions through biofeedback.
   d. Naturopathy is based on the premise that like cures like.

9. Factors that contribute to a long life and successful aging include all of the following *except*
   a. healthy weight
   b. moderate smoking
   c. regular exercise
   d. social involvement

10. When should concern change to intervention?
    a. Uncle Charlie is 85 and continues to drive himself to the grocery store and to the Senior Center during the daytime.
    b. Nana takes pills at breakfast, lunch, and dinner but sometimes mixes them up.

c. Mom's hot flashes have become a family joke.

d. Your older brother can never remember where he put his car keys.

Answers to these questions can be found on page 376.

Critical Thinking

1. Jocelyn has been experiencing a great deal of fatigue and frequent headaches for the past couple of months. She doesn't have health insurance and doesn't want to spend money on a doctor visit. So she did some research on the Internet about ways to relieve her symptoms and was considering taking a couple of herbal supplements that were touted as potential treatments. If she asked you for your advice, what would you tell her? Do you think that self-care is appropriate in this situation?

2. Have you used any complementary or alternative approaches to health care? If so, were you satisfied with the results? How did your experience with the CAM therapist compare with your most recent experience with a traditional medical practitioner? Do you feel confident that you know the difference between alternative care and quackery?

3. If you're young and healthy, you'll have little problem getting health insurance. However, if you develop a chronic illness, sustain serious injuries in an accident, or simply get older, you may find insurance harder to get and more expensive to keep. What is your insurance coverage? Do you believe insurance companies have the right to turn down applicants with preexisting conditions, such as high blood pressure? Do they have the right to require screening for potentially serious health problems, such as HIV infection, or to cancel the policies of individuals who have run up high medical bills in the past?

Media Menu

Health ⊛ Now™

Don't forget to check out the wealth of resources on the HealthNow website at **http://healthnow.brookscole.com/itw** that will:
- Help you evaluate your knowledge of the material
- Allow you to take an exam-prep quiz
- Provide a Personalized Learning Plan targeting resources that address areas you should study
- Coach you through identifying target goals for behavior change and creating and monitoring your personal change plan throughout the semester.

INTERNET CONNECTIONS

National Health Information Center
www.health.gov/nhic/
This excellent site, sponsored by the National Health Information Center (NHIC) of the U.S. Office of Disease Prevention and Health Promotion, is a health information referral service providing health professionals and consumers with a database of various health organizations. The site provides a searchable database, publications, and a list of toll-free numbers for health information.

National Center for Complementary and Alternative Medicine
nccam.nih.gov
This National Institutes of Health site features a variety of fact sheets on alternative therapies and dietary supplements, research, current news, and databases for the public as well as for practitioners.

MedicineNet.com
www.medicinenet.com
This comprehensive site is written for the consumer by board-certified physicians and contains medical news, a directory of procedures, a medical dictionary, and first aid and pharmacologic information. You can use the information at MedicineNet.com to prepare for a doctor visit, learn more about a diagnosis, or understand a prescribed treatment or procedure.

RealAge.com
www.realage.com
This site features diet and exercise assessment tools—such as a body mass index (BMI) calculator, exercise estimator, and RealAge assessment quizzes on a variety of health topics—to help you determine your risk of disease and what you can do to reduce this risk. The main feature is an interactive personal lifestyle assessment that also suggests options for "growing younger."

 InfoTrac College Edition Activities Schneider, Mary Ellen. "Safety, efficacy testing of CAM needed," *Internal Medicine News,* Feb 15, 2005 v38 i4 p2 (1)

1. Why did the Institute of Medicine recommend that complementary and alternative therapies be held to the same standards for safety and effectiveness as traditional ones?

2. How much do comsumers spend on CAM annually?

3. How many patients tell their physicians that they use CAM? Why do you think more patients do not confide this information to their doctors?

You can find additional readings related to personal health with InfoTrac College Edition, an online library of more than 900 journals and publications. Follow the instructions for accessing InfoTrac College Edition that were packaged with your textbook; then search for articles using a keyword search.

For additional links, resources, and suggested readings on the InfoTrac College Edition, visit our Health and Wellness Resource Center at **http://health.wadsworth.com.**

Key Terms

The terms listed are used on the page indicated. Definitions of the terms are in the Glossary at the end of the book.

Avoiding Substance Abuse

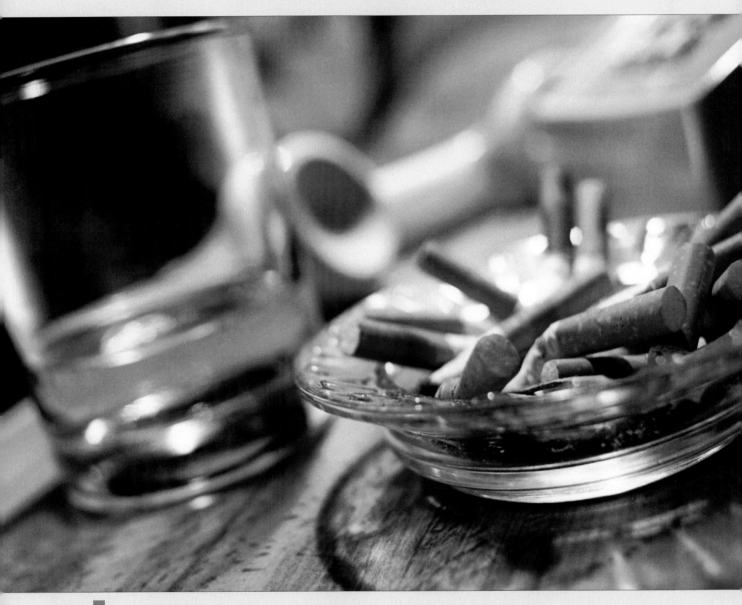

Jason doesn't do drugs. That's what he says to anyone who asks. Sure, he and his friends occasionally pass a joint around while listening to music. He's chugged his share of beers at frat parties. He's tried a tab or two of ecstasy. And when he was stressed out after finals, he took some of his roommate's Vicodin. But he thinks of alcoholics and drug users as desperate addicts craving a fix. He's not like that. That's what he tells himself.

Although he doesn't realize it, Jason is at risk of drug-related problems—physical, psychological, and legal—and of developing a substance abuse disorder. Like Jason, the people who use substances such as alcohol, tobacco, or illicit drugs don't think they'll ever lose control. But with continued use, these substances produce changes in an individual's body, mind and behavior.

Alcohol causes more disability and premature death than any medical condition other than heart disease. Despite widespread awareness of the dangers of tobacco, smoking continues to kill more people than AIDS, alcohol, drug abuse, car crashes, murders, suicides, and fires combined. Although heroin and cocaine use has stabilized and even declined in some countries, marijuana and illicit synthetic or designer drugs are more widespread.

Even if you never drink to excess, don't smoke and stay away from drugs, you live with the consequences of others' substance abuse. That's why it's important for everyone to know about these harmful habits. This chapter provides information that can help you understand, avoid, and change behaviors that could destroy your health, happiness, and life.

Tom Hussey GETTY

After studying the material in this chapter, you should be able to:

▌ **Distinguish** between drug misuse, drug abuse, and addiction.

▌ **Describe** how substance abuse affects each of the dimensions of wellness.

▌ **Define** BAC and alcohol poisoning.

▌ **Describe** the common drinking problems on college campuses and the actual and potential consequences for all students.

▌ **List** the health effects of tobacco use for all individuals and those specific to men and women.

▌ **Describe** some of the tobacco-control policies on college campuses.

▌ **Name** the negative physical effects of marijuana, club drugs, and amphetamines.

Health Now™

Don't forget to check out the wealth of resources on the HealthNow website at **http://healthnow.brookscole.com/itw** that will:

• Help you evaluate your knowledge of the material
• Allow you to take an exam-prep quiz
• Provide a Personalized Learning Plan targeting resources that address areas you should study
• Coach you through identifying target goals for behavior change and creating and monitoring your personal change plan throughout the semester.

✚ Understanding Drugs and Their Effects

A **drug** is a chemical substance that affects the way you feel and function. In some circumstances, taking a drug can help the body heal or relieve physical and mental distress. In other circumstances, taking a drug can distort reality, undermine well-being, and threaten survival. No drug is completely safe; all drugs have multiple effects that vary greatly in different people at different times. Knowing how drugs affect the brain, body, and behavior is crucial to understanding their impact and making responsible decisions about their use.

Drug misuse is the taking of a drug for a purpose or by a person other than that for which/whom it was medically intended. Borrowing a friend's prescription for penicillin when your throat feels scratchy is an example of drug misuse. The World Health Organization defines **drug abuse** as excessive drug use that's inconsistent with accepted medical practice. Taking prescription painkillers to get high is an example of drug abuse.

Risks are involved with all forms of drug use. Even medications that help cure illnesses or soothe symptoms have side effects and can be misused. Some substances that millions of people use every day, such as caffeine, pose some health risks. Others—like the most commonly used drugs in our society, alcohol and tobacco—can lead to potentially life-threatening problems. With some illicit drugs, any form of use can be dangerous.

Many factors determine the effects a drug has on an individual. These include how the drug enters the body, the dosage, the drug action, and the presence of other drugs in the body—as well as the physical and psychological makeup of the person taking the drug and the setting in which the drug is used.

✚ Substance Use Disorders

People have been using mind-altering, or **psychoactive,** chemicals for centuries. Citizens of ancient Mesopotamia and Egypt used opium. More than 3,000 years ago Hindus included cannabis products in religious ceremonies. For centuries the Inca in South America have chewed the leaves of the coca bush. Today millions of people regularly turn to drugs to pick them up, bring them down, alter perceptions, or ease psychological pain.

The word **addiction,** as used by the general population, refers to the compulsive use of a substance, loss of control, negative consequences, and denial. Mental health professionals describe drug-related problems in terms of *dependence* and *abuse.*

Individuals may develop **psychological dependence** and feel a strong craving for a drug because it produces pleasurable feelings or relieves stress and anxiety. **Physical dependence** occurs when a person develops *tolerance* to the effects of a drug and needs larger and

larger doses to achieve intoxication or another desired effect. Individuals who are physically dependent and have a high tolerance to a drug may take amounts many times those that would produce intoxication or an overdose in someone who was not a regular user.

Individuals with drug dependence become intoxicated or high on a regular basis—whether every day, every weekend, or several binges a year. They may try repeatedly to stop using a drug and yet fail, even though they realize their drug use is interfering with their health, family life, relationships, and work.

Some drug users do not develop the symptoms of tolerance and withdrawal that characterize dependence, yet they use drugs in ways that clearly have a harmful effect on them. These individuals are diagnosed as having a *psychoactive substance abuse disorder.* They continue to use drugs despite their awareness of persistent or repeated social, occupational, psychological, or physical problems related to drug use, or they use drugs in dangerous ways or situations (before driving, for instance).

Intoxication refers to maladaptive behavioral, psychological, and physiologic changes that occur as a result of substance use. **Withdrawal** is the development of symptoms that cause significant psychological and physical distress when an individual reduces or stops drug use.

✚ Addictive Behaviors and Wellness

Substance abuse and other self-destructive behaviors, such as gambling or compulsive shopping, can affect every dimension of wellness. Yet often individuals are unaware of the harmful effects of their unhealthy choices:

▮ **Physical wellness.** As shown in this chapter, the abuse of alcohol, tobacco, and drugs takes a toll on every organ system in the body, increasing the likelihood of disease, disability, and premature death.

▮ **Psychological wellness.** Sometimes people begin abusing substances as a way of "self-medicating" symptoms of anxiety or depression. However, alcohol or drugs provide only temporary relief. As abuse continues, shame and guilt increase, and coping with daily stressors becomes more difficult. Depression and anxiety are as likely to be the consequences as the causes of substance abuse.

▮ **Spiritual wellness.** Substance abuse blocks the pursuit of meaning and inner fulfillment. As they rely more and more on a chemical escape, individuals lose their sense of self and of connection with others and with a higher power.

▮ **Social wellness.** Substance abuse strains and, in time, severs the ties that bind an individual to family, friends, colleagues, and classmates. The primary relationship in the life of alcoholics or addicts is with a drug. They withdraw from others and become increasingly isolated.

▌ **Intellectual wellness.** The brain is one of the targets of alcohol and drugs. Under their influence, logic and reasoning break down. Impulses become more difficult to control. Judgment falters. Certain substances, such as ecstasy, can lead to permanent changes in brain chemistry.

▌ **Environmental wellness.** The use of some substances, such as tobacco, directly harms the environment. Abusers of alcohol and drugs also pose indirect threats because their behavior can lead to injury and damage.

Caffeine and Its Effects

Caffeine, which has been drunk, chewed, and swallowed since the Stone Age, is the most widely used **psychotropic** (mind-affecting) drug in the world. Eighty percent of Americans drink coffee, our principal caffeine source —an average of 3.5 cups a day. Coffee contains 100 to 150 milligrams of caffeine per cup; tea, 40 to 100 milligrams; cola, about 45 milligrams. Most medications that contain caffeine are one-third to one-half the strength of a cup of coffee. However, some, such as Excedrin, are very high in caffeine (**Table 13–1**).

Despite 20 years of reassuring research, many people still avoid caffeinated coffee because they worry about its

TABLE 13-1 ▌ Caffeine Counts

Substance (typical serving)	Caffeine (milligrams)
No Doz, one pill	200
Coffee (drip), one 5-ounce cup	130
Excedrin, two pills	130
Espresso, one 2-ounce cup	100
Energy drink, one can	80
Instant coffee, one 5-ounce cup	74
Coca-Cola, 12 ounces	46
Tea, one 5-ounce cup	40
Dark chocolate, 1 ounce	20
Milk chocolate, 1 ounce	6
Cocoa, 5 ounces	4
Decaffeinated coffee, one 5-ounce cup	3

health effects. In moderation—a few cups a day—coffee is a safe beverage that may offer some health benefits, including lowering the risk for type 2 diabetes.[1] Coffee also may reduce the likelihood of gallstones, Parkinson's disease, and colon cancer.

As a **stimulant,** caffeine relieves drowsiness, helps in the performance of repetitive tasks, and improves the capacity for work. Caffeine improves performance and endurance during prolonged, exhaustive exercise, and to a lesser degree, enhances short-term, high-intensity athletic performance. Additional benefits include improved concentration, reduced fatigue, and sharpened alertness. Major sports organizations ban excessive use of caffeine, but these policies remain controversial. Caffeinated energy drinks, such as Red Bull, which typically contain sugar, caffeine, and an amino acid called taurine, are popular on campus. Health experts caution that they should not be mixed with alcohol. Also do not drink them before intense exercise because of the increased risk of dehydration.

Consumption of high doses of caffeine can lead to dependence, anxiety, insomnia, rapid breathing, upset stomach and bowels, and dizziness. In a study of college men and women who normally consumed fewer than three caffeinated beverages per day, caffeine boosted anxiety but did not significantly affect performance on various low-intensity tasks, except for hand-eye coordination, which improved.[2]

You'll stay more alert, particularly if you are fighting sleep deprivation, if you spread your coffee consumption over the course of the day. For instance, rather than drinking two 8-ounce cups in the morning, try consuming smaller 2-to-3-ounce servings in the course of the day.

Alcohol and Its Effects

Pure alcohol is a colorless liquid obtained through the fermentation of a liquid containing sugar. **Ethyl alcohol,** or *ethanol,* is the type of alcohol in alcoholic beverages. Another type—methyl, or wood, alcohol—is a poison that should never be drunk. Any liquid containing 0.5 to 80 percent ethyl alcohol by volume is an alcoholic beverage. However, different drinks contain different amounts of alcohol (**Figure 13–1**).

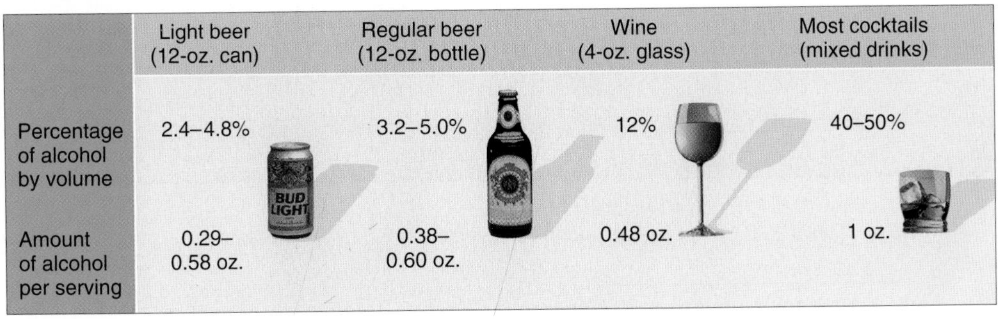

	Light beer (12-oz. can)	Regular beer (12-oz. bottle)	Wine (4-oz. glass)	Most cocktails (mixed drinks)
Percentage of alcohol by volume	2.4–4.8%	3.2–5.0%	12%	40–50%
Amount of alcohol per serving	0.29–0.58 oz.	0.38–0.60 oz.	0.48 oz.	1 oz.

FIGURE 13-1 ▌ The Alcohol Content of Different Drinks

One drink can be any of the following:

- One bottle or can (12 ounces) of beer, which is 5 percent alcohol.
- One glass (4 ounces) of table wine, such as burgundy, which is 12 percent alcohol.
- One small glass (2½ ounces) of fortified wine, which is 20 percent alcohol.
- One shot (1 ounce) of distilled spirits (such as whiskey, vodka, or rum), which is 50 percent alcohol.

All of these drinks contain close to the same amount of alcohol—that is, if the number of ounces in each drink is multiplied by the percentage of alcohol, each drink contains the equivalent of approximately ½ ounce of 100 percent ethyl alcohol. With distilled spirits (such as bourbon, scotch, vodka, gin, and rum), alcohol content is expressed in terms of **proof,** a number that is twice the percentage of alcohol: 100 proof bourbon is 50 percent alcohol; 80 proof gin is 40 percent alcohol.

But the words *bottle* and *glass* can be deceiving in this context. Drinking a 16-ounce bottle of malt liquor, which is 6.4 percent alcohol, is not the same as drinking a 12-ounce glass of 3.2 percent beer. Two bottles of high-alcohol wines (such as Cisco), packaged to resemble much less powerful wine coolers, can lead to alcohol poisoning, especially in those who weigh less than 150 pounds. This is one reason alcoholic drinks are a serious danger for young people.

How Much Alcohol Can I Drink?

The best way to figure how much you can drink safely is to determine the amount of alcohol in your blood at any given time, or your **blood-alcohol concentration (BAC).** BAC is expressed in terms of the percentage of alcohol in the blood and is often measured from breath or urine samples.

Law enforcement officers use BAC to determine whether a driver is legally drunk. Most states have followed the recommendation of the federal Department of Transportation to set 0.08 percent—the BAC that a 150-pound man would have after consuming about three mixed drinks within an hour—as the threshold at which a person can be cited for drunk driving (**Figure 13-2**). In the past, 0.1 percent was often the legal limit.

A BAC of 0.05 percent indicates approximately 5 parts alcohol to 10,000 parts other blood components. Most people reach this level after consuming one or

Men	Approximate blood alcohol percentage								
	Body weight in pounds								
Drinks	100	120	140	160	180	200	220	240	
0	.00	.00	.00	.00	.00	.00	.00	.00	Only safe driving limit
1	.04	.03	.03	.02	.02	.02	.02	.02	Impairment begins
2	.08	.06	.05	.05	.04	.04	.03	.03	
3	.11	.09	.08	.07	.06	.06	.05	.05	Driving skills significantly affected
4	.15	.12	.11	.09	.08	.08	.07	.06	Possible criminal penalties
5	.19	.16	.13	.12	.11	.09	.09	.08	
6	.23	.19	.16	.14	.13	.11	.10	.09	
7	.26	.22	.19	.16	.15	.13	.12	.11	
8	.30	.25	.21	.19	.17	.15	.14	.13	Legally intoxicated
9	.34	.28	.24	.21	.19	.17	.15	.14	Criminal penalties
10	.38	.31	.27	.23	.21	.19	.17	.16	

Subtract .01% for each 40 minutes of drinking.
One drink is 1.25 oz. of 80 proof liquor, 12 oz. of beer, or 5 oz. of table wine.

Women	Approximate blood alcohol percentage									
	Body weight in pounds									
Drinks	90	100	120	140	160	180	200	220	240	
0	.00	.00	.00	.00	.00	.00	.00	.00	.00	Only safe driving limit
1	.05	.05	.04	.03	.03	.03	.02	.02	.02	Impairment begins
2	.10	.09	.08	.07	.06	.05	.05	.04	.04	Driving skills significantly affected
3	.15	.14	.11	.10	.09	.08	.07	.06	.06	
4	.20	.18	.15	.13	.11	.10	.09	.08	.08	Possible criminal penalties
5	.25	.23	.19	.16	.14	.13	.11	.10	.09	
6	.30	.27	.23	.19	.17	.15	.14	.12	.11	
7	.35	.32	.27	.23	.20	.18	.16	.14	.13	
8	.40	.36	.30	.26	.23	.20	.18	.17	.15	Legally intoxicated
9	.45	.41	.34	.29	.26	.23	.20	.19	.17	Criminal penalties
10	.51	.45	.38	.32	.28	.25	.23	.21	.19	

Subtract .01% for each 40 minutes of drinking.
One drink is 1.25 oz. of 80 proof liquor, 12 oz. of beer, or 5 oz. of table wine.

FIGURE 13-2 | Alcohol Impairment Chart

Source: Adapted from data supplied by the Pennsylvania Liquor Control Board.

two drinks and experience all the positive sensations of drinking—relaxation, euphoria, and well-being—without feeling intoxicated. If they continue to drink past the 0.05 percent BAC level, they start feeling worse rather than better, gradually losing control of speech, balance, and emotions. At a BAC of 0.2 percent, they may pass out. At a BAC of 0.3 percent, they could lapse into a coma; at 0.4 percent, they could die.

For some people, even very low blood alcohol concentrations can cause a headache, upset stomach, or dizziness. These reactions often are inborn. People who have suffered brain damage, often as a result of head trauma or encephalitis, may lose all tolerance for alcohol, either temporarily or permanently, and behave abnormally after drinking small amounts. The elderly, as well as those who are unusually fatigued or have a debilitating physical illness, may also have a low tolerance for alcohol and respond inappropriately to a small amount.

Federal health authorities at the National Institute of Alcohol Abuse and Alcoholism (NIAAA) recommend that men have no more than two drinks a day and women, no more than one. The American Heart Association (AHA) advises that alcohol account for no more than 15 percent of the total calories consumed by an individual every day, up to an absolute maximum of 1.75 ounces of alcohol a day—the equivalent of three beers, two mixed drinks, or three and a half glasses of wine.

Your own limit may well be less, depending on your gender, size, and weight. Some people—such as women who are pregnant or trying to conceive; individuals with problems, such as ulcers, that might be aggravated by alcohol; those taking medications such as sleeping pills or antidepressants; and those driving or operating any motorized equipment—shouldn't drink at all.

The dangers of alcohol increase along with the amount you drink. Heavy drinking destroys the liver, weakens the heart, elevates blood pressure, damages the brain, and increases the risk of cancer. Individuals who drink heavily have a higher mortality rate than those who have two or fewer drinks a day. However, the boundary between safe and dangerous drinking isn't the same for everyone. For some people, the upper limit of safety is zero: Once they start, they can't stop.

Intoxication

If you drink too much, the immediate consequence is that you get drunk—or, more precisely, intoxicated. Alcohol intoxication, which can range from mild inebriation to loss of consciousness, is characterized by at least one of the following signs: slurred speech, poor coordination, unsteady gait, abnormal eye movements, impaired attention or memory, stupor, or coma.

Medical risks of intoxication include falls, hypothermia in cold climates, and increased risk of infections be-

cause of suppressed immune function. Time and a protective environment are the recommended treatments for alcohol intoxication.

Alcohol Poisoning

Every year an estimated 1,400 college students between the ages of 18 and 24 die from an alcohol overdose. Because federal law requires colleges to publish all student deaths, the stories of young lives ended by alcohol poisoning have gained national attention. Yet many students remain unaware that alcohol, in large enough doses, can and does kill.

Alcohol depresses nerves that control involuntary actions, such as breathing and the gag reflex (which prevents choking). A fatal dose of alcohol will eventually suppress these functions. Because alcohol irritates the stomach, people who drink an excessive amount often vomit. If intoxication has led to a loss of consciousness, a drinker is in danger of choking on vomit, which can cause death by asphyxiation. Blood alcohol concentration can rise even after a drinker has passed out because alcohol in the stomach and intestine continues to enter the bloodstream and circulate throughout the body.

The critical signs of alcohol poisoning are:

▍ **Mental confusion,** lack of responsiveness, stupor, coma.
▍ **Vomiting.**
▍ **Seizures.**
▍ **Slow breathing** (fewer than eight breaths per minute).
▍ **Irregular breathing** (10 seconds or more between breaths).
▍ **Hypothermia** (low body temperature), bluish skin color, paleness.

Alcohol poisoning is a medical emergency requiring immediate treatment. Black coffee, a cold shower, or letting a person "sleep it off" does not help. Without medical treatment, breathing slows, becomes irregular, or stops. The heart beats irregularly. Body temperature falls, which can cause cardiac arrest. Blood sugar plummets, which can lead to seizures. Vomiting creates severe dehydration, which can cause seizures, permanent brain damage, or death. Even if the victim lives, an alcohol overdose can result in irreversible brain damage.

Rapid binge drinking is especially dangerous because the victim can ingest a fatal dose before becoming unconscious. If you suspect alcohol poisoning, call 911 for help. Don't try to guess the level of drunkenness. Keep the victim from choking on vomit. Tell emergency medical technicians the symptoms and, if you know, how much alcohol the victim drank. Prompt action may save a life.

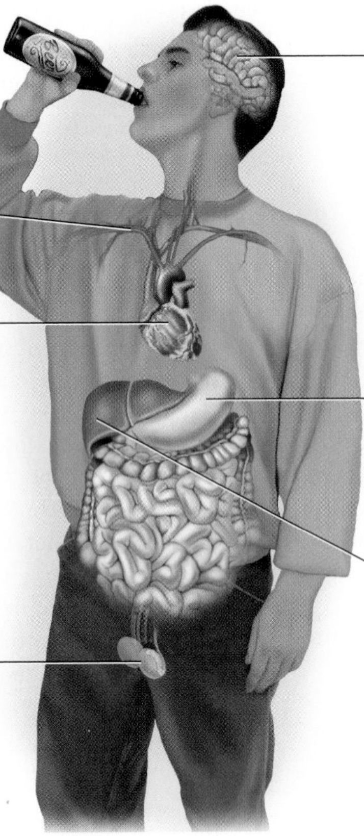

Brain
- Damages and eventually destroys brain cells
- Impairs memory
- Dulls senses
- Impairs physical coordination

Immune system
- Lowers resistance to diseases

Heart
- Weakens heart muscle
- May raise blood pressure
- Causes irregular heartbeat

Stomach and intestines
- Causes bleeding and inflammation
- May trigger cancer

Liver
- Damages and eventually destroys liver cells
- Displace important nutrients which can cause malnutrition

Reproductive system
- In men, hormone levels may be altered; impotence may occur
- In women, menstrual cycles become irregular; pregnant women have an increased risk of bearing children with birth defects

FIGURE 13-3 ▌ The Effects of Alcohol Abuse on the Body

Alcohol has a major effect on the brain, where it damages brain cells and impairs judgment and perceptions, often leading to accidents and altercations. Alcohol also damages the digestive system, especially the liver.

The Impact of Alcohol

Unlike drugs in tablet form or food, alcohol is directly and quickly absorbed into the bloodstream through the stomach walls and upper intestine. The alcohol in a typical drink reaches the bloodstream in 15 minutes and rises to its peak concentration in about an hour. The bloodstream carries the alcohol to the liver, heart, and brain (**Figure 13-3**).

Most of the alcohol you drink can leave your body only after metabolism by the liver, which converts about 95 percent of the alcohol to carbon dioxide and water. The other 5 percent is excreted unchanged, mainly through urination, respiration, and perspiration.

Alcohol is a diuretic, a drug that speeds up the elimination of fluid from the body, so drink water when you drink alcohol to maintain your fluid balance. And alcohol lowers body temperature, so you should never drink to get or stay warm.

Alcohol is responsible for 100,000 deaths each year and is the third leading cause of death after tobacco and improper diet and lack of exercise. The leading alcohol-related cause of death is injury. Alcohol plays a role in at least half of all traffic fatalities, half of all homicides, and a quarter of all suicides. The second leading cause of alcohol-related deaths is cirrhosis of the liver, a chronic disease that causes extensive scarring and irreversible damage. In addition, as many as half of patients admitted to hospitals and 15 percent of those making office visits seek or need medical care because of the direct or indirect effects of alcohol.

Young drinkers—teens and those in their early twenties—are at highest risk of dying from injuries, mostly car accidents. Older drinkers over age 50 face the greatest danger of premature death from cirrhosis of the liver, hepatitis, and other alcohol-linked illnesses.

Fetal Alcohol Effects and Syndrome

An estimated 15 percent of women drink alcohol while pregnant, most having one drink or less per day. Even light consumption of alcohol can lead to **Fetal Alcohol**

Effects (FAE): low birthweight, irritability as newborns, and permanent mental impairment.

The babies of women who consume three or more ounces of alcohol (the equivalent of six or seven cocktails) are at risk of more severe problems. One of every 750 new-borns has a cluster of physical and mental defects called **Fetal Alcohol Syndrome (FAS):** small head, abnormal facial features, jitters, poor muscle tone, sleep disorders, sluggish motor development, failure to thrive, short stature, delayed speech, mental retardation, and hyperactivity.[3]

Weight and Waists

At 7 calories per gram, alcohol has nearly as many calories as fat (9 calories per gram) and significantly more than carbohydrates or protein (which have 4 calories per gram). Since a standard drink contains 12–15 grams of alcohol, the alcohol in a single drink adds about 100 calories to your daily intake. A glass of wine contains as many calories as some candy bars; you would have to walk a mile to burn them off. In addition to being a calorie-dense food, alcohol stimulates the appetite so you're likely to eat more.

"Beer bellies" earn their name. In a study of men and women over age 20 in Copenhagen, those who drank the most beer or spirits had wider waists on a ten-year followup. Wine did not have a similar impact. In another study of the waist-hip ratio and body mass index of French adults who consumed varying amounts of alcohol, drinking was linked to an increase in both waist circumference and waist-to-hip ratio in both men and women.[4]

Interaction with Other Drugs

Alcohol can interact with other drugs—prescription and nonprescription, legal and illegal. Of the 100 most frequently prescribed drugs, more than half contain at least one ingredient that interacts adversely with alcohol. Because alcohol and other psychoactive drugs may work on the same areas of the brain, their combination can produce an effect much greater than that expected of either drug by itself. The consequences of this synergistic interaction can be fatal. (See Savvy Consumer: "Alcohol and Drug Interactions.") Alcohol is particularly dangerous when combined with depressants and antianxiety medications.

✚ Drinking in America

According to the most recent statistics available from the National Institute on Alcohol Abuse and Alcoholism, about 60 percent of American adults use alcohol, although

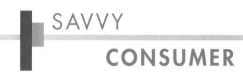

ALCOHOL AND DRUG INTERACTIONS

Drug	Possible Effects of Interaction
Analgesics (painkillers)	
Narcotic (Codeine, Demerol, Percodan)	Increase in central nervous system depression, possibly leading to respiratory failure and death.
Nonnarcotic (aspirin, acetaminophen)	Irritation of stomach resulting in bleeding and increased susceptibility to liver damage.
Antabuse (disulfiram; an aid to quit drinking)	Nausea, vomiting, headache, high blood pressure, and erratic heartbeat.
Antianxiety drugs (Valium, Librium)	Increase in central nervous system depression; decreased alertness and impaired judgment.
Antidepressants (Prozac, Zoloft)	Increase in central nervous system depression; certain antidepressants in combination with red wine could cause a sudden increase in blood pressure.
Antihistamines (Actifed, Dimetap, and other cold medications)	Increase in drowsiness; driving more dangerous.
Antibiotics	Nausea, vomiting, headache; some medications rendered less effective.
Central nervous system stimulants (caffeine, Dexedrine, Ritalin)	Stimulant effects of these drugs may reverse depressant effect of alcohol but do not decrease its intoxicating effects.
Diuretics (Diuril, Lasix)	Reduction in blood pressure resulting in dizziness upon rising.
Sedatives (Dalmane, Nembutal, Quaalude)	Increase in central nervous system depression, possibly leading to coma, respiratory failure, and death.

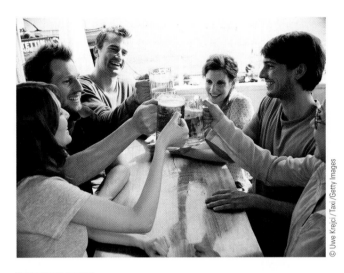

▌ Drinking is often part of the college social scene.

they vary in how much and how often they drink. Whites are more likely to be daily or near-daily drinkers than nonwhites. Men tend to drink more and more often than women.

The median age of first alcohol use is 15. Drinking typically accelerates in the late teens, peaks in the early 20s, and decreases as people age.[5] The median age of onset for alcohol-use disorders is 19 to 20.

Abstinence

Because of concern about alcohol's health effects, increasing numbers of Americans are choosing not to drink. With alcohol consumption in the United States at its lowest level in 30 years, nonalcoholic beverages have grown in popularity. Under federal law, these drinks can contain some alcohol, but a much smaller amount than regular beer or wine. Nonalcoholic beers and wines on the market also are lower in calories than alcoholic varieties.

Why People Drink

The most common reason people drink alcohol is to relax. Because it depresses the central nervous system, alcohol can make people feel less tense. Some psychologists theorize that men engage in *confirmatory drinking;* that is, they drink to reinforce the image of masculinity associated with alcohol consumption. Both genders may engage in *compensatory drinking,* consuming alcohol to heighten their sense of masculinity or femininity.

Here are some other reasons why men, women, or both drink:

▌ **Inherited susceptibility.** In both women and men, genetics accounts for 50 to 60 percent of a person's vulnerability to a serious drinking problem. Female alcoholics are more likely than males to have a parent who abused drugs or alcohol, who had psychiatric problems, or who attempted suicide.

▌ **Childhood traumas.** Female alcoholics often report that they were physically or sexually abused as children or suffered great distress because of poverty or a parent's death.

▌ **Depression.** Women are more likely than men to be depressed prior to drinking and to suffer from both depression and a drinking problem at the same time.

▌ **Relationship issues.** Single, separated, or divorced men and women drink more and more often than married ones.

▌ **Psychological factors.** Both men and women may drink to compensate for feelings of inadequacy. Women who tend to ruminate, or mull over, bad feelings may find that alcohol increases this tendency and makes them feel more distressed.

▌ **Self-medication.** More so than men, some women feel it's permissible to use alcohol as if it were a medicine. As long as they're taking it for a reason, it seems acceptable to them, even if they're drifting into a drinking problem.

▌ **Social ease.** When people use alcohol, they may seem bolder, wittier, sexier. At the same time, they become more relaxed and seem to enjoy each other's company more. Because alcohol lowers inhibitions, some people see it as a prelude to seduction.

▌ **Role models.** Athletes, some of the most admired celebrities in our country, have a long history of appearing in commercials for alcohol. Many advertisements feature glamorous women holding or sipping alcoholic beverages.

▌ **Advertising.** Brewers and beer distributors spend $15 to $20 million a year promoting the message: If you want to have fun, have a drink. Adolescents may be especially responsive to such sales pitches.

Binge Drinking

An alcohol binge consists of having five or more drinks at a single sitting for a man or four drinks at a single sitting for a woman. Binge drinkers are 14 times more likely to drive drunk than non−binge-drinkers. They also are at risk for a long list of adverse health outcomes, including injuries from falls, drowning, hypothermia, and burns; heart attack; suicide; violence to others; unplanned pregnancy; and sexually transmitted infection.

The prevalence of binge drinking among young adults decreased from the mid-1980s to the late 1990s but may be rising among current drinkers. In a recent survey, 31 percent of 12th graders and 40 percent of college students reported at least one episode of binge drinking during the previous two weeks.[6] While drinking is a problem nationwide, the percentage of U.S. adults who binge drink varies substantially from one city to another. According to a study of 120 metropolitan areas, Chattanooga, Tennessee, has the lowest rate and San Antonio, Texas, the highest.[7]

Binge drinking among women ages 18 to 44 has increased nationally by 13 percent since 1999.[8] This may endanger not only a woman's health but that of her unborn child. Binge drinking during pregnancy, not the total amount of alcohol consumed, doubles the risk of mental retardation and delinquent behavior in children.[9]

✚ Drinking on Campus

About eight in ten college students drink, at least occasionally. For most, alcohol usually does not interfere with their school and work responsibilities. However, an increasing number—about two in five—engage in the dangerous practice of binge drinking.[10] A single binge combined with poor judgment or bad luck, can lead to life-altering and sometimes life-threatening consequences.

How Common Is Drinking in College?

In the last decade, patterns in college drinking have changed in some ways but not in others. More students abstain—19.3 percent, up from 16.4 percent in 1993. However, more students now say that they drink primarily for the purpose of getting drunk. While fewer students attend or drink heavily at fraternity and sorority parties than a decade ago, more are drinking heavily at off-campus parties.

College drinkers drink more, more often, and more dangerously than young people not in college. According to a study that included 3,000 students from California, young adults of the same age who aren't enrolled in college may have 12 or more drinks on about 10 percent of the occasions they have alcohol. College drinkers may have 12 or more drinks on 20 percent of such occasions. This level of drinking greatly increases both immediate and long-term risks related to alcohol use. The heaviest drinking occurs among male freshmen and at the beginning of each academic year. By senior year, drinking moderates.

College men drink more frequently and in greater quantities and drink to intoxication more than women. About half of college men and a third of college women report drinking to excess. Male athletes drink more often, consume more alcohol, and drink to intoxication more than other students, while female athletes consume the lowest quantities of alcohol. Of all students, male athletes are the most likely to drink for social reasons and to drink to get high. College women (athletes or not) and men who are not athletes are more likely to drink as a way of coping, for instance, to feel better or "get through it." [11]

African-American students are more likely than white undergraduates to abstain and to report never having had an alcoholic drink and not having a drink in the past 30 days. They also drink less frequently and consume fewer drinks per occasion than whites. Black undergraduates experience fewer negative consequences of drinking and more regularly use strategies to prevent problem drinking, such as eating before drinking and keeping track of how many drinks they consume.[12]

Students drink more at certain colleges, such as those located along the Mexican border,[13] and in certain locations, such as off-campus parties and bars and fraternity and sorority parties. Heavy drinking is most likely to occur at events where many people become intoxicated, illicit drugs are available, and drinking games are played. More college sports fans drink alcohol, engage in binge drinking, have a heavy drinking style, and report alcohol-related problems compared with nonfans.

Why College Students Drink

Most college students drink for the same reasons undergraduates have always turned to alcohol: Away from home, often for the first time, many are excited by and

---

STUDENT SNAPSHOT

Drinking and Smoking on Campus

Undergraduates Who . . .	
Consumed alcohol in the past year	85%
Consumed alcohol in the past 30 days	70%
Consumed five or more drinks at least once within the past two weeks	43%
Currently smoke cigarettes	28%
Currently use tobacco	33%
Used a tobacco product in the last year	46%

Sources: Foote, Jeffrey, et al. "A National Survey of Alcohol Screening and Referral in College Health Centers." *Journal of American College Health*, Vol. 52, No. 4, January–February 2004, p. 149. Mitchell, Rebecca, et al. "Alcohol Policies on College Campuses." *Journal of American College Health*, Vol. 53, No. 4, January–February 2005, p. 149. Obermayer, Jami, et al. "College Smoking-Cessation Using Cell Phone Text Messaging." *Journal of American College Health*, Vol. 53, No. 2, September–October 2004, p. 71.

apprehensive about their newfound independence. When new pressures seem overwhelming, when they feel awkward or insecure, when they just want to let loose and have a good time, they reach for a drink.

Freshmen may be especially vulnerable to dangerous drinking as they struggle to adapt to an often bewildering new world. Many who were nondrinkers as high school seniors start to drink in college. They are less likely to do so if friends discourage them from drinking.

About 5 percent of college students are experiencing depression or poor mental health at any given time, and they are more vulnerable to alcohol abuse. Depressed young women are at the highest risk. About eight in ten students who report poor mental health or depression drink alcohol. They are more likely to drink to get drunk and to report high levels of harm from alcohol.[14]

In a recent study of 137 undergraduates, factors such as family history and sensation-seeking influenced student drinking. For some, drinking occasions were times to discuss problems with friends, regardless of the day's stress. On average, students tended to drink more on days when they were feeling good—possibly because of what the researchers called the "celebratory and social" nature of college drinking. Drinking—and positive emotions— also peaked on weekends.[15]

Binge Drinking on Campus

Binge drinking—defined as the consumption of five or more alcoholic drinks in a row by men and four or more by women—is the leading cause of preventable death among undergraduates and the most serious threat to their intellectual, physical, and psychological development. In spite of great efforts across U.S. college campuses to decrease binge drinking, the national average—two out of five students report binging—has remained steady for the last 15 to 20 years.

Frequent binge drinkers account for almost 70 percent of all alcohol consumed by college students. Students in four-year colleges are more likely to binge than those in two-year colleges.

Binge drinkers are most likely to be white, fraternity and sorority members, under 24 years of age, involved in athletics, and frequent socializers. White males binge drink the most; African-American women, the least. Students who study a great deal or are involved in community service or the arts are less likely to binge drink.

More women now binge. At coed schools, 41.2 percent report at least one binge within the previous two weeks; 17.4 percent are frequent bingers. At all-female colleges, binge drinking has jumped from one in four to almost one in three. In one recent study, women who reported binge drinking were more likely to have greater weight concerns than those who did not binge, and the women who were more physically active binged more than those who were the least active. Women who thought their peers drank

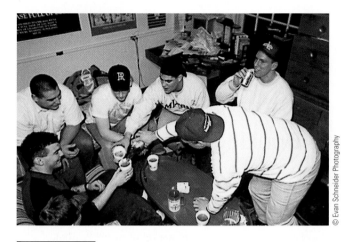

Binge drinkers can get into—and cause—trouble. Dangerously large amounts of alcohol can lead to death, and heavy party drinking often results in violence and accidents.

frequently engaged in more binge drinking episodes than others.[16] Unplanned sexual activities, date rape, and sexual assault are 150 percent more likely among women who drink than among those who do not. Sophomore, junior, and senior women are much less likely to engage in heavy episodic drinking than freshman women.

Surveys consistently show that students who engage in binge drinking, particularly those who do so more than once a week, experience a far higher rate of problems than other students. Frequent binge drinkers are likely to miss classes, vandalize property, and drive after drinking. Frequent binge drinkers are also more likely to experience five or more different alcohol-related problems and to use other substances, including nicotine, marijuana, cocaine, and LSD.

Why Do Students Binge?

Young people who came from, socialized within, or were exposed to "wet" environments—settings in which alcohol is cheap and accessible and drinking is prevalent— are more likely to engage in binge drinking. Students who reported drinking at least once a month during their final year of high school were over three times more likely to binge drink in college than those who drank less frequently in high school.

The factors that most influence students to binge drink are:

▌ **Low price** for alcohol.
▌ **Easy access to alcohol.** In one study, the density of alcohol outlets (such as bars) near campus affected the drinking of students.
▌ **Attending a school** or living in a residence with many binge drinkers.
▌ **Belief** that close friends were likely to binge.
▌ **Drinking games**—such as tongue twisters or drinking whenever a certain phrase is mentioned in a song or on a TV program—are dangerous because they can

result in high levels of intoxication in a short period of time.

▪ **Parents who drank** or did not disapprove of their children drinking.

▪ **Recreational drinking** before age 16.

Some educators view binging as a product of the college environment. More students binge drink at the beginning of the school year and then cut back as the semester progresses and academic demands increase. Binge drinking also peaks following exam times, during home football weekends, and during spring break. Many new students engage in binge drinking for the first time very soon after they arrive on campus. Binges become less common in their subsequent years at school and almost always end following college. Real life, one educator notes, is "a strong disincentive" to this type of drinking.

Underage Drinking on Campus

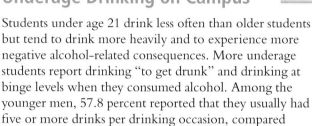

Students under age 21 drink less often than older students but tend to drink more heavily and to experience more negative alcohol-related consequences. More underage students report drinking "to get drunk" and drinking at binge levels when they consumed alcohol. Among the younger men, 57.8 percent reported that they usually had five or more drinks per drinking occasion, compared with 41.9 percent of older students. Similar rates were found among female students, with 32.4 of underage women versus 20.5 percent of those over 21 reporting binge drinking.

Underage students are more likely than students of legal age to experience a host of negative drinking-related consequences, including doing something they regretted; forgetting where they were or what they did; causing property damage; getting into trouble with police; and being hurt or injured. The drinking behavior of underage students also depends on their living arrangements. Those in controlled settings, such as their parents' home or a substance-free dorm, are less likely to binge drink. Students living in fraternities or sororities were most likely to binge drink, regardless of age.

Students under age 21 in states with tough laws against underage drinking are less likely to drink than those in states with fewer restrictions. When they drink, underage students are more likely to drink to excess than older ones—possibly because they feel greater pressure to drink quickly before some authority cuts off their alcohol supply or they get caught.

The Toll of College Drinking

Each year more than 2 million college students aged 18 to 24 drive after drinking; more than 3 million ride in motor vehicles with drinking drivers; over one half million are injured because of drinking; and 1,400 die.

According to the Commission on Substance Abuse at Colleges and Universities, alcohol is involved in two-

TABLE 13-2 ▪ The Consequences of College Drinking

Consequence	Number of Students per Year
Assault by another student	600,000
Unintentional injury	500,000
Unprotected sex after drinking	400,000
Arrest for alcohol-related violations	110,000
Sexual assault or date rape	70,000
Death	1,400

Source: www.collegedrinkingprevention.gov

thirds of college student suicides, nine of ten rapes, and 95 percent of violent crimes on campus (**Table 13-2**). According to a national survey released by the Higher Education Center for Alcohol and Other Drug Prevention, 75 to 90 percent of all violence on college campuses is alcohol-related. About 300,000 of today's college students will eventually die from alcohol-related causes, including drunk-driving accidents, cirrhosis of the liver, various cancers, and heart disease, estimates the Core Institute, an organization that studies college drinking.

In one study at a large public university, nearly 55 percent of college women had experienced at least one alcohol-related problem in the previous 12 months. The most common were doing something they later regretted, forgetting where they were or what they did, physically injuring themselves, and having unprotected sex.

About two-thirds of college men reported one or more alcohol-linked problems in the same time period. In addition to the same negative consequences as the women, more men developed academic difficulties.[17]

Heavy drinking has been correlated with increased casual sex without condoms, an increased number of sex partners, and sexual attacks on women. Alcohol and drug use can lead to earlier sexual initiation, unprotected sexual intercourse, multiple sex partners, and increased risk of sexually transmitted infections.

Smart choices can help you avoid many of the negative consequences of drinking. Various "self-protective" behaviors, such as designating a driver, eating before or during drinking, and keeping track of the number of drinks consumed, have proved effective in reducing alcohol-related problems. Women employ these strategies more often when partying or socializing than men; black students use them more often than white men. The students who used these strategies most often had the fewest problem behaviors.[18]

"Secondhand" Drinking Problems

Heavy alcohol use can endanger both drinkers and others. Secondhand problems caused by other's alcohol use include loss of sleep, interruption of studies, assaults, vandalism, and unwanted sexual advances. Students living on campuses with high rates of binge drinking are two or more times as likely to experience these secondhand effects as those living on campuses with low rates.

In a recent study, nearly three-quarters of campus rapes happened when the victims were so intoxicated that they were unable to consent or refuse. Women from colleges with medium and high binge-drinking rates had more than a 1.5-fold increased chance of being raped while intoxicated than those from schools with low binge-drinking rates.[19]

Over two academic years at a large university medical center, 13 percent of emergency visits by undergraduates were related to alcohol. Injuries accounted for 53 percent of all visits, and acute intoxication accounted for 34 percent. Men aged 21 years and older had the highest odds of visiting the emergency department, mostly as the result of accidents and fights.[20]

Changing Drinking Patterns on Campus

At many schools, a growing number of students almost never engage in heavy drinking. Even those who drank heavily as freshmen often curtail their alcohol use either before or after graduation. This is the result both of personal changes in behavior and in college policies.

Stages of Personal Change

In a study at Ohio State University, researchers classified student heavy drinkers according to four stages of change:[21]

1. **Precontemplation.** Nearly two-thirds of the students continued to drink heavily and had no intention of changing their behavior. These students drank an average of 12.5 alcoholic beverages a week.
2. **Contemplation.** 12 percent of the students were still drinking heavily but considering changing their drinking behavior.
3. **Action.** 14 percent of the students had stopped their pattern of heavy drinking.
4. **Maintenance.** 9 percent of the students had avoided heavy alcohol use for at least six months. They drank an average of one alcoholic drink a month. These students no longer drank heavily, even though they felt that such drinking was the norm on their campus. However, they saw more risks and fewer benefits associated with alcohol use.

Such change is not unusual, even among students who continued heavy drinking throughout their college years. Despite their heavy drinking as undergraduates, within three years of graduation, students who had been members of fraternities and sororities drink no more than students who did not join Greek houses. Heavy drinking may be the result of students' perceptions that excessive

---

STRATEGIES *for* PREVENTION

Protecting Yourself from Dangerous Drinking

If you drink, the following "self-protective" strategies can help you avoid drinking too much:

▌ Alternate alcoholic and nonalcoholic beverages.

▌ Decide in advance not to exceed a set number of drinks.

▌ Choose not to drink at some occasions.

▌ Use a designated driver.

▌ Eat before or during drinking.

▌ Ask a friend to let you know when you've had enough.

▌ Keep track of how many drinks you're consuming.

▌ Pace your drinks to one or fewer per hour.

▌ Avoid drinking games.

▌ Drink an alcohol look-alike (such as nonalcoholic beer).

---

alcohol use is normal in Greek houses, along with the encouragement of peers.

College Alcohol Policies

The majority of college administrators—described students' alcohol use as a problem or a major problem on their campus. All schools report some action to manage campus drinking, although policies vary greatly. Some colleges, particularly small schools, southern schools, and historically black colleges ban alcohol. Others prohibit alcohol use or possession or restrict alcohol at events such as concerts or athletic contests and games. (**Table 13-3**).[22] Many provide alcohol education for freshmen, fraternity and sorority members, or athletes.

TABLE 13-3 ▌ Restricting Alcohol on Campus

Schools That Prohibit:

Alcohol use on campus	32%
Alcohol possession	38%
Beer kegs	78%
Use at sporting events	14%
Use at home games	85%
Greek alcohol use	25%

Based on a survey of 73 colleges in Minnesota and Wisconsin.

Source: Mitchell, Rebecca, et al. "Alcohol Policies on College Campuses." *Journal of American College Health,* Vol. 53, No. 4, January–February 2005, p. 149.

Colleges and universities are required to provide a copy of their alcohol policies to students. Some schools post their policies online, but in many cases they are difficult to find among all of the other information on a school's website. Can you find the policy for your school?

A recent survey found that 32 percent of colleges—mostly urban, public, and large institutions—routinely screen students for alcohol use. Other schools screen only about 10 percent of students. When screening reveals a potential drinking problem, schools are most likely to refer students to a campus counseling center, a substance abuse treatment provider in the community, or to a 12-step program. In one study at a large northeastern university, only 15 percent of college drinkers reported that a health-care professional had ever asked them about their drinking. But nine in ten of student drinkers said they would cut down on alcohol consumption if a physician advised them to do so.[23]

Fewer than 10 percent of frequent binge drinkers experience any disciplinary action as a result of their drinking. Support for tougher campus restrictions has grown among students, particularly those who do not binge drink and who have experienced the negative consequences of others' drinking, such as violence and vandalism. According to studies of schools that have lowered binge-drinking rates, a combination of social and environmental approaches has the greatest impact on reducing binge drinking.[24] Key elements are involvement of students and development of alternatives, such as alcohol-free parties and events.

The U.S. Department of Education has begun highlighting innovative antidrinking practices on campus; Mothers Against Drunk Driving (MADD) is planning to rank colleges based on how well they curb student drinking. There has been an increase in on-campus chapters of national support groups such as AA, Al-Anon, Adult Children of Alcoholics, and a peer-education program called BACCHUS: Boost Alcohol Consciousness Concerning the Health of University Students.

Drinking and Driving

Alcohol impairs driving-related skills regardless of the age of the driver or the time of day it is consumed. However, younger drinkers and drivers are at greatest risk. Underage drinkers are more likely to drive after drinking, to ride with intoxicated drivers, and to be injured after drinking—at least in part because they believe that people can drive safely and legally after drinking. Drunk driving is the most frequently committed crime in the United States.

In a recent survey, 29 percent of students drove after drinking some alcohol; 10 percent after five or more drinks; 23 percent with a driver who was high or drunk. The rates of drinking and driving are higher at larger schools and schools in the southern and north-central regions.[25]

STRATEGIES for PREVENTION

How to Prevent Drunk Driving

▪ When going out in a group, always designate one person who won't drink at all to serve as the driver.

▪ Never get behind the wheel if you've had more than two drinks within two hours, especially if you haven't eaten.

▪ Never let intoxicated friends drive home. Call a taxi, drive them yourself, or arrange for them to spend the night in a safe place.

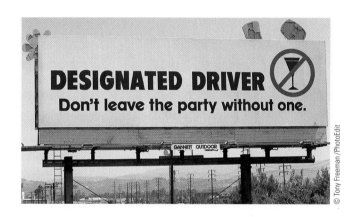

© Tony Freeman/PhotoEdit

Public awareness campaigns like this one for designated drivers can help prevent the high incidence of fatalities caused by drunk drivers.

In the last two decades, families of the victims of drunk drivers have organized to change the way the nation treats its drunk drivers. Because of the efforts of MADD (Mothers Against Drunk Driving), SADD (Students Against Destructive Decisions), and other lobbying groups, cities, counties, and states are cracking down on drivers who drink. Since courts have held establishments that serve alcohol liable for the consequences of allowing drunk customers to drive, many bars and restaurants have joined the campaign against drunk driving. Many communities also provide free rides home on holidays and weekends for people who've had too much to drink. Designated drivers can help save lives—if they refrain from drinking. In one study of college students, female designated drivers had lower blood alcohol concentrations than males.[26]

Alcohol Problems

By the simplest definition, problem drinking is the use of alcohol in any way that creates difficulties, potential difficulties, or health risks for an individual. Like alcoholics,

STRATEGIES for **PREVENTION**

How to Recognize the Warning Signs of Alcoholism

▮ Experiencing the following symptoms after drinking: frequent headaches, nausea, stomach pain, heartburn, gas, fatigue, weakness, muscle cramps, irregular or rapid heartbeats.

▮ Needing a drink in the morning to start the day.

▮ Denying any problem with alcohol.

▮ Doing things while drinking that are regretted afterward.

▮ Dramatic mood swings, from anger to laughter to anxiety.

▮ Sleep problems.

▮ Depression and paranoia.

▮ Forgetting what happened during a drinking episode.

▮ Changing brands or going on the wagon to control drinking.

▮ Having five or more drinks a day.

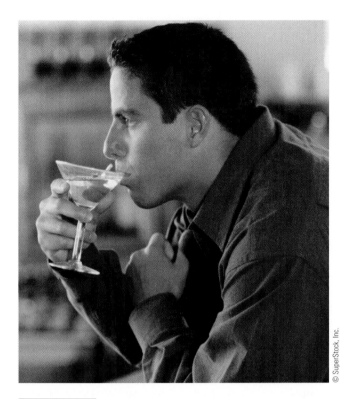

▮ Alcohol dependence may spring from the perception that alcohol relieves stress or creates a pleasant feeling. Daytime drinking and drinking alone can be signs of a serious problem, even though the drinker may otherwise appear to be in control.

problem drinkers are individuals whose lives are in some way impaired by their drinking. The only difference is one of degree. Alcohol becomes a problem, and a person becomes an alcoholic, when the drinker can't "take it or leave it." He or she spends more and more time anticipating the next drink, planning when and where to get it, buying and hiding alcohol, and covering up secret drinking. As many as one in six adults in the United States may have a problem with drinking.[27]

Alcohol abuse involves continued use of alcohol despite awareness of social, occupational, psychological, or physical problems related to drinking, or drinking in dangerous ways or situations (before driving, for instance). A diagnosis of alcohol abuse is based on one or more of the following occurring at any time during a 12-month period:

▮ **A failure to fulfill major role obligations** at work, school, or home (such as missing work or school).

▮ **The use of alcohol in situations in which it is physically hazardous** (such as before driving).

▮ **Alcohol-related legal problems** (such as drunk-driving arrests).

▮ **Continued alcohol use despite persistent or recurring social or interpersonal problems** caused or exacerbated by alcohol (such as fighting while drunk).

Alcohol dependence is a separate disorder in which individuals develop a strong craving for alcohol because it produces pleasurable feelings or relieves stress or anxiety. Over time they experience physiological changes that lead to *tolerance* of its effects; this means that they must consume larger and larger amounts to achieve intoxication. If they abruptly stop drinking, they suffer *withdrawal,* a state of acute physical and psychological discomfort. A diagnosis of alcohol dependence is based on three or more of the following symptoms occurring during any 12-month period:

▮ **Tolerance,** as defined by either a need for markedly increased amounts of alcohol to achieve intoxication or desired effect, or a markedly diminished effect with continued drinking of the same amount of alcohol as in the past.

▮ **Withdrawal,** including at least two of the following symptoms: sweating, rapid pulse, or other signs of autonomic hyperactivity; increased hand tremor; insomnia; nausea or vomiting; temporary hallucinations or illusions; physical agitation or restlessness; anxiety; or grand mal seizures.

▮ **Drinking to avoid** or relieve the symptoms of withdrawal.

▮ **Consuming larger amounts of alcohol,** or drinking over a longer period than was intended.

▮ **Persistent desire** or unsuccessful efforts to cut down or control drinking.

■ **A great deal of time spent** in activities necessary to obtain alcohol, drink it, or recover from its effects.

■ **Important social, occupational, or recreational activities given up** or reduced because of alcohol use.

■ **Continued alcohol use** despite knowledge that alcohol is likely to cause or exacerbate a persistent or recurring physical or psychological problem.

According to a survey of more than 14,000 undergraduates at four-year colleges, 6 percent of college students met criteria for a diagnosis of alcohol dependence or alcoholism, 31 percent for alcohol abuse. More than two of every five students reported at least one symptom of these conditions and were at increased risk of developing a true alcohol disorder. Few reported seeking treatment since coming to college.

Alcoholism, as defined by the National Council on Alcoholism and Drug Dependence and the American Society of Addiction, is a primary, chronic disease in which genetic, psychosocial, and environmental factors influence its development and manifestations. The disease is often progressive and fatal. Its characteristics include an inability to control drinking, a preoccupation with alcohol, continued use of alcohol despite adverse consequences, and distorted thinking, most notably denial. Like other diseases, alcoholism is not simply a matter of insufficient will-power but a complex problem that causes many symptoms, can have serious consequences, yet can improve with treatment.

A lack of obvious signs of alcoholism can be deceiving. A person who doesn't drink in the morning but feels that he or she must always have a drink at a certain time of the day may have lost control over his or her drinking. A person who never drinks alone but always drinks socially with others may be camouflaging loss of control. A person who is holding a job or taking care of the family may still spend every waking hour thinking about that first drink at the end of the day (preoccupation).

Alcoholism Treatments

Almost 600,000 Americans undergo treatment for alcohol-related problems every year. Until recent years, the only options for professional alcohol treatment were, as one expert puts it, "intensive, extensive, and expensive," such as residential programs at hospitals or specialized treatment centers. Today individuals whose drinking could be hazardous to their health may choose from a variety of approaches. Treatment that works well for one person may not work for another. As research into the outcomes of alcohol treatments has grown, more attempts have been made to match individuals to approaches tailored to their needs and more likely to help them overcome their alcohol problems.

Men and women who have seriously remained sober for more than a decade credit a variety of approaches, including Alcoholics Anonymous (AA), individual psycho-

STRATEGIES for CHANGE

If Someone Close to You Drinks Too Much

■ Try to remain calm, unemotional, and factually honest in speaking about the drinker's behavior. Include the drinker in family life.

■ Discuss the situation with someone you trust: a member of the clergy, social worker, friend, or someone who has experienced alcoholism directly.

■ Never cover up or make excuses for the drinker, or shield him or her from the consequences of drinking. Assuming the drinker's responsibilities undermines his or her dignity and sense of importance.

■ Refuse to ride with the drinker if he or she is driving while intoxicated.

■ Encourage new interests and participate in leisure-time activities that the drinker enjoys.

■ Try to accept setbacks and relapses calmly.

therapy, and other groups, such as Women for Sobriety. There is no one sure path to sobriety—a wide variety of treatments may offer help and hope to those with alcohol-related problems.

Tobacco and Its Effects

One in four Americans age 12 and older—some 56 million persons—smoked part or all of a cigarette during the past month. Smoking rates have dropped dramatically among young teens in the last decade.[28] However, college-age young adults have the highest percentage of smokers. The more and the longer they smoke, the greater their risks of heart disease, respiratory problems, several types of cancer, and a shortened lifespan. Nationally, smoking results in more than 5 million years of potential life lost each year.

Figure 13-4 shows a summary of the physiological effects of tobacco and the other chemicals in tobacco smoke. If you're an adult smoker who inhales deeply and started smoking before the age of 15, you're trading a minute of future life for every minute you now spend smoking. On average smokers die nearly seven years earlier than nonsmokers. Smoking not only eventually kills, it also ages you: Smokers get more wrinkles than nonsmokers.

But the effects of smoking are far more than skin-deep. A cigarette smoker is 10 times more likely to de-

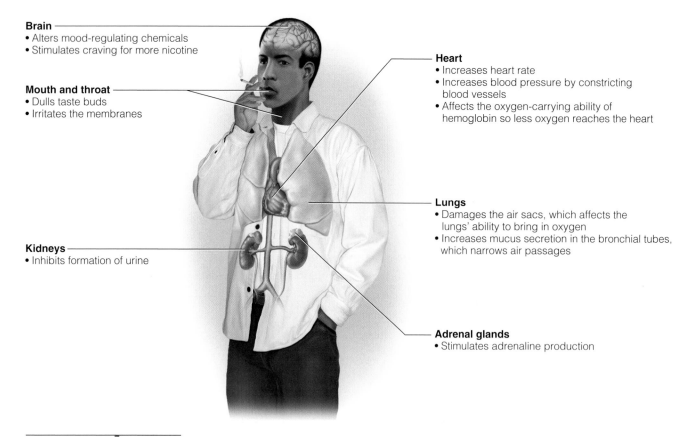

Brain
• Alters mood-regulating chemicals
• Stimulates craving for more nicotine

Mouth and throat
• Dulls taste buds
• Irritates the membranes

Kidneys
• Inhibits formation of urine

Heart
• Increases heart rate
• Increases blood pressure by constricting blood vessels
• Affects the oxygen-carrying ability of hemoglobin so less oxygen reaches the heart

Lungs
• Damages the air sacs, which affects the lungs' ability to bring in oxygen
• Increases mucus secretion in the bronchial tubes, which narrows air passages

Adrenal glands
• Stimulates adrenaline production

FIGURE 13-4 ▮ Some Effects of Smoking on the Body
Smoking harms the respiratory system and the cardiovascular system. The leading cause of death for smokers is heart attack.

STRATEGIES for PREVENTION

Why Not to Light Up

Before you start smoking—before you ever face the challenge of quitting—think of what you have to gain by not smoking.

▮ A significantly reduced risk of cancer of the lungs, larynx, mouth, esophagus, pancreas, and bladder.

▮ Half the risk of heart disease that smokers face.

▮ A lower risk of stroke, chronic obstructive lung disease (COLD), influenza, ulcers, and pneumonia.

▮ A lower risk of having a low-birthweight baby.

▮ A longer lifespan.

▮ Potential savings of tens of thousands of dollars that you would otherwise spend on tobacco products and medical care.

velop lung cancer than a nonsmoker and 20 times more likely to have a heart attack.

Smoking accounts for more than 430,000 death per year. The annual costs to society total more than $100 billion in lost productivity, medical problems, and morality issues.[29]

Tobacco Use on Campus

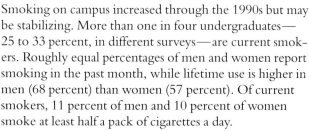

Smoking on campus increased through the 1990s but may be stabilizing. More than one in four undergraduates—25 to 33 percent, in different surveys—are current smokers. Roughly equal percentages of men and women report smoking in the past month, while lifetime use is higher in men (68 percent) than women (57 percent). Of current smokers, 11 percent of men and 10 percent of women smoke at least half a pack of cigarettes a day.

White students report the highest rates of smoking: 36 percent, compared with 16 percent for African Americans, 26 percent for Hispanics, and 23 percent for Asian Americans. Although black students have the lowest smoking rates, these students had the greatest percentage increase in smoking rates in the last decade.[30] Smoking is more common in students who live in housing where smoking is permitted, use alcohol and other drugs, and have a lower psychological sense of well-being.[31]

In a survey of more than 17,000 college students from 140 schools, fewer men involved in athletics were current smokers: 15 percent of those who participated in athletics every day, compared with 20 percent of those who were less involved and 26 percent of men not involved in athletics.[32]

Marijuana and alcohol use and weekend exposure to smoke increase the likelihood of being a tobacco user.[33]

College students smoke for many reasons, including defiance of their parents and relaxed smoking standards in their dorms. Many students who had never tried smoking may experiment with cigarettes in colleges. Students who were occasional smokers in high school are more likely to become more frequent, heavier smokers once in college.

Many college students say they smoke as a way of managing depression or stress. Studies consistently link smoking with depression and low life satisfaction. Smokers are significantly more likely to have higher levels of perceived stress than nonsmokers. In one study, students who had been diagnosed or treated for depression were seven times as likely as other students to use tobacco.[34]

Male students who smoke are more likely to say that smoking makes them feel more masculine and less anxious. More than half of female smokers feel that smoking helps them control their weight. Overweight female students are more likely to smoke to lose weight and to see weight gain as a barrier to quitting.

The tobacco industry regularly targets college students with marketing strategies such as providing free samples of cigarettes at campus parties or in bars or clubs. This approach seems to have a particularly strong effect on nonsmokers. In a group of about 8,500 students who did not smoke prior to college, one in four of those who attended a promotional event became a smoker, twice the rate of those who did not attend such events.[35]

College Tobacco-Control Policies

Other than religious institutions, colleges and universities have traditionally had few smoking restrictions. This has changed. Several national health organizations, including the American College Health Association and National Center on Addiction and Substance Abuse, have recommended that colleges ban smoking in and around all campus buildings, including student housing, and prohibit the sale, advertisement, and promotion of tobacco products on campus. Although some schools, particularly large public universities, have made progress in adopting such policies, most still fall short of the national recommendations.

A growing number of public and private schools provide completely smoke-free student housing, a dramatic increase from a decade ago. Two-thirds do not allow tobacco sales on campus; a third of student newspapers do not allow tobacco advertising. None have specifically banned tobacco industry sponsorships and promotions on college property. In general, schools in the West have done the most to implement tobacco policies. Those in the South, particularly in the major tobacco-growing states, have done the least.

An estimated 44 percent of students live in smoke-free dorms, while another 29 percent who don't would like to move into one. Freshmen who did not smoke regularly in high school and who live in smoke-free dorms are 40 percent less likely to take up smoking than those in unrestricted housing, according to a study of the smoking behavior of 4,495 students at 101 schools.[36]

Despite concern about student smoking, more than 40 percent of schools do not offer smoking cessation programs to students who want to quit. Those that do primarily refer students to campus support groups or community-based programs like Nicotine Anonymous; they report little student demand for these options.

Smoking, Race, and Gender

Cigarette smoking is a major cause of disease and death in all population groups. However, tobacco use varies within and among racial and ethnic minority groups. Among adults, Native Americans and Alaska Natives have the highest rates of tobacco use—37.9 percent of the men smoke cigarettes, compared with about 25 percent of adults in the overall U.S. population. African-American men (32.1 percent) and Southeast Asian men also have a high smoking rate. Asian-American and Hispanic women have the lowest rates of smoking. Tobacco use is significantly higher among white college students than among Hispanic, African-American, and Asian students.

Tobacco is the substance most abused by Hispanic youth, whose smoking rates have soared in the last ten years. In general, smoking rates among Hispanic adults increase as they adopt the values, beliefs, and norms of American culture. Recent declines in the prevalence of smoking have been greater among Hispanic men with at least a high school education than among those with less education.

On average, girls who begin smoking during adolescence continue smoking for 20 years, four years longer than boys. Women are at greater risk for developing smoking-related illnesses compared with men who smoke the same amount.

According to the U.S. Surgeon General, women account for 39 percent of smoking-related deaths each year, a proportion that has doubled since 1965. Each year, American women lose an estimated 2.1 million years of life due to premature deaths attributable to smoking. If she smokes, a woman's annual

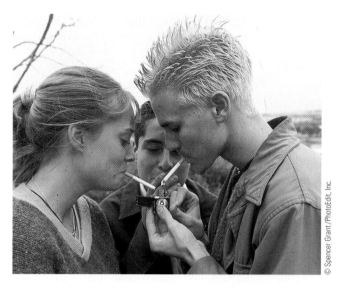

▌ Smoking doubles your risk of heart disease and stroke.

risk of dying more than doubles after age 45 compared with a woman who has never smoked.

Lung cancer now claims more women's lives than breast cancer. In men, cigarette smoking increases the risk of aggressive prostate cancer.

Smoking is a risk factor for developing rheumatoid arthritis for men, but not for women. Women who smoke are more likely to develop osteoporosis, a bone-weakening disease. They tend to be thin, which is a risk factor for osteoporosis, and they enter menopause earlier, thus extending the period of jeopardy from estrogen loss.

High nicotine intake may affect male hormones, including testosterone. Smoking also can reduce blood flow to the penis, impairing a man's sexual performance and increasing the likelihood of erectile dysfunction.[37] Smoking directly affects women's reproductive organs and processes. Women who smoke are less fertile and experience menopause one or two years earlier than women who don't smoke. Smoking also greatly increases the possible risks associated with taking oral contraceptives. Older women who smoke are weaker, have poorer balance, and are at greater risk of physical disability than nonsmokers. Women who smoke during pregnancy increase their risk of miscarriage and pregnancy complications, including bleeding, premature delivery, and birth defects such as cleft lip or palate.

✚ Other Forms of Tobacco

Some 10.7 million Americans smoke cigars; 7.6 million use smokeless tobacco, and 2.1 million smoke pipes. Ingesting tobacco may be less deadly than smoking cigarettes, but it is dangerous. Smoking cigars, clove cigarettes, and pipes, and chewing or sucking on smokeless tobacco

all put the user at risk of cancer of the lip, tongue, mouth, and throat, as well as other diseases and ailments.

Cigars

Cigar use has declined in the last few years. However, after cigarettes, cigars are the tobacco product most widely used by college students. According to the first national survey to report on undergraduate cigar use, more than a third reported ever smoking a cigar (more than half of men and a quarter of women); 23 percent had smoked a cigar within the past year and 8.5 percent had smoked one within the previous 30 days. About one in five students smoked both cigars and cigarettes. Most cigar use was occasional; fewer than 1 percent of current cigar users on campus smoked daily.

Cigar smoking is as dangerous even though smokers do not inhale. Cigars are known to cause cancer of the lung and the digestive tract. The risk of death related to cigars approaches that of cigarettes, as the number of cigars smoked and the amount of cigar smoke inhaled increases. Cigar smoking can lead to nicotine addiction, even if the smoke is not inhaled. The nicotine in the smoke from a single cigar can vary from an amount roughly equivalent to that in a single cigarette to that in a pack or more of cigarettes.

Clove Cigarettes

Sweeteners have long been mixed with tobacco, and clove, a spice, is the latest ingredient to be added to the recipe for cigarettes. Clove cigarettes typically contain two-thirds tobacco and one-third clove. Consumers of these cigarettes are primarily teenagers and young adults.

Many users believe that clove cigarettes are safer because they contain less tobacco, but this isn't necessarily the case. The Centers for Disease Control and Prevention (CDC) reports that people who smoke clove cigarettes may be at risk of serious lung injury. Smoking clove cigarettes during a mild upper respiratory tract illness can lead to severe breathing difficulty. And clove cigarette smokers, like other cigarette smokers, can become addicted to the tobacco.

Clove cigarettes deliver twice as much nicotine, tar, and carbon monoxide as moderate-tar American brands. Eugenol, the active ingredient in cloves (which dentists have used as an anesthetic for years), deadens sensation in the throat, allowing smokers to inhale more deeply and hold smoke in their lungs for a longer time. Chemical relatives of eugenol can produce the kind of damage to cells that may lead to cancer.

What Are Bidis?

Skinny, sweet-flavored cigarettes called **bidis** (pronounced "beedees") have become a smoking fad among teens and young adults. For centuries, bidis were popular in India,

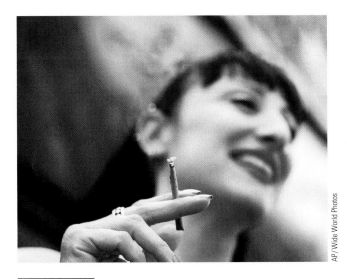

The smoke produced by bidis—skinny, flavored cigarettes—can contain higher concentrations of toxic chemicals than the smoke from regular cigarettes.

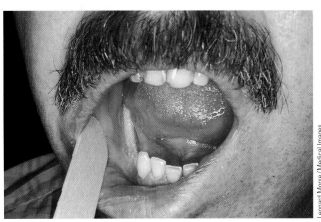

Chewing smokeless tobacco can damage the tissues of the mouth and lead to cancer of the larynx, esophagus, kidney, pancreas, and bladder.

where they are known as the poor man's cigarette and sell for less than five cents a pack. They look strikingly like clove cigarettes or marijuana joints and are available in flavors like grape, strawberry, and mandarin orange. Bidis are legal for adults and even minors in some states and are sold on the Internet as well as in stores.

Although bidis contain less tobacco than regular cigarettes, their unprocessed tobacco is more potent. Smoke from bidis has about three times as much nicotine and carbon monoxide and five times as much tar as smoke from regular filtered cigarettes. Because bidis are wrapped in nonporous brownish leaves, they don't burn as easily as cigarettes, and smokers have to inhale harder and more often to keep them lit. In one study, smoking a single bidi required 28 puffs, compared to 9 puffs for cigarettes.

Smokeless Tobacco

The consumption of smokeless tobacco products is rising, particularly among young males. These substances include snuff, finely ground tobacco that can be sniffed or placed inside the cheek and sucked, and chewing tobacco, tobacco leaves mixed with flavoring agents such as molasses. With both, nicotine is absorbed through the mucous membranes of the nose or mouth.

Smokeless tobacco can cause cancer and noncancerous oral conditions and lead to nicotine addiction and dependence. Smokeless tobacco users are more likely than nonusers to become cigarette smokers.

More than 7 million people, many of them young, use snuff and chewing tobacco. This number may include as many as one in five college men. Use is highest in the south-central United States. Even when users spot lesions in their mouths, most do not seek medical help but continue to use smokeless tobacco.

Environmental Tobacco Smoke

Maybe you don't smoke—never have, never will. That doesn't mean you don't have to worry about the dangers of smoking, especially if you live or work with people who smoke. **Environmental tobacco smoke,** or secondhand cigarette smoke, the most hazardous form of indoor air pollution, ranks behind cigarette smoking and alcohol as the third-leading preventable cause of death.

On average, a smoker inhales what is known as **mainstream smoke** eight or nine times with each cigarette, for a total of about 24 seconds. However, the cigarette burns for about 12 minutes, and everyone in the room (including the smoker) breathes in what is known as **sidestream smoke.**

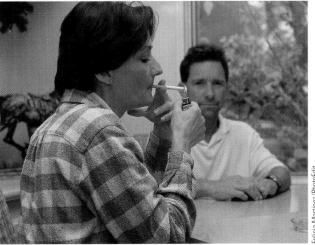

Secondhand smoke is the most common and hazardous form of indoor air pollution.

According to the American Lung Association, incomplete combustion from the lower temperatures of a smoldering cigarette makes sidestream smoke dirtier and chemically different from mainstream smoke. It has twice as much tar and nicotine, five times as much carbon monoxide, and 50 times as much ammonia. And because the particles in sidestream smoke are small, this mixture of irritating gases and carcinogenic tar reaches deeper into the lungs. If you're a nonsmoker sitting next to someone smoking seven cigarettes an hour, even in a ventilated room, you'll take in almost twice the maximum amount of carbon monoxide set for air pollution in industry—and it will take hours for the carbon monoxide to leave your body.

What Are the Risks of Secondhand Smoke?

Even a little secondhand smoke is dangerous. According to the CDC, every year environmental tobacco smoke causes 3,000 deaths from lung cancer. In a ten-year Harvard University study that tracked 10,000 healthy women who never smoked, regular exposure to other people's smoke at home or work almost doubled the risk of heart disease. On the basis of their findings, the researchers estimated that up to 50,000 Americans may die every year of heart attacks from environmental tobacco smoke, and another 3,000 to 4,000 die of other forms of heart disease caused by secondhand smoke. As a cancer-causing agent, secondhand smoke may be twice as dangerous as radon gas and more than a hundred times more hazardous than outdoor pollutants regulated by federal law. Secondhand smoke also increases sick leave rates among employees.

✚ Quitting

Smoking is a remarkably difficult habit to kick. About 70 percent of smokers want to quit, but only about 5 percent succeed, according to the American Lung Association.

About half of whites who have smoked were able to kick the habit, compared with 45 percent of Asian Americans, 43 percent of Hispanics, and 37 percent of African Americans. Men and women with college and graduate degrees were much more likely to quit successfully than high-school dropouts.[38]

Compared with men, women seem to have a higher behavioral dependence on cigarettes. For them, wearing a nicotine patch or chewing nicotine gum does not substitute for the "hand-to-mouth" behaviors associated with smoking, such as lighting a cigarette, inhaling, and

---

STRATEGIES for PREVENTION

How Nonsmokers Can Clear the Air

∎ Let people know your feelings in advance by putting up "No Smoking" signs in your office, home, or car. If you're in a car and someone pulls out a cigarette, ask politely if the smoker can hold off until you reach your destination or stop for a break.

∎ When giving a party, designate a smoking room. Suggest that friends do the same for parties at their houses.

∎ If you're about to participate in a long meeting or class, suggest regular smoking breaks to avoid a smoke-filled room.

∎ At restaurants, always ask for a table in the nonsmoking section or, if there is none, one in a well-ventilated part of the restaurant.

∎ If someone's smoke is bothering you, speak up. Be polite, not pushy. Say something like, "Excuse me, but smoke bothers me."

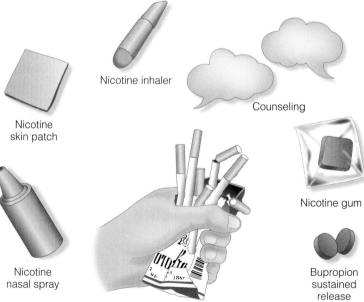

FIGURE 13-5 ∎ How to Quit

Combining one of the four nicotine replacement therapies (or bupropion/Zyban) with counseling is the most effective strategy to quit smoking.

Source: Department of Medicine, Center for Tobacco Research and Intervention, University of Wisconsin Medical School, Madison.

handling the cigarette. Some investigators have found that women are more likely to quit successfully when they receive a combination of nicotine replacement and the use of a device like a nicotine inhaler to substitute for smoking behaviors.

Although a large proportion of students have made an attempt to quit, only a minority succeed. Among current smokers, 59 percent report ever making an attempt to quit. Among those who ever smoked daily, 82 percent have tried to quit, while 75 percent are still smokers. The barriers to quitting in college include fears of weight gain, inability to manage stress without nicotine, and denial of nicotine addiction.[39]

One campus-based program that employed peer facilitators to help smokers quit and avoid relapse reported a success rate of 88 percent. Being "in the group" was the single most powerful contributor to quitting, and participants said their sense of connectedness helped them quit and stay smoke-free.[40]

Nicotine withdrawal symptoms can behave like characters in a bad horror flick: Just when you think you've killed them, they're back with a vengeance. In recent studies, some people who tried to quit smoking reported a small improvement in withdrawal symptoms over two weeks, but then their symptoms leveled off and persisted. Others found that their symptoms intensified rather than lessened over time. For reasons scientists cannot yet explain, former smokers who start smoking again put their lungs at even greater jeopardy than smokers who never quit.

Once a former smoker takes a single puff, the odds of a relapse are 80 to 85 percent. Smokers are most likely to quit in the third, fourth, or fifth attempt.[41] The good news is that half of all living Americans who ever smoked have managed to quit. Sooner is better than later, but later is better than not at all. And thanks to new products and programs, it may be easier now than ever before to become an ex-smoker.

Drugs and Their Effects

People who try illegal drugs don't think they'll ever lose control. Even regular drug users are convinced that they are smart enough, strong enough, lucky enough not to get caught and not to get hooked. But with continued use, drugs produce changes in an individual's body, mind, and behavior. In time, a person's need for a drug can outweigh everything else, including the values, people, and relationships he or she once held dearest.

After growing significantly in the past half century, the spread of drugs has slowed: 95 percent of the world's people do not use illegal drugs, according to the United Nations. In the last year, fewer than one in every 30 people between ages 15 to 64 used an illicit drug.[42]

In the United States, drug use by young teenagers has dropped dramatically—from 24 percent in 1996 to 15 percent in 2004.[43] Fewer young people report that they use or have ever used marijuana, ecstasy, amphetamines, methamphetamine, PCP, ketamine, and steroids (discussed in Chapter 5). Among college students, the most widely used drugs are marijuana and "club drugs," including ecstasy.

WELLNESS COACH

Developing Positive Addictions

When you're anxious, bored, restless, or confused, when drugs seem all too appealing as a "quick fix," there are real solutions, "positive addictions" that can help you solve your problems without creating new and bigger ones. A positive addiction—whether it is exercising, mountain-climbing, or listening to music— can produce very real "highs." But there's a crucial difference between this sort of stimulation and drug dependency: one is real, the other is chemical. With one, you're in control; with the other, drugs are.

Here are some examples:

▮ **If you feel a need for physical relaxation,** if you want more energy or distraction from physical discomforts, you can turn to athletics, exercise (including walking and hiking), dance, or outdoor hobbies.

▮ **If you want to stimulate your senses,** enhance sexual stimulation, or magnify the sensations of sight, sound, and touch, train yourself to be more sensitive to nature and beauty. Take time to appreciate the sensations you experience when you're walking in the woods or embracing a person you love. Through activities like sailing or sky-diving, you can literally fill up your senses without relying on chemicals.

▮ **If you have psychological troubles,** if you're anxious or depressed, if you feel inhibited or uptight, if you don't know how to solve complex personal problems and want relief from emotional pain, turn to people who can offer lasting help: in some cases, friends; in others, professional counselors or support groups.

▮ **If you want peer acceptance,** if you'd like to overcome your shyness, if you want to communicate and relate more effectively, you can join expertly managed sensitivity or encounter groups, enroll in confidence-building seminars, seek counseling, or volunteer in programs in which you can assist others and not focus only on your self-consciousness.

▮ **If you want to escape mental boredom,** gain new understanding of the world around you, study better, experiment with your levels of awareness, or indulge your intellectual curiosity, challenge your mind through reading, classes, creative games, discussion groups, memory training, or travel.

█ **If you want to enhance your creativity** or your appreciation of the arts, pursue training in music, art, singing, gardening, or writing. Sign up for a nongraded course in art history or music appreciation. Attend more concerts, ballets, museum shows.

█ **If you want to promote political or social change,** defy the establishment, change drug legislation, or gain power, you can volunteer in political campaigns, work on nonpartisan projects, or join lobbying and political action groups.

█ **If you want to find meaning in life,** to understand the nature of the universe, or expand your personal awareness, explore various philosophical theories through classes, seminars, and discussion groups. Study different religious orientations, including mysticism, or try yoga and meditation.

█ **If you're looking for kicks,** adventure, danger, and excitement, sign up for an Outward Bound wilderness survival course. Take up an adventurous sport, like hang-gliding or parachuting. Set a challenging professional or personal goal and direct your energies to meeting it.

█ Drug Use on Campus

Drug use on campus has increased since 1993, with the steepest rise in the mid-1990s. Almost half of undergraduates say they have used marijuana; 30 percent report its use in the last year and 17 percent in the last 30 days. Seven percent report that they've used another illicit

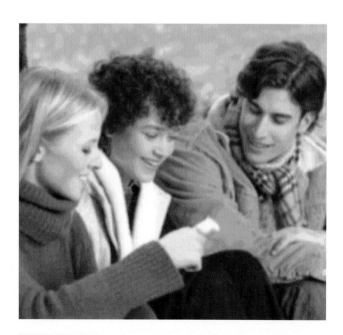

█ Spend time with friends who don't need alcohol or drugs to enjoy themselves.

TABLE 13-4 █ Who Drinks Alcohol?[1]

	Percentage of Students	Days per Week	Drinks per Occasion
By sex			
Women	79%	2.2	4.3
Men	87%	2.7	6.7
By race			
Caucasian	89%	2.6	5.95
African American	55%	1.6	3.4
Asian	62%	2.2	4.7
By fraternity/sorority membership			
Members	93%	2.98	6.2
Non-members	78%	2.2	5.4

Who Uses Drugs?[1]

	Percentage of Students	Days per Week
By sex		
Women	16.5%	3.99
Men	27.5%	3.3
By race		
Caucasian	23.9%	3.5
African American	10.7%	3.1
Asian	14.6%	2.5
By fraternity/sorority membership		
Members	29.2%	3.4
Non-members	18.1%	3.5

[1] Based on a study of 740 undergraduates

Source: Shinew, Kimberly and Diana Parry. "Examining College Students' Participation in the Leisure Pursuits of Drinking and Illegal Drug Use," *Journal of Leisure Research,* Summer 2005 Vol. 37, No. 3, p. 364(23)

drug in the last 30 days; 14 percent did so in the last year (**Table 13-4**).

Drug use has increased most dramatically among minority students, particularly African Americans and Asian–Pacific Islanders. However, white students still have the highest rates of drug use. More than 9 in 10 of students who used marijuana and other illicit drugs also used other substances, smoked cigarettes, and/or were binge drinkers.[44]

In recent years, ecstasy use more than doubled on campus. The Harvard College Alcohol Study revealed an increase of almost 70 percent in ecstasy use by undergraduates over a two-year period.

There is a large gap between actual drug use on campus and how prevalent students believe drug use to be. When researchers have compared students' self-reports of frequency of drug use with what students perceived to be the frequency of drug use by "the average student," findings show they greatly overestimate the use of a variety of drugs.

Why Students Use Drugs

Various factors influence which students use drugs, including the following:

- **Race /ethnicity.** In general, white students have higher levels of alcohol and drug use than do African-American students. In a comparison of African-American students at predominantly white and predominantly black colleges, those at historically black colleges had lower rates of alcohol and drug use than did either white or African-American students at white schools. The reason, according to the researchers, may be that these colleges provide a greater sense of self-esteem, which helps prevent alcohol and drug use.

- **Perception of risk.** Students seem most likely to try substances they perceive as being "safe," or low risk. Of these, the top three are caffeine, alcohol, and tobacco; marijuana is listed fourth in terms of perceived safety. Other agents—barbiturates, heroin, cocaine, PCP, speed, LSD, crack, and inhalants—are viewed as more risky and are used much less often.

- **Alcohol use.** Often individuals engage in more than one "risk behavior," and researchers have documented correlations among smoking, drinking, and drug use. Among college students, researchers have found that those who report binge drinking are much more likely than other students to report current or past use of marijuana, cocaine, or other illegal drugs.

- **Environment.** As with alcohol use, students are influenced by their friends, their residence, the general public's attitude toward drug use, and even the Internet. College health officials are realizing that rather than simply trying to change students' substance abuse, they also must change the environment to promote healthier lifestyle choices. One successful innovation is substance-free dorms.

- **Sexual identity.** In a recent survey of 3,607 undergraduate students, self-identified lesbian women were significantly more likely than heterosexual women to use marijuana, ecstasy, and other drugs.[45] Gay and bisexual men were significantly less likely than heterosexual men to drink heavily but were more likely to use some drugs.[46] In another survey, college women with both male and female sex partners were up to three times more likely to smoke cigarettes, binge drink, and use marijuana than exclusively heterosexual women.[47]

- **Gambling.** In a study at four Connecticut universities, one in nine students had a gambling problem significantly connected to a substance-related issue. Problem/pathological gamblers report a higher number of drug and alcohol problems than nongamblers or social gamblers.[48]

▌ Common Drugs of Abuse

Table 13-5 describes the common drugs of abuse within these categories: cannabis, club drugs, stimulants, depressants, hallucinogens, and inhalants.

Cannabis

Marijuana (pot) and **hashish** (hash)—the most widely used illegal drugs—are derived from the cannabis plant. The major psychoactive ingredient in both is *THC (delta-9-tetrahydrocannabinol)*. Marijuana is the most widely abused substance, with more than 150 million people reporting they've used it at least once in the last year. Some 12 million Americans use cannabis; more than 1 million cannot control this use. Although fewer teens smoke marijuana, recent research has found that significantly more 45-to-64-year-old men and women are using marijuana.[49]

The incidence of marijuana use disorders, including dependence and abuse, has increased, particularly in young black men and women and young Hispanic men. Marijuana use disorders among young white men and women have remained stable over the last decade.

Different types of marijuana have different percentages of THC. Because of careful cultivation, the strength of today's marijuana is much greater than that used in the 1970s. Today a marijuana joint contains 150 mg of THC, compared to 10 mg in the 1960s.

Usually, marijuana is smoked in a joint (hand-rolled cigarette) or pipe; it may also be eaten as an ingredient in other foods (as when baked in brownies), though with a less predictable effect. The drug high is enhanced by holding the marijuana smoke in the lungs, and experienced smokers learn to hold the smoke for longer periods to increase the amount of drug diffused into the bloodstream. The circumstances in which marijuana is smoked, the communal aspects of its use, and the user's experience all can affect the way a marijuana-induced high feels.

Marijuana produces a range of effects in different bodily systems, such as diminished immune responses and impaired fertility in men. Other risks include damage to the brain, lungs, and heart, and to babies born to mothers who use marijuana during pregnancy or while nursing (**Figure 13-6**, page 316).

Marijuana has shown some medical benefits, including boosting appetite in patients who are HIV-positive or undergoing chemotherapy, alleviating cancer and neck pain, helping reduce pressure on the eyeball in glaucoma patients, and helping people with spasticity (extreme muscle tension) due to multiple sclerosis or injuries.[50]

Support for the legalization of marijuana for medicinal purposes has grown in recent years, although the majority of Americans still oppose such legislation. Several states allow marijuana to be grown and distributed to people with a doctor's recommendation.

TABLE 13-5 ▌ Common Drugs of Abuse

Type of Drug	Drug Name	Street Name	Description	How It's Used	Related Paraphernalia	Signs and Symptoms of Use
Cannabis	**Marijuana**	Pot, grass, reefer, weed, Colombian hash, joints, sinsemilla, blunts, Acapulco gold, Thai sticks	Like dried oregano leaves, dark green or brown	Usually smoked in hand-rolled cigarettes, pipes, or thin cigars, or eaten	Rolling papers, pipes, bongs, baggies, roach clips	Sweet burnt odor, neglect of appearance, loss of motivation, slow reactions, red eyes, memory lapses
Club Drugs/ Designer Drugs (stimulants, depressants, and/or hallucinogens)	**MDMA, MDA, MDEA**	Ecstasy, XTC, X, Adam, clarity	Tablet or capsule; colorless, tasteless, and odorless	Swallowed, can be added to beverages by individuals who want to intoxicate others	Pacifiers, glow sticks (used at all-night dance parties, raves, or trances)	Agitated state, confusion, sleep problems, paranoia
	Date-rape drug Rohypnol	Roofies, roche, forget-me pill, love drug	Tasteless, odorless, dissolves easily in all beverages	Swallowed, can be added to beverages by individuals who want to sedate others	Drinks, soda cans	1 milligram can impair a victim for 8 to 12 hours, can cause amnesia, decreased blood pressure, urinary retention
	GHB	Liquid ecstasy, grievous bodily harm, G	Clear liquid, tablet, capsule	Swallowed, dissolved in drinks	Drinks, soda cans	Can relax or sedate
Stimulants (stimulate the nervous system)	**Amphetamines** amphetamine, dextroamphetamine, methamphetamine	Speed, uppers, pep pill, bennies, dexies, meth, crank, crystal, black beauties, white crosses	Variety of tablets, capsules, and crystal-like rock salt	Swallowed in pill or capsule form, or injected	Syringe, needles	Excess activity, irritability, nervousness, mood swings, needle marks, dilated pupils, talkativeness then depression
	Cocaine	Coke, snow, toot, white lady	White odorless powder	Usually inhaled; can be injected, swallowed, or smoked	Razor blade, straws, glass surfaces	Restlessness, dilated pupils, oily skin, talkativeness; euphoric short-term high, followed by depression
	Tobacco/Nicotine	Smokes, butts, cigs, cancer sticks, snuff, dip, chew, plug	Dried brown organic material, bidis (skinny, sweet-flavored cigarettes); smokeless is moist	Smoked in cigarettes, pipes, cigars, cigarillos; chewed; or inhaled through the nose as snuff	Rolling papers, pipes, spit cups, cigar cutters, lighters, matches	Shortness of breath, respiratory illnesses; oral, lung, and other cancers
Depressants (depress the nervous system)	**Alcohol**	Booze, hooch, juice, brew, alcopops (hard lemonade or fruit juices)	Clear or amber-colored liquid; sweet, fruit-flavored or malt-based drinks	Swallowed in liquid form	Flask, bottles, cans, use of food color to disguise it; colorful, innocent-looking labels	Impaired judgment, poor muscle coordination, lowered inhibitions

TABLE 13-5 | Common Drugs of Abuse (*continued*)

Type of Drug	Drug Name	Street Name	Description	How It's Used	Related Paraphernalia	Signs and Symptoms of Use
	Barbiturates Amyl, Seconal, Nembutal, Butisol, Tuinal	Barbs, downers, yellow jackets, red devils, blue devils	Variety of tablets, capsules, powder	Swallowed in pill form or injected into the veins	Syringe, needles	Drowsiness, confusion, impaired judgment, slurred speech, needle marks, staggering gait
	Tranquilizers/ Benzodiazepines Valium, Librium, Miltown, Xanax	V's, blues, downers, candy	Variety of tablets	Swallowed in pill form or injected	Syringe, pill bottles, needles	Drowsiness, faulty judgment, disorientation
	Narcotics/ Opioids heroin, morphine	Dreamer, junk, smack, horse	White or brown powders, tablets, capsules, liquid	Injected, smoked, may be blended with marijuana	Syringes, spoon, lighter, needles, medicine dropper	Lethargy, loss of skin color, needle marks, constricted pupils, decreased coordination
Hallucinogens (alter perceptions of reality)	**PCP** (phencyclidine)	Angel dust, killer weed, supergrass, hog, peace pill	White powder or tablet	Usually smoked, can be inhaled (snorted), injected, or swallowed in tablets	Tinfoil	Slurred speech, blurred vision, lack of coordination, confusion, agitation, violence, unpredictability, "bad trips"
	LSD (lysergic acid diethylamide)	Acid, cubes, purple haze, white lightning	Odorless, colorless, tasteless powder	Injected, or swallowed in tablets or capsules	Blotter papers, tinfoil	Dilated pupils, illusions, hallucinations, disorientation, mood swings, nausea, flashbacks
	Mescaline caps, psilocybin, psilocin, mushrooms	Mesc, cactus, caps, magic mushrooms, shrooms	Capsules, tablets, mushrooms	Ingested in its natural form, smoked, or brewed as tea	Dried mushrooms	Same as LSD
Inhalants (substances abused by sniffing)	**Solvents, aerosols** airplane glue, gasoline, dry cleaning solution, correction fluid		Chemicals that produce mind-altering vapors	Inhaled or sniffed, often with the use of paper or plastic bags	Cleaning rags, empty spray cans, tubes of glue, baggies	Poor motor coordination; bad breath; impaired vision, memory, and thoughts; violent behavior
	Nitrates amyl and butyl	Poppers, locker room, rush, snappers	Clear yellowish liquid	Inhaled or sniffed from gauze or single-dose glass vials	Cloth-covered bulb that pops when broken, small bottles	Slowed thought, headache
	Nitrous oxide	Laughing gas, whippets	Colorless gas with sweet taste and smell	Inhaled or sniffed by mask or cone	Aerosol cans such as whipped cream, small canisters	Light-headedness, loss of motor control

Source: "A Parent's Guide for the Prevention of Alcohol, Tobacco and Other Drug Use." Copyright © 2000 Lowe Family Foundation, Inc., Revised 2001 (Lowe Family Foundation, 3339 Stuyvesant Pl. NW, Washington, DC, 20015, 202-362-4883). Used with permission.

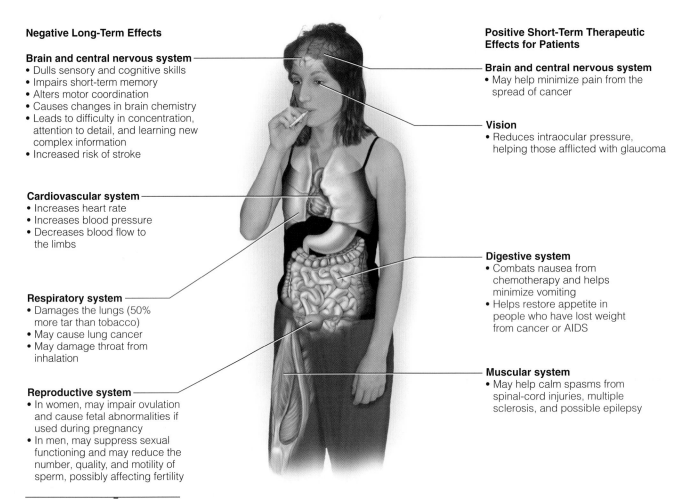

Negative Long-Term Effects

Brain and central nervous system
• Dulls sensory and cognitive skills
• Impairs short-term memory
• Alters motor coordination
• Causes changes in brain chemistry
• Leads to difficulty in concentration, attention to detail, and learning new complex information
• Increased risk of stroke

Cardiovascular system
• Increases heart rate
• Increases blood pressure
• Decreases blood flow to the limbs

Respiratory system
• Damages the lungs (50% more tar than tobacco)
• May cause lung cancer
• May damage throat from inhalation

Reproductive system
• In women, may impair ovulation and cause fetal abnormalities if used during pregnancy
• In men, may suppress sexual functioning and may reduce the number, quality, and motility of sperm, possibly affecting fertility

Positive Short-Term Therapeutic Effects for Patients

Brain and central nervous system
• May help minimize pain from the spread of cancer

Vision
• Reduces intraocular pressure, helping those afflicted with glaucoma

Digestive system
• Combats nausea from chemotherapy and helps minimize vomiting
• Helps restore appetite in people who have lost weight from cancer or AIDS

Muscular system
• May help calm spasms from spinal-cord injuries, multiple sclerosis, and possible epilepsy

FIGURE 13-6 ❚ Some Effects of Marijuana on the Body

Marijuana may have some positive short-term therapeutic effects for people with cancer, glaucoma, or AIDS, but the long-term effects for healthy users are all negative.

Club Drugs (Designer Drugs)

The National Institute on Drug Abuse identifies a variety of drugs—alcohol, LSD (acid), MDMA (ecstasy), GHB, GBL, Ketamine (Special-K), Fentanyl, Rohypnol, amphetamines, and methamphetamine—as **"club drugs,"** popular among teens and young adults at nightclubs, bars, or raves and trances—night-long dances often held in warehouses or other unusual settings.

Although many who attend raves do not generally use drugs, they may be told that club drugs are cheap, energizing, and safe. As scientists are demonstrating, this is not true. Brain scans reveal changes in critical parts of the brain from use of club drugs (**Figure 13-7**, page 317). In high doses most of these drugs can cause a sharp increase in body temperature (a condition called malignant hyperthermia), leading to muscle breakdown, kidney and cardiovascular system failure, and possible death.

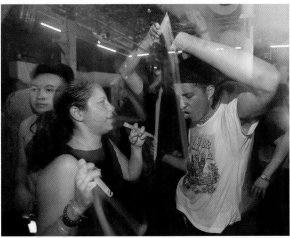

Club drugs are often used at raves, even those that are alcohol-free, and can pose unexpected risks.

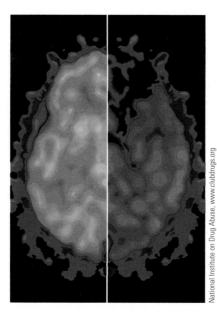

FIGURE 13-7 ▌ Effects of Ecstasy on the Brain

On the brain scan for an individual who has never used drugs (left), the bright reddish color shows active serotonin sites in the brain. Serotonin is a critical neurochemical that regulates mood, emotion, learning, memory, sleep, and pain. In the scan of an individual who used the club drug ecstasy many times but had not used any drugs for at least three weeks before the scan (right), the dark sections indicate areas where serotonin is not present even after three weeks without any drugs.

National Institute on Drug Abuse, www.clubdrugs.org

Ecstasy

Ecstasy (Adam, XTC, X, hug, beans, love drug) is the common street name for methylene-dioxymethamphetamine (MDMA), a synthetic compound with both stimulant and mildly hallucinogenic properties. MDMA is spreading beyond the young white populations frequenting raves to mainstream dance clubs and house parties, with use increasing among African Americans, Hispanics, and people in their thirties.

Students who use ecstasy do not differ from others in terms of academic achievement (as measured by GPA) or commitment to community service. In one study, they were found significantly more likely to be white, to belong to a fraternity/sorority, and to have used other drugs of abuse during the previous year.[51] Ecstasy users are more likely to use marijuana, binge drink, spend more time socializing and less time studying, have more sexual partners, smoke cigarettes, rate parties as more important than academics, and view religion as less important.[52]

Stimulants

Central nervous system stimulants are drugs that increase activity in some portion of the brain or spinal cord. Some increase motor activity and enhance mental alert-

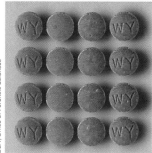

▌ Ya-ba/Thai Tabs are a new, powerful form of methamphetamine that tastes sweet like candy.

DEA/Office of Forensic Sciences

ness, and some combat mental fatigue. Amphetamine, methamphetamine, caffeine, cocaine, and khat are stimulants.

Amphetamine and Methamphetamine

Amphetamines trigger the release of epinephrine (adrenaline), which stimulates the central nervous system. They were once widely prescribed for weight control because they suppress appetite, but they have emerged as a global danger. Amphetamines are sold under a variety of names: amphetamine (brand name Benzedrine, streetname bennies), dextroamphetamine (Dexedrine, dex), methamphetamine (Methedrine, meth, speed), and Desoxyn (copilots). Related *uppers* include the prescription drugs methylphenidate (Ritalin), pemoline (Cylert), and phenmetrazine (Preludin). Amphetamines are available in tablet or capsule form.

Methamphetamine (meth, crank, crystal, fast, glass, speed, beanies, black beauties, blade, christmas tree meth, cinnamon, sugar, crys, shabu, tic, wash) is a powerful addictive stimulant that comes in three forms—powder, crystal, and pills—and can be ingested by mouth, injected, or snorted. "Ice," the slang name for crystallized methamphetamine hydrochloride, is smokeable methamphetamine, highly addictive and toxic.

A new form of methamphetamine, Ya-ba/Thai Tabs, may seem less dangerous but is actually more powerful and dangerous than other forms of methamphetamine. It has hallucinogenic effects and may cause increased heart rate, dehydration, paranoia, and depression.

Unlike cocaine, which is quickly removed from the brain, methamphetamine remains in the central nervous system and the body, producing prolonged stimulant effects. Chronic abuse produces a psychosis similar to schizophrenia, characterized by paranoia, picking at the skin, preoccupation with one's thoughts, and auditory and visual hallucinations. Symptoms can persist for months or even years after discontinuing use.

Methamphetamine "laboratories," created to meet the black-market demand for stimulants, have spread across the country. Using a relatively simple process, meth "cooks" in kitchens, basements, and garages make powder amphetamines in makeshift laboratories. Fires and explosions are common because of the volatile chemicals involved. Large amounts of methamphetamines are also smuggled into the United States from Mexico.

Cocaine

Cocaine (coke, snow, lady) is a white crystalline powder extracted from the leaves of the South American coca plant. Usually mixed with various sugars and local anesthetics like lidocaine and procaine, cocaine powder is generally inhaled. When sniffed or snorted, cocaine anesthetizes the nerve endings in the nose and relaxes the lung's bronchial muscles.

Cocaine can be dissolved in water and injected intravenously. The drug is rapidly metabolized by the liver, so the high is relatively brief, typically lasting only about 20 minutes. This means that users will commonly inject the drug repeatedly, increasing the risk of infection and damage to their veins. Many intravenous cocaine users prefer the practice of *speedballing,* the intravenous administration of a combination of cocaine and heroin.

Cocaine alkaloid, or *freebase,* is obtained by removing the hydrochloride salt from cocaine powder. *Freebasing* is smoking the fumes of the alkaloid form of cocaine. *Crack,* pharmacologically identical to freebase, is a cheap, easy-to-use, widely available, smokeable, and potent form of cocaine named for the popping sound it makes when burned. Because it is absorbed rapidly into the bloodstream and large doses reach the brain very quickly, it is particularly dangerous. However, its low price and easy availability have made it a common drug of abuse in poor urban areas.

Khat (Kat, Catha, Chat, Abyssinian Tea)

For centuries people in East Africa and the Arabian peninsula consumed the fresh young leaves of the *Catha edulis* shrub in ways similar to our drinking coffee. Its active ingredients are two controlled substances, cathinone and cathine. Chewing alleviates fatigue and reduces appetite. Compulsive use may result in manic behavior, grandiose illusions, paranoia, and hallucinations.[53]

Depressants

Depressants depress the central nervous system, reduce activity, and induce relaxation, drowsiness, or sleep. They include the benzodiazepines and the barbiturates, the opioids, and alcohol.

Benzodiazepines and Barbiturates

These depressants are the sedative-hypnotics, also known as anxiolytic or antianxiety drugs. The **benzodiazepines**—the most widely used drugs in this category—are commonly prescribed for tension, muscular strain, sleep problems, anxiety, panic attacks, anesthesia, and in the treatment of alcohol withdrawal. They include such drugs as *chlordiazepoxide* (Librium), *diazepam* (Valium), *oxazepam* (Serax), *lorazepam* (Ativan), *flurazepam* (Dalmane), and *alprazolam* (Xanax). They differ widely in their mechanism of action, absorption rate, and metabolism, but all produce similar intoxication and withdrawal symptoms.

Rohypnol, a trade name for flunitrazepam, is one of the benzodiazepines, and it has been of particular concern for the last few years because of its abuse in date rape. When mixed with alcohol, Rohypnol can incapacitate victims and prevent them from resisting sexual assault. It produces "anterograde amnesia," which means individuals may not remember events they experienced while under the effects of the drug. Rohypnol may be lethal when mixed with alcohol or other depressants.

Benzodiazepine sleeping pills have largely replaced the **barbiturates,** which were used medically in the past for inducing relaxation and sleep, relieving tension, and treating epileptic seizures.

Opioids

The **opioids** include *opium* and its derivatives (*morphine, codeine,* and *heroin*) and nonopioid synthetic drugs that have similar sleep-inducing and pain-relieving properties. The opioids come from a resin taken from the seedpod of the Asian poppy. **Nonopioids,** such as *meperidine* (Demerol), *methadone,* and *propoxyphene* (Darvon), are chemically synthesized. Whether natural or synthetic, these drugs are powerful *narcotics,* or painkillers.

Heroin (also known as horse, junk, smack, or downtown), the most widely abused opioid, is illegal in this country. In other nations it is used as a potent painkiller for conditions such as terminal cancer. There are an estimated 600,000 heroin addicts in the United States, with men outnumbering women addicts by three to one. Among people aged 18 to 25, the percentage of heroin users who inject the drug has doubled in the last decade. While the number of young heroin users in major cities has dropped by 50 percent, their numbers almost tripled in suburban and rural areas.[54]

Heroin users typically inject the drug into their veins. Individuals who experiment with recreational drugs often prefer *skin-popping* (subcutaneous injection) rather than *mainlining* (intravenous injection); they also may snort heroin as a powder or dissolve it and inhale the vapors. To try to avoid addiction, some users begin by *chipping,* taking small or intermittent doses. Regardless of the method of administration, tolerance can develop rapidly.

Morphine, used as a painkiller and anesthetic, acts primarily on the central nervous system, eyes, and digestive tract. By producing mental clouding, drowsiness, and euphoria, it does not decrease the physical sensation of pain as much as it alters a person's awareness of the pain; in effect, he or she no longer cares about it.

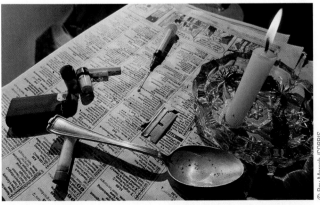

❚ Opioid drugs, made from the Asian poppy, come in both legal and illegal forms. All are highly addictive.

Two semisynthetic derivatives of morphine are *hydromorphone* (Dilaudid, little D), with two to eight times the painkilling effect of morphine, and *oxycodone* (OxyContin, Percocet, Percodan, perkies), similar to codeine but more potent. The synthetic narcotic *meperidine* (Demerol, demies) is now probably second only to morphine for use in relieving pain. It is also used by addicts as a substitute for morphine or heroin.

Codeine, a weaker painkiller than morphine, is an ingredient in liquid products prescribed for relieving coughs and in tablet and injectable form for relieving pain. The synthetic narcotic *propoxyphene* (Darvon), a somewhat less potent painkiller than codeine, is no more effective than aspirin in usual doses. It has been one of the most widely prescribed drugs for headaches, dental pain, and menstrual cramps. At higher doses, Darvon produces a euphoric high, which may lead to misuse.

Prescription opioids are taken orally in pill form but can also be injected intravenously. Some individuals first take a medically prescribed opioid for pain relief or cough suppression, then gradually increase the dose and frequency of use on their own, often justifying this because of their symptoms rather than for the sensations the drug induces. They expend increasing efforts to obtain the drug, frequently seeking out several doctors to write prescriptions.

Hallucinogens

The drugs known as **hallucinogens** produce vivid and unusual changes in thought, feeling, and perception. Hallucinogens do not produce dependence in the same way as cocaine or heroin. Individuals who have an unpleasant experience after trying a hallucinogen may stop using the drug completely without suffering withdrawal symptoms. Others continue regular or occasional use because they enjoy the effects.

LSD and Mescaline

LSD (*lysergic acid diethylamide*, acid) was initially developed as a tool to explore mental illness. It became popular in the 1960s and resurfaced among teenagers in the 1990s.

LSD is taken orally, either blotted onto pieces of paper that are held in the mouth or chewed along with another substance, such as a sugar cube. Peyote (containing the active ingredient *mescaline*) is another hallucinogen, but it is much less commonly used in this country.

Phencyclidine (PCP)

PCP (phencyclidine, brand name Sernyl; street names angel dust, peace pill, lovely, and green) is an illicit drug manufactured as a tablet, capsule, liquid, flake, spray, or crystal-like white powder that can be swallowed, smoked, sniffed, or injected. Sometimes it is sprinkled on crack, marijuana, tobacco, or parsley, and smoked. A fine-powdered form of PCP can be snorted or injected. Once PCP was thought to have medicinal value as an anesthetic, but its side effects, including delirium and hallucinations, now make it unacceptable for medical use.

PCP use peaked in the 1970s, but it remains a popular drug of abuse in both inner-city ghettos and suburban high schools. Users often think that the PCP they take together with another illegal psychoactive substance, such as amphetamines, coke, or hallucinogens, is responsible for the highs they feel, so they seek it out specifically.

Inhalants

Inhalants or **deleriants** are chemicals that produce vapors with psychoactive effects. The most commonly abused inhalants are solvents, aerosols, model-airplane glue, cleaning fluids, and petroleum products like kerosene and butane. Some anesthetics and nitrous oxide (laughing gas) are also abused.

Young people who have been treated for mental health problems, have a history of foster care, or who already abuse other drugs have an increased risk of abusing or becoming dependent on inhalants. In addition, adolescents who first begin using inhalants at an early age are more likely to become dependent on them. Approximately 9 percent of adolescents nationwide report having used inhalants in their lifetime. Teens with inhalant use disorders report coexisting multiple drug abuse and dependence, mental health treatment, and delinquent behaviors.[55]

✚ Prescription Drug Abuse

According to the National Institute on Drug Abuse, 9 million American use prescription drugs for "nonmedical" purposes every year—up drastically from about half a million in 1988. This problem, experts stress, often is not one of "bad" drugs or "bad" people but of dangerous misperceptions about the power and process of addiction.

STRATEGIES for PREVENTION

How to Say No

If people offer you a drug, here are some ways to say no:

▌ Let them know you're not interested. Change the subject. If the pressure seems threatening, just walk away.

▌ Have something else to do: "No, I'm going for a walk now."

▌ Be prepared for different types of pressure. If your friends tease you, tease them back.

▌ Keep it simple. "No, thanks," "No," or "No way" all get the point across.

▌ Hang out with people who won't offer you drugs.

Prescription drug abuse has increased most dramatically among 12 to 25 year olds. The most widely abused medications among teens and young adults are the painkillers Vicodin and OxyContin and sedatives.[56]

The abuse of stimulant medications such as Ritalin for attention-deficit hyperactivity disorder has surged. In a recent study at a Midwestern university, 17 percent of the men and 11 percent of the women surveyed reported illicit use of prescribed stimulants. The primary reason for taking these drugs was to increase energy and alertness.[57]

Like other addictions, a prescription drug "habit" is a treatable brain disease. Recovery usually requires carefully supervised detoxification, appropriate medications (similar to those used for opioid dependence), behavior therapy, and ongoing support.

✚ Treating Substance Dependence and Abuse

An estimated 6.1 million Americans are in need of drug treatment, but the vast majority—some 5 million—never get treatment.[58] The most difficult step for a drug user is to admit that he or she *is* in fact an addict. If drug abusers are not forced to deal with their problem through some unexpected trauma, such as being fired or going bankrupt, those who care—family, friends, coworkers, doctors —may have to confront them and insist that they do some-thing about their addiction. Often this *intervention* can be the turning point for addicts and their families. Treatment has proved equally successful for young people and for older adults.

Treatment may take place in an outpatient setting, a residential facility, or a hospital. Increasingly, treatment thereafter is tailored to address coexisting or dual diagnoses. A personal treatment plan may consist of individual psychotherapy, marital and family therapy, medication, and behavior therapy. Once an individual has made the decision to seek help for substance abuse, the first step usually is detoxification, which involves clearing the drug from the body.

Medications are used in detoxification to alleviate withdrawal symptoms and prevent medical and psychiatric complications. Once withdrawal is complete, these medications are discontinued, so the individual is in a drug-free state. However, individuals with mental disorders may require appropriate psychiatric medication to manage their symptoms and reduce the risk of relapse. For example, a person suffering from major depression or panic disorder may require ongoing treatment with antidepressant medication.

The aim of chemical dependence treatment is to help individuals establish and maintain their recovery from alcohol and drugs of abuse. Recovery is a dynamic process of personal growth and healing in which the drug user makes the transition from a lifestyle of active substance use to a drug-free lifestyle.

✚ MAKING HEALTHY CHOICES

For Responsible Substance Use

As you decide about the role alcohol should play in your life, you might want to follow these guidelines proposed by BACCHUS, a volunteer college student organization that promotes responsible alcohol-related behavior:

▮ **Set a limit on how many drinks you're going to have** ahead of time—and stick to it.

▮ **When you're mixing a drink, measure the alcohol.**

▮ **Drink slowly;** don't guzzle.

▮ **Develop alternatives to drinking** so you don't turn to alcohol whenever you're depressed or upset. Exercise is a wonderful release for tension; meditation or relaxation techniques can also help you cope.

▮ **Avoid performing tasks that require skilled reactions** during or after drinking.

▮ **Don't encourage or reinforce others' irresponsible behavior.**

Above all, keep in mind that drinking should not be the primary focus of any activity. Responsible drinking is a matter of you controlling your drinking rather than the drinking controlling you.

If you smoke—even just a few cigarettes a few times a week—you are at risk of nicotine addiction. Here is how to get back into control:

▮ **Use delaying tactics.** Have your first cigarette of the day 15 minutes later than usual, then 15 minutes later than that the next day, and so on.

▮ **Distract yourself.** When you feel a craving for a cigarette, talk to someone, drink a glass of water, or get up and move around.

▮ **Establish nonsmoking hours.** Instead of lighting up at the end of a meal, for instance, get up immediately, brush your teeth, wash your hands, or take a walk.

▮ **Never smoke two packs of the same brand in a row.** Buy cigarettes only by the pack, not by the carton.

▮ **Make it harder to get to your cigarettes.** Lock them in a drawer, wrap them in paper, or leave them in your coat or car.

▮ **Spend more time in places where you can't smoke.** Take up bike-riding or swimming. Shower often. Go to movies or other places where smoking isn't allowed.

▮ **Stop completely for just one day at a time.** Promise yourself 24 hours of freedom from cigarettes; when the day's over, make the same commitment for one more day. At the end of any 24-hour period, you can go back to smoking and not feel guilty.

SELF-SURVEY 1

Do You Have a Drinking Problem?

The self-assessment, the Michigan Alcoholism Screening Test (MAST), is widely used to identify potential problems. This test screens for the major psychological, sociological, and physiological consequences of alcoholism. To complete it, simply answer Yes or No to the following questions, and add up the points shown in the right column for your answers.

	Yes	No	Points
1. Do you enjoy a drink now and then?			(0 for either)
2. Do you think that you're a normal drinker? (By normal, we mean that you drink less than or as much as most other people.)			(2 for no)
3. Have you ever awakened the morning after some drinking the night before and found that you couldn't remember part of the evening?			(2 for yes)
4. Does your wife, husband, a parent, or other near relative ever worry or complain about your drinking?			(1 for yes)
5. Can you stop drinking without a struggle after one or two drinks?			(2 for no)
6. Do you ever feel guilty about your drinking?			(1 for yes)
7. Do friends or relatives think that you're a normal drinker?			(2 for no)
8. Do you ever try to limit your drinking to certain times of the day or to certain places?			(0 for either)
9. Have you ever attended a meeting of Alcoholics Anonymous?			(2 for yes)
10. Have you ever gotten into physical fights when drinking?			(1 for yes)
11. Has your drinking ever created problems for you and your wife, husband, a parent, or other relative?			(2 for yes)
12. Has your wife, husband, or other family members ever gone to anyone for help about your drinking?			(2 for yes)
13. Have you ever lost friends because of your drinking?			(2 for yes)
14. Have you ever gotten into trouble at work or school because of your drinking?			(2 for yes)

	Yes	No	Points
15. Have you ever lost a job because of your drinking?			(2 for yes)
16. Have you ever neglected your obligations, your family, or your work for two or more days in a row because of drinking?			(2 for yes)
17. Do you drink before noon fairly often?			(1 for yes)
18. Have you ever been told you have liver trouble? Cirrhosis?			(2 for yes)
19. After heavy drinking, have you ever had delirium tremens (DTs) or severe shaking, or heard voices or seen things that weren't actually there?			(2 for yes★)
20. Have you ever gone to anyone for help about your drinking?			(5 for yes)
21. Have you ever been in a hospital because of your drinking?			(5 for yes)
22. Have you ever been a patient in a psychiatric hospital or on a psychiatric ward of a general hospital where drinking was part of the problem that resulted in hospitalization?			(2 for yes)
23. Have you ever been seen at a psychiatric or mental health clinic or gone to any doctor, social worker, or clergyman for help with any emotional problem where drinking was part of the problem?			(2 for yes)
24. Have you ever been arrested for drunk driving, driving while intoxicated, or driving under the influence of alcoholic beverages?			(2 for yes)
25. Have you ever been arrested, or taken into custody, even for a few hours, because of drunken behavior?			(2 for yes)

(If Yes, how many times? _____★★)

★ Five points for delirium tremens
★★ Two points for each arrest

Scoring

In general, five or more points places you in an alcoholic category, four points suggests alcoholism; while three or fewer points indicates that you're *not* alcoholic.

ACTION PLAN 1

Your Action Plan for Responsible Drinking

▮ **Don't drink alone.** Cultivate friendships with non-drinkers and responsible moderate drinkers.
▮ **Don't use alcohol as a medicine.** Rather than reaching for a drink to put you to sleep, help you relax, or relieve tension, develop alternative means of

unwinding, such as exercise, meditation, or listening to music.

▌ **Develop a party plan.** Set a limit on how many drinks you'll have before you go out—and stick to it.

▌ **Alternate alcoholic and nonalcoholic drinks.** At a social occasion, have a nonalcoholic beverage to quench your thirst.

▌ **Drink slowly.** Never have more than one drink an hour.

▌ **Eat before and while drinking.** Choose foods high in protein (cheese, meat, eggs, or milk) rather than salty foods, like peanuts or chips, that increase thirst.

▌ **Be wary of mixed drinks.** Fizzy mixers, like club soda and ginger ale, speed alcohol to the blood and brain.

▌ **Don't make drinking the primary focus of any get-together.** Cultivate other interests and activities that you can enjoy on your own or with friends.

▌ **Learn to say no.** A simple "Thank you, but I've had enough" will do.

▌ **Stay safe.** During or after drinking, avoid any tasks, including driving, that could be affected by alcohol.

SELF-SURVEY 2

Are You Addicted to Nicotine?

Answer the following questions as honestly as you can by placing a check mark in the appropriate column:

	Yes	No
1. Do you smoke every day?	_____	_____
2. Do you smoke because of shyness and to build up self-confidence?	_____	_____
3. Do you smoke to escape from boredom and worries or while under pressure?	_____	_____
4. Have you ever burned a hole in your clothes, carpet, furniture, or car with a cigarette?	_____	_____
5. Have you ever had to go to the store late at night or at another inconvenient time because you were out of cigarettes?	_____	_____
6. Do you feel defensive or angry when people tell you that your smoke is bothering them?	_____	_____
7. Has a doctor or dentist ever suggested that you stop smoking?	_____	_____
8. Have you ever promised someone that you would stop smoking, then broken your promise?	_____	_____

	Yes	No
9. Have you ever felt physical or emotional discomfort when trying to quit?	_____	_____
10. Have you ever successfully stopped smoking for a period of time, only to start again?	_____	_____
11. Do you buy extra supplies of tobacco to make sure you won't run out?	_____	_____
12. Do you find it difficult to imagine life without smoking?	_____	_____
13. Do you choose only those activities and entertainments during which you can smoke?	_____	_____
14. Do you prefer, seek out, or feel more comfortable in the company of smokers?	_____	_____
15. Do you inwardly despise or feel ashamed of yourself because of your smoking?	_____	_____
16. Do you ever find yourself lighting up without having consciously decided to?	_____	_____
17. Has your smoking ever caused trouble at home or in a relationship?	_____	_____
18. Do you ever tell yourself that you can stop smoking whenever you want to?	_____	_____
19. Have you ever felt that your life would be better if you didn't smoke?	_____	_____
20. Do you continue to smoke even though you are aware of the health hazards posed by smoking?	_____	_____

If you answered Yes to one or two of these questions, there's a chance that you are addicted or are becoming addicted to nicotine. If you answered Yes to three or more of these questions, you are probably already addicted to nicotine.

Source: Nicotine Anonymous World Services, San Francisco.

ACTION PLAN 2

Your Action Plan for Kicking the Habit

Here's a six-point program to help you or someone you love quit smoking. (*Caution:* Don't undertake the quit-smoking program until you have a two-to-four-week period of relatively unstressful work and study schedules or social commitments.)

1. *Identify your smoking habits.* Keep a daily diary (a piece of paper wrapped around your cigarette pack with a

rubber band will do) see Wellness Journal 1 for a sample diary. Record the time you smoke, the activity associated with smoking (after breakfast, in the car), and your urge for a cigarette (desperate, pleasant, or automatic). For the first week or two, don't bother trying to cut down; just use the diary to learn the conditions under which you smoke.

2. *Get support.* It can be tough to go it alone. Phone your local chapter of the American Cancer Society or otherwise get the names of some ex-smokers who can give you support.

3. *Begin by tapering off.* For a period of one to four weeks, aim at cutting down to, say, 12 or 15 cigarettes a day; or change to a lower-nicotine brand, and concentrate on not increasing the number of cigarettes you smoke. As indicated by your diary, begin by cutting out those cigarettes you smoke automatically. In addition, restrict the times you allow yourself to smoke. Throughout this period, stay in touch, once a day or every few days, with your ex-smoker friend(s) to discuss your problems.

4. *Set a quit date.* At some point during the tapering-off period, announce to everyone—friends, family, and ex-smokers—when you're going to quit. Do it with flair. Announce it to coincide with a significant date, such as your birthday or anniversary.

5. *Stop.* A week before Q-day, smoke only five cigarettes a day. Begin late in the day, say after 4:00 P.M. Smoke the first two cigarettes in close succession. Then, in the evening, smoke the last three, also in close succession, about 15 minutes apart. Focus on the negative aspects of cigarettes, such as the rawness in your throat and lungs. After seven days, quit and give yourself a big reward on that day, such as a movie or a fantastic meal or new clothes.

6. *Follow up.* Stay in touch with your ex-smoker friend(s) during the following two weeks, particularly if anything stressful or tense occurs that might trigger a return to smoking. Think of the person you're becoming—the very person cigarette ads would have you believe smoking makes you. Now that you're quitting smoking, you're becoming healthier, sexier, more sophisticated, more nature, and better looking —and you've earned it!

Sources: American Cancer Society: National Cancer Institute.

SELF-SURVEY 3

Do You Have a Substance Use Disorder?

Individuals with a substance dependence or abuse disorder may

■ Use more of an illegal drug or a prescription medication or use a drug for a longer period of time than they desire or intend. _____

■ Try, repeatedly and unsuccessfully, to cut down or control their drug use _____

■ Spend a great deal of time doing whatever is necessary in order to get drugs, taking them, or recovering from their use. _____

■ Be so high or feel so bad after drug use that they often cannot do their job or fulfill other responsibilities. _____

■ Give up or cut back on important social, work, or recreational activities because of drug use. _____

■ Continue to use drugs even though they realize that they are causing or worsening physical or mental problems. _____

■ Use a lot more of a drug in order to achieve a "high" or desired effect or feel fewer such effects than in the past. _____

■ Use drugs in dangerous ways or situations. _____

■ Have repeated drug-related legal problems, such as arrests for possession. _____

■ Continue to use drugs, even though the drug causes or worsens social or personal problems, such as arguments with a spouse. _____

■ Develop hand tremors or other withdrawal symptoms if they cut down or stop drug use. _____

■ Take drugs to relieve or avoid withdrawal symptoms. _____

The more blanks that you or someone close to you checks, the more reason you have to be concerned about drug use. The most difficult step for anyone with a substance use disorder is to admit that he or she has a problem. Sometimes a drug-related crisis, such as being arrested or fired, forces individuals to acknowledge the impact of drugs. If not, those who care—family, friends, boss, physician—may have to confront them and insist that they do something about it. This confrontation, planned beforehand, is called an *intervention* and can be the turning point for drug users and their families.

ACTION PLAN 3

Your Action Plan for Recognizing Substance Abuse

How can you tell if a friend or loved one has a substance use disorder? Look for the following warning signs:

■ **An abrupt change in attitude.** Individuals may lose interest in activities they once enjoyed or in being with friends they once valued.

▮ **Mood swings.** Drug users may often seem withdrawn or "out of it," or they may display unusual temper flareups.

▮ **A decline in performance.** Students may start skipping classes, stop studying, or not complete assignments; their grades may plummet.

▮ **Increased sensitivity.** Individuals may react intensely to any criticism or become easily frustrated or angered.

▮ **Secrecy.** Drug users may make furtive telephone calls or demand greater privacy concerning their personal possessions or their whereabouts.

▮ **Physical changes.** Individuals using drugs may change their pattern of sleep, spending more time in bed or sleeping at odd hours. They also may change their eating habits and lose weight.

▮ **Money problems.** Drug users may constantly borrow money, seem short of cash, or begin stealing.

▮ **Changes in appearance.** As they become more involved with drugs, users often lose regard for their personal appearance and look disheveled.

▮ **Defiance of restrictions.** Individuals may ignore or deliberately refuse to comply with deadlines, curfews, or other regulations.

▮ **Changes in relationships.** Drug users may quarrel more frequently with family members or old friends and develop new, strong allegiances with new acquaintances, including other drug users.

SETTING GOALS

Setting Goals for Personal Substance Abuse Avoidance

Your Personal Substance Abuse Avoidance Goal:

Is It S.M.A.R.T.?
   Specific? _____
   Measurable? _____
   Achievable? _____
   Rewarding? _____
   Time Defined? _____

Strategies for Success
   1. _____
   2. _____
   3. _____

Potential Obstacles
   1. _____
   2. _____
   3. _____

Ways Around Them
   1. _____
   2. _____
   3. _____

Daily Report

The Week that Was:

What Went Right?
What Could I Do Better?

WELLNESS JOURNAL 1

Daily Cigarette Smoking Log

Today's Date: Quit Date: Decision Date:

Cigarettes to be smoked today: Brand:

No.	Time	Activity	Rating[a]	Amount Smoked[b]	Remarks/Substitutes
1.					
2.					
3.					
4.					
5.					
6.					
7.					
8.					

9. _____

10. _____

    a Rating: 1 = desperately needed, 2 = moderately needed, 3 = no real need
    b Amount Smoked: entire cigarette, two-thirds, half, etc.

Additional comments, list of friends and/or activities to avoid.

_____
_____
_____

Conclusion

In a few sentences indicate your feelings about cigarette smoking and what you have learned from Self-Survey 2.

_____
_____
_____
_____
_____
_____
_____
_____
_____
_____

WELLNESS JOURNAL 2

Substance Abuse Values Clarification

Our values help guide our decisions. However, when we act in ways that are contrary to our value system we create stress in our lives and that often leads us to participate in negative health behaviors. How true are you to your values? Are there some areas in which you are willing to compromise your values and other areas in which you wouldn't even think of it? Express your thoughts regarding the following:

    To me, substance abuse is . . .

    My family's attitude toward substance use is . . .

When I see drugs being used at a party I . . .

If my friends were drinking and/or smoking marijuana in my presence I would . . .

Driving home after having a few beers at a friend's house is . . .

Experimenting with different drugs while at college is something that . . .

When faced with peer pressure to do drugs I would . . .

Alcohol and tobacco advertisements targeted to adolescents should be . . .

If I felt I had a problem with substance abuse I would . . .

CHAPTER

13 Making This Chapter Work for You

1. In most states the blood-alcohol concentration at which a person is legally drunk is
   a. 0.06 percent.
   b. 0.08 percent.
   c. 0.10 percent.
   d. 0.12 percent.

2. Which of the following statements about the effects of alcohol on the body system is *true?*
   a. In most individuals, alcohol sharpens the responses of the brain and nervous system, enhancing sensation and perception.

b. Many prescription drugs contain an ingredient that interacts adversely with alcohol.

c. Alcohol reaches your bloodstream in 45 minutes.

d. The leading alcohol-related cause of death is liver damage.

3. Which of the following statements about drinking on college campuses is true?

a. The percentage of students who abstain from alcohol has increased.

b. The number of women who binge drink has decreased.

c. Because of peer pressure, students in fraternities and sororities tend to drink less than students in dormitories.

d. Students who live in substance-free dormitories tend to binge drink when alcohol is available.

4. Mark drinks beer with his buddies three or four nights a week, but he has thought about cutting down and just drinking on Saturday nights. What stage of change is Mark in?

a. precontemplation

b. contemplation

c. preparation

d. action

5. Tobacco use on college campuses

a. is more prevalent among athletes than nonathletes.

b. is linked with depression.

c. has decreased in the past 10 years because almost all schools have adopted a no-smoking policy on their premises.

d. is considered a minor problem by most student health center directors, since fewer than a third of students smoke.

6. Which of the following statements is *false?*

a. Using chewing tobacco can lead to damage to the mucous membranes of the mouth.

b. Bidis come in several flavors.

c. The active ingredient in cloves lowers sensation in the throat, so clove-cigarette smokers inhale more deeply.

d. Smoking cigars is safe if you don't inhale.

7. Environmental tobacco smoke

a. is smoke emitted by tobacco-processing factories.

b. is not dangerous to nonsmokers.

c. is the most hazardous form of indoor air pollution.

d. is responsible for 1 million heart attacks per year.

8. Which of the following statements about marijuana is *false?*

a. Marijuana today contains much more THC than the marijuana of 40 years ago.

b. Marijuana has shown some effectiveness in treating chemotherapy-related nausea.

c. Unlike long-term use of alcohol, regular use of marijuana does not have any long-lasting health consequences.

d. Circumstances affect a user's response to marijuana.

9. Which of the following statements about club drugs is true?

a. Club drugs can produce many unwanted effects, including hallucinations and paranoia.

b. Most club drugs do not pose the same health dangers as "hard" drugs such as heroin.

c. MDMA is the street name for ecstasy.

d. When combined with extended physical exertion, club drugs can lead to hypothermia (lowered body temperature).

10. More than physical wellness is affected by addiction. The primary relationship in the life of addicts is with the addictive substance or behavior, which impairs this dimension of wellness:

a. psychological wellness

b. spiritual wellness

c. social wellness

d. environmental wellness

Answers to these questions can be found on p. 376.

Critical Thinking

1. Driving home from his high school graduation party, 18-year-old Rick has had too much to drink. As he crosses the dividing line on the two-lane road, the driver of an oncoming car—a young mother with two young children in the backseat—swerves to avoid an accident. She hits a concrete wall and dies instantly, but her children survive. Rick has no record of drunk driving. Should he go to prison? Is he guilty of manslaughter? How would you feel if you were the victim's husband? If you were Rick's friend?

2. Have you ever been around people who have been intoxicated when you have been sober? What did you think of their behavior? Were they fun to be around? Was the experience not particularly enjoyable, boring, or difficult in some way? Have you ever been intoxicated? How do you behave when you are drunk? Do you find the experience enjoyable? What do the people around you think of your actions when you are drunk?

3. Has smoking become unpopular among your friends or family? What social activities continue to be associated with smoking? Can you think of any situation in which smoking might be frowned upon?

4. Some argue that marijuana should be a legal drug like alcohol and tobacco. What is your opinion on this issue? Defend your position.

Media Menu

Health Now™

Don't forget to check out the wealth of resources on the HealthNow website at **http://healthnow.brookscole.com/itw** that will:

• Help you evaluate your knowledge of the material

• Allow you to take an exam-prep quiz

- Provide a Personalized Learning Plan targeting resources that address areas you should study
- Coach you through identifying target goals for behavior change and creating and monitoring your personal change plan throughout the semester.

INTERNET CONNECTIONS

Tobacco Information and Prevention Source (TIPS)
www.cdc.gov/tobacco/
This comprehensive feature on the Centers for Disease Control and Prevention (CDC) website provides educational information, research, a report from the U.S. Surgeon General, tips on how to quit smoking, and much more.

Facts on Tap: Alcohol and Your College Experience
www.factsontap.org
This excellent site is geared to college students. It features links to the following topics and more: Risky Relationship: Alcohol and Sex, College Experience: Alcohol and Student Life, The Naked Truth: Alcohol and Your Body, When Someone Else's Drinking Gives You a Hangover.

National Institute on Drug Abuse
www.nida.nih.gov
This government site—a virtual clearinghouse of information for students, parents, teachers, researchers, and health professionals—features current treatments and research, as well as a comprehensive database on common drugs of abuse.

Joe Chemo
www.joechemo.org
Based on the character Joe Chemo, an antismoking parody of Joe Camel, this site is highly interactive and allows visitors to test their Tobacco IQ, get a personalized Smoke-o-Scope, and send free Joe Chemo e-cards. There is also extensive information for teachers, antismoking activists, health-care providers, journalists, and smokers who wish to quit.

College Drinking: Changing the Culture
www.collegedrinkingprevention.gov
This website, sponsored by the National Institute of Alcohol Abuse and Alcoholism, focuses on the college alcohol culture with information for students, parents, college and health administrators and more. The site features information about alcohol prevention, college alcohol policies, research topics, and facts on the consequences of alcohol abuse and alcoholism.

InfoTrac College Edition Activities Sheffield, Felicia et al. "Binge drinking and alcohol-related problems among community college students: implications for prevention policy," *Journal of American College Health,* Nov–Dec 2005 v54 i3 p137 (5)

1. What are some of the consequences of binge-drinking by college students?

2. Describe the most common patterns of drinking among the community college students in this study.

3. What are some reasons why binge-drinking rates may be lower at community colleges than at four-year universities?

Gerson, Megan. "Impact of smoke-free residence hall policies: the views of administrators at 3 state universities," *Journal of American College Health,* Nov–Dec 2005 v54 i3 p157 (9)

1. Has smoking by college students increased or decreased in recent years?

2. Why do some college administrators hesitate to ban smoking in residence halls?

3. What have been some of the positive impacts of smoke-free housing in this study?

You can find additional readings related to personal health with InfoTrac College Edition, an online library of more than 900 journals and publications. Follow the instructions for accessing InfoTrac College Edition that were packaged with your textbook; then search for articles using a keyword search.

For additional links, resources, and suggested readings on the InfoTrac College Edition, visit our Health and Wellness Resource Center at **http://health .wadsworth.com.**

Key Terms

The terms listed are used on the page indicated. Definitions of the terms are in the Glossary at the end of the book.

addiction 292
alcohol abuse 304
alcohol dependence 304
alcoholism 305
amphetamines 317
barbiturates 318
benzodiazepines 318
bidis 308
binge drinking 300
blood–alcohol concentration (BAC) 294
club drugs 315
cocaine 317
deleriants 319
drug 292
drug abuse 292
drug misuse 292
ecstasy 315
environmental tobacco smoke 309
ethyl alcohol 299
Fetal Alcohol Effects (FAE) 296
Fetal Alcohol Syndrome (FAS) 297
hallucinogens 319
hashish 313
inhalants 319
intoxication 292
mainstream smoke 309
marijuana 313
nonopioids 318
opioids 318
PCP 319
physical dependence 292
proof 294
psychoactive 292
psychological dependence 292
psychotropic 293
sidestream smoke 309
stimulant 293
withdrawal 292

Protecting Your Sexual Health

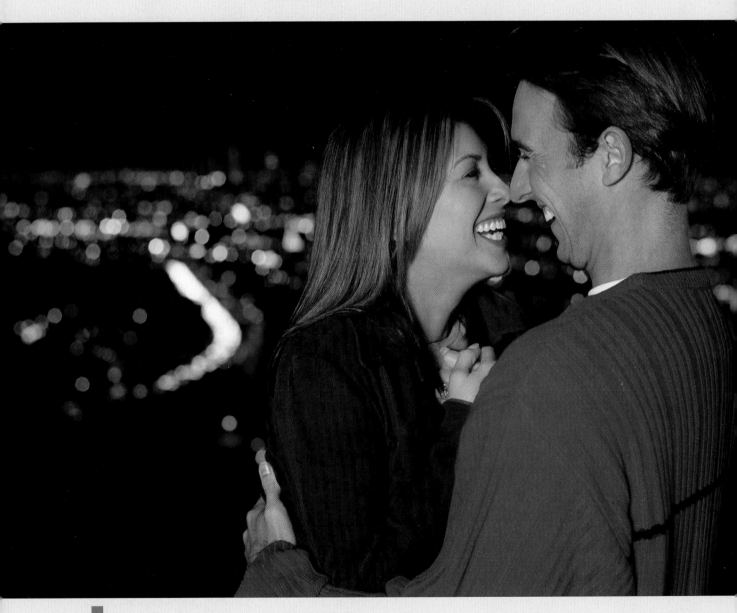

 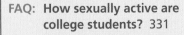

"There's something I have to tell you." Anise knew, just by the sound of her boyfriend's voice, that the "something" wasn't good news.

"My herpes is back."

Stunned, Anise tried to absorb all the information packed into this short sentence: She'd had no idea that the man she'd been sleeping with for several months had a sexually transmitted infection (STI). How did he get it? What else hadn't he told her about his past? What did he mean that it was "back"? Could she have caught it? And, finally, she asked the all-too-human question: How could this have happened to me?

Some of today's most common and dangerous infectious illnesses spread primarily through sexual contact, and their incidence has skyrocketed. The federal government estimates that 65 million Americans have a sexually transmitted infection.[1] These diseases cannot be prevented in the laboratory. Only you, by your behavior, can prevent and control them.

This chapter is a lesson in self-defense. The information it provides can help you protect yourself from sexually transmitted infections and realize when to seek help.

After studying the material in this chapter, you should be able to:

▌ **Name** the five characteristics of a sexually healthy relationship.

▌ **Discuss** the dimensions of wellness as they relate to human sexuality.

▌ **Describe** the levels of safer sex and how to use a condom.

▌ **Name** the sexually transmitted infections and the means of transmission for each.

▌ **Discuss** behaviors that increase the risk of HIV infection.

Health Now™

Don't forget to check out the wealth of resources on the HealthNow website at **http://healthnow.brookscole.com/itw** that will:

• Help you evaluate your knowledge of the material

• Allow you to take an exam-prep quiz

• Provide a Personalized Learning Plan targeting resources that address areas you should study

• Coach you through identifying target goals for behavior change and creating and monitoring your personal change plan throughout the semester.

Responsible Sexuality

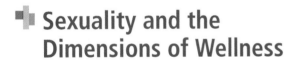

Understanding sexuality is a lifelong process. While you may think you know a great deal about **sex,** many people grow up with a lot of myths and misconceptions. Certain concepts, such as what sex means to a man or a woman, may be influenced by religious, cultural, and racial beliefs. Among Hispanic college students, for instance, researchers have found surprising differences between men and women, such as the widespread male belief in the acceptability of forcing one's spouse to have sex and the female belief that if you are sexually aroused, you must have sex.[2]

A sexually healthy relationship, as defined by the Sexuality Information and Education Council of the United States (SIECUS), is based on shared values and has five characteristics: It is consensual, nonexploitative, honest, mutually pleasurable, and protected against unintended pregnancy and **sexuality transmitted infections (STIs),** including HIV/AIDS. All individuals also have sexual rights, which include the right to the information, education, skills, support, and services they need to make responsible decisions about their sexuality consistent with their own values, as well as the right to express their sexual orientation without violence or discrimination.

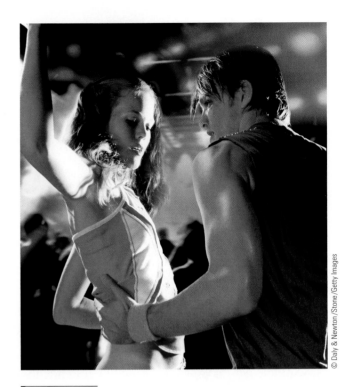

Have your sexual relationships been healthy and responsible? How would you rate yourself on the dimensions of wellness related to sexuality?

Sexuality and the Dimensions of Wellness

Our sexuality both affects and is affected by the various dimensions of wellness. Responsible sexuality and high-level sexual health contribute to the fullest possible functioning of body, mind, spirit, and social relationships. In turn, other aspects of wellness enhance our sexuality. Here are some examples:

- **Physical.** As described later in this chapter, safer sex practices reduce the risk of sexually transmitted infections that can threaten sexual health, physical health, and even survival. When our bodies are healthy and well, we feel better about how we look and move —which enhances both self-esteem and healthy sexuality.

- **Emotional.** By acknowledging and respecting the intimacy of a sexual relationship, responsible sexuality builds trust and commitment. When our emotional wellness is high, we can better understand and cope with the complex feelings related to being sexual.

- **Social.** From dating to mating, we express and fulfill our sexual identities in the context of families, friends, and society as a whole. Having strong friendships, intimate relationships, and caring partnerships enables us to explore our sexuality in safe and healthy ways.

- **Intellectual.** Our most fulfilling relationships involve a meeting of minds as well as bodies. High-level intellectual wellness enables us to acquire and understand sexual information, analyze it critically, and make healthy sexual decisions.

- **Spiritual.** At its deepest, most fulfilling level, sexuality uplifts the soul by allowing us to connect to something greater than oneself. Individuals who have developed their spiritual wellness bring to their most intimate relationships an awareness and appreciation that lifts them beyond the physical.

- **Environmental.** Responsible sexuality makes people more aware of the impact of their decisions on others. Protecting yourself from sexual threats and creating a supportive environment in which to study and work are crucial to high-level wellness and to healthy sexuality.

Choosing Celibacy or Abstinence

A celibate person does not engage in sexual activity. Complete **celibacy** means that the person doesn't masturbate (stimulate himself or herself sexually) or engage in sexual activity with a partner. In partial celibacy, the person masturbates but doesn't have sexual contact with

+ STRATEGIES
for CHANGE

How to Say No to Sex

▮ First of all, recognize your own values and feelings. If you believe that sex is something to be shared only by people who've already become close in other ways, be true to that belief.

▮ If you're at a loss for words, try these responses: "I like you a lot, but I'm not ready to have sex." "You're a great person, but sex isn't something I do to prove I like someone." "I'd like to wait until I'm married to have sex."

▮ If you're feeling pressured, let your date know that you're uncomfortable. Be simple and direct. Watch out for emotional blackmail. If your date says, "If you really liked me, you'd want to make love," point out that if he or she really liked you, he or she wouldn't try to force you to do something you don't want to do.

▮ If you're a woman, monitor your sexual signals. Men impute more sexual meaning to gestures (such as casual touching) that women perceive as friendly and innocent.

▮ Communicate your feelings to your date sooner rather than later. It's far easier to say, "I don't want to go to your apartment" than to fight off unwelcome advances once you're there.

▮ Remember that if saying no to sex puts an end to a relationship, it wasn't much of a relationship in the first place.

others. Many people decide to be celibate at certain times of their lives. Some don't have sex because of concerns about pregnancy or STIs; others haven't found a partner for a permanent, monogamous relationship. Many simply have other priorities, such as finishing school or starting a career, and realize that sex outside of a committed relationship is a threat to their physical and psychological well-being.

The CDC defines **abstinence** as "refraining from sexual activities which involve vaginal, anal, and oral intercourse." The definition of abstinence remains a subject of debate and controversy, with some emphasizing positive choices and others avoidance of specific behaviors.[3] In reality abstinence means different things to different people, cultures, and religious groups.

Increasing numbers of adolescents and young adults are choosing to remain virgins and abstain from sexual intercourse until they enter a permanent, committed relationship.

＋■ How Sexually Active 🔲 Are College Students?

According to federal statistics, about two-thirds of never-married 18- to 19-year-olds—69 percent of women and 64 percent of men—have had intercourse.[4] In a recent national survey of 1,051 students ages 18 to 24, about 25 percent said they had never engaged in sexual intercourse: 34 percent of men and 18 percent of women. One in four said they had passed on an opportunity to have sex during the previous year. Three in four agreed that sex and contraception should be discussed in advance. The average number of sex partners reported by the students during the previous year was 1.2. Two in three women and one in three men described themselves as being in committed relationships.[5]

Sexual behavior on campus has changed dramatically in the last 25 years. Surveys conducted in the United States and in Canada since 1980 reveal a steady increase in the number of students who have had intercourse and an increase in safer sex practices among sexually active ones. Today's undergraduates are more likely to question potential partners about their past, use condoms with a new partner, and maintain fairly long-term monogamous relationships.[6] They also engage in behaviors that weren't widespread in the past, such as using the Internet to search for sexually explicit material and potential sex partners. (See Savvy Consumer: "X-Rated Online Sites.")

College students see sexual activity as normal behavior for their peer group. When researchers at Pennsylvania State University conducted focus groups with undergraduates, most agreed that the majority of college

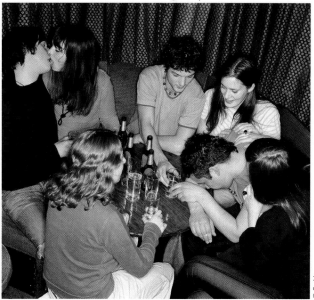

▮ Drinking games often lead to sexually risky behavior.

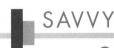

SAVVY CONSUMER

X-RATED ONLINE SITES

Sex is the number-one word searched for online. About 15 percent of Americans logging onto the Internet visit sexually oriented sites. Men are the largest consumers of sexually explicit material and outnumber women by a ratio of six to one. However, while men look for visual erotica, women are more likely to visit chat rooms, which offer more interactions. Most people who check out sex sites on the Internet do not suffer any negative impact, but psychologists warn of some potential risks, including the following:

▪ **Dependence.** Individuals who spend eleven hours or more a week online in sexual pursuits show signs of psychological distress and admit that their behavior interferes with some areas of their lives.

▪ **Interference with work and study.** While most individuals use their home computers when surfing the Internet for sex-related sites, one in ten has used a school computer. Some universities have strict policies barring such practices and may take

punitive actions against employees who violate the rules.

▪ **Sexual compulsivity.** A small but significant number of users are at risk of a serious problem as a result of their heavy Internet use.

▪ **Dishonesty.** Most Internet surfers admit that they occasionally "pretend" about their age on the Internet. Most keep secret how much time they spend on sexual pursuits in cyberspace.

---

students (80 to 90 percent, in their estimate) are sexually active and that alcohol and drug use make sexual activity more likely.

College students who binge drink or participate in drinking games, which often involve physical skills (such as bouncing a coin into a glass) or word play, increase their odds of sexually risky behavior. Both men and women report being taken advantage of sexually, including someone having sex with them when they were too drunk to give consent, after such games.[7]

Annual spring breaks provide what researchers describe as "ideal conditions for the potentially lethal interaction between alcohol, drugs, and sexual risk-taking."[8] Students typically engage in binge drinking, illicit drug use, and unsafe sexual practices. The likelihood of casual sex depends on several factors, including peer influences, prior experiences with casual sex, alcohol consumption prior to sex, and impulsivity.

✚ Safer Sex

Having sex is never completely safe; the only 100 percent risk-free sexual choice is abstinence. By choosing not to be sexually active with a partner, you can safeguard your physical health, your fertility, and your future.

For men and women who are sexually active, a mutually faithful sexual relationship with just one healthy partner is the safest option. For those not in such relationships, safer-sex practices are essential for reducing risks.

STRATEGIES for PREVENTION

Seven Steps of Correct Male Condom Use

▪ Use a new condom at each act of intercourse.

▪ Handle the condom carefully to avoid damage from fingernails, teeth, or other sharp objects.

▪ Put the condom on after the penis is erect and before any genital contact with a partner.

▪ Make sure that air is trapped in the tip of the condom.

▪ Ensure adequate lubrication during intercourse.

▪ Use only water-based lubricants with latex condoms.

▪ Withdraw the penis while it is still erect to prevent slippage. Hold the condom firmly against the base of the penis during withdrawal.

If you are sexually active, condoms can reduce your risk of STIs—if you use them correctly and consistently. Unless you are allergic, always use latex condoms, which block more STI organisms than natural membrane condoms. Although condoms do not provide 100 percent protection, they can reduce the risk of transmission of an STI by 50 to 80 percent.[9]

Condoms prevent direct contact between the penis and the vagina, cervix, mouth, or rectum, thereby protecting against lesions, discharges, and infected semen. Condoms are more effective against STIs transmitted by bodily fluids (chlamydia, gonorrhea, trichomoniasis, HIV) than those transmitted by skin-to-skin contact (herpes, HPV, chancroid, syphilis).

How can you tell if someone you're dating or hope to date has been exposed to an STI? The bad news is you can't. But the good news is it doesn't matter—as long as you avoid sexual activity that could put you at risk of infection. Ideally, before engaging in any such behavior, both of you should talk about your prior sexual history (including number of partners and sexually transmitted infections) and other high-risk behavior, such as the use of injection drugs.

Why Don't College Students Practice Safer Sex?

Decades of education about sexual risks has had an impact. Most young Americans between the ages of 18 and 24 agree that "it's smart to carry condoms," according to a recent national survey. However, their words and actions often differ. Although nine in ten say they take personal responsibility for their sexual health, only half ask potential partners about sexually transmitted infections. Less than half always or often use a condom during sexual activity.[10]

Heterosexual students—male and female—are more likely to say they always use condoms than gay men. Of those engaging in heterosexual sex, 52 percent of men and 43 percent of women report consistent condom use, compared with 32 percent of men with only male partners.[11]

Researchers explain that the college environment "provides students with a sense of new independence, self-determination, and strong peer pressure to experiment with a variety of sexual behaviors." Yet by engaging in sex with multiple partners and not regularly using condoms, college students put themselves at high risk of contracting HIV and other sexually transmitted infections (Table 14-1).

In a study of African-American undergraduates, male and female students identified barriers to their use of safer sex practices. Negative views of condoms rank first. But the reason men and women don't like condoms is not reduced sensitivity or pleasure, but a sense that not wearing a condom provides a sense of greater intimacy.[12]

Latino students are less likely to use condoms than African Americans. In a recent analysis, 30 percent of Latino undergraduates reported

TABLE 14-1 ▌ Risky Sex on Campus		
	Percent	
Men	**1 or 2 partners**	**3 or more partners**
Not using condom (last time)	51	37
Sex with a stranger (ever)	28	72
Active anal intercourse (ever)	27	43
Multiple partners during same act (ever)	12	28
Unwise sex after alcohol/drugs (ever)	45	89

	Percent	
Women	**1 or 2 partners**	**3 or more partners**
Not using condom (last time)	62	46
Sex with a stranger (ever)	16	42
Active anal intercourse (ever)	27	35
Multiple partners during same act (ever)	3	23
Unwise sex after alcohol/drugs (ever)	49	84

Based on a survey of 630 students (247 men and 383 women) at Okanagan University College in British Columbia.

Source: Netting, N. S., and Matthew Burnett. "Twenty Years of Student Sexual Behavior: Subcultural Adaptations to a Changing Health Environment." *Adolescence,* Vol. 39, No. 153, Spring 2004, p. 19.

condom use in the previous three months, compared with 43 percent of African Americans. Those who had ever had a test for HIV following oral sex and who had had anal sex partners of both genders reported more condom use.[13]

Providing information on sexual health does not influence condom use, nor does teaching specific communication skills. In one experiment, 106 heterosexual college students in sexually active relationships were taught specifically how to make direct requests for condom use and how to counter refusals from a partner. Nonetheless, the students did not change their subsequent communication or use condoms more consistently.[14]

Trust is another issue that affects safer sex practices. Men tend to trust a woman as safe and healthy on the basis of the way she looks. Women trust a man because they believe they are in a monogamous relationship after a period of time (one month on average) or number of encounters (twelve). Neither men nor women base their feelings of trust on a discussion with a partner. They simply assume that a partner can be trusted and that condoms are not necessary.

Race and ethnicity affect risk in the young. Young African-American men, who are more likely to be sex-

STRATEGIES
for PREVENTION

Before You Have Sex

Here are some questions to consider as you think and talk about the significance of becoming sexually intimate with a partner.

▮ What role do we want relationships and sex to have in our life at this time?

▮ What are my values and my potential partner's values as they pertain to sexual relationships? Does each of us believe that intercourse should be reserved for a permanent partnership or committed relationship?

▮ Will a decision to engage in sex enhance my positive feelings about myself or my partner? Does either of us have questions about sexual orientation or the kinds of people we are attracted to?

▮ Do I and my partner both want to have sex? Is my partner pressuring me in any way? Am I pressuring my partner? Am I making this decision for myself or my partner?

▮ Have my partner and I discussed our sexual histories and risk factors? Have I spoken honestly about any STIs I've had in the past? Am I sure that neither my partner nor I have a sexually transmitted infection?

▮ Have we taken precautions against unwanted pregnancy and STIs?

ually active and to have more partners than young white men, also have higher STI infection rates. While the chlamydia rate for Hispanics is almost three times that of whites, the rate for blacks is ten times that of whites. The gonorrhea rate for African-American males aged 20 to 24 is 40 times that of whites. Although HIV infection rates have declined for all men, they are falling at a slower rate for African-American men.

WELLNESS COACH

Making Healthy Sexual Choices

Sexual decision making always takes place within the context of an individual's values and perceptions of right and wrong behavior. Making sexually responsible decisions means considering all the possible consequences of sexual behavior for both yourself and your partner. It must always take into account, not just personal preferences and desires, but the very real risks of unwanted pregnancy, sexually transmitted infections (STIs), and long-term medical consequences (such as impaired fertility). You also must consider the emotional consequences of a sexual relationship—not just for yourself but also for your partner.

Only human beings have the unique ability to choose to conceive or not to conceive. And only human beings have the capacity to protect themselves from sexually transmitted infections. Not recognizing this responsibility is in itself a choice, one that could have profound consequences for your future.

Some forms of contraception, such as condoms, provide protection against both pregnancy and STIs. Others, like the birth control pill, are highly effective in preventing pregnancy but offer no protection against STIs. You should consider these factors in making healthy choices for birth control and for protecting your sexual health.

Talking About Sex

Prior to any sexual activity that involves a risk of sexually transmitted infection or pregnancy, both partners should talk about their prior sexual histories (including number of partners and exposure to STIs) and other high-risk behavior, such as the use of injection drugs. They should also discuss the issue of birth control and which methods might be best for them to use. If you know some-

© Medio Images/PictureQuest

▮ Making healthy sexual choices includes talking with a potential partner about sexual histories and risk factors before having sex.

one well enough to consider having sex with that person, you should be able to talk about such sensitive subjects. If a potential partner is unwilling to talk or hedges on crucial questions, you shouldn't be engaging in sex.

Choose a time and place that is relaxed and comfortable. Arm yourself with facts so you can answer any questions or objections your partner raises. Start on a positive note—for instance, by saying how much you care for your partner and saying that this is the reason you want to discuss something important. This is the time for you to be honest about any STIs you might have had or still carry. Give your partner time to take in what you've said. If you find out about a partner's STI, you may feel a range of emotions. You also will need to acquire information about symptoms, treatment, and how the disease is spread.

➕ Sexually Transmitted Infections

Venereal diseases (from the Latin *venus,* meaning *love* or *lust*) are called sexually transmitted infections (STIs). Around the world, some 50 million cases of curable STIs occur each year (not including HIV and herpes). Almost 700,000 people are infected every day with one of the over 20 STIs tracked by world health officials. The highest rates of sexually transmitted infections occur among 16- to 24-year-olds, particularly older teenagers.[15] STIs are much more widespread in developing nations because of lack of adequate health standards, prevention practices, and access to treatment.

More Americans are infected with STIs now than at any other time in history. According to the Institute of Medicine, the odds of acquiring an STI during a lifetime are one in four. STIs are among the top ten most frequently reported diseases in the United States. The major cause of preventable sterility in America, STIs have tripled the rate of ectopic (tubal) pregnancies, which can be fatal if not detected early. STI complications, including miscarriage, premature delivery, and uterine infections after delivery, annually affect more than 100,000 women. Moreover, infection with an STI greatly increases the risk of HIV transmission (discussed later in this chapter). The incidence of STIs is highest in young adults and homosexual men. Others affected by STIs include unborn and newborn children who can "catch" potentially life-threatening infections in the womb or during birth.

Although each STI is a distinct disease, all STI pathogens like dark, warm, moist body surfaces, particularly the mucous membranes that line the reproductive organs; they hate light, cold, and dryness (**Figure 14-1**). It is possible to catch or have more than one STI at a time. Curing one doesn't necessarily cure another, and treatments don't prevent another bout with the same STI (**Table 14-2** on page 336).

Many STIs, including early HIV infection and gonorrhea in women, may not cause any symptoms. As a result, infected individuals may continue their usual sexual activity without realizing that they're jeopardizing others' well-being.

How Common Are STIs in Young Adults?

Fewer teens are engaging in sexual activity than in the past, and those that do are more likely to use contraceptives, according to the National Center for Health Statistics.[16] Nonetheless, young people account for about half of new cases of sexually transmitted infections (STIs). Three infections—chlamydra, human papilloma virus (HPV), and trichomoniasis—account for 88 percent of all new cases of STIs among young people.[17] Some reportable STIs declined during the 1990s, but as many as

Tough outer skin covers the outside of your body, including hands and lips. Viruses and bacteria enter when skin is chapped, or through a hangnail, cut, scrape, sore, or needle puncture.

Tough outer skin

Blood

Vaginal fluid

Semen

Other body fluids: saliva, urine, feces, breast milk

HIV and other STIs

Fragile inner skin lines the inside of your vagina or penis, anus, and mouth. Viruses and bacteria can enter when skin is torn during sexual contact that involves rubbing, stretching, or not enough lubrication (wetness).

Fragile inner skin

Body fluids

Latex condom

Spermicide or lubricant

Barrier protection made of latex helps prevent body fluids from entering your body. Latex condoms are recommended for intercourse. Spermicides help kill many STI microbes. They also reduce friction so latex condoms are less likely to break.

FIGURE 14-1 ▮ How HIV Infection and Other STIs Are Spread

Most STIs are spread by viruses or bacteria carried in certain body fluids.

TABLE 14-2 █ Common Sexually Transmitted Infections (STIs): Mode of Transmission, Symptoms, and Treatment

STI	Transmission	Symptoms	Treatment
Chlamydia	*Chlamydia trachomatis* bacterium transmitted primarily through sexual contact (can also be spread by fingers from one body site to another)	**Women:** usually no symptoms: leading cause of PID (pelvic inflammatory disease) **Men:** discharge, burning feeling during urination, but often no symptoms	Doxycycline, azithromycin, ofloxacin, levofloxacin
Gonorrhea ("clap")	*Neisseria gonorrhoeae* bacterium (gonococcus) spread through genital, oral-genital, or genital-anal contact	**Men:** cloudy discharge from the penis and burning sensations during urination. If disease is untreated, complications may include inflammation of scrotal skin and swelling at base of the testicle. **Women:** some green or yellowish discharge but commonly remains undetected. Later, PID may develop.	Ceftriaxone, cefixime, or spectinomycin
Nongonococcal urethritis (NGU)	Most commonly transmitted through coitus	**Men:** discharge from the penis and irritation during urination **Women:** mild discharge of pus from the vagina but often no symptoms	A single dose of azithromycin or doxycycline for seven days
Syphilis	*Treponema pallidum* bacterium (spirochete) transmitted from open lesions during genital, oral-genital, or genital-anal contact	*Primary stage:* painless chancre at the site where the spirochetes entered the body *Secondary stage:* generalized skin rash *Latent stage:* no visible symptoms *Tertiary stage:* heart failure, blindness, mental disturbance	Benzathine penicillin G, doxycycline, erythromycin, or ceftriaxone
Herpes simplex	Genital herpes virus (HSV-2) transmitted primarily by vaginal, anal, or oral-genital intercourse. Oral herpes virus (HSV-1) transmitted primarily by kissing	Small, painful red bumps (papules) in the genital region (genital herpes) or mouth (oral herpes). The papules become painful blisters that eventually rupture to form wet, open sores.	No known cure. A variety of treatments may reduce symptoms; acyclovir, famcyclovir, or valacyclovir promote healing and suppress recurrent outbreaks.
Chancroid	*Haemophilus ducrevi* bacterium transmitted by sexual interaction	Small bumps (papules) in genital regions eventually rupture and form painful, soft, crater-like ulcers that emit a foul-smelling discharge.	Single doses of either ceftriaxone or azithromycin, or seven days of erythromycin
Human papilloma virus (HPV) (genital warts)	Spread primarily through vaginal, anal, or oral-genital sexual interaction	Hard and yellow-gray on dry skin areas; soft, pinkish-red, and cauliflowerlike on moist areas	Freezing; application of topical agents like trichloroacetic acid or podofilox; cauterization, surgical removal, or vaporization by carbon dioxide laser
Pubic lice ("crabs")	*Phthirus pubis,* spread easily through body contact or through shared clothing or bedding	Persistent itching. Visible lice may often be located in pubic hair or other body hair.	1% permethrin cream for body areas; 1% Lindane shampoo for hair
Scabies	*Sarcoptes scabiei,* highly contagious, transmitted by close physical contact, sexual and nonsexual	Small bumps and a red rash that itch intensely, especially at night	5% permethrin lotion or cream
Acquired immune deficiency syndrome (AIDS)	Blood and semen are the major vehicles for transmitting HIV, passed primarily through sexual contact, or needle sharing among injection drug users	Vary with the type of cancer or opportunistic infections that afflict an infected person. Common symptoms: fevers, night sweats, weight loss, chronic fatigue, swollen lymph nodes, diarrhea and/or bloody stools, atypical bruising or bleeding, skin rashes, headache, chronic cough, and a whitish coating on the tongue or throat	Combination of three or more antiretroviral drugs (HAART) plus other specific treatment of opportunistic infections and tumors

TABLE 14-2 ▍ Common Sexually Transmitted Infections (STIs), (*continued*)

STI	Transmission	Symptoms	Treatment
Viral hepatitis	Hepatitis A primarily spread via the fecal-oral route, but oral-anal sexual contact a common mode. Hepatitis B virus transmitted by blood, semen, vaginal secretions, and saliva. Manual, oral, or penile stimulation of the anus are strongly associated with the spread of this virus.	Vary from nonexistent to mild, flulike symptoms to an incapacitating illness characterized by high fever, vomiting, and severe abdominal pain	Bed rest and adequate fluid intake. Combination therapy with interferon and ribavarin may be effective for hepatitis C infections.
Bacterial vaginosis	Most common causative agent, *Gardnerella vaginalis* bacterium, sometimes transmitted through coitus	**Women:** fishy- or musty-smelling, thin discharge, like flour paste in consistency and usually gray **Men:** mostly asymptomatic	Metronidazole (Flagyl) by mouth or intravaginal applications of topical metronidazole gel or clindamycin cream
Candidiasis (yeast infection)	*Candida albicans* fungus may accelerate growth when the chemical balance of the vagina is disturbed; it may also be transmitted through sexual interaction.	White, "cheesy" discharge; irritation of vaginal and vulval tissues	Vaginal suppositories or topical cream, such as clotrimazole and miconazole, or oral fluconazole
Trichomoniasis	Protozoan parasite *Trichomonas vaginalis* usually passed through genital sexual contact	White or yellow vaginal discharge with an unpleasant odor; sore and irritated vulva	Metronidazole (Flagyl) for both women and men

Sources: Crooks, Robert L., and Karla Baur. *Our Sexuality,* 8th ed. Pacific Grove, CA: Wadsworth, 2002; Miller, Karl, et al. "Update on Prevention and Treatment of Sexually Transmitted Diseases." *American Family Physician,* Vol. 67, No. 9, May 1, 2003, p. 1915.

20 to 50 percent of other infections, including gonorrhea and syphilis, are not diagnosed and reported.

The college years are a prime time for contracting STIs. According to the American College Health Association, chlamydia and HPV have reached epidemic levels at many schools—although many of those infected aren't even aware of it. Contracting STIs may increase the risk of being infected with HIV, and half of new HIV infections occur in people under age 25. Because college students have more opportunities to have different sexual partners and may use drugs and alcohol more often before sex, they are at greater risk.

More than half of 13- to 24-year-old women with HIV are infected heterosexually.

Risk Factors and Risk Continuums

Various factors put young people at risk of STIs, including:

▍ **Feelings of invulnerability,** which lead to risk-taking behavior. Even when they are well informed of the risks, adolescents may remain unconvinced that anything bad can or will happen to them.

▍ **Multiple partners.** Figure 14-2 illustrates how STI risks increase as relationships become less familiar and

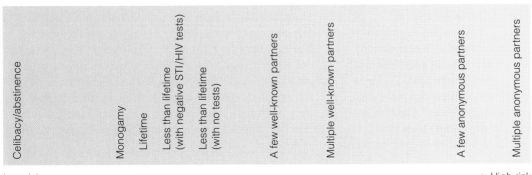

FIGURE 14-2 ▍ A Continuum of Risk for Sexual Relationships
STI risks increase as relationships become less familiar and exclusive.

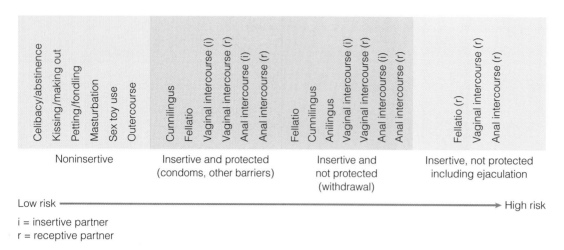

FIGURE 14-3 ▎ A Continuum of Risk for Sexual Behaviors

STI risks increase as sexual activities become unprotected and receptive.

exclusive. In surveys of students, a significant minority report having had four or more sexual partners during their lifetime.

- **Failure to use condoms.** Among those who reported having had sexual intercourse in the previous three months, fewer than half reported condom use. **Figure 14-3** shows the risk continuum for protected and unprotected sexual behaviors. STI risks increase as sexual activities become unprotected and receptive. Students who'd had four or more sexual partners were significantly less likely to use condoms than those who'd had fewer partners.
- **Substance abuse.** Teenagers who drink or use drugs are more likely to engage in sexually risky behaviors, including sex with partners whose health status and history they do not know, and unprotected intercourse.

Rate your own sexual health risk by taking the Self-Survey on page 347.

Chlamydia

The most widespread sexually transmitted bacterium in the United States is *Chlamydia trachomatis,* which causes an estimated 3 million cases of **chlamydia** each year.[18] One in 25 young Americans is infected with chlamydia, according to a recent nationwide study. Chlamydia is six times more prevalent in young black adults than in young white adults, with almost 14 percent of young black women and more than 11 percent of black men testing positive.[19] Chlamydial infections are more common in younger than in older women, and they also occur more often in both men and women with gonorrhea.

Those at greatest risk of chlamydial infection are individuals 25 years old or younger who engage in sex with more than one new partner within a two-month period and women who use birth control pills or other nonbarrier contraceptive methods. The U.S. Preventive Services Task Forces recommend regular screening for chlamydia for all sexually active women under age 25 and for older women with multiple sexual partners, a history of STIs, or inconsistent use of condoms.

As many as 75 percent of women and 50 percent of men with chlamydia have no symptoms or symptoms so mild that they don't seek medical attention. Without treatment, up to 40 percent of cases of chlamydia can lead to pelvic inflammatory disease, a serious infection of a woman's fallopian tubes that can also damage the ovaries and uterus. Also, women infected with chlamydia may have three to five times the risk of getting infected with HIV if exposed. Babies exposed to chlamydia in the birth canal during delivery can be born with pneumonia or with an eye infection called conjunctivitis, both of which can be dangerous unless treated early with antibiotics. Symptom-less women who are screened and treated for chlamydial infection are almost 60 percent less likely than unscreened women to develop pelvic inflammatory disease. Chlamydia may also be linked to cervical cancer.[20]

The use of condoms with spermicide can reduce, but not eliminate, the risk of chlamydial infection. Sexual partners should be examined and treated if necessary. The CDC, in its most recent guidelines, recommends that all women with chlamydia be rescreened three to four months after treatment is completed. The reason is that re-infection, which often happens because a patient's sex partners were not treated, increases the risk of pelvic inflammatory disease and other complications. Immediately treating the partners of people infected with gonorrhea or chlamydia can reduce rates of recurrence of these infections.[21]

Pelvic Inflammatory Disease

Infection of a woman's fallopian tubes or uterus, called **pelvic inflammatory disease (PID),** is not actually an STI, but rather a complication of STIs. About one in

STRATEGIES for PREVENTION

What You Can Do to Lower the Risk of STIs

▌ Use a new condom each and every time you engage in any form of intercourse. Men should try different brands to find the ones they like best.

▌ Do not use spermicide containing nonoxynol-9. Contrary to past advice, experts now advise against choosing safer-sex products with nonoxynol-9. According to recent research, nonoxynol-9 without condoms is ineffective against HIV transmission. Even with condoms, it does not protect women from the bacteria that cause gonorrhea and chlamydia.

▌ If a condom fails during vaginal or anal intercourse, carefully remove it and use another one.

▌ After potential exposure to an STI, men may give themselves a little extra protection by urinating and washing their genitals with an antibacterial soap.

▌ Oral sex can transmit various STIs, including herpes, gonorrhea, syphilis, and HIV. A latex condom (without nonoxynol-9) for fellatio can lower the risk.

▌ Because bacteria can be transmitted by hand, wash your hands with hot water and antibacterial soap after sex.

▌ Make sure the package says that the condoms are meant to prevent disease. If not, the condoms may not provide adequate protection, even though they may be the most expensive ones you can buy.

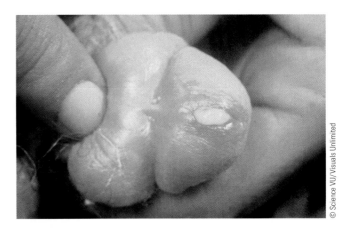

▌ A cloudy discharge is symptomatic of gonorrhea.

traced to some IUDs that are no longer on the market. Several studies have shown that women with PID are more likely to have used douches than those without the disease. Consistent condom use may decrease PID risk.

PID is a silent disease that in half of all cases produces no noticeable symptoms as it progresses and causes scarring of the fallopian tubes. Experts are encouraging women with mild symptoms, such as abdominal pain or tenderness, to seek medical evaluation and are encouraging physicians to test these patients for infections. Urine testing is a cost-effective method of detecting gonorrhea and chlamydia in young women and can prevent development of PID. For women with symptoms, magnetic resonance imaging (MRI) is highly accurate in establishing a diagnosis of PID and detecting other diseases that may be responsible for the symptoms. Treatment may require hospitalization and intensive antibiotics therapy. PID causes an estimated 15 to 30 percent of all cases of infertility every year and about half of all cases of ectopic pregnancy.

Gonorrhea

Gonorrhea (sometimes called "the clap" in street language) is one of the most common STIs in the United States. After steady declines from the 1970s to the late 1990s, gonorrhea infections have increased, with about 60 percent of new cases occurring in young adults.[22] The incidence is highest among teenagers and young adults. Sexual contact, including oral-genital sex, is the primary means of transmission.

Most men who have gonorrhea know it. Thick, yellow-white pus oozes from the penis and urination causes a burning sensation. These symptoms usually develop two to nine days after the sexual contact that infected them. Men have a good reason to seek help: It hurts too much not to. Women also may experience discharge and burning on urination. However, as many as eight out of ten infected women have no symptoms.

Gonococcus, the bacterium that causes gonorrhea, can live in the vagina, cervix, and fallopian tubes for

every seven women of reproductive age has PID; half of all adult women may have had it. Each year, about 1 million new cases are reported.

Ten to 20 percent of initial episodes of PID lead to scarring and obstruction of the fallopian tubes severe enough to cause infertility. Other long-term complications are ectopic pregnancy and chronic pelvic pain. The risk of these complications rises with subsequent PID episodes, bacterial vaginosis, and use of an IUD. Smoking also may increase the likelihood of PID. Two bacteria —gonococcus (the culprit in gonorrhea) and chlamydia —are responsible for one-half to one-third of all cases of PID. Other organisms are responsible for the remaining cases.

Most cases of PID occur among women under age 25 who are sexually active. Gonococcus-caused cases tend to affect poor women; those caused by chlamydia range across all income levels. One-half to one-third of all cases are transmitted sexually, and others have been months, even years, and continue to infect the woman's sexual partners. Approximately 5 percent of sexually active American women have positive gonorrhea cultures but are unaware that they are silent carriers.

If left untreated in men or women, gonorrhea spreads through the urinary-genital tract. In women, the inflammation travels from the vagina and cervix, through the uterus, to the fallopian tubes and ovaries. The pain and fever are similar to those caused by stomach upset, so a woman may dismiss the symptoms. Eventually these symptoms diminish, even though the disease spreads to the entire pelvis. Pus may ooze from the fallopian tubes or ovaries into the peritoneum (the lining of the abdominal cavity), sometimes causing serious inflammation. However, this, too, can subside in a few weeks. Gonorrhea, the leading cause of sterility in women, can cause PID. In pregnant women, gonorrhea becomes a threat to the newborn. It can infect the infant's external genitals and cause a serious form of conjunctivitis, an inflammation of the eye that may lead to blindness. As a preventive step, newborns may have penicillin dropped into their eyes at birth.

In men, untreated gonorrhea can spread to the prostate gland, testicles, bladder, and kidneys. Among the serious complications are urinary obstruction and sterility caused by blockage of the vas deferens (the excretory duct of the testis). In both sexes, gonorrhea can develop into a serious, even fatal, bloodborne infection that can cause arthritis in the joints, attack the heart muscle and lining, cause meningitis, and attack the skin and other organs.

Although a blood test has been developed for detecting gonorrhea, the tried-and-true method of diagnosis is still a microscopic analysis of cultures from the male's urethra, the female's cervix, and the throat and anus of both sexes.

Because gonorrhea often occurs along with chlamydia, practitioners often prescribe an agent effective against both, such as ofloxacin. In some parts of the United States, gonorrhea has become so resistant to certain antibiotics such as fluoroguinolone that they are no longer advised for use in its treatment.[23] Antibiotics taken for other reasons may not affect or cure the gonorrhea because of their dosage or type. And you can't develop immunity to gonorrhea; within days of recovering from one case, you can catch another.

Nongonococcal Urethritis (NGU)

The term **nongonococcal urethritis (NGU)** refers to any inflammation of the urethra that is not caused by gonorrhea. NGU is the most common STI in men, accounting for 4 to 6 million visits to a physician every year. Three microorganisms—*Chlamydia trachomatis, Ureaplasma urealyticum,* and *Mycoplasma genitalium*—are the primary causes; the usual means of transmission is sexual intercourse. Other infectious agents, such as fungi or bacteria, allergic reactions to vaginal secretions, or irritation by soaps or contraceptive foams or gels may also lead to NGU.

In the United States, NGU is more common in men than gonococcal urethritis. The symptoms in men are similar to those of gonorrhea, including discharge from the penis (usually less than with gonorrhea) and mild burning during urination. Women frequently develop no symptoms or very mild itching, burning during urination, or discharge. Symptoms usually disappear after two or three weeks, but the infection may persist and cause cervicitis or PID in women and, in men, may spread to the prostate, epididymis, or both. Treatment usually consists of doxycycline or azithromycin and should be given to both sexual partners after testing.

Syphilis

A corkscrew-shaped, spiral bacterium called *Treponema pallidum* causes **syphilis.** This frail microbe dies in seconds if dried or chilled but grows quickly in the warm, moist tissues of the body, particularly in the mucous membranes of the genital tract. Entering the body through any tiny break in the skin, the germ burrows its way into the bloodstream. Sexual contact, including oral sex or intercourse, is a primary means of transmission. Genital ulcers caused by syphilis may increase the risk of HIV infection, while individuals with HIV may be more likely to develop syphilis.

Public education programs, expanded screening and surveillance, increased tracing of contacts, and condom promotion have helped control the spread of syphilis in some areas. Syphilis rates have fallen to the lowest ever reported in the United States. The decline has been particularly significant in African Americans and people living in the South.

Syphilis has clearly identifiable stages:

▪ **Primary syphilis.** The first sign of syphilis is a lesion, or *chancre* (pronounced "shanker"), an open lump or crater the size of a dime or smaller, teeming with bacteria. The incubation period before its appearance ranges from 10 to 90 days; three to four weeks is average. The chancre appears exactly where the bacteria entered the body: in the mouth, throat, vagina, rectum, or penis. Any contact with the chancre is likely to result in infection.

▪ **Secondary syphilis.** Anywhere from one to twelve months after the chancre's appearance, secondary-stage symptoms may appear. Some people have no symptoms. Others develop a skin rash or a small, flat rash in moist regions on the skin; whitish patches on the mucous membranes of the mouth or throat; temporary baldness; low-grade fever; headache; swollen glands; or large, moist sores around the mouth and genitals. These are loaded with bacteria; contact with them, through kissing or intercourse, may transmit the infection. Symptoms may last for several days or several months. Even without treatment, they eventually disappear as the syphilis microbes go into hiding.

▌**Latent syphilis.** Although there are no signs or symptoms, no sores or rashes at this stage, the bacteria are invading various organs inside the body, including the heart and brain. For two to four years, there may be recurring infectious and highly contagious lesions of the skin or mucous membranes. However, syphilis loses its infectiousness as it progresses: After the first two years, a person rarely transmits syphilis through intercourse.

After four years, even congenital syphilis is rarely transmitted. Until this stage of the disease, however, a pregnant woman can pass syphilis to her unborn child. If the fetus is infected in its fourth month or earlier, it may be disfigured or even die. If infected late in pregnancy, the child may show no signs of infection for months or years after birth but may then become disabled with the symptoms of tertiary syphilis.

▌**Tertiary syphilis.** Ten to 20 years after the beginning of the latent stage, the most serious symptoms of syphilis emerge, generally in the organs in which the bacteria settled during latency. Syphilis that has progressed to this stage has become increasingly rare. Victims of tertiary syphilis may die of a ruptured aorta or of other heart damage, or may have progressive brain or spinal cord damage, eventually leading to blindness, insanity, or paralysis. About a third of those who are not treated during the first three stages of syphilis enter the tertiary stage later in life.

Health experts are urging screening for syphilis for everyone who seeks treatment for an STI, especially adolescents; for everyone using illegal drugs; and for the partners of these two groups. They also recommend that anyone diagnosed with syphilis be screened for other STIs and be counseled about voluntary testing for HIV.

Penicillin is the drug of choice for treating primary, secondary, and latent syphilis. The earlier treatment begins, the more effective it is. Those allergic to penicillin may be treated with doxycycline, ceftriaxone, or erythromycin. An added danger of not getting treatment for syphilis is an increased risk of HIV transmission.

Herpes

Herpes (from the Greek word that means to *creep*) collectively describes some of the most common viral infections in humans. Characteristically, **herpes simplex** causes blisters on the skin or mucous membranes. Herpes simplex exists in several varieties. *Herpes simplex virus 1 (HSV-1)* generally causes cold sores and fever blisters around the mouth. *Herpes simplex virus 2 (HSV-2)* may cause blisters on the penis, inside the vagina, on the cervix, in the pubic area, on the buttocks, or on the thighs. With the increase of oral-genital sex, some doctors report finding type 2 herpes lesions in the mouth and throat.

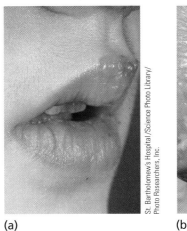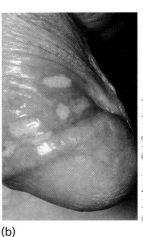

(a)   (b)

▌(a) Herpes simplex virus (HSV-1) as a mouth sore
(b) Herpes simplex virus (HSV-2) as a genital sore.

Genital herpes has skyrocketed during the last three decades, yet only a minority of infections with HSV-2 are recognized by those infected. About 40 percent of new cases of genital herpes occur in young people ages 15 to 24. An estimated 4.2 million young adults in this age range—11 percent of the population—have been infected.[24]

Research has shown that individuals without any obvious symptoms shed the virus subclinically, whether or not they have lesions. Most people with herpes contract it from partners who were not aware of any symptoms or of their own contagiousness. Standard methods of diagnosing genital herpes in women, which rely primarily on physical examination and viral cultures, may miss as many as two-thirds of all cases. Newly developed blood tests are more effective in detecting unrecognized and subclinical infections with HSV-2.

In the past, patients and most doctors thought people with herpes could safely have unprotected sex when they had no symptoms. The herpes virus is present in genital secretions even when patients do not notice any signs of the disease, and people infected with genital herpes can spread it even between flare-ups when they have no symptoms. There is growing evidence that genital herpes promotes the spread of HIV.

HSV transmission occurs through close contact with mucous membranes or abraded skin. Condoms help prevent infection but aren't foolproof. When herpes sores are present, the infected person is highly contagious and should avoid bringing the lesions into contact with someone else's body through touching, sexual interaction, or kissing.

A newborn can be infected with genital herpes while passing through the birth canal, and the frequency of mother-to-infant transmission seems to be increasing. Most infected infants develop typical skin sores, which can be cultured to confirm a herpes diagnosis. Some physicians recommend treatment with acyclovir. Because of the risk of severe damage and possible death, caesarean delivery may be advised for a woman with active herpes lesions.

The virus that causes herpes never entirely goes away; it retreats to nerves near the lower spinal cord, where it remains for the life of the host. Herpes sores can return without warning weeks, months, or even years after their first occurrence, often during menstruation or times of stress, or with sudden changes in body temperature. Of those who experience HSV recurrence, 10 to 35 percent do so frequently—that is, about six or more times a year. In most people, attacks diminish in frequency and severity over time. Herpes, like other STIs, can trigger feelings of shame, guilt, and depression.

Antiviral drugs, such as acyclovir (Zovirax), have proved effective in treating and controlling herpes. Available as an ointment, in capsules, and in injection form, acyclovir relieves the symptoms but doesn't kill the virus. Whereas the ointment works only for the initial bout with herpes, acyclovir in injectable and pill form dramatically reduces the length and severity of herpes outbreaks. Continuing daily oral acyclovir can reduce recurrences by about 80 percent. However, its safety in pregnant women has not been established. Infection with herpes viruses resistant to acyclovir is a growing problem, especially in individuals with immune-suppressing disorders.

Various treatments—compresses made with cold water, skim milk, or warm salt water; ice packs; or a mild anesthetic cream—can relieve discomfort. Herpes sufferers should avoid heat, hot baths, or nylon underwear. Some physicians have used laser therapy to vaporize the lesions. Clinical trials of an experimental vaccine to protect people from herpes infections are underway.

What Is Human Papilloma Virus (HPV)?

Infection with **human papilloma virus (HPV),** a pathogen that can cause *genital warts,* is the most common viral STI. By some estimates, 20 million or more women in the United States are infected with HPV, as are three out of four their male sexual partners. Young women who engage in sexual intercourse at an early age are more likely than those with later sexual debuts to become infected with HPV. Their risk also increases if they have multiple sexual partners or a history of a sexually transmitted disease, use drugs, or have partners with multiple sexual partners.[25]

Three in four new infections with genital human papilloma virus occur among 15- to 24-years-olds. An estimated 9.2 million young adults have been infected with HPV and could spread the virus.[26] College-age women are among those at greatest risk of acquiring HPV infection. In various studies conducted in college health centers, 10 to 46 percent of female students (mean age 20 to 22) had a cervical HPV in-

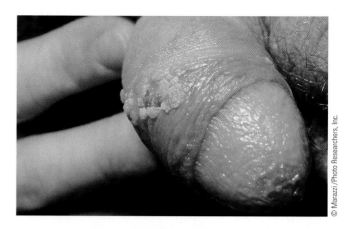

Human papilloma virus, which causes genital warts, is the most common viral STI.

fection—and increased risk of precancerous cell changes. Risk factors include smoking, use of oral contraceptives, multiple sex partners, anal as well as vaginal intercourse, alcohol consumption at the time of engaging in vaginal intercourse, and sex partners with a history of HPV.

HPV infections in young women tend to be of short duration. In a three-year study, 60 percent of 608 college women became infected with the virus; the average duration of infection was eight months. According to the researchers, many young women who get HPV may not require treatment because the condition often regresses on its own.

HPV is transmitted primarily through vaginal, anal, and oral-genital sex. More than half of HPV-infected individuals do not develop any symptoms. After contact with an infected individual, genital warts may appear from three weeks to eighteen months, with an average period of about three months. The warts are treated by freezing, cauterization, chemicals, or surgical removal. Recurrences are common because the virus remains in the body.

HPV infection may invade the urethra and cause urinary obstruction and bleeding. It greatly increases a woman's risk of developing a precancerous condition called *cervical intraepithelial neoplasia,* which can lead to cervical cancer. There also is a strong association between HPV infections and cancer of the vagina, vulva, urethra, penis, and anus.

HPV may be the single most important risk factor in 95 percent of all cases of cervical cancer. Adolescent girls infected with HPV appear to be particularly vulnerable to developing cervical cancer. It is not known if HPV itself causes cancer or acts in conjunction with cofactors (such as other infections, smoking, or suppressed immunity). HPV transmission may be the reason women are five to eleven times as likely to get cervical cancer if their steady sexual partner has had 20 or more previous partners.

Women who have had an HPV infection should examine their genitals regularly and get an annual Pap smear. However, this standard diagnostic test for cervical cancer doesn't identify HPV infection. A new laboratory test can detect the presence of HPV, including the high-risk types associated with the development of cervical cancer. The HPV DNA test does not test for cancer but for the HPV viruses that can cause cell changes in the cervix. If left untreated, these changes can eventually lead to cancer in some women. Surgery or laser therapy can prevent further damage.

HPV may also cause genital warts in men and increase the risk of cancer of the penis. HPV-infected men, who may not develop any symptoms, can spread the infection to their partners. People with visible genital warts also may have asymptomatic or subclinical HPV infections that are extremely difficult to treat.

No form of therapy has been shown to completely eradicate HPV, nor has single treatment been uniformly effective in removing warts or preventing their recurrence. CDC guidelines suggest treatments that focus on the removal of visible warts—cryotherapy (freezing) and topical applications of podofilox, podophyllin, or trichloroacetic acid—and then eradication of the virus. At least 20 to 30 percent of treated individuals experience recurrence. In experimental studies, interferon, a biologic substance produced by virus-infected cells that inhibits viral replication, has proved helpful.

Chancroid

A **chancroid** is a soft, painful sore or localized infection caused by the bacterium *Haemophilus ducrevi* and usually acquired through sexual contact. Half of the cases heal by themselves. In other cases, the infection may spread to the lymph glands near the chancroid, where large amounts of pus can accumulate and destroy much of the local tissue. The incidence of this STI, widely prevalent in Africa and tropical and semitropical regions, is rapidly increasing in the United States, with outbreaks in several states, including Louisiana, Texas, and New York. Chancroids, which may increase susceptibility to HIV infection, are believed to be a major factor in the heterosexual spread of HIV. This infection is treated with antibiotics (ceftriaxone, azithromycin, or erythromycin) and can be prevented by keeping the genitals clean and washing them with soap and water in case of possible exposure.

Pubic Lice and Scabies

These infections are sometimes, but not always, transmitted sexually. *Pubic lice* (or "crabs") are usually found in the pubic hair, although they can migrate to any hairy areas of the body. Lice lay eggs called nits that attach to the base of the hair shaft. Irritation from the lice may produce intense itching. Scratching to relieve the itching can produce sores. *Scabies* is caused by a mite that burrows under the skin, where they lay eggs that hatch and undergo many changes in the course of their life cycle, producing great discomfort, including intense itching.

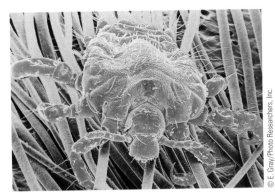

© E. Gray/Photo Researchers, Inc.

Actual size

A pubic louse, or "crab."

Lice and scabies are treated with applications of permethrin cream and Lindane shampoo to all the areas of the body where there are concentrations of body hair (genitals, armpits, scalp). You must repeat treatment in seven days to kill any newly developed adults. Wash or dry-clean clothing and bedding.

✚ HIV and AIDS

Thirty years ago, no one knew about **human immuno-deficiency virus (HIV)**. No one had ever heard of **acquired immune deficiency syndrome (AIDS)**. Once seen as an epidemic affecting primarily gay men and injection drug users, AIDS has taken on a very different form. Today, heterosexuals in developing countries have the highest rates of infection and mortality. And HIV infection continues to spread, doubling at an estimated rate of every ten years. About 40 million people worldwide are infected with HIV; 15,000 more individuals are infected every day. AIDS now claims about 3 million lives around the world a year.[27] According to the CDC, 800,000 to 900,000 Americans are infected with HIV, with about 40,000 new infections every year.

At least half of new HIV infections occur in people under age 25, mainly by sexual contact. HIV is the fifth leading cause of death for Americans between the ages of 25 and 44. Among African-American women in this age group, HIV infection is the third leading cause of death, and among African-American men, it's the leading cause of death.[28]

Federal health officials fear that a new generation may not be using adequate safer sex precautions because they have grown complacent about the dangers of HIV/AIDS.[29] Efforts to prevent sexual transmission of HIV have taken a new focus: counseling those who already have HIV in an attempt to get them to stop spreading it.

Breakthrough drugs are indeed allowing HIV-infected people to live longer. However, new dangers have emerged. Up to 15 percent of new HIV cases in the country may stem from drug-resistant strains of the virus. "Superinfection" with more than one strain of

HIV seems more common than previously thought. As a result, HIV-infected people who initially were doing well without drugs may become ill after contracting a second strain of the AIDS virus.

Efforts to prevent nonsexual forms of HIV transmission have been very effective. Screening the blood supply has reduced the rate of transfusion-associated HIV transmission by 99.9 percent. Treatment with antiretroviral drugs during pregnancy and birth has reduced transmission by about 90 percent in optimal conditions. Among drug users in some settings, programs that combine addiction treatment and needle exchange reduced the incidence of HIV infection by 30 percent.

The percentage of individuals who acquired HIV through heterosexual contact has increased. However, many heterosexual adults are not aware of their partners' HIV status and may not see themselves as at risk of HIV infection. According to the CDC, about a third of the HIV-infected individuals in the United States have not been diagnosed.

Although HIV/AIDS is often seen as a threat to men, 30 percent of new HIV infections in the United States occur among women. About a quarter of Americans living with HIV/AIDS are women. Women of color, particularly African Americans, have been hardest hit. While African-American women make up just 13 percent of the female population of the United States, they account for 63 percent of newly diagnosed cases. HIV/AIDS is most prevalent among women in their child-bearing years.[30]

Reducing the Risk of HIV Transmission

HIV/AIDS can be so frightening that some people have exaggerated its dangers, whereas others understate them. The fact is that although no one is immune to HIV, you can reduce the risk if you abstain from sexual activity, remain in a monogamous relationship with an uninfected partner, and do not inject drugs.

If you're not in a long-term monogamous relationship with a partner you're sure is safe, and you're not willing to abstain from sex, there are things you can do to lower your risk of HIV infection. Remember that the risk of HIV transmission depends on sexual behavior, not sexual orientation. Among young men, the prevalence and frequency of sexual risk behaviors are similar regardless of sexual orientation, ethnicity, or age. Homosexual, heterosexual, and bisexual individuals all need to know about the kinds of sexual activity that increase their risk.

Here's what you should know about HIV transmission:

▌ Casual contact does *not* spread HIV infection. You cannot get HIV infection from drinking from a water fountain, contact with a toilet seat, or touching an infected person.

STUDENT SNAPSHOT
HIV Testing and Telling

	Percentage
Say a partner had never asked about HIV status	79%
Rarely or never ask partners about HIV status	51%
Have been tested for HIV	21%
Of these, told partners the results	73%
Told a partner they were HIV-negative without being tested	5%

Based on a study of 246 sexually active heterosexuals at two universities in Southern California.
Source: Marelich, William, and Tonya Clark. "Human Immunodeficiency Virus (HIV) Testing and False Disclosures in Heterosexual College Students." *Journal of American College Health,* Vol. 53, No. 3, November–December 2004, p. 109.

▌ Compared to other viruses, HIV is extremely difficult to get.

▌ HIV can live in blood, semen, vaginal fluids, and breast milk.

▌ Many chemicals, including household bleach, alcohol, and hydrogen peroxide, can inactivate HIV.

▌ In studies of family members sharing dishes, food, clothing, and frequent hugs with people with HIV infection or AIDS, those who have contracted the virus have shared razor blades, toothbrushes, or had other means of blood contact.

▌ You cannot tell visually whether a potential sexual partner has HIV. A blood test is needed to detect the antibodies that the body produces to fight HIV, thus indicating infection.

▌ HIV can be spread in semen and vaginal fluids during a single instance of anal, vaginal, or oral sexual contact between heterosexuals, bisexuals, or homosexuals. The risk increases with the number of sexual encounters with an infected partner.

▌ Teenage girls may be particularly vulnerable to HIV infection because the immature cervix is easily infected.

▌ Anal intercourse is an extremely high-risk behavior because HIV can enter the bloodstream through tiny breaks in the lining of the rectum. HIV transmission is much more likely to occur during unprotected anal intercourse than vaginal intercourse.

▌ Other behaviors that increase the risk of HIV infection include having multiple sexual partners, engaging in sex without condoms or virus-killing spermicides, sexual contact with persons known to be at high risk (for example, prostitutes or injection drug users), and sharing injection equipment for drugs.

- Individuals are at greater risk if they have an active sexual infection. Sexually transmitted infections, such as herpes, gonorrhea, and syphilis, facilitate transmission of HIV during vaginal or rectal intercourse.

- No cases of HIV transmission by deep kissing have been reported, but it could happen. Studies have found blood in the saliva of healthy people after kissing; other lab studies have found HIV in saliva. Social (dry) kissing is safe.

- Oral sex can lead to HIV transmission. The virus in any semen that enters the mouth could make its way into the bloodstream through tiny nicks or sores in the mouth. A man's risk in performing oral sex on a woman is smaller because an infected woman's genital fluids have much lower concentrations of HIV than does semen.

- HIV infection is not widespread among lesbians, although there have been documented cases of possible female-to-female HIV transmission. In each instance, one partner had had sex with a bisexual man or male injection drug user or had injected drugs herself.

HIV Testing

Nearly 50 percent of American adults younger than 65 have been tested for HIV. In general, women are more likely to have sought testing than men.[31] In one study of 246 sexually active heterosexual college students, 21 percent had been tested for HIV, and most had disclosed the results to their intimate partners. Five percent admitted to telling a potential partner that they were HIV-negative, even though they had not been tested.[32] (See Student Snapshot "HIV Testing and Telling.") About 10,000 facilities provide publicly funded HIV testing and counseling in the United States; approximately 2.6 million tests are performed annually at these sites.

All HIV tests measure antibodies, cells produced by the body to fight HIV infection. A negative test indicates no exposure to HIV. It can take three to six months for the body to produce the telltale antibodies, however, so a negative result may not be accurate, depending on the timing of the test.

HIV testing can be either confidential or anonymous. In confidential testing, a person's name is recorded along with the test results, which are made available to medical personnel and, in 32 states, the state health department. In anonymous testing, no name is associated with the test results. Anonymous testing is available in 39 states.

Different groups of individuals at risk prefer different tests. Asian–Pacific Islander and white men who have sex with men are most likely to choose anonymous testing; African-American men who have sex with men are much more likely to choose

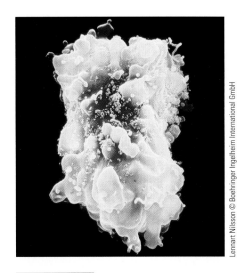

Electron micrograph of a white blood cell being attacked by HIV (*blue light particles*), the virus that causes AIDS.

Lennart Nilsson © Boehringer Ingelheim International GmbH

confidential testing. Consumers must be wary of bogus HIV tests offered via the Internet.

The following HIV tests are currently available in the United States:

- **EIA** (enzyme immune assay) or **ELISA** (enzyme-linked immunosorbent assay). These standard blood tests are the most commonly used HIV screens. A health-care provider draws a blood sample, which is analyzed for antibodies produced to fight against HIV particles. Results are available within a few days to two weeks.

- **Oral HIV tests.** These tests have become available in some doctors' offices and health clinics. A health-care worker swabs a tissue sample from the inside of the mouth. The only oral test approved by the Food and Drug Administration (FDA) is the OraSure.

- **Rapid tests.** Different types, such as the OraQuick Rapid HIV-1 Antibody Test, can detect HIV antibodies in blood or oral fluid. The advantage is fast results—usually in 20 or 30 minutes.

- **Western blot.** This more accurate and expensive test is used to confirm the results of a positive HIV test.

- **HomeAccess.** This test—the only home HIV test approved by the FDA—is available in drug stores for $40 to $50. An individual draws a blood sample by pricking a finger and sends it to a laboratory along with a personal identification number. Results are given over the phone by a trained counselor, usually within several days.

- **Urine test.** This alternative to a blood test must be ordered by a physician. A urine sample is screened by a laboratory. Results are generally available in a few days to two weeks.[33]

Newly developed blood tests can determine how recently a person was infected with HIV and distinguish between long-standing infections and those contracted within the previous four to six months. Health officials recommend HIV testing for the following individuals:

▮ Men who have had sex with other men, regardless of whether they consider themselves homosexual.

▮ Anyone who uses injection drugs or has shared needles.

▮ Anyone who has had sex with someone who uses injection drugs or has shared needles.

▮ Women who have had sex with bisexual men.

▮ Anyone who has had sex with someone from an area with a high incidence of HIV infection.

▮ Individuals who have had sex with people they do not know well.

▮ Anyone who received blood transfusions or blood products between 1978 and 1985, their sexual partners, and, if they are new mothers, their infants.

Diagnosing and Treating HIV/AIDS

A diagnosis of AIDS applies to anyone with HIV whose immune system is severely impaired, as indicated by a test of the immune system's strength based on T-4, or T-helper, cells. A CD4 count of less than 200 cells per cubic millimeter of blood, compared to normal CD4 cell counts in healthy people not infected with HIV of 800 to 1,200 per cubic millimeter of blood indicates AIDS. In addition, AIDS is diagnosed in persons with HIV infection who experience recurrent pneumonia, invasive cervical cancer, or pulmonary tuberculosis.

People with AIDS also may experience persistent fever, diarrhea that persists for more than one month, or involuntary weight loss of more than 10 percent of normal body weight. Neurological disease—including dementia (confusion and impaired thinking) and other problems with thinking, speaking, movement, or sensation—may occur. Secondary infectious diseases that may develop in people with AIDS include *Pneumocystis carinii* pneumonia, tuberculosis, or oral candidiasis (thrush). Secondary cancers associated with HIV infection include Kaposi's sarcoma and cancer of the cervix.

New forms of therapy have been remarkably effective in boosting levels of protective T cells and reducing *viral load*—the amount of HIV in the bloodstream. People with high viral loads are more likely to progress rapidly to AIDS than people with low levels of the virus.

The current "gold-standard" approach to combating HIV is known as HAART (highly active antiretroviral therapies), which dramatically reduces viral load even though it does not eradicate the virus. This complex regimen uses one of 250 different combinations of three or more anti-retroviral drugs. Since the development of HAART, the number of deaths among persons with AIDS in the United States has declined substantially, and the number of those living with AIDS has risen.

✚ MAKING HEALTHY CHOICES

For Safer, Smarter Sex

We remain sexual beings throughout life. At different ages and stages, sexuality can take on different meanings. As you forge relationships and explore your sexuality, you may encounter difficult situations and unfamiliar feelings. But sex is never just about hormones and body parts. People describe the brain as the sexiest of our organs. Using your brain to make responsible sexual decisions leads to both a smarter and a more fulfilling sex life.

▮ **Communicate openly.** If you or your partner cannot talk openly and honestly about your sexual histories and contraception, you should avoid having sex. For the sake of protecting your sexual health, you have to be willing to ask—and answer—questions that may seem embarrassing.

▮ **Share responsibility in a sexual relationship.** Both partners should be involved in protecting themselves and each other from STIs and, if heterosexual, unwanted pregnancy.

▮ **Respect sexual privacy.** Revealing sexual activities violates the trust between two partners. Bragging about a sexual conquest demeans everyone involved.

▮ **Be prepared.** If there's any possibility that you may be engaging in sex, be sure you have the means to protect yourself against unwanted pregnancy and sexually transmitted infections.

▮ **In sexual situations, always think ahead.** For the sake of safety, think about potential dangers—parking in an isolated area, going into a bedroom with someone you hardly know, and the like—and options to protect yourself.

▮ **Be aware of your own and your partner's alcohol and drug intake.** The use of such substances impairs judgment and reduces the ability to say no. While under their influence, you may engage in sexual behavior you'll later regret.

▮ **Be sure sexual activity is consensual.** Coercion can take many forms: physical, emotional, and verbal. All cause psychological damage and undermine trust and respect. At any point in a relationship, whether the couple is dating or married, either individual has the right to say no.

Source: Adapted from Robert Hatcher et al. *Sexual Etiquette 101 and More.* Atlanta, GA: Emory University School of Medicine, 2002.

SELF-SURVEY

Assessing Your STI Risk

Many factors must be considered in assessing your health and fitness. Among these are (a) your risk of acquiring or transmitting any sexually transmitted infection (STI) and (b) your use of psychoactive chemicals in connection with sexual activity, a practice that can increase your risk of acquiring an STI.

The first two questions are biographical in nature and are not part of the risk assessment score. The remaining 11 are the scored behavioral risk assessment. Please be honest in responding to the questions.

Please check the one single answer that best describes your preferences or activities.

A. How long have you been sexually active? _____

B. Your most recent consistent sexual partner experience male _____ female _____ both male and female _____

1. How many sexual partners *per month* in the last year?
    3 _____ 5 or more
    2 _____ 2–4
    1 _____ 0–1

2. How many partners *per month* in the year previous?
    3 _____ 5 or more
    2 _____ 2–4
    1 _____ 0–1

3. The kinds of sexual contacts I have are
    3 _____ one-time or anonymous "tricks," "one night stands," groups, or prostitutes
    2 _____ multiple times with two or more partners
    1 _____ exclusively with one partner

4. I have sexual encounters or contacts most frequently
    3 _____ bookstores, parties, "massage parlors," "spas," public restrooms, autos
    1 _____ in my or my partner's home

5. The frequency with which I use drugs or alcohol to enhance my sexual encounters:
    3 _____ frequently
    2 _____ occasionally
    1 _____ rarely/never

Please circle drug used: "poppers" (amyl or butyl nitrates), alcohol, marijuana, hallucinogens (LSD, mushrooms), "angel dust" (PCP), amphetamines, barbiturates, Quaaludes, ecstasy, eve, cocaine, crack, or (please fill in others).

6. I have injected myself with one or more of the preceding drugs (see Question 5) in the past 5 years.
    4 _____ yes
    1 _____ no

7. I have sexual encounters most frequently in
    3 _____ New York, Los Angeles, San Francisco, Miami, Washington, Dallas, Houston, Newark, Atlanta
    2 _____ other large urban areas (Boston, Philadelphia, St. Louis, Seattle, San Diego, etc.)
    1 _____ small cities, towns, rural areas

8. Those kinds of sexual activities I practice most frequently are (please circle specific activities)
    4 _____ vaginal or anal intercourse without a condom, oral-anal contact ("rimming"), direct fecal or urine contact ("scat" or "water sports"), or manual anal contact ("fisting")
    3 _____ "protected" vaginal or anal intercourse (use of condoms and spermicides)
    2 _____ oral-genital contact (fellatio or cunnilingus)
    1 _____ masturbation, massage, body rubbing, kissing

9. My current sexual partner and I have discussed our previous sexual behavior and experiences with each other.
    4 _____ No
    1 _____ Yes

10. I negotiate with sexual partners for safer sexual practices.
    4 _____ No
    2 _____ Sometimes
    1 _____ Yes

11. I ask potential sexual partners about their use of drugs and steroids, especially their use of needles.
    4 _____ No
    2 _____ Sometimes
    1 _____ Yes

Add up the numbers from each question (1–11) and see the key below to determine your level of risk.

My score is _____
If you answered "1" (the last option) for question 8, deduct 3 points.

Total Adjusted Score: _____

Key:

17 or more: You appear to be at high risk for developing STIs, including HIV infection, and for possibly developing dependence on psychoactive substances. You should visit your health-care provider immediately to discuss your risk of these dangers.

12–16 points: You appear to be at moderate risk for developing either an STI or chemical dependence and are encouraged to lower your overall risk by altering the behaviors that resulted in high scores on some of the questions. See your health-care provider for any questions or concerns you may have regarding your risk.

11 points: You are at low risk for problems and are encouraged to continue your healthy behavior.

Source: Reprinted (excerpted) from the special report, "AIDS on the College Campus" (no longer in print), by Leland G. Wessell, M.D., M.P.H., with permission from the American College Health Association, PO Box 28937, Baltimore, MD 20840–8937.

ACTION PLAN

Your Action Plan for Coping with STIs

What to Do If You Have an STI

▪ If you suspect that you have an STI, don't feel too embarrassed to get help through a physician's office or a clinic. Treatment relieves discomfort, prevents complications, and halts the spread of the disease.

▪ Following diagnosis, take oral medication (which may be given instead of or in addition to shots) exactly as prescribed.

▪ Try to figure out from whom you got the STI. Be sure to inform that person, who may not be aware of the problem.

▪ If you have an STI, never deceive a prospective partner about it. Tell the truth—simply and clearly. Be sure your partner understands exactly what you have and what the risks are.

Telling a Partner You Have an STI

Even though the conversation can be awkward and embarrassing, you need to talk honestly about any STI that you may have been exposed to or contracted. What you don't say can be hazardous to your partner's health. Here are some guidelines:

▪ **Talk before you become intimate.** A good way to start is simply by saying, "*There is something we need to talk over first.*"

▪ **Be honest.** Don't downplay any potential risks.

▪ **Don't blame.** Even if you suspect that your partner was the source of your infection, focus on the need for medical attention.

▪ **Be sensitive to your partner's feelings.** Anger and resentment are common reactions when someone feels at risk. Try to listen without becoming defensive.

▪ **Seek medical attention.** Do not engage in sexual intimacies until you obtain a doctor's assurance that you are no longer contagious.

Source: From www.smartersex.org, the Bacchus and Gamma Peer Education Network.

SETTING GOALS

Personal Safer Sex

Your Personal Safer Sex Goal

Is It S.M.A.R.T.?

   Specific? _____

   Measurable? _____

   Achievable? _____

   Rewarding? _____

   Time Defined? _____

Strategies for Success

   1. _____

   2. _____

   3. _____

Potential Obstacles

   1. _____

   2. _____

   3. _____

Ways Around Them

   1. _____

   2. _____

   3. _____

Daily Report

The Week that Was:

What Went Right?

What Could I Do Better?

WELLNESS JOURNAL

What If?

Like many people, you may think that you aren't at risk for sexually transmitted infections or that the choices you make are good enough to keep you safe. But what if you were to discover that a partner had an STI? Write down the reaction you might have. Describe the feelings you might experience.

Imagine how you would cope with a diagnosis of an STI. Think of whom you would tell and how you would tell them. Write down, maybe in dialogue form, what you would say. Describe how you would feel about seeking treatment. What would you tell future potential sexual partners?

What if the STI you were exposed to was HIV? On a page in your journal, write a description that begins, "As soon as I realized I might be HIV-positive. . . ." Record the thoughts and emotions you might experience. What would be your regrets? Your fears? Your plans? How would your life and future be different?

CHAPTER 14

Making This Chapter Work for You

1. A sexually healthy relationship is based on shared values and has these five characteristics: consensual, mutually pleasurable, honest, protected against unintended pregnancy and STIs, and
   a. always available.
   b. exclusive.
   c. willing to try anything.
   d. nonexploitative.

2. According to the Centers for Disease Control, abstinence is defined as
   a. refraining from all sexual behaviors that result in arousal.
   b. refraining from all sexual activities that involve vaginal, anal, and oral intercourse.
   c. having sexual intercourse with only one partner exclusively.
   d. refraining from drinking alcohol before sexual activity.

3. Jake is sexually active but doesn't want to use a condom. His other choices to protect himself against STIs include all of these *except*
   a. abstinence.
   b. a sexual relationship with a longtime friend.
   c. a sexual relationship with one STI-free partner.
   d. masturbation only.

4. Which statement about college students is *not* true?
   a. They consider sexual activity as normal for their peer group.
   b. They agree that sex and contraception should be discussed before having sex.
   c. More than 80 percent always or often use a condom during sexual activity.
   d. Men trust a woman as safe and healthy on the basis of the way she looks.

5. Talking about his prior sexual history makes Mark uncomfortable, so he wrote out all the instances where he had put himself at risk for an STI. Thinking about e-mailing the list to a prospective partner made him even more uncomfortable, and he decided that talking was preferable. And it was the _____ thing to do.
   a. responsible
   b. honest
   c. caring
   d. all of the above

6. Sexually transmitted infections:
   a. are the major cause of preventable sterility in the United States.
   b. can result in a severe kidney disease called pylonephritis.
   c. have declined in incidence in developing nations due to improving health standards.
   d. do not increase the risk of being infected with HIV.

7. Bacterial agents cause all of the following STIs *except*
   a. genital warts.
   b. syphilis.
   c. chlamydia.
   d. gonorrhea.

8. Viral agents cause all of the following STIs *except*
   a. herpes.
   b. genital warts.
   c. hepatitis B.
   d. candidiasis.

9. Which of the following statements about HIV transmission is *true?*
   a. Individuals are not at risk for HIV if they are being treated for chlamydia or gonorrhea.
   b. HIV can be transmitted between lesbians.
   c. Heterosexual men who do not practice safe sex are at less risk for contracting HIV than homosexual men who do practice safe sex.
   d. HIV cannot be spread in a single instance of sexual intercourse.

10. A person with AIDS
    a. has a low viral load and a high number of T4 helper cells.
    b. can no longer pass HIV to a sexual partner.
    c. may suffer from secondary infectious diseases and cancers.
    d. will not respond to treatment.

Answers to these questions can be found on page 376.

Critical Thinking

1. Bill has told his girlfriend, Anita, that he has never taken any sexual risks. But when she suggested that they get tested for STIs, he became furious and refused. Now Anita says she doesn't know what to believe. Could Bill be telling the truth, or is he hiding something? If he is telling the truth, why is Bill so upset? Anita doesn't want to take any risks, but she doesn't want to lose him either. What would you advise her to say or do? What would you advise Bill to say or do?

2. The U.S. military and some employers routinely screen personnel for HIV. Some hospitals test patients

and note their HIV status on their charts. Some insurance companies test for HIV before selling a policy. Do you believe that an individual has the right to refuse to be tested for HIV? Should a physician be able to order an HIV test without a patient's consent? Can a surgeon refuse to operate on an HIV-infected patient or one who refuses HIV testing? Do patients have the right to know if their doctors, dentists, or nurses are HIV-positive?

3. A man who developed herpes sued his former girlfriend. A woman who became sterile as a result of pelvic inflammatory disease (PID) took her ex-husband to court. A woman who contracted HIV infection from her dentist, who had died of AIDS, filed suit against his estate. Do you think that anyone who knowingly transmits a sexually transmitted disease should be held legally responsible? Do you think such an act should be a criminal offense?

Media Menu

Health⊗Now™

Don't forget to check out the wealth of resources on the HealthNow website at **http://healthnow.brookscole.com/itw** that will:

- Help you evaluate your knowledge of the material
- Allow you to take an exam-prep quiz
- Provide a Personalized Learning Plan targeting resources that address areas you should study
- Coach you through identifying target goals for behavior change and creating and monitoring your personal change plan throughout the semester.

INTERNET CONNECTIONS

HIV InSite: Gateway to AIDS Knowledge

http://hivinsite.ucsf.edu
This site, sponsored by the University of California, San Francisco (UCSF), School of Medicine, provides statistics, education, prevention, and new developments related to HIV/AIDS.

Go Ask Alice

www.goaskalice.columbia.edu/index.html
Sponsored by the health education and wellness program of the Columbia University Health Service, this site features educator's answers to questions on a wide variety of topics, including those related to relationships, marriage, and family. The site promotes family planning worldwide and provides referrals to local chapters.

Human Rights Campaign

www.hrc.org
The Human Rights Campaign is America's largest gay, lesbian, bisexual, and transgender civil rights organization. Its website features up-to-date information on issues related to gay rights and suggests courses of action to change government policies.

National Center for HIV, STD, and TB Prevention

www.cdc.gov/hiv/dhap.htm
This site, sponsored by the Centers for Disease Control and Prevention (CDC) features current information, fact sheets, conferences, media campaigns, publications, the 20-year history of HIV/AIDS, information on prevention and treatment, a FAQ section, as well as the most current HIV/AIDS statistics.

The Alan Guttmacher Institute

www.agi-usa.org
This site offers excellent resources on teen pregnancy rates and sexual health for teens and young adults along with a discussion on contraceptives versus abstinence.

 InfoTrac College Edition Activities Grosby, Richard et al. "Condom discomfort and associated problems with their use among university students," *Journal of American College Health,* Nov–Dec 2005 v54 i3 p143 (5)

1. In this study, what percentage of students reported discomfort when using a condom?

2. What can condom users do to avoid discomfort?

3. Is there an association between discomfort and condom breakage? What can be done to prevent this problem?

You can find additional readings related to personal health with InfoTrac College Edition, an online library of more than 900 journals and publications. Follow the instructions for accessing InfoTrac College Edition that were packaged with your textbook; then search for articles using a keyword search.

For additional links, resources, and suggested read-ings on the InfoTrac College Edition, visit our Health and Wellness Resource Center at **http://health.wadsworth.com.**

Key Terms

The terms listed are used on the page indicated. Definitions of the terms are in the Glossary at the end of the book.

abstinence 330	**celibacy** 330
acquired immune deficiency syndrome (AIDS) 343	**chancroid** 343
	chlamydia 338
	gonorrhea 339

CHAPTER

15

Protecting Your Safety and Your Environment

"This can't be happening to me!" This was the phrase that first ran through Parker's mind when the car swerved out of control. He kept repeating it to himself as he heard the sickening sound of metal hitting metal and felt a terrible crushing pain shoot up through his legs. Later at the hospital, when he woke up after surgery, it was his first thought. And all through the long months of rehabilitation, on the days when he thought life would never go back to normal, he'd try to tell himself that this too couldn't be happening to him.

Most young people think the same way. Accidents, injuries, assaults, crimes—all seem like things that happen only to other people, only in other places. The same is true for environmental issues, which may seem so enormous that nothing any individual can do will have an effect.

Recognizing the threat of intentional and unintentional injury and of environmental threats is the first step to ensuring your personal safety. You may think that the risk of something bad happening is simply a matter of chance, of being in the wrong place at the wrong time. That's not the case. Certain behaviors, such as using alcohol or drugs or not buckling your seat belt, greatly increase the risk of harm. Ultimately, you have more control over your safety than anyone or anything else in your life.

This chapter is a primer in self-protection that could help safeguard—perhaps even save—your life. It also explores the complex interrelationships between your world and your well-being, discusses major threats to the environment, and provides specific guidance on what you can do about them.

© Jason Hosking/zefa/Corbis

After studying the material in this chapter, you should be able to:

▌ List and explain factors that increase the likelihood of an accident.

▌ Describe how to be a safe driver and a safe cyclist.

▌ Define nonvolitional sex, sexual coercion, rape, and list five factors that contribute to date rape.

▌ Discuss the health effects of indoor and outdoor pollution.

▌ List some actions that individuals can take to protect our environment.

▌ Describe ways to protect your ears from noise-induced hearing loss.

Health💮Now™

Don't forget to check out the wealth of resources on the HealthNow website at **http://healthnow.brookscole.com/itw** that will:

• Help you evaluate your knowledge of the material
• Allow you to take an exam-prep quiz
• Provide a Personalized Learning Plan targeting resources that address areas you should study
• Coach you through identifying target goals for behavior change and creating and monitoring your personal change plan throughout the semester.

✚ The Dimensions of Wellness and Your Safety and Environment

You cannot separate your individual wellness from the security and health of the world in which you live. Here are some examples of the ways in which protecting yourself and your environment can enhance various dimensions of wellness:

- **Physical.** Preventing injuries, intentional or unintentional, protects your physical well-being. The quality of the air you breathe, the water you drink, the chemicals you use all have an impact on your physical wellness.
- **Emotional.** Watching out for yourself, for others, and for your world calls for a commitment that goes beyond words. Only in a safe setting can you explore and express your emotions fully. And working for a healthier environment demands a commitment that goes beyond words to emotions and actions.
- **Social.** You live in a "micro-environment" made up of family, friends, and acquaintances and a larger "macro-environment" that encompasses your campus, city, country, and the entire globe. Your own wellness depends on the well-being of these larger worlds.
- **Intellectual.** The challenges of living in an unsafe world and on a planet at risk in many ways demand—and sharpen—your highest intellectual skills. By developing your intellectual wellness, you gain skills and insights to find solutions to problems that may at first seem overwhelming.
- **Occupational.** Depending on which career you choose, you may confront safety and environmental issues on the job. You have to take responsibility for your personal safety, but you also have to work to ensure that your coworkers are safe.
- **Spiritual.** A sense of personal security enables us to focus on deeper issues. A belief in a higher value commits us to working toward the greater well-being of all people on Earth.
- **Environmental.** Creating a safe, healthy, supportive environment promotes wellness in its most global sense. Our fate is inevitably tied to the fate of our planet. The lifestyle choices we make, the products we use, the efforts we undertake to clean up a beach or save wetlands ultimately affect our own future.

✚ Personal Safety

The major threat to the lives of college students isn't illness but injury. Almost 75 percent of deaths among Americans 15 to 24 years old are caused by "unintentional injuries" (a term public health officials prefer), suicides, and homicides. The odds of dying from an injury in any given year are about 1 in 765; over a lifetime they rise to 1 in 23.[1] In all, injuries—intentional and unintentional—claim almost 150,000 lives a year. Accidents, especially motor vehicle crashes, kill more college-age men and women than all other causes combined; the greatest number of lives lost to accidents is among those 25 years of age.

Unintentional Injury

Some of the many factors that influence an individual's risk of accident or injury are these:

- **Age.** Injury is the leading cause of death in the United States during the first four decades of life. Most victims of fatal accidents are males, often in their teens and twenties. Feeling full of life and energy, they may take dangerous risks because they think they're invulnerable.
- **Alcohol.** An estimated 40 percent of Americans are involved in an alcohol-related accident sometime during their lives. Alcohol plays a role in about a quarter of fatal motor vehicle accidents and half of fatal motorcycle crashes.[2]
- **Stress.** When we're tense and anxious, we all pay less attention to what we're doing. One common result is an increase in accidents. If you find yourself having a series of small mishaps or near-misses, do something to lower your stress level, rather than wait for something more harmful to happen (see Chapter 7).
- **Situational factors.** Some situations—such as driving on a curvy, wet road in a car with worn tires—are so inherently dangerous that they greatly increase the odds of an accident. But even when there's greater risk, you can lower the danger: For instance, you can make sure your tires and brakes are in good condition.
- **Thrill seeking.** To some people, activities that others might find terrifying—such as skydiving or parachute jumping—are stimulating. These thrill seekers may have lower-than-normal levels of the brain chemicals that regulate excitement. Because the stress of potentially hazardous sports may increase the levels of these chemicals, they feel pleasantly aroused rather than scared.

Safety on the Road

With more drivers and more vehicles on the roads than ever before, the fatality rate per 100 million vehicle miles of travel has fallen to an all-time low of 1.51.[3] However, despite the progress that has been made, our streets and highways remain dangerous. Eight nations now have lower fatality rates than the United States.

An average of 120 people die in motor vehicle crashes every day in the United States. Alcohol use is a factor in about 50 of these crashes; speeding, in about 40. Rollovers caused by drivers who lose control of their vehicles kill about 25 people daily. Crashes involving teen drivers result in about 25 fatalities each day.[4]

Motor vehicle accidents in the United States annually claim about 42,800 lives and injure almost three million people, more than any other form of unintentional injury. They are the leading cause of all deaths for people ages 2 to 33; only cancer and heart attacks claim more American lives. Driving accidents have killed more Canadians in the last 50 years than both World Wars.[5]

Race, gender, and education affect a person's risk on the road. African-Americans, particularly men, are at increased risk of dying compared to whites. Hispanic men, but not Hispanic women, are at greater risk of dying than whites, but less so than blacks.[6] However, education has a strong influence. Whites without high school degrees have the highest death rates per 10 million road trips. People with no education beyond high school are less likely to use seat belts and more likely to drink and drive.

WELLNESS COACH

✚ Becoming a Safer Driver

Most road accidents don't just happen. A variety of factors—alcohol, speed, aggressive driving, age, and inexperience—increase the danger. Drunk driving is the number one cause of serious motor vehicle accidents. In recent years, there has been a decline in the number of fatalities caused by drunk driving, particularly among young people. The National Highway Traffic Safety Administration (NHTSA) attributes this decline to increases in the drinking age, to educational programs aimed at reducing nighttime driving by teens, to the formation of Students Against Destructive Decisions (SADD) and similar groups, and to changes in state laws that lowered the legal blood-alcohol concentration level for drivers under age 21 (some states have zero tolerance blood alcohol content (BAC) for drivers under 21).

Falling asleep at the wheel is second only to alcohol as a cause of serious motor-vehicle accidents. About half of drivers in the United States drive while drowsy. Nearly 14 million have fallen asleep at the wheel in the past year, according to the National Sleep Foundation. Men and young adults between the ages of 18 and 29 are at the highest risk for driving while drowsy or falling asleep at the wheel.

Speed literally kills, claiming more than 12,000 lives a year. Among male drivers 15 to 20 years old, 39 percent of those involved in fatal crashes were speeding.

College students aren't necessarily safer drivers than others their age. According to national data, full-time college students drink and drive more often than part-time students and other

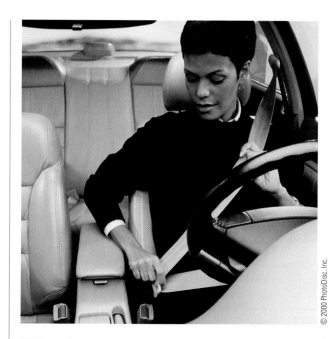

▌ Buckling up is one of the simplest and most effective ways of protecting yourself from injury.

young adults, but they also are more likely to wear seat belts while driving and riding in cars.[7] (See Student Snapshot: "Student Drivers.")

The vehicles drivers choose affect their safety. Equipment such as air bags, padded dashboards, safety glass windows, a steel frame, and side-impact bags help protect against fatal injuries. Size and make also matter—to those in your vehicle and in other vehicles. Per vehicle mile, motorcyclists are 26 times as likely as car passengers to die in a traffic crash.

How can you increase your odds of staying safe on the road? Three key factors are using your seat belt, making sure your vehicle has working air bags, and controlling road rage.

Buckle Up

Seat belt use has reached an all-time high, with three in four Americans buckling up. States with seat belt-laws have even higher rates of use: 80 percent. However, young people are less likely to use seat belts. By official estimates, two-thirds of 15- to 20-year-olds killed in motor vehicle accidents were not wearing seat belts.[8]

Seat belts save an estimated 9,500 lives in the United States each year. When lap-shoulder belts are used properly, they reduce the risk of fatal injury to front-seat passengers by 45 percent and the risk of moderate-to-critical injury by 50 percent. Because an unrestrained passenger can injure others during a crash, the risk of death is lowest when all occupants wear seat belts, according to federal analysts.[9] Seat belt use by everyone in a car may prevent about one in six deaths that might otherwise occur in a crash.[10]

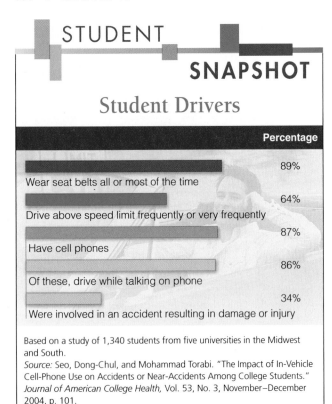

STUDENT SNAPSHOT

Student Drivers

	Percentage
Wear seat belts all or most of the time	89%
Drive above speed limit frequently or very frequently	64%
Have cell phones	87%
Of these, drive while talking on phone	86%
Were involved in an accident resulting in damage or injury	34%

Based on a study of 1,340 students from five universities in the Midwest and South.
Source: Seo, Dong-Chul, and Mohammad Torabi. "The Impact of In-Vehicle Cell-Phone Use on Accidents or Near-Accidents Among College Students." *Journal of American College Health,* Vol. 53, No. 3, November–December 2004, p. 101.

Check for Air Bags

An air bag, either with or without a seat belt, has proved the most effective means of preventing adult death, somewhat more so for women than for men. However, they do not lower the risk of serious injury. A study of 15 million people involved in crashes found that seat belts provided the most protection. Air bags used in conjunction with seat belts did not significantly reduce the risk of injury; without seat belts, they increased the risk of injury, particularly to the head and legs.[11]

Because there is controversy over the potential hazard they pose to children, the American Academy of Pediatrics recommends that children be placed in the backseat, whether or not the car is equipped with a passenger air bag.

Rein in Road Rage

The emotional outbursts known as road rage are a factor in as many as two-thirds of all fatal car crashes and one-third of nonfatal accidents, according to the NHTSA. Psychologist Arnold Nerenberg of Whittier, California, a specialist in motorway mayhem, estimates 1.78 billion episodes of road rage a year, resulting in more than 28,000 deaths and 1 million injuries.[12]

Some strategies for reducing road rage include the following:

- **Lower the stress in your life.** Take a few moments to breathe deeply and relax your shoulders before putting the key in the ignition.

- **Consciously decide not to let other drivers get to you.** Decide that whatever happens, it's not going to make your blood pressure go up.
- **Slow down.** If you're going five or ten miles over the speed limit, you won't have the time you need to react to anything that happens.
- **Modify bad driving habits one at a time.** If you tend to tailgate slow drivers, spend a week driving at twice your usual following distance. If you're a habitual horn honker, silence yourself.
- **Be courteous—even if other drivers aren't.** Don't dawdle in the passing lane. Never tailgate or switch lanes without signaling. Don't use your horn or high beams unless absolutely necessary.
- **Never retaliate.** Whatever another driver does, keep your cool. Count to ten. Take a deep breath. If you yell or gesture at someone who's upset with you, the conflict may well escalate.

STRATEGIES *for* PREVENTION

How to Drive Safely

- Don't drive while under the influence of alcohol or other drugs, including medications that may impair your reflexes, cause drowsiness, or affect your judgment. Never get into a car if you suspect the driver may be intoxicated or affected by a drug.

- Remain calm when dealing with drivers who are reckless or rude. Be alert and anticipate possible hazards. Don't let yourself be distracted by conversations, children's questions, arguments, food or drink, or scenic views.

- Don't get too comfortable. Alertness matters. Use the rearview mirror often. Don't let passengers or packages obstruct your view. Use turn signals when changing lanes or making a turn. If someone cuts you off, back off to a safe distance.

- Watch out for warning signs of fatigue, such as difficulty focusing, frequent blinking or heavy eyelids, trouble keeping one's head up; repeated yawning; trouble remembering the last few miles driven; and drifting from the lane or hitting the shoulder rumble strip.

- Drive more slowly if weather conditions are bad. Avoid driving at all during heavy rain, snow, or other conditions that affect visibility and road conditions. If you must drive in hazardous conditions, make sure that your car has the proper equipment, such as chains or snow tires, and that you know how to respond in case of a skid.

- Maintain your car properly, replacing windshield wipers, tires, and brakes when necessary. Keep flares and a fire extinguisher in your car for use in emergencies.

▌ **If you do something stupid, show that you're sorry.** On its website, the AAA Foundation for Traffic Safety solicited suggestions for automotive apologies. The most popular: slapping yourself on your forehead or the top of your head to indicate that you know you goofed. Such gestures can soothe a miffed motorist—and make the roads a slightly safer place for all of us.

Is It Safe to Talk on the Phone While Driving?

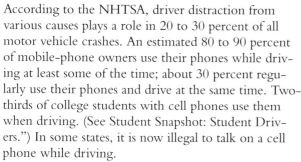

According to the NHTSA, driver distraction from various causes plays a role in 20 to 30 percent of all motor vehicle crashes. An estimated 80 to 90 percent of mobile-phone owners use their phones while driving at least some of the time; about 30 percent regularly use their phones and drive at the same time. Two-thirds of college students with cell phones use them when driving. (See Student Snapshot: Student Drivers.") In some states, it is now illegal to talk on a cell phone while driving.

Although many believe that hands-free car phones are less hazardous, researchers have shown this is not the case. Talking on a wireless phone while driving a car is just as dangerous with a hands-free or a handheld phone. The reason is that talking while driving distracts the brain as well as the eyes—much more so than talking to another person in the vehicle. Conversation on any type of phone disrupts a driver's attention to the visual environment, leading to what researchers call "inattention blindness," the inability to recognize objects encountered in the driver's visual field. This form of cog-nitive impairment may distract drivers for up to two minutes after the phone conversation has ended.[13]

On the other hand, mobile phones are helpful in alerting authorities to road hazards, congestion, or problem drivers and in summoning help in case of a breakdown or another emergency.

Here are some car phone safety tips you can follow:

▌ Find out if cell phone use while driving is legal in your state.
▌ Do not dial new calls until you're stopped or are in a safe, low-traffic environment.
▌ Keep calls short, less than 1 or 2 minutes.
▌ When you're on the phone, avoid difficult maneuvers, such as changing lanes, that require a lot of attention.
▌ Have a passenger send or receive calls.
▌ Invest in a hands-free model, especially if you use your phone regularly. While the cognitive distraction is the same, it helps to avoid the mechanical distraction.

Safe Cycling

Mile for mile, motorcycling is far more risky than automobile driving. The most common motorcycle injury

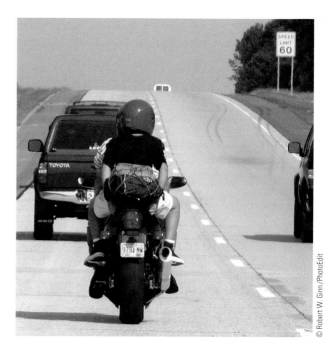

▌ In states with motorcycle helmet laws, motorcyclist deaths and injuries have decreased drastically.

is head trauma, which can lead to physical disability, including paralysis and general weakness, as well as problems reading and thinking. It can also cause personality changes and psychiatric problems, such as depression, anxiety, uncontrollable mood swings, and anger. Complete recovery from head trauma can take four to six years, and the costs can be staggering. Head injury can also result in permanent disability, coma, and death. To help prevent head trauma, motorcycle helmets are required in most states.

Approximately 80.6 million people ride bicycles. Each year, bicycle crashes kill about 900 of these individuals; about 200 of those killed are children under age 15. Men are more likely to suffer cycling injuries. Bicycle injuries are the most common cause of serious head injury in children, and most of these injuries are preventable.[14]

According to a national survey, 50 percent of all bicycle riders in the United States regularly wear bike helmets—43 percent every time they ride and 7 percent more than half the time. (See Savvy Consumer: "Buying a Bicycle Helmet.")

Intentional Injury

In the Americas, more than 300,000 people die each year as a result of violence, suicide, or accidental injury. Interpersonal violence is the third-leading cause of death among people 15 to 44 years old. Some studies show that a third of women age 16 to 49 have, at some point in their lives, been victims of sexual abuse.

Crime on Campus

Once considered havens from the meanness of America's streets, colleges and universities have seen a dramatic rise in crime in recent years. However, crime rates in these

SAVVY CONSUMER

BUYING A BICYCLE HELMET

What should you look for when buying a helmet? Here are some basic guidelines:

▪ A government regulation requires all helmets produced after 1999 meet the Consumer Product Safety Commission standard; look for a CPSC sticker inside the helmet. The ASTM (American Society for Testing and Materials) standard is comparable to CPSC. The Snell Memorial Foundation's B-90 standard is even better.

▪ **Check the fit.** The helmet should sit level on your head, touching all around, comfortably snug but not tight. The helmet should not move more than about an inch in any direction, regardless of how hard you tug at it.

▪ **Pick a bright color for visibility.** Avoid dark colors, thin straps, or a rigid visor that could snag in a fall.

▪ **Look for a smooth plastic outer shell,** not one with alternating strips of plastic and foam.

▪ **Watch out for excessive vents,** which put less protective foam in contact with your head in a crash.

▪ **Mirrors should have a breakaway mount;** the wire type mounted on eyeglasses can gouge an eye in a fall.

---

institutions are lower than in the general community. Property crimes, such as burglary and theft, account for most crimes on campus. However, the rates of murder and hate crimes have risen in recent years. According to the U.S. Department of Education, the criminal homicide rate on campus is 0.07 per 100,000 students—compared with a criminal homicide rate of 5.7 per 100,000 persons overall in the United States and of 14.1 per 100,000 for young people ages 17 to 29.

Colleges must compile annual security reports with statistics on violent crime, as well as drug and alcohol violations. The most recent crime statistics for the nation's 6,269 colleges, universities, and career schools are posted on the Internet at http://ope.ed.gov/security. Under the Jeanne Clery Disclosure of Campus Security Policy and Campus Statistics Act, all colleges and universities receiving federal funds must publish and make readily available the number of campus killings, assaults, sexual assaults, robberies, burglaries, and other crimes, and their security policies.

Because of concerns about safety on campus, more schools are taking tougher stands on student behavior. Many have established codes of conduct barring the use of alcohol and drugs, fighting, and sexual harassment. Many also have instituted policies requiring suspension or expulsion for students who violate this code.

Sexual Victimization and Violence on Campus

Sexual victimization refers to any situation in which a person is deprived of free choice and forced to comply with sexual acts. This is not only a woman's issue; in fact, men also are victimized. In recent years, researchers have come to view acts of sexual victimization along a continuum, ranging from street hassling, stalking, and obscene telephone calls to rape, battering, and incest.

A national survey found that the most common forms of sexual victimization on campus involved sexual or sexist remarks, catcalls, and whistles. One in five women reported obscene phone calls or being asked intrusive questions about her sex or romantic life. One in ten had false rumors spread about her sex life. About 6 percent confronted pornographic pictures, while 5 percent encountered a man exposing his sexual organs.[15]

Nonvolitional sex is sexual behavior that violates a person's right to choose when and with whom to have sex and what sexual behaviors to engage in. The more

▪ A peaceful scene like this doesn't mean there is no crime on a campus. Do you know the crime statistics for your college?

extreme forms of this behavior include sexual coercion or forced sex, rape, childhood sexual abuse, and violence against people with nonconventional sexual identities. Other forms, such as engaging in sex to keep one's partner or to pass as heterosexual, are so common that many think of them as normal.

Sexual coercion can take many forms, including exerting peer pressure, taking advantage of one's desire for popularity, threatening an end to a relationship, getting someone intoxicated, stimulating a partner against his or her wishes, or insinuating an obligation based on the time or money one has expended. Men may feel that they need to live up to the sexual stereotype of taking advantage of every opportunity for sex. Women are far more likely than men to encounter physical force.

Rape refers to sexual intercourse with an unconsenting partner under actual or threatened force. Sexual intercourse between a male over the age of 16 and a female under the age of consent (which ranges from 12 to 21 in different states) is called *statutory rape*. In *acquaintance rape,* or *date rape,* the victim knows the rapist. In *stranger rape,* the rapist is an unknown assailant. Both stranger and acquaintance rapes are serious crimes that can have a devastating impact on their victims.

Over the course of five years (the national average for a college career), including summers and vacations, one of every four or five female students is raped. In a single academic year, 2.7 percent of coeds are raped— 35 rapes for every 1,000 women.

In nine surveys of male university students, between 3 and 6 percent had been raped by other men; up to 25 percent had been sexually assaulted. Like female rape victims, male victims suffer long-term psychological problems and physical injuries and are at risk of contracting a sexually transmitted infection.[16]

Acquaintance or Date Rape

Both women and men report having been forced into sexual activity by someone they know. Many college students are in the age group most likely to face this threat: women aged 16 to 25 and men under 25. Women are most vulnerable and men are most likely to commit assaults during their senior year of high school and their first year of college.

Women who describe incidents of sexual coercion that meet the legal definition of rape often don't label it as such. They may have a preconceived notion that true rape consists of a blitzlike attack by a stranger. Or they may blame themselves for getting into a situation in which they couldn't escape. They may feel some genuine concern for others who would be devastated if they knew the truth (for example, if the rapist were the brother of a good friend or the son of a neighbor).

According to various studies, 25 to 60 percent of college men have engaged in some form of sexual coercion. Most often these men ignored a woman when she said no or protested. In addition, many college men reported engaging in sexual activity against their own wishes, most often because of male peer pressure or a desire to be popular.

Certain factors can set the stage for date rape: Socialization into an aggressive role, acceptance of rape myths, and a view that force is justified in certain situations increase the likelihood of a man's committing date rape. Other factors can also play a role, including the following:

- **Personality and early sexual experiences.** Certain factors may predispose individuals to sexual aggression, including first sexual experience at a very young age, earlier and more frequent than usual childhood sexual experiences (both forced and voluntary), hostility toward women, irresponsibility, lack of social consciousness, and a need for dominance over sexual partners.
- **Situational variables (what happens during the date).** Men who initiate a date, pay all expenses, and provide transportation are more likely to be sexually aggressive, perhaps because they feel they can call all the shots.
- **Rape-tolerant attitudes.** As several studies have confirmed, college men hold more rape-tolerant attitudes than do college women. For example, college men are significantly more likely than college women to agree with statements such as, "Some women ask to be raped and may enjoy it" and "If a woman says 'no' to having sex, she means 'maybe' or even 'yes.'"[17]

Some social groups, such as fraternities and athletic teams, may encourage the use of alcohol; reinforce stereo-

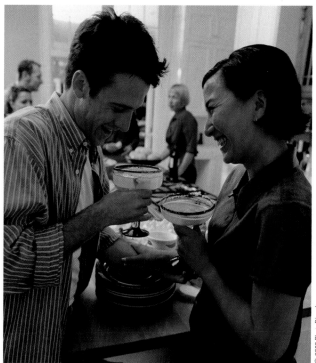

Acquaintance rape and alcohol use are very closely linked. Both men and women may find their judgment impaired or their communications unclear as a result of drinking.

types about masculinity; and emphasize violence, force, and competition. The group's shared values, including an acceptance of sexual coercion, may keep individuals from questioning their behavior.

▌ **Drinking.** Alcohol use is one of the strongest predictors of acquaintance rape. Men who've been drinking may not react to subtle signals, may misinterpret a woman's behavior as a come-on, and may feel more sexually aroused. At the same time, drinking may impair a woman's ability to effectively communicate her wishes and to cope with a man's aggressiveness.

▌ **Date rape drugs.** Drugs such as Rohypnol (flunitrazepam) and GHB (gamma hydroxybutrate) have been implicated in cases of acquaintance or date rape. Since both are odorless and tasteless, victims have no way of knowing whether their drink has been tampered with. The subsequent loss of memory leaves victims with no explanation for where they've been or what's happened.

Rohypnol—which can cause impaired motor skills and judgment, lack of inhibitions, dizziness, confusion, lethargy, very low blood pressure, coma, and death—has been outlawed in this country. Deaths also have been attributed to GHB overdoses.

▌ **Gender differences in interpreting sexual cues.** In research comparing college men and women, the men typically overestimated the woman's sexual availability and interest, seeing friendliness, revealing clothing, and attractiveness as deliberately seductive. In one study of date rape, the men reported feeling "led on," in part because their female partners seemed to be dressed more suggestively than usual.

How Can I Prevent Date Rape?

For men:

▌ **Remember that it's okay not to "score" on a date.**

▌ **Don't assume that a sexy dress or casual flirting is an invitation to sex.**

▌ **Be aware of your partner's actions.** If she pulls away or tries to get up, understand that she's sending you a message—one you should acknowledge and respect.

▌ **Restrict drinking, drug use, or other behaviors** (such as hanging out with a group known to be sexually aggressive in certain situations) that could affect your judgment and ability to act responsibly.

▌ **Think of the way you'd want your sister or a close woman friend to be treated** by her date. Behave in the same manner.

For women:

▌ **If the man pays for all expenses, he may think he's justified in using force** to get "what he paid for." If you cover some of the costs, he may be less aggressive.

▌ **Back away from a man who pressures you** into other activities you don't want to engage in on a date, such as chugging beer or drag racing with his friends.

▌ **Avoid misleading messages and avoid behavior that may be interpreted as sexual teasing.** Don't tell him to stop touching you, talk for a few minutes, and then resume petting.

▌ **Despite your clearly stated intentions, if your date behaves in a sexually coercive manner,** use a strategy of escalating forcefulness—direct refusal, vehement verbal refusal, and, if necessary, physical force.

▌ **Avoid using alcohol or other drugs when you definitely do not wish to be sexually intimate with your date.**

What to Do in Case of Rape

Women who are raped should call a friend or a rape crisis center. A rape victim should not bathe or change her clothes before calling. Semen, hair, and material under her fingernails or on her apparel all may be useful in identifying the man who raped her.

A rape victim who chooses to go to a doctor or hospital should remember that she may not necessarily have to talk to police. However, a doctor can collect the necessary evidence, which will then be available if she later decides to report the rape to police. All rape victims should talk with a doctor or health-care worker about testing and treatment for sexually transmitted infections and postintercourse conception.

Even an unsuccessful rape attempt should be reported because the information a woman may provide about the attack—the assaulter's physical characteristics, voice, clothes, car, even an unusual smell—may prevent another woman from being raped.

✚ The Environment and Your Health

The planet Earth—once taken for granted as a ball of rock and water that existed for our use for all time—now is seen as a single, fragile **ecosystem** (a community of organisms that share a physical and chemical environment). Our environment is a closed ecosystem, powered by the sun. The materials needed for the survival of this planet must be recycled over and over again. Increasingly, we're realizing just how important the health of this ecosystem is to our own well-being and survival.

Our environment affects our well-being both directly and indirectly. Changes in temperature and rainfall patterns disturb ecological processes in ways that can be hazardous to health. The environment may account for 25 to 40 percent of diseases worldwide. Children are the most vulnerable because of their greater sensitivity to toxic threats. In response to this trend, Congress has approved funding to create a nationwide system to track environmental links to chronic diseases.

No individual is immune to environmental health threats. Depletion of the ozone layer has already been implicated in the increase in skin cancers and cataracts. Global warming, according to some theorists, might lead to changes in one-third to one-half of the world's vegetation types and to the extinction of many plant and animal species. A warmer world is expected to produce more severe flooding in some places and more severe droughts in others, jeopardizing natural resources and the safety of our water supply. Warmer weather—a consequence of changes in atmospheric gases and climate—worsens urban industrial air pollution and, if the air also is moist, increases concentrations of allergenic pollens and fungal spores. These are truly problems without borders.

▙ Pollution

Any change in the air, water, or soil that could reduce its ability to support life is a form of **pollution.** Natural events, such as smoke from fires triggered by lightning, can cause pollution. The effects of pollution depend on the concentration (amount per unit of air, water, or soil) of the **pollutant,** how long it remains in the environment, and its chemical nature. An *acute effect* is a severe immediate reaction, usually after a single, large exposure. For example, pesticide poisoning can cause nausea and dizziness, even death. A *chronic effect* may take years to develop or may be a recurrent or continuous reaction, usually after repeated exposures. The development of cancer after repeated exposure to a pollutant such as asbestos is an example of a chronic effect.

Environmental agents that trigger changes, or **mutations,** in the genetic material (the DNA) of living cells are called **mutagens.** The changes that result can lead to the development of cancer. A substance or agent that causes cancer is a *carcinogen:* All carcinogens are mutagens; most mutagens are carcinogens. Furthermore, when a mutagen affects an egg or a sperm cell, its effects can be passed on to future generations. Mutagens that can cross the placenta of a pregnant woman and cause a spontaneous abortion or birth defects in the fetus are called **teratogens.**

Pollution is a hazard to all who breathe. Deaths caused by air pollution exceed those from motor vehicle injuries. Those with respiratory illnesses are at greatest risk during days when smog or allergen counts are high. However, even healthy joggers are affected; carbon monoxide has been shown to impair their exercise performance. The effects of carbon monoxide are much worse in smokers, who already have higher levels of the gas in their blood.

Toxic substances in polluted air can enter the human body in three ways: through the skin, through the digestive system, and through the lungs. The combined interaction of two or more hazards can produce an effect greater than that of either one alone. Pollutants can affect an organ or organ system directly or indirectly.

Among the health problems that have been linked with pollution are the following:

▮ Headaches and dizziness.
▮ Eye irritation and impaired vision.
▮ Nasal discharge.

▮ Cough, shortness of breath, and sore throat.
▮ Constricted airways.
▮ Constriction of blood vessels and increased risk of heart disease.
▮ Chest pains and aggravation of the symptoms of colds, pneumonia, bronchial asthma, emphysema, chronic bronchitis, lung cancer, and other respiratory problems.
▮ Birth defects and reproductive problems.
▮ Nausea, vomiting, and stomach cancer.
▮ Allergy and asthma from diesel fumes in polluted air.

Smog

A combination of smoke and fog, **smog** is made up of chemical vapors from auto exhaust, industrial and commercial pollutants (volatile organic compounds, carbon monoxide, nitrogen oxides, sulfur oxides, particulates), and ozone. The most obvious sources of these pollutants are motor vehicles, industrial factories, electric utility plants, and wood-burning stoves.

Gray-air, or *sulfur-dioxide,* smog, often seen in Europe and much of the eastern United States, is produced by burning oil of high sulfur content. Among the cities that must deal with gray-air smog are Chicago, Baltimore, Detroit, and Philadelphia. Like cigarette smoke, gray-air smog affects the cilia in the respiratory passages; the lungs are unable to expel particulates, such as soot, ash, and dust, which remain and irritate the tissues. This condition is hazardous to people with chronic respiratory problems.

Brown-air, or *photochemical* smog, is found in large traffic centers such as Los Angeles, Salt Lake City, Denver, Mexico City, and Tokyo. This type of smog results

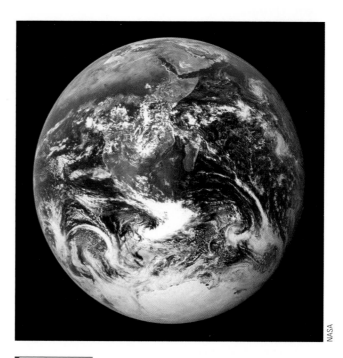

NASA

▮ As a citizen of Earth, remember that you are responsible for safeguarding the future of the planet.

principally from nitric oxide in car exhaust reacting with oxygen in the air, forming nitrogen dioxide, which produces a brownish haze and, when exposed to sunlight, other pollutants.

One of these, *ozone,* the most widespread pollutant, can impair the body's immune system and cause long-term lung damage. (Ozone in the upper atmosphere protects us by repelling harmful ultraviolet radiation from the sun, but ozone in the lower atmosphere is a harmful component of air pollution.) Automobiles also produce carbon monoxide, a colorless and odorless gas that diminishes the ability of red blood cells to carry oxygen. The resulting oxygen deficiency can affect breathing, hearing, and vision in humans and stunt the growth of plants and trees.[18]

Indoor Pollutants

Because people in industrialized nations spend more than 90 percent of their time in buildings, the quality of the air they breathe inside can have an even greater impact on their well-being than outdoor pollution.

Indoor pollution accounts for 2.2 million deaths and costs the world between $150 billion and $750 billion per year—0.5 to 2.5 percent of the world's gross national product—mainly in lost production through sickness and death.[19]

The most hazardous form of indoor air pollution is cigarette smoke. Passive smoking—inhaling others' cigarette smoke—may rank just behind active smoking and alcohol use as the third-leading preventable cause of death. Each year secondhand cigarette smoke kills 53,000 nonsmokers.

Toxic Threats

Unlike outdoor contaminants from exhaust pipes or smokestacks, indoor pollutants come from the very materials the buildings are made of and from the appliances

STRATEGIES for CHANGE

Doing Your Part for Cleaner Air

❙ Drive a car that gets high gas mileage and produces low emissions. Keep your speed at or below the speed limit.

❙ Keep your tires inflated and your engine tuned. Recycle old batteries and tires. (Most stores that sell new ones will take back old ones.)

❙ Turn off your engine if you're going to be stopped for more than a minute.

❙ Collect all fluids that you drain from your car (motor oil, antifreeze) and recycle or properly dispose of them.

inside them. For instance, formaldehyde, commonly used in building materials, carpet backing, furniture, foam insulation, plywood, and particle board, can cause nausea, dizziness, headaches, heart palpitations, stinging eyes, and burning lungs. Formaldehyde gas, which is colorless and odorless, has been shown to cause cancer in animals.

Asbestos, a mineral widely used for building insulation, has been linked to lung and gastrointestinal cancer among asbestos workers and their families, although it may take 20 to 30 years for such cancers to develop. Fibers from asbestos home insulation or fireproofing that become airborne can cause progressive and deadly lung diseases, including cancer. More than 200,000 lawsuits have been filed for asbestos-related injuries, and as many as 300,000 American workers may have died from asbestos-linked diseases, including lung cancer. The danger may be greatest for those who smoke and are also exposed to asbestos.

A danger both inside and outside our homes is lead, which lurks in some 57 million American homes, most built before 1960, with walls, windows, doors, and banisters coated with more than 3 million metric tons of lead-based paint. The percentage of children aged one to five with elevated levels of lead in their blood has dropped to 2.2 percent, half of what it was in the early 1990s.[20]

Adults exposed to low levels of lead (which once were thought to be safe) may develop headaches, high blood pressure, irritability, tremors, and insomnia. Health effects increase with exposure to higher levels and include anemia, stomach pain, vomiting, diarrhea, and constipation. Long-term exposure can impair fertility and damage the kidneys. Workers exposed to lead may become sterile or suffer irreversible kidney disease, damage to their central nervous system, stillbirths, or miscarriages.

Carbon monoxide (CO) gas, which is tasteless, odorless, colorless, and nonirritating, can be deadly. Produced by the incomplete combustion of fuel in space heaters, furnaces, water heaters, and engines, CO reduces the delivery of oxygen in the blood. Every year an estimated 10,000 Americans seek treatment for CO inhalation; at least 250 die because of this silent killer. Those most at risk are the chronically ill, the elderly, pregnant women, and infants. Typical symptoms of CO poisoning, which is most common in winter, are headache, nausea, vomiting, fatigue, and dizziness. More severe poisoning can damage the heart and cause respiratory distress, confusion, and coma. A blood test can measure CO levels; inhaling pure oxygen speeds re-moval of the gas from the body. Most people who don't lose consciousness as a result of CO poisoning recover completely.

Radioactive radon—which diffuses from rock, brick, concrete building materials, and natural soil deposits under some homes—produces charged decay products that cling to dust particles. Once trapped inside a building, radon can reach levels that may increase the risk of lung cancer. The EPA estimates that the inhalation of indoor radon is responsible for approximately 14,000 lung cancer deaths per year. Radon levels tend to be highest in areas with granite and black shale topped with porous soil.

An estimated 10 million homes and over 30 million people are at risk from high levels of radon.[21] If you live in a high-radon area, don't panic. Your hypothetical risk of dying from radon-caused lung cancer is about equal to the known risk of dying in a home fire or fall.

Is Mold Dangerous?

One of the oldest and most widespread substances on earth, mold—a type of fungus that decomposes organic matter and provides plants with nutrients—has emerged as a major health concern. Common molds include *Aspergillus, Penicillium,* and *Stachybotrys,* a slimy, dark green mold that has been blamed for infant deaths and various illnesses, from Alzheimer's disease to cancer, in adults that breathe in its spores. Faulty ventilation systems and airtight buildings have been implicated as contributing to the increased mold problem.[22]

Experts agree that mold may trigger or worsen a number of health problems, including allergic reactions, dizziness, breathing problems, nausea, and asthma attacks. Individuals with preexisting health conditions or suppressed immunity are at greater risk. In the last decade, high-profile lawsuits have resulted in multimillion dollar judgments, despite minimal scientific evidence linking mold exposure and cancer or brain damage.[23]

Mold problems can range from small patches to large infestations of entire rooms or even a whole building. The first step to reduce mold exposure is moisture control, which may require new methods of keeping rainwater and ground water away from the interior and maintaining the heating ventilation and air conditioning systems appropriately. Bleach or soap and water can clean up small infestations. Larger ones may require appropriate protective respiratory equipment or professionally trained, licensed, and experienced contractors.

What Health Risks Are Caused by Pesticides?

High quantities of toxic chemical waste from unused or obsolete pesticides are posing a continuing and worsening threat to people and the environment in eastern Europe, Africa, Asia, the Middle East, and Latin America.[24] In the United States, the FDA estimates that 33 to 39 percent of our food supply contains residues of pesticides that may pose a long-term danger to our health. Scientists have detected traces of pesticides in groundwater in both urban and rural areas.

Exposure to pesticides may, however, pose a risk to pregnant women and their unborn children. Men whose jobs routinely expose them to pesticides may be at increased risk of prostate cancer. Parental exposure does not increase the likelihood of childhood brain cancer.[25]

Chlorinated hydrocarbons include several high-risk substances—such as DDT, kepone, and chlordane —that have been restricted or banned because they may cause cancer, birth defects, neurological disorders, and damage to wildlife and the environment. They are extremely resistant to breakdown.

Organic phosphates, including chemicals such as malathion, break down more rapidly than the chlorinated hydrocarbons. Most are highly toxic, causing cramps, confusion, diarrhea, vomiting, headaches, and breathing difficulties. Higher levels in the blood can lead to convulsions, paralysis, coma, and death.

Farmworkers and those in the communities surrounding agricultural land are at greatest risk for pesticide exposure. However, even city dwellers aren't out of range. About half (52 percent) of the nation uses insect repellents, including some made with potent insecticides.

"Going Green"

Simple steps can help save energy, lower carbon dioxide (CO_2) emissions, and cut down on energy costs. Here are some recommendations from the Environmental Defense and World Wildlife Fund:

- Wash laundry in warm or cold water, not hot. *Average annual CO_2 reduction: up to 500 pounds for two loads of laundry a week.*
- Buy products sold in the simplest possible packaging. Carry a tote bag or recycle shopping bags. *Average annual CO_2 reduction: 1,000 pounds because garbage is reduced 25 percent.*
- Switch from standard light bulbs to energy-efficient fluorescent ones. *Average annual CO_2 reduction: about 500 pounds per bulb.*

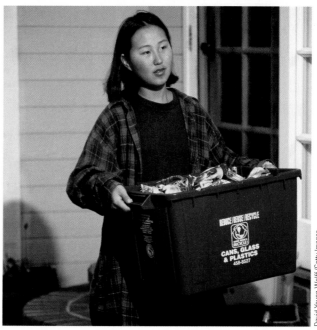

Recycling helps save energy and conserve resources.

▮ Set room thermostats lower in winter and higher in summer. *Average annual CO_2 reduction: about 500 pounds for each two-degree reduction.*

▮ Run dishwashers only when full, and choose the energy-saving mode rather than the regular setting. *Average annual CO_2 reduction: 200 pounds.*

▮ Bike, carpool, or take mass transit whenever possible. *Average annual CO_2 reduction: 20 pounds for each gallon of gasoline saved.*

✚ Your Hearing Health

Hearing loss is the third most common chronic health problem, after high blood pressure and arthritis, among older Americans. Approximately 25 to 40 percent of adults older than age 65 have some degree of hearing loss, as do 40 to 66 percent of people age 75 and older. Loud noises cause hearing loss in an estimated 10 million Americans every year. Only about one-fifth of the 28 million Americans suffering from hearing loss have sought professional help.[26]

How Loud Is That Noise?

Loudness, or the intensity of a sound, is measured in **decibels (dB).** A whisper is 20 decibels; a conversation in a living room is about 50 decibels. On this scale, 50 isn't two and a half times louder than 20, but 1,000 times louder: Each 10-dB rise in the scale represents a tenfold increase in the intensity of the sound. Very loud but short bursts of sounds (such as gunshots and fireworks)

STRATEGIES for **CHANGE**

Protecting Your Ears

▮ If you must live or work in a noisy area, wear hearing protectors to prevent exposure to blasts of very loud noise. Don't think cotton or facial tissue stuck in your ears can protect you; foam or soft plastic earplugs are more effective. Wear them when operating lawn mowers, weed trimmers, or power tools.

▮ Soundproof your home by using draperies, carpets, and bulky furniture. Put rubber mats under washing machines, blenders, and other noisy appliances. Seal cracks around windows and doors.

▮ When you hear a sudden loud noise, press your fingers against your ears. Limit your exposure to loud noise. Several brief periods of noise appear to be less damaging than one long exposure.

▮ Be careful if you wear Walkman-type headphones. The volume is too high if you can feel the vibrations.

▮ Beware of large doses of aspirin. Researchers have found that eight aspirin tablets a day can aggravate the damage caused by loud noise; twelve a day can cause ringing in the ears (tinnitus).

▮ Don't drink in noisy environments. Alcohol intensifies the impact of noise and increases the risk of life-long hearing damage.

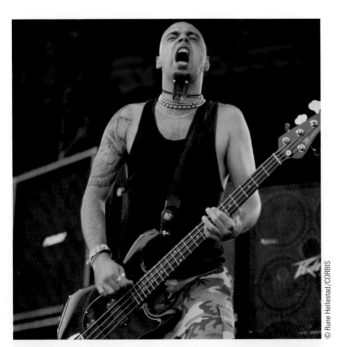

▮ Besides listening to the music at your next concert, tune in to the noise level and how your ears are feeling.

© Rune Hellestad/CORBIS

and quieter but longer-lasting sounds (such as power tools) can induce hearing loss.

Sounds under 75 dB don't seem harmful. However, prolonged exposure to any sound over 85 dB (the equivalent of a power mower or food blender) or brief exposure to louder sounds can harm hearing. The noise level at rock concerts can reach 110 to 140 dB, about as loud as an air raid siren. Personal sound systems (boom boxes) can blast sounds of up to 115 dB. Cars with extremely loud music systems, known as boom cars, can produce an earsplitting 145 dB—louder than a jet engine or thunderclap (**Figure 15-1**).

Effects of Noise

Noise-induced hearing loss is 100 percent preventable—and irreversible. Hearing aids are the only treatment, but they do not correct the problem; they just amplify sound to compensate for hearing loss.

The healthy human ear can hear sounds within a wide range of frequencies (measured in hertz), from the low-frequency rumble of thunder at 50 hertz to the high-frequency overtones of a piccolo at nearly 20,000 hertz.

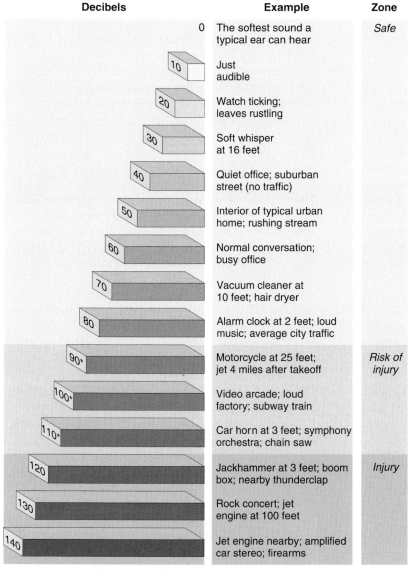

Decibels	Example	Zone
0	The softest sound a typical ear can hear	Safe
10	Just audible	
20	Watch ticking; leaves rustling	
30	Soft whisper at 16 feet	
40	Quiet office; suburban street (no traffic)	
50	Interior of typical urban home; rushing stream	
60	Normal conversation; busy office	
70	Vacuum cleaner at 10 feet; hair dryer	
80	Alarm clock at 2 feet; loud music; average city traffic	
90*	Motorcycle at 25 feet; jet 4 miles after takeoff	Risk of injury
100*	Video arcade; loud factory; subway train	
110*	Car horn at 3 feet; symphony orchestra; chain saw	
120	Jackhammer at 3 feet; boom box; nearby thunderclap	Injury
130	Rock concert; jet engine at 100 feet	
140	Jet engine nearby; amplified car stereo; firearms	

*Note: The maximum exposure allowed on the job by federal law, in hours per day: 90 decibels, 8 hours; 100 decibels, 2 hours; 110 decibels, ¹/₂ hour.

FIGURE 15-1 ▮ Loud and Louder

The human ear perceives a 10-decibel increase as a doubling of loudness. Thus, the 100 decibels of a subway train sound much more than twice as loud as the 50 decibels of a rushing stream.

High-frequency noise damages the delicate hair cells that serve as sound receptors in the inner ear. Damage first begins as a diminished sensitivity to frequencies around 4,000 hertz, the highest notes of a piano.

Early symptoms of hearing loss include difficulty understanding speech and *tinnitus* (ringing in the ears). Brief, very loud sounds, such as an explosion or gunfire, can produce immediate, severe, and permanent hearing loss. Longer exposure to less intense but still hazardous sounds, such as those common at work or in public places, can gradually impair hearing, often without the individual's awareness.

Conductive hearing loss, often caused by ear infections, cuts down on perception of low-pitched sounds.

Sensorineural loss involves damage or destruction of the sensory cells in the inner ear that convert sound waves to nerve signals.

✚ The Quality of Your Drinking Water

Worldwide 2.2 million people die annually as a result of contaminated water and poor sanitation.[27] Fears about the public water supply have led many Americans to turn off their taps. About two-thirds take steps to drink purer water, either by using filtration and distillation methods or by drinking bottled water. However, Consumer Union, a nonprofit advocacy group, maintains that the United States has the safest water supply in the world. The Environmental Protection Agency has set standards for some 80 contaminants. These include many toxic chemicals and heavy metals—including lead, mercury, cadmium, and chromium—that can cause kidney and nervous system damage and birth defects.

Each year the CDC reports an average of 7,400 cases of illness related to the water people drink. The most common culprits include parasites, bacteria, viruses, chemicals, and lead. Health officials suggest having your water tested if you live near a hazardous waste dump or industrial park, if the pipes in your house are made of lead or joined together with lead solder, if your water comes from a well, or if you purchase water from a private company. Check to see if your state health department or local water supplier will provide free testing. If not, use a state-certified laboratory that tests water in accordance with EPA standards.

Is Bottled Water Better?

Is bottled water better? That's what consumers have often assumed. Bottled water sales have tripled in the past ten years. Women and college-age Americans make up the majority of bottled-water drinkers. Yet in the past, the Food and Drug Administration (FDA) simply defined bottled water as "sealed in bottles or other containers and intended for human consumption." Bottled water wasn't required to be "pure" or even to be tested for toxic chemicals. One survey found chemical contaminants associated with cancer in 22 of 100 brands tested.

The FDA has called for federal monitoring of the purity of bottled water. Some states, including California and New York, have their own bottled-water safety standards to ensure that bottled water is at least as safe as drinking water.

Chemicals in Water

About half (53 percent) of Americans drink water containing fluoride, an additive to water and toothpaste that helps teeth resist decay. According to the American Dental Association, the incidence of tooth decay is 50 to 70 percent lower in areas with fluoridated water. However, laboratory rats given fluoridated water have shown a high rate of bone cancer. The more fluoride they drank in their water, the more likely they were to develop this cancer. But this type of cancer is extremely rare in humans, and the estimated lifetime risk to any individual from drinking fluoridated water is less than one in 5,000.

Federal health officials have found no evidence that fluoride causes cancer in humans and have concluded that its benefits far outweigh any risks. However, excessive fluoride can increase bone loss and fractures in pre- and post-menopausal women. Health professionals advise consumers to use only small amounts of fluoridated toothpaste, rinse thoroughly after brushing, and use fluoride supplements only when the home water supply is known to be deficient.

✚ Invisible Threats

Among the unseen threats to health are various forms of *radiation,* energy radiated in the form of waves or particles. Any electrically charged conductor generates two kinds of invisible fields: electric and magnetic. Together they're called **electromagnetic fields (EMFs).** For years, these fields, produced by household appliances, home wiring, lighting fixtures, electric blankets, and overhead power lines, were considered harmless. However, epidemiological studies have revealed a link between exposure to high-voltage lines and cancer (especially leukemia, a blood cancer) in electrical workers and children.

Laboratory studies on animals have shown that alternating current, which changes strength and direction 60 times a second (and electrifies most of North America), emits EMFs that may interfere with the normal functioning of human cell membranes, which have their own electromagnetic fields. The result may be mood disorders, changes in circadian rhythms (our inner sense of time), miscarriage, developmental problems, or cancer. Researchers have documented increases in breast cancer deaths in women who worked as electrical engineers, electricians, or in other high-exposure jobs, and a link between EMF exposure and an increased risk of leukemia and possibly brain cancer.

After six years of congressionally mandated research, the National Institute of Environmental Health Sciences concluded that the evidence of a risk of cancer and other human disease from the electric and magnetic fields around power lines is "weak." This finding applies to the extremely-low-frequency electric and magnetic fields surrounding both the big power lines that distribute power and the smaller but closer electric lines in homes and appliances. However, the researchers also noted that EMF exposure "cannot be recognized as entirely safe."

Are Cell Phones Safe to Use?

Since cellular phone service was introduced in the United States in 1984, mobile and handheld phones have become ubiquitous. More than 86 million people use cell phones, and concern has grown about their possible health risks. The federal government sets upper exposure limits to electromagnetic energy from cell phones known as the specific absorption rate, or SAR. A phone emits the most radiation during a call, but it also emits small amounts periodically whenever it's turned on.

Can exposure to low levels of electromagnetic energy that the body absorbs from a cell phone be harmful? More than 70 research papers on the potentially harmful effects of cell phone use have raised concerns about cancer, neurological disorders, sleep problems, or headaches; others have shown no association or were inconclusive. The Food and Drug Administration (FDA) and Federal Communications Commission (FCC) have stated that "the available scientific evidence does not

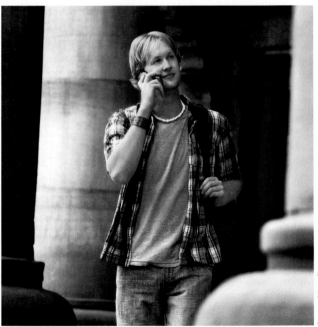

Cell phones do emit electromagnetic energy, and research has yet to prove whether they are completely safe or pose a possible risk.

show that any health problems are associated with using wireless phones. There is no proof, however, that wireless phones are absolutely safe." Additional studies are underway.

Swedish and Finnish researchers have found no "consistent evidence" of increased risk of cancer from use for up to five years, but they did document protein changes in human cells exposed to cell phone radiation and an increased rate of benign brain tumors. Health experts in Britain, France, and Germany have discouraged children from using cell phones largely because of concerns that their developing nervous systems may be especially vulnerable.

A headset can keep the phone's antenna away from your head and body. Shields that claim to reduce exposure generally don't work as advertised, say the FDA and FCC.[28]

▌ MAKING HEALTHY CHOICES

To Safeguard Yourself and Your World

Just as many diseases of the previous century have been eradicated, so in time we may be able to remove or reduce many environmental threats. Your future—and our planet's future—may depend on it.

▌ **Plant a tree.** Even a single tree helps absorb carbon dioxide and produces cooling that can reduce the need for air-conditioning.

▌ **Look for simply packaged items.** Whenever possible, choose items packed in recycled materials or something recyclable.

▌ **Bring your own bag.** Whenever possible, avoid using plastic or paper bags for items you could carry in a cloth or string carryall.

▌ **Hit the switch.** Turn off all electrical appliances (TVs, CD players, radios, lights) when you're not in the room or paying attention to them.

▌ **Avoid disposables.** Use a mug instead of a paper or Styrofoam cup, a sponge instead of a paper towel, a cloth napkin instead of a paper one.

▌ **Be water wise.** Turn off the tap while you shave or brush your teeth. Install water-efficient faucets and showerheads. Wash clothes in cold water.

▌ **Cancel junk mail.** It consumes 100 million trees a year. To get off mailing lists, write: Direct Mail Association, Mail Preference Service, P.O. Box 9008, Farmingdale, NY 11735-9008.

▌ **Don't buy products made of endangered substances.** Examples include coral, ivory, tortoise shell, or wood from endangered forests (teak, mahogany, ebony, rosewood).

▌ **Speak out.** E-mail your senators and congressional representatives, who vote on pollution controls, budgets for the enforcement of safety regulations, and the preservation of forests and wildlife. Identify the particular bill or issue you're addressing. Be as specific, brief, and to the point as possible. Go to www.senate.gov and click on "Senators" to find the e-mail addresses. To find your congressional representative, go to www.house.gov and click on "Write Your Representative."

SELF-SURVEY 1

How Safe Is Your Campus, Dorm Room, or Home?

Place a ✔ in the column that corresponds to your answer to each statement. At the end of the survey make some notes about how you can improve your safety at school and at home.

Dormitory Security

Yes	No	Students:
_____	_____	card swipe (like hotels)
_____	_____	patented keys
_____	_____	standard keys
_____	_____	propped doors
_____	_____	doors locked at night
_____	_____	doors never locked
_____	_____	doors always locked
_____	_____	guards on duty (24 hours)
_____	_____	police patrols nightly
_____	_____	security patrols nightly
_____	_____	parking lots patrolled

Yes	No	Visitors:
_____	_____	intercom at entrance
_____	_____	show ID
_____	_____	sign-in guests

Dorm Features:

Yes	No	
_____	_____	single sex dorms
_____	_____	freshman dorms
_____	_____	coed dorms
_____	_____	senior dorms
_____	_____	alcohol prohibited
_____	_____	drugs prohibited
_____	_____	substance-free
_____	_____	propped door alarms
_____	_____	panic alarms in rooms
_____	_____	fire sprinklers
_____	_____	peep hole in room door
_____	_____	dead bolt in door
_____	_____	safety chain on room door
_____	_____	toilet in room
_____	_____	shower in room
_____	_____	bathrooms down the hallway
_____	_____	single sex bathrooms
_____	_____	female hall bathrooms locked
_____	_____	single sex floors locked
_____	_____	secure windows (1st and 2nd floor)

Campus Security

Campus Security Force:

Yes	No	
_____	_____	sworn police force
_____	_____	arrest power
_____	_____	patrolling day
_____	_____	patrolling night
_____	_____	carry firearms
_____	_____	security guards
_____	_____	bicycle patrols
_____	_____	surveillance cameras
_____	_____	emergency phones
_____	_____	student amateurs
_____	_____	escort services
_____	_____	shuttle services

Health Services:

_____	_____	rape crisis center
_____	_____	alcohol/drug counselors
_____	_____	AA meetings on campus

Campus Judicial System:

_____	_____	open campus judicial hearings
_____	_____	reveal campus sex offender names

Parental Involvement

Yes	No	**Parental Notification:**
_____	_____	for underage drinkers
_____	_____	for alcohol poisoning
_____	_____	for illegal drug use
_____	_____	for acts of violence
_____	_____	for public drunkenness
_____	_____	for housing firearms
_____	_____	for sexual assault
_____	_____	for hate crimes or speech
_____	_____	for academic probation
_____	_____	for disciplinary probation
_____	_____	for residence hall violations
_____	_____	for DUI convictions

Roommates Quickly Transferred by Dean for:

_____	_____	using illegal drugs
_____	_____	underage drinking
_____	_____	noisy parties
_____	_____	hate crimes or speech
_____	_____	physical abuse

Obtain campus crime statistics for the last 3 years from the campus security office for:

Aggravated assault _____   Arson _____
Motor vehicle crimes _____   Murder _____
Forcible sex offenses _____   Burglary _____
Nonforcible sex offenses _____   Robbery _____
Hate crimes _____
Vandalism _____

Total criminal offenses _____

For Students Living Off-campus

Yes	No	Home:
_____	_____	working smoke alarms
_____	_____	working fire extinguisher
_____	_____	emergency fire escape plan
_____	_____	posted emergency phone numbers
_____	_____	all windows have locks
_____	_____	exterior doors have deadbolts
_____	_____	peep hole in front door
_____	_____	shrubs trimmed near windows
_____	_____	firearms stored unloaded, locked up
_____	_____	interior stairwells/hallways well lit
_____	_____	non-slip treads on stairs
_____	_____	carpets firmly secured to floors
_____	_____	exterior lighting at entry doors
_____	_____	exterior lighting on walkways
_____	_____	monitored home security system
_____	_____	all appliances in good working order
_____	_____	never open the door to a stranger
_____	_____	member of neighborhood watch

Vehicle Maintenance Tips:

Keeping the correct tire pressure, checking brake pads and tire tread wear, getting regular oil and filter changes and monitoring coolant and other fluid levels will help keep your car in good working condition, running smoothly and decrease the chance of a breakdown.

More Safety Tips:

- Always park in well-lit areas, especially at overnight parking lots.
- Don't keep valuables in plain sight in your car. Lock them in the trunk *before* you arrive at your destination and make sure nobody sees you doing this.
- Stay alert when approached by strangers while waiting for a bus or a train.
- Don't share a taxi ride with a stranger.
- Don't pick up hitchhikers.
- Limit driving time when eating, searching the radio stations or talking on a cell phone. Concentrate on the road and other cars.

Source: Security on Campus, Inc., www.securityoncampus.org. Security on Campus assists victims of campus crime.

ACTION PLAN 1

Your Action Plan for Personal Safety on Campus

Fundamentals

- Freshmen should "respectfully decline" to have photo and personal information published for distribution to the campus community. Fraternities and upperclassmen have abused this type of publication to "target" naive freshmen.
- Study the campus and neighborhood with respect to routes between your residence and class/activities scheduled. Know where emergency phones are located.
- Share your class/activities schedule with parents and a network of close friends, effectively creating a type of "buddy" system. Give network telephone numbers to your parents, advisors, and friends.
- Always travel in groups. Use a shuttle service after dark. Never walk alone at night. Avoid shortcuts.
- Survey the campus, academic buildings, residence halls, and other facilities while classes are in session and after dark to see that buildings, walkways, quadrangles, and parking lots are adequately secured, lit, and patrolled. Are emergency phones, escorts, and shuttle services adequate?
- To gauge the social scene, drive down fraternity row on weekend nights and stroll through the student hangouts. Are people behaving responsibly, or does the situation seem reckless and potentially dangerous?

Remember, alcohol and/or drug abuse is involved in about 90 percent of campus crime. Carefully evaluate off-campus student apartment complexes and fraternity houses if you plan to live off-campus.

Residence

- Doors and windows to your residence hall should be equipped with quality locking mechanisms. Room doors should be equipped with peep holes and deadbolts. Always lock them when you are absent. Do not loan out your key. Rekey locks when a key is lost or stolen.
- Card access systems are far superior to standard metal key and lock systems. Card access enables immediate lock changes when keys are lost, stolen, or when housing arrangements change. Most hotels and hospitals have changed to card access systems for safety reasons. Higher education institutions need to adopt similar safety features.
- Always lock your doors and 1st and 2nd floor windows at night. Never compromise your safety for a roommate who asks you to leave the door unlocked.
- Dormitories should have a central entrance/exit lobby where nighttime access is monitored, as well as an outside telephone which visitors must use to gain access.
- Dormitory residents should insist that residential assistants and security patrols routinely check for propped doors—day and night.
- Do not leave your identification, wallets, check-books, jewelry, cameras, and other valuables in open view.
- Program your phone's speed dial memory with emergency numbers that include family and friends.
- Know your neighbors and don't be reluctant to report illegal activities and suspicious loitering.

Off-Campus Residents

Off-campus residents should contact their student legal aid representative to draft leases that stipulate minimum standards of security and responsibility. Students and parents should also consult any "Neighborhood Watch" association active in the community or the municipal police regarding local crime rates.

Security on Campus assists victims of campus crime.

Source: Reprinted with permission by Security on Campus, Inc., www.securityoncampus.org.

SETTING GOALS 1

Personal Safety

Your Personal Safety Goal

Is It S.M.A.R.T.?
  Specific? _____
  Measurable? _____

Achievable? _____

Rewarding? _____

Time Defined? _____

Strategies for Success

1. _____

2. _____

3. _____

Potential Obstacles

1. _____

2. _____

3. _____

Ways Around Them

1. _____

2. _____

3. _____

Daily Report

The Week That Was:

What Went Right?

What Could I Do Better?

WELLNESS JOURNAL 1

Personal Safety

Everyone should be aware of the crime trends that are occurring in their area and take action to reduce the risk of becoming a victim. Denial, fear, or hiding from crime will not make crime disappear. Your best defense is to understand criminal activity and take personal action to reduce your exposure to crime. Developing a "Personal Safety Attitude" can help you become more aware of your surroundings and stay safe. The Personal Safety Attitude consists of three major actions:

▌ Walking with your head up and staying alert.

▌ Walking like you are on a mission

▌ Making eye contact with people you walk past.

How often do you do these three things when you are on campus or walking around in town? Jot down your observations for a week and, in your Wellness Journal, assess your "Attitude".

1. Walking with Your Head Up and Staying Alert

Criminals want easy prey; someone they can surprise, who will offer little resistance and have trouble identifying them. Observe your surroundings and where you are going. Note potential hazards and have an "escape" plan in mind every time you go out in public. Don't be an easy target!

2. Walking Like You Are on a Mission

Think of this as walking like you have to be somewhere and, perhaps, you are a bit late! This sends a message to people that you know where you are going and that you are not a person to mess around with.

3. Making Eye Contact with People You Walk Past

Criminals like to be anonymous and blend in with society. Being noticed is not in their best interest. Look at the people walking toward you and make eye contact. Try not to stare, however, as this might result in a confrontation. Just send the message that you see who is around you and that you are not intimidated.

Other Safety Considerations

▌ Don't walk near poorly lit areas or on trails that appear to be deserted or rarely used.

▌ Use a variety of routes so nobody can anticipate your chances of showing up at a certain place and time.

▌ Wearing headphones can decrease your ability to hear a car, dog, or another person approaching you.

▌ If you are harassed from someone in a car, quickly turn and walk in the other direction.

How to Deal with a Dog

▌ Always look ahead for any potential problems in the street or on the trail. Turn around or cross over to the other side of the street, if necessary, to avoid a confrontation.

▌ Know warning signs of an aggressive dog. Head down, ears back, tail low, and snarling while coming toward you, are signs of aggression and you should be very alert for an attack.

▌ Don't run (dogs are born to "chase.") Face the dog and speak quietly but in an authoritative voice. Terms such as "no", "stop" and "stay" are words that may get a response. Back away slowly if you have to.

▌ Don't stare at the dog (this is viewed as a threat.) Keep the dog in your view in a sideways glance as you walk away.

SELF-SURVEY 2

Are You Doing Your Part for the Planet?

You may think that there is little you can do, as an individual, to save Earth. But everyday acts can add up and make a difference in helping or harming the planet on which we live.

	Almost Never	Sometimes	Always
1. Do you walk, cycle, carpool, or use public transportation as much as possible to get around?	____	____	____
2. Do you recycle?	____	____	____
3. Do you reuse plastic and paper bags?	____	____	____
4. Do you try to conserve water by not running the tap as you shampoo or brush your teeth?	____	____	____
5. Do you use products made of recycled materials?	____	____	____
6. Do you drive a car that gets good fuel mileage and has up-to-date emission control equipment?	____	____	____
7. Do you turn off lights, televisions, and appliances when you're not using them?	____	____	____
8. Do you avoid buying products that are elaborately packaged?	____	____	____
9. Do you use glass jars and waxed paper rather than plastic wrap for storing food?	____	____	____
10. Do you take brief showers rather than baths?	____	____	____
11. Do you use cloth towels and napkins rather than paper products?	____	____	____
12. When listening to music, do you keep the volume low?	____	____	____
13. Do you try to avoid any potential carcinogens, such as asbestos, mercury, or benzene?	____	____	____
14. Are you careful to dispose of hazardous materials (such as automobile oil or antifreeze) at appropriate sites?	____	____	____
15. Do you follow environmental issues in your community and write your state or federal representative to support "green" legislation?	____	____	____

Count the number of items you've checked in each column. If you've circled 10 or more in the "always" column, you're definitely helping to make a difference. If you've circled 10 or more in the "never" column, read this chapter carefully and "Your Action Plan for Protecting the Planet" to find out what you can do. If you've mainly circled "sometimes," you're moving in the right direction, but you need to be more consistent and more conscientious.

ACTION PLAN 2

Your Action Plan for Protecting the Planet

By the choices you make and the actions you take, you can improve the state of the world. No one expects you to sacrifice every comfort or spend great amounts of money. However, for almost everyone, there's plenty of room for improvement. If enough people make small individual changes, they can have an enormous impact.

One basic environmental action is *precycling*: buying products packaged in recycled materials. According to Earthworks, a consumer group, packaging makes up a third of what people in the United States throw away. When you precycle, you consider how you're going to dispose of a product and the packaging materials before purchasing it. For example, you might choose eggs in recyclable cardboard packages rather than in plastic cartons and look for juice and milk in refillable bottles.

Recycling—collecting, reprocessing, marketing, and using materials once considered trash—has become a ne-

cessity for several reasons: We've run out of space for all the garbage we produce; waste sites are often health and safety hazards; recycling is cheaper than landfill storage or incineration (a major source of air pollution); and recycling helps save energy and natural resources. Different communities take different approaches to recycling. Many provide regular curbside pickup of recyclables, which is so convenient that a majority of those eligible for such services participate. Most programs pick up bottles, cans, and newspapers—either separated or mixed together. Other communities have drop-off centers where consumers can leave recyclables. Conveniently located and sponsored by community organizations (such as charities or schools), these centers accept beverage containers, newspapers, cardboard, metals, and other items.

Buyback centers, usually run by private companies, pay for recyclables. Many centers specialize in aluminum cans, which offer the most profit. Some operate in supermarket parking lots; other centers have regular hours and staff members who carefully weigh and evaluate recyclables. In some places, reverse vending machines accept returned beverage containers and provide deposit refunds, in the form of either cash or vouchers.

Discarded computers and other electronic devices should also be recycled, by donating them to schools or charitable organizations. "Tech trash" buried in landfills is creating a new hazard because trace amounts of potentially hazardous agents, such as lead and mercury, can leak into the ground and water.

With *composting*—which some people describe as nature's way of recycling—the benefits can be seen as close as your backyard. Organic products, such as leftover food and vegetable peels, are mixed with straw or other dry material and kept damp. Bacteria eat the organic material and turn it into a rich soil. Some people keep a compost pile (which should be stirred every few days) in their backyard; others take their organic garbage (including mowed grass and dead leaves) to community gardens or municipal composting sites.

SETTING GOALS 2

Personal Environmental Protection Goals

Understanding all of the potential environmental hazards you face on a daily basis may seem like a daunting task. Controlling the massive amounts of the toxic pollutants that work their way into the environment is, for the most part, beyond your control. There are, however, some steps you can take to help reduce the amount of pollutants you contribute to this problem. Setting and working toward some personal goals for improving the environment and protecting yourself can be a rewarding experience.

What can you realistically do? Examples of goals might be to recycle more products, spend less time driving, reduce your electric and gas bills or more effectively control your water usage. Create some goals, develop some strategies to achieve them and get started on your way to a cleaner environment.

Your Personal Environmental Protection Goal

Is It S.M.A.R.T.?
Specific? _____
Measurable? _____
Achievable? _____
Rewarding? _____
Time Defined? _____

Strategies for Success
1. _____
2. _____
3. _____

Potential Obstacles
1. _____
2. _____
3. _____

Ways Around Them
1. _____
2. _____
3. _____

Daily Report

The Week That Was:

What went right?
What could I do better?

WELLNESS JOURNAL 2

Thinking about Environmental Protection

Environmental health risks are all around us. Air, water, noise and land pollution are becoming more prevalent in our world as we try to meet the demands of a constantly rising world population and fuel an increasing appetite for goods and services. Forty percent of deaths worldwide are now attributed to factors related to the environment. American manufacturers alone emit over 2.5 billion pounds of toxic pollutants into the atmosphere each year, and over 220 million tons of municipal solid waste each day. Health care costs of exposure to outdoor air pollutants in our country have risen to $50 billion per year.

This short quiz will test your knowledge about environmental pollution. In your Wellness Journal, discuss your feelings about the environment. What can you do limit, or just minimize, pollution and overconsumption in your day-to-day activities? In what ways can you make the world a cleaner and better place to live? How do you feel about the future of the environment, both locally and globally?

How Does the Environment Affect Your Health?

1. Which kind of food generally contains the highest levels of toxic chemicals?
   a. fish   c. produce
   b. red meat   d. dairy

2. Overexposure to the sun can suppress our immune system.
   a. true   b. false

3. How many Americans become ill each year from eating contaminated food?
   a. 175   c. 75,000
   b. 750   d. 750,000

4. The amount of second hand smoke has decreased during the past decade.
   a. true   b. false

5. Air pollution has been shown to cause which of the following ailments?
   a. decreased bone density
   b. kidney and liver damage

c. infertility
d. all of the above

6. Which of the following diseases is not linked to environmental causes?
   a. autism
   b. arthritis
   c. irritable bowel syndrome
   d. diabetes

7. What is the leading cause of death for women in the workplace?
   a. cancer
   b. poor air quality
   c. violence
   d. none of the above

8. During the past decade, by what percentage have pesticide poisonings increased?

a. 25 percent
b. 50 percent
c. 75 percent
d. 100 percent

9. How many gallons of gas are spilled nationwide each year by people refueling their lawnmowers?
   a. 1,700
   b. 17,000
   c. 170,000
   d. 17 million

10. Scenic views can help you recover more quickly from surgery.
    a. true
    b. false

Answers: 1. a, 2. a, 3. d, 4. a, 5. b, 6. d, 7. c, 8. d, 9. d, 10. a.

Source: Natural Health Magazine (July 2001).

WELLNESS JOURNAL 3

The Five R's of Recycling

We live in a disposable society. Unfortunately, most of the material we throw away ends up in our landfills, sewers, lakes, and rivers. Only about 10% of our garbage is now being recycled, with about 80% going to landfills and the remaining 10% being incinerated. With an estimated combined daily household and business waste exceeding 4 pounds for every U.S. citizen, the amount of disposable material is filling up available landfill space at an alarming rate.

You can help this problem by utilizing the 5 R's of recycling:

REDUCE the amount of waste products you produce.
REUSE products a second and third time or as many times as possible.
RECYCLE whatever can be recycled in your town.
REJECT excessively packaged products and products hazardous to the environment.
REACT by voicing your concerns to manufacturers and elected government leaders.

Use the chart to help you list what you are willing to do to improve the environment.

What Can I Do to Help the Environment?

Reduce
Buy only what you really need
Buy recycled products and products with less packaging

1.
2.
3.

Reuse
Boxes, grocery bags, wrapping paper, plastic and metal containers

1.
2.
3.

Recycle
Paper, aluminum, tin, steel, glass, cardboard, plastic, newspapers, motor oil, and computer paper

1.
2.
3.

Reject
Aerosol cans, non-recyclable products, 6 pack rings, blister packs, over-packaged products, and products harmful to the environment

1.
2.
3.

React
Call manufacturer 800 numbers to voice your opinions
Write manufacturers to recommend more use of recycled materials and less packaging
Call your elected leaders and request them to support environmental protection legislation

1.
2.
3.

CHAPTER 15
Making This Chapter Work for You

1. Which of the following factors affects an individual's risk of accident or injury?
   a. hunger level
   b. stress level
   c. amount of automobile insurance coverage
   d. knowledge of CPR

2. Safe-driving tips include all of the following except:
   a. Avoid driving at night for the first year after getting a license.
   b. Make sure your car has snow tires or chains before driving in hazardous snowy conditions.
   c. If riding with an intoxicated driver, keep talking to him so that he doesn't fall asleep at the wheel.
   d. Don't let packages or people obstruct the rear or side windows.

3. Which statement about violence of college campuses is *false*?
   a. Property crimes account for most crimes on campus.
   b. Crime rates at colleges and universities are higher than in the general community.
   c. Many campuses have codes of conduct on alcohol, drugs, fighting, and sexual harassment.
   d. Crime statistics for colleges and universities are posted on the Internet.

4. Sexual victimization
   a. includes sexual harassment, sexual coercion, and rape.
   b. is gender-specific, affecting women who are violated emotionally or physically by men.
   c. is rare in academic environments such as college campuses.
   d. most commonly takes the form of physical assault and stalking.

5. Which of the following statements about rape is *true*?
   a. When a person is sexually attacked by a stranger, it is referred to as *rape*. When a person is sexually attacked by an acquaintance, it is referred to as *sexual coercion*.
   b. Statutory rape is defined as sexual intercourse initiated by a woman under the age of consent.
   c. Men who rape other men usually consider themselves heterosexuals.
   d. Women who flirt and dress provocatively are typically more willing to participate in aggressive sex than women who dress conservatively and do not flirt.

6. Ways to protect or prevent rape include:
   a. Use alcohol and drugs only in familiar surroundings.
   b. Take a self-defense class.
   c. To avoid angering a sexually aggressive person, become passive and quiet.

   d. Do not discuss your sexual limits on a first or second date, because just talking about sex will encourage your date to think you are interested in a sexual relationship.

7. Threats to the environment include
   a. an open ecosystem.
   b. depletion of the oxygen layer.
   c. ecological processes.
   d. global warming.

8. One of the most important things you can do to help protect the environment is
   a. recycle paper, bottles, cans, and unwanted food.
   b. use as much water as possible to help lower the ocean water levels.
   c. avoid energy-depleting fluorescent bulbs.
   d. use plastic storage containers and plastic wrap to save trees from being cut down.

9. You can protect your hearing by
   a. avoiding prolonged exposure to sounds under 75 decibels.
   b. using foam earplugs when operating noisy tools or attending rock concerts.
   c. limiting noise exposure to short bursts of loud sounds such as fireworks.
   d. drinking alcohol in noisy environments to mute the sounds.

10. Indoor pollutants include
    a. lead, which is often found in paint and can result in nervous system damage in adults and impaired fertility and kidney damage in children.
    b. radon, which is found in building materials and can cause heart disease.
    c. asbestos, which may be found in building insulation and can cause lung diseases.
    d. carbon monoxide, which can be produced by furnaces and engines and can result in chronic illnesses such as emphysema.

Answers to these questions can be found on page 376.

Critical Thinking

1. Can you name two risk factors in your daily life that might increase the likelihood of accidental injury? What actions have you taken to keep yourself safe? Are there other risk factors you could minimize or eliminate? What might you do about them?

2. A friend of yours, Eric, frequently makes crude or derogatory comments about women. When you finally call him on this, his response is, "I didn't say anything wrong. I like women." What might you say to him?

3. At one college, women raped by acquaintances or dates scrawled the names of their assailants on the walls of women's restrooms on campus. Several

young men whose names appeared on the list objected, protesting that they were innocent and were being unfairly accused. How do you feel about this method of fighting back against date rape? Do you think it violates the rights of men? How do you feel about naming women who've been raped in news reports? Are there circumstances in which a woman's identity should be revealed? Would fewer women report a rape if not assured of privacy?

4. In one Harris poll, 84 percent of Americans said that, given a choice between a high standard of living (but with hazardous air and water pollution and the depletion of natural resources) and a lower standard of living (but with clean air and drinking water), they would prefer clean air and drinking water and a lower standard of living. What about you? What exactly would you be willing to give up: air conditioning, convenience packaging and products, driving your own car rather than using public transportation? Do you think most people are willing to change their lifestyles to preserve the environment?

Media Menu

Health⟨⟩Now™

Don't forget to check out the wealth of resources on the HealthNow website at **http://healthnow.brookscole.com/itw** that will:
- Help you evaluate your knowledge of the material
- Allow you to take an exam-prep quiz
- Provide a Personalized Learning Plan targeting resources that address areas you should study
- Coach you through identifying target goals for behavior change and creating and monitoring your personal change plan throughout the semester.

INTERNET CONNECTIONS

RAINN-Rape Assault Incest National Network
www.rainn.org
This site provides great information from an organization fighting against rape, assault, and incest.

The Rape Crisis Center
www.rapecrisis.com
This private nonprofit organization provides support to victims of sexual violence and their families, including a 24/7 crisis hotline and several advocacy programs.

National Safety Council
www.nsc.org
The mission of the NSC is to educate and influence society to adopt safety, health, and environmental policies, practices, and procedures that prevent human suffering and economic losses arising from preventable causes.

Envirolink
www.envirolink.org
Envirolink is a nonprofit organization that brings together individuals and groups concerned about the environment and provides access to a wealth of online environmental resources.

Student Environmental Action Coalition
www.seac.org
Since 1988, the Student Environmental Action Coalition has been empowering students and youth to fight for environmental and social justice in our schools and communities.

InfoTrac College Edition Activities Moreira, Naila. "The Wind and the Fury: Has Climate Change Made Hurricanes Fiercer, or Are Such Claims Hot Air?" *Science News,* Sept 17, 2005 v168 i12 p184(3)

1. What do scientists believe are some possible causes for the increase in the number and intensity of hurricanes in recent years?

2. How might global warming contribute to this increase?

3. What are some of the consequences of more frequent and severe hurricanes for the United States?

You can find additional readings related to personal health with InfoTrac College Edition, an online library of more than 900 journals and publications. Follow the instructions for accessing InfoTrac College Edition that were packaged with your textbook; then search for articles using a keyword search.

For additional links, resources, and suggested readings on the InfoTrac College Edition, visit our Health and Wellness Resource Center at **http://health .wadsworth.com.**

Key Terms

The terms listed are used on the page indicated. Definitions of the terms are in the Glossary at the end of the book.

Making This Chapter Work for You

Answers to Multiple-Choice Questions

Chapter 1

1. a; 2. b; 3. d; 4. d; 5. d; 6. c; 7. c; 8. c; 9. d; 10. d

Chapter 2

1. b; 2. c; 3. c; 4. c; 5. d; 6. a; 7. c; 8. d; 9. a; 10. c

Chapter 3

1. c; 2. d; 3. a; 4. b; 5. c; 6. d; 7. b; 8. d; 9. c; 10. d

Chapter 4

1. b; 2. b; 3. c; 4. a; 5. b; 6. c; 7. d; 8. c; 9. a; 10. c

Chapter 5

1. a; 2. c; 3. c; 4. d; 5. b; 6. c; 7. c; 8. a; 9. b; 10. d

Chapter 6

1. a; 2. c; 3. b; 4. b; 5. d; 6. b; 7. c; 8. a; 9. d; 10. b

Chapter 7

1. b; 2. a; 3. a; 4. a; 5. c; 6. d; 7. b; 8. a; 9. c; 10. d

Chapter 8

1. c; 2. a; 3. d. 4. a; 5. d; 6. c; 7. a; 8. c; 9. a; 10. b

Chapter 9

1. c; 2. b; 3. c; 4. c; 5. d; 6. a; 7. c; 8. c; 9. a; 10. c

Chapter 10

1. c; 2. a; 3. c; 4. d; 5. b; 6. a; 7. b; 8. c; 9. d; 10. b

Chapter 11

1. d; 2. a; 3. d; 4. a; 5. d; 6. d; 7. c; 8. b; 9. c; 10. b

Chapter 12

1. c; 2. c; 3. b; 4. c; 5. b; 6. a; 7. d; 8. d; 9. b; 10. b

Chapter 13

1. b; 2. b; 3. a; 4. b; 5. b; 6. d; 7. c; 8. c; 9. a; 10. c

Chapter 14

1. d; 2. b; 3. b; 4. c; 5. d; 6. a; 7. a; 8. d; 9. b; 10. c

Chapter 15

1. b; 2. c; 3. b; 4. a; 5. c; 6. b; 7. d; 8. a; 9. b; 10. c

References

Chapter 1

1. Travis, John, and Regina Sara Ryan. *The Wellness Workbook,* 3rd ed. Berkeley, CA: Celestial Arts, 2004.
2. "Constitution of the World Health Organization." *Chronicle of the World Health Organization.* Geneva, Switzerland: WHO, 1947.
3. Travis, John. Personal interview.
4. Smith, Roger. Personal interview.
5. Mathews, Dale. Personal interview.
6. Kochanek, Kenneth, and Betty Smith. "Deaths: Preliminary Data for 2002." *National Vital Statistics Reports,* Vol. 52, No. 13, February 11, 2004.
7. Terry, Anna. "Osteoporosis May Threaten Young Women." University of Arkansas Press Release, June 21, 2004.
8. Preston, Samuel. "Deadweight? The Influence of Obesity on Longevity." *New England Journal of Medicine,* Vol. 352, No. 1, March 17, 2005, p. 1135.
9. Olshansky, S. Jay, et al. "A Potential Decline in Life Expectancy in the United States in the 21st Century." *New England Journal of Medicine,* Vol. 352, No. 1, March 17, 2005, p. 1138.
10. Healthy People 2010, www.healthypeople.gov.
11. "Summary Health Statistics for U.S. Adults: National Health Interview Study, 2002." *Vital and Health Statistics,* Series 10, No. 222. Hyattsville, MD: Centers for Disease Control and Prevention, National Center for Health Statistics, July 2004.
12. "Health Behaviors of Adults: United States, 1999–2001." *Vital and Health Statistics,* Series 10, No. 219. Hyattsville, MD: Centers for Disease Control and Prevention, National Center for Health Statistics, February 2004.
13. "Cancer Facts for Minorities in the United States." National Center for Chronic Disease Prevention and Health Promotion. www.cdc.gov/cancer/minorityawareness.htm.
14. National Eye Institute. News release. *U.S. Latinos Have High Rates of Eye Disease and Visual Impairment.* www.nei.nih.gov/latinoeyestudy/.
15. "Treatments, Outcomes Differ Widely Among Women of Different Races, Ethnicities." *Women's Health Weekly,* February 13, 2003, p. 14.
16. Knapp, Laura. "Postsecondary Enrollment." *Education Statistics Quarterly,* Vol. 5, No. 4, August 2004, p. 85.
17. Hanauer, David, et al. "Internet Use among Community College Students: Implications in Designing Healthcare Interventions." *Journal of American College Health,* Vol. 52, No. 5, March–April 2004, p. 197.
18. Battle, Delores. "Project Success: Assuring College Students with Disabilities a Quality Higher Education." *ASHA* (American Speech-Language-Hearing Association) *Leader,* Vol. 9, No. 2, February 3, 2004, p. 6.
19. Green, John, et al. "Heart Disease Risk Perception in College Men and Women." *Journal of American College Health,* Vol. 51, No. 5, March 2003, p. 207.
20. Sax, Linda, et al. *The American Freshman: National Norms for Fall 2004.* Los Angeles: UCLA Higher Education Research Institute, 2004.
21. Travis, and Ryan, *The Wellness Workbook.*
22. Yoon, Paula. Personal interview.

Chapter 2

1. Prochaska, James, et al. *Changing for Good.* New York: Quill, 1994.
2. van Sluijs, E. M., et al. "Stage-based Lifestyle Interventions in Primary Care: Are They Effective?" *American Journal of Preventive Medicine,* Vol. 26, No. 4, May 2004, p. 330.
3. Dalton, C. C., and L. N. Gottlieb. "The Concept of Readiness to Change." *Journal of Advances in Nursing,* Vol. 42, No. 2, April 2003, pp. 108–117.
4. Jacobs, A. D., et al. "Effects of a Tailored Follow-up Intervention on Health Behaviors, Beliefs, and Attitudes." *Journal of Women's Health,* Vol. 13, No. 4, June 2004, p. 557.
5. Prokhorov, A., et al. "Self-Reported Health Status, Health Vulnerability, and Smoking Behavior in College Students: Implications for Intervention." *Nicotine and Tobacco Research,* Vol. 5, No. 4, August 2003, p. 545.
6. Steinman, K. J. "College Students' Early Cessation from Episodic Heavy Drinking: Prevalence and Correlates." *Journal of American College Health,* Vol. 51, No. 5, March 2003, p. 197.
7. Seligman, Martin. Personal interview.
8. Fadiman, James. Personal interview.
9. "More Than Good Intentions: Realistic Goals Help You Lose Weight and Get Fit." *Healthy Women,* January 2005.
10. Christian, Kenneth W. Personal interview.

Chapter 3

1. Suminski, Richard, et al. "Physical Activity Among Ethnically Diverse College Students." *Journal of American College Health,* Vol. 51, September 2002, p. 75.
2. "Biology Shows Women and Men Are Different." *Mayo Clinic Women's Healthsource,* September 2002.
3. Lavie, C., et al. "Exercise Capacity in Adult African-Americans Referred for Exercise Stress Testing: Is Fitness Affected by Race?" *Chest,* Vol. 126, No. 6, December 2004, pp. 1962–68.
4. Hunter, G. R., et al. "Aerobic Fitness, Physiologic Difficulty and Physical Activity in Black and White Women." *International Journal of Obesity and Related Metabolic Disorders,* Vol. 28, No. 9, September 2004, pp. 1111–1117.
5. "Physical Activity and Health: Adults." A Report of the Surgeon General, President's Council on Physical Fitness and Sports, www.cdc.gov.
6. "Information From Your Family Doctor. Physical Activity For Healthy Weight." *American Family Physician,* Vol. 67, No. 6, March 15, 2003, p. 1266.
7. "How Fit You Are Determines Your Life Span." *Tufts University Health & Nutri-*

tion Letter, Vol. 20, No. 5, July 2002, p. 6.

8. Mokdad, A., et al. "Actual Causes of Death in the United States, 2004." *Journal of the American Medical Association,* Vol. 291, 2004, p. 1238.

9. Marshall, E. "Public Enemy Number One: Tobacco or Obesity?" *Science,* Vol. 7, No. 304(5672), May 2004, p. 804.

10. Wallace, Lorraine, et al. "Promoting Physical Activity in the Family Practice Setting." *American Family Physician,* Vol. 67, No. 6, March 15, 2003, p. 1196.

11. MacIntosh, D. "Getting the Facts on Physical Activity." *Canadian Family Physician,* Vol. 49, January 2003, p. 23.

12. College of Family Physicians of Canada, www.cfpc.ca.

13. Buckworth, Janet, and Claudio Nigg. "Physical Activity, Exercise, and Sedentary Behavior in College Students." *Journal of American College Health,* Vol. 53, No. 1, July–August 2004, p. 28.

14. Suminski, "Physical Activity Among Ethnically Diverse College Students."

15. Mack, Mick, et al. "Changes in Short-term Attitudes Toward Physical Activity and Exercise of University Personal Wellness Students." *College Student Journal,* Vol. 38, No. 4, December 2004, p. 587.

16. Bray, Steven, and Heidi Born. "Transition to University and Vigorous Physical Activity: Implications for Health and Psychological Well-Being." *Journal of American College Health,* Vol. 52, No. 4, January–February 2004, p. 181.

17. Sparling, Phillip, and Teresa Snow. "Physical Activity Patterns in Recent College Alumni." *Research Quarterly for Exercise and Sport,* Vol. 73, No. 2, June 2002, p. 200.

18. "Poor Fitness in Young Adults Associated with Later Cardiovascular Problems." *FDA Consumer,* Vol. 38, No. 1, January–February 2004, p. 7.

19. Marcus, Bess, and Beth Lewis. "Physical Activity and the Stages of Motivational Readiness for Change Model." *President's Council on Physical Fitness and Sports Research Digest,* Series 4, No. 1, March 2003, p. 1.

20. Marcus, H., and L. J. Forsyth. *Motivating People to Be Physically Active.* Champaign, IL: Human Kinetics, 2003.

21. Cardinal, Bradley, and Maria Kosma. "Self-Efficacy and the Stages and Process of Change Associated with Adopting and Maintaining Muscular Fitness-Promoting Behavior." *Research Quarterly for Exercise and Sport,* Vol. 78, No. 2, June 2004, p. 186.

22. Mack, et al. "Changes in Short-Term Attitudes Toward Physical Activity and Exercise of University Personal Wellness Students."

23. DeVoe, Dale, and Cathy Kennedy. "Physical Activity Stages-of-Change and Activity Self-Efficacy of College Students

Enrolled in a University-Required Fitness and Wellness Course." *Research Quarterly for Exercise and Sport,* Vol. 72, No. 1, March 2001, p. A-28.

24. Thomas, D. Q., et al. "Physiologic Profile of the Fitness Status of Collegiate Cheerleaders." *Journal of Strength Conditioning Research,* Vol. 18, No. 2, May 2004, p. 252.

25. Bauman, A. E., et al. "Updating the Evidence That Physical Activity Is Good for Health: An Epidemiological Review 2000–2003." *Journal of the Science of Medicine and Sport,* Vol. 7, No. 1 (Suppl.), April 2004, pp. 6–19.

26. Yu, S., et al. "What Level of Physical Activity Protects Against Premature Cardiovascular Death? The Caerphilly Study." *Heart,* Vol. 89, April 2003, p. 502.

27. Aronson, D., et al. "C-Reactive Protein Is Inversely Related to Physical Fitness in Middle-aged Subjects." *Atherosclerosis,* Vol. 176, No. 1, September 2004, pp. 173–179.

28. Katzmarzyk, P. T., et al. "Cardiorespiratory Fitness Attenuates the Effects of the Metabolic Syndrome on All-cause and Cardiovascular Disease Mortality in Men." *Archives of Internal Medicine,* Vol. 164, No. 10, May 24, 2004, p. 1092.

29. Ortlepp, J. R., et al. "Relationship Between Physical Fitness and Lifestyle Behaviour in Healthy Young Men." *European Journal of Cardiovascular Prevention and Rehabilitation,* Vol. 11, No. 3, June 2004, p. 192.

30. Scranton, R., et al. "Predictors of 14-year Changes in the Total Cholesterol to High-Density Lipoprotein Cholesterol Ratio in Men." *American Heart Journal,* Vol. 147, No. 6, June 2004, p. 1033.

31. Arbab-Zadeh, Armin, et al. "Effect of Aging and Physical Activity on Left Ventricular Compliance." *Circulation,* Vol. 110, 2004, www.circulationaha.org.

32. Bauman, "Updating the Evidence That Physical Activity Is Good for Health."

33. Stevens, J., et al. "Fitness and Fatness as Predictors of Mortality From All Causes and From Cardiovascular Disease in Men and Women in the Lipid Research Clinics Study." *American Journal of Epidemiology,* Vol. 156, No. 9, November 1, 2002, p. 832.

34. Bauman, "Updating the Evidence That Physical Activity Is Good for Health."

35. van Gelder, B. M., et al. "Physical Activity in Relation to Cognitive Decline in Elderly Men: The FINE Study." *Neurology,* Vol. 63, No. 12, December 28, 2004, pp. 2316–2321.

36. Colcombe, S. J., et al. "Neurocognitive Aging and Cardiovascular Fitness: Recent Findings and Future Directions." *Journal of Molecular Neuroscience,* Vol. 24, No. 1, 2004, pp. 9–14.

37. Ford, M. A., et al. "Past and Recent Physical Activity and Bone Mineral Density

in College-aged Women." *Journal of Strength and Conditioning Research,* Vol. 18, No. 3, August 2004, p. 405.

38. Mayo, M. J., et al. "Exercise-Induced Weight Loss Preferentially Reduces Abdominal Fat." *Medicine and Science in Sports and Exercise,* Vol. 35, No. 2, 2003, pp. 207–213.

39. Penhollow, Tina, and Michael Young. "Sexual Desirability and Sexual Performance: Does Exercise and Fitness Really Matter?" *Electronic Journal of Human Sexuality,* Vol. 7, October 5, 2004, www.ejhs.org.

40. Molaison, E. F. "Linking Decisional Balance to Participation in Physical Activity in College Students." *Journal of the American Dietetic Association,* Vol. 104, No. 8, August 2004, p. A57(1).

41. Hu, F. B., et al. "Adiposity as Compared with Physical Activity in Predicting Mortality Among Women." *New England Journal of Medicine,* Vol. 351, No. 26, December 23, 2004, pp. 2694–2703.

42. *Dietary Guidelines for Americans.* Washington, D.C.: Departments of Health and Human Services and Agriculture, 2005.

43. Wessel, Timothy, et al. "Relationship of Physical Fitness vs. Body Mass Index with Coronary Artery Disease and Cardiovascular Events in Women." *Journal of the American Medical Association,* Vol. 292, No. 10, September 8, 2004, p. 1179.

44. Weinstein, Amy, et al. "Relationship of Physical Activity vs. Body Mass Index with Type 2 Diabetes in Women." *Journal of the American Medical Association,* Vol. 292, No. 10, September 8, 2004, p. 1188.

45. Blair, S. N., et al. "The Evolution of Physical Activity Recommendations: How Much is Enough?" *American Journal of Clinical Nutrition,* Vol. 79, No. 5, May 2004, p. 913S.

46. 2005 Dietary Guidelines Advisory Committee, *Report of the Dietary Guidelines Advisory Committee on the Dietary Guidelines for Americans, 2005.* Washington, DC: Health and Human Services and U.S. Department of Agriculture, 2004, www.health.gov/dietary guidelines/dga2005/report.

47. Blair, Steven, and Tim Church. "The Fitness, Obesity, and Health Equation." *Journal of the American Medical Association,* Vol. 292, No. 10, September 8, 2004, p. 1232.

48. White, K., et al. "EMG Power Spectra of Intercollegiate Athletes and Anterior Cruciate Ligament Injury Risk in Females." *Medicine and Science in Sports and Exercise,* Vol. 35, No. 3, 2003, pp. 371–376.

49. Fagenbaum, R., and W. G. Darling, "Jump Landing Strategies in Male and Female College Athletes and the Implications of Such Strategies for Anterior Cruciate Ligament Injury." *American*

Journal of Sports Medicine, Vol. 31, No. 2, March–April 2003, p. 233.

50. Garman, F., et al. "Occurrence of Exercise Dependence in a College-Aged Population." *Journal of American College Health,* Vol. 52, No. 5, March–April 2004, p. 221.

Chapter 4

1. Hussey, J. M., et al. "Physical Activity Behavior and Knowledge of Effects of Physical Activity and Exercise Recommendations among University Students." *Journal of Sports Sciences,* March 2004, Vol. 22, No. 3, p. 282.
2. Hammett, C. J., et al. "Effect of Six Months' Exercise Training on C-Reactive Protein Levels in Healthy Elderly Subjects." *Journal of the American College of Cardiology,* Vol. 44, No. 12, December 21, 2004, pp. 2411–2413.
3. "Aerobic Exercise: Why and How." Mayo Clinic: www.mayoclinic.com/invoke .cfm?id=EP00002
4. "Measuring Exercise Intensity." *IDEA Personal Trainer,* Vol. 13, No. 9, October 2002, p. 60.
5. "Variety of Preparticipation Activities, Not Just Stretching, Recommended to Prevent Injuries in Sports." *American College of Sports Medicine,* News Release, March 3, 2004.
6. Molaison, E. F. "Linking Decisional Balance to Participation in Physical Activity in College Students." *Journal of the American Dietetic Association,* August 2004, Vol. 104, No. 18 p. A57(1).
7. Grubbs, Laurie, and Jason Carter. "The Relationship of Perceived Benefits and Barriers to Reported Exercise Behaviors in College Undergraduates." *Family and Community Health,* Vol. 25, No. 2, July 2002, p. 78.
8. Bauman, A. E. "Updating the Evidence that Physical Activity is Good for Health." *Journal of Science and Medicine in Sport,* Vol. 7, No. 1 (Suppl.), April 2004, p. 6.
9. Lange, R. M., and M. A. Nies. "Benefits of Walking for Obese Women in the Prevention of Bone and Joint Disorders." *Orthopedic Nursing,* Vol. 23, No. 3, May–June 2004, p. 211.
10. "College Students Walk Less than Younger Children." American College of Sports Medicine, News Release, June 2, 2004.
11. "Number of Daily Steps Impacts Obesity Factors in Women." American College of Sports Medicine, News Release, May 5, 2004.
12. "Pedometer-Based Walking Programs Can Help Achieve Physical Activity Recommendations." American College of Sports Medicine, News Release, January 12, 2004.
13. "Women with Pedometers Step Up Exercise Levels." American College of Sports Medicine, News Release, April 5, 2005.
14. "Spin It." "Fit Facts," American Council on Exercise. www.acefitness.org
15. "Kick Your Way to Fitness." "Fit Facts," American Council on Exercise: www .acefitness.org
16. "Running." American Orthopaedic Society for Sports Medicine: http://orthoinfo .aaos.org

Chapter 5

1. Cardinal, Bradley, and Maria Kosma. "Self-Efficacy and the Stages and Process of Change Associated with Adopting and Maintaining Muscular Fitness-Promoting Behaviors." *Research Quarterly for Exercise and Sport,* Vol. 78, No. 2, June 2004, p. 186.
2. Cardinal and Kosma. "Self-Efficacy and the Stages and Process of Change Associated with Adopting and Maintaining Muscular Fitness-Promoting Behaviors."
3. Cardinal and Kosma. "Self-Efficacy and the Stages and Process of Change Associated with Adopting and Maintaining Muscular Fitness-Promoting Behaviors."
4. Fontera, Walter, and Bean, Jonathan. *Strength and Power Training.* Boston: Harvard Health Publications, 2004.
5. Galvao, D. A., and D. R. Taaffe. "Single- vs. Multiple-Set Resistance Training: Recent Developments in the Controversy." *Strength Conditioning Research,* Vol. 18, No. 3, 2004, p. 660.
6. Pollock, Michael, et al. "The Recommended Quantity and Quality of Exercise for Developing and Maintaining Cardiorespiratory and Muscular Fitness and Flexibility in Healthy Individuals." *Medicine & Science in Sports and Exercise,* Vol. 30, No. 6, June 1998, www .acsm.org
7. Witvrous, E., et al. "Stretching and Injury Prevention: An Obscure Relationship." *Sports Medicine,* Vol. 34, No. 7, 2004, p. 443.
8. "The Truth About Steroids." *Fit Facts,* American Council on Exercise, www .acefitness.org
9. Mayo Clinic staff. "Strength Training in Women." www.mayoclinic.com

Chapter 6

1. Thacker, Stephen, et al. "The Impact of Stretching on Sports Injury Risk: A Systematic Review of the Literature." *Medicine and Science in Sports and Exercise,* Vol. 36, No. 3, March 2004, pp. 371–378.
2. "Yoga Becomes Big Business." *Sporting Good Business,* Vol. 38, No. 3, March 2005, p. 16.
3. Dykema, Ravi, *Yoga for Fitness and Wellness.* Belmont, CA: Brooks/Cole, 2005.
4. McCall, Timothy. "Count on Yoga." *Yoga Journal,* January/February 2005, p. 96.
5. "Yoga Should Heal, Not Hurt, Says ACSM Expert." News Release, American College of Sports Medicine, April 1, 2005.
6. "Pilates Research Offers New Information on Popular Technique." News Release, American College of Sports Medicine, March 30, 2005.
7. "T'ai Chi Training Improves Balance Control in Elderly." News Release, American College of Sports Medicine, April 5, 2004.
8. Cutts, Steven. "Back Pain—and Its Management." *Practice Nurse,* December 17, 2004, p. 38(5).
9. Malanga, Gerard, and Robin Dennis. "Treatment of Acute Low Back Pain: Use of Medications: Reduction and Control of Pain and Return of Function Are the Goals." *The Journal of Musculoskeletal Medicine,* Vol. 22, No. 2, February 2005, p. 79.
10. Margo, Katherine. "Spinal Manipulative Therapy for Low Back Pain." *American Family Physician,* Vol. 71, No. 3, February 1, 2005, p. 464.
11. Wendling, Patrice. "Surgery No Better than Rehab for Low Back Pain." *American Family Physician,* Vol. 71, No. 3, February 1, 2005, p. 558.

Chapter 7

1. Segerstrom, Suzanne, and Gregory E. Miller, "Psychological Stress and the Human Immune System: A Meta-Analytic Study of 30 Years of Inquiry." *Psychological Bulletin,* Vol. 130, No. 4, July 2004, p. 601.
2. Lazarus, R., and R. Launier. "Stress-Related Transactions Between Person and Environment." In *Perspectives in Interactional Psychology,* New York: Plenum, 1978.
3. Young, D. R., et al. "Health Status Among Urban African American Women: Associations Among Well-Being, Perceived Stress, and Demographic Factors." *Journal of Behavioral Medicine,* Vol. 27, No. 1, February 2004, p. 63.
4. Bovier, P.A., et al. "Perceived Stress, Internal Resources, and Social Support as Determinants of Mental Health Among Young Adults." *Quality of Life Research,* Vol. 13, No. 7, February 2004, p. 161.
5. Epel, Eliisa, et al. "Accelerated Telomere: Shortening in Response to Life Stress." Proceedings of the National Academy of Sciences, Vol. 101, No. 49, December 7, 2004, p. 17312.
6. Schmeelk-Cone, K. H., et al. "The Buffering Effects of Active Coping on the Relationship Between SES and Cortisol Among African American Young Adults." *Behavioral Medicine,* Vol. 29, No. 2, Summer 2003, p. 85.
7. Dickerson, Sally, and Margaret Kemeny. "Acute Stressors and Cortisol Responses: A Theoretical Integration and Synthesis of Laboratory Research." *Psychological Bulletin,* Vol. 130, No. 3, May 2004, p. 355.
8. Ketterer, Mark. "Stressed Out Men May Have Inherited Risk for Early Heart Dis-

ease." Presentation, American Psycho-somatic Society, March 2003.

9. Matthews, Karen, et al. "Blood Pressure Reactivity to Psychological Stress Predicts Hypertension in the CARDIA Study." *Circulation,* Vol. 110, No. 1, July 6, 2004, p. 74.

10. "Stress and the Heart." *Harvard Men's Health Watch,* February 2005.

11. Ibid.

12. Wittstein, Ilan, et al. "Neurohumoral Features of Myocardial Stunning Due to Sudden Emotional Stress." *New England Journal of Medicine,* Vol. 352, No. 6, February 10, 2005, pp. 539–548.

13. Segerstrom and Miller, "Psychological Stress and the Human Immune System."

14. Freeman, L. M., and K. M. Gil. "Daily Stress, Coping, and Dietary Restraint in Binge Eating." *International Journal of Eating Disorders,* Vol. 36, No. 2, September 2004, p. 204.

15. Sax, Linda, et al. *The American Freshman: National Norms for Fall 2004.* Los Angeles, CA: University of California, Los Angeles Higher Education Research Institute, December 2004.

16. ACHA-National College Health Assessment (NCHA). Baltimore, MD: American College Health Association (ACHA), www.acha.org.

17. Dusselier, Lauri, et al. "Personal, Health, Academic, and Environmental Predictors of Stress for Residence Hall Students." *Journal of American College Health,* Vol. 54, No. 1, July–August 2005, p. 15.

18. Ibid.

19. Bartlett, Thomas. "Freshmen Pay, Mentally and Physically, As They Adjust to Life in College." *Chronicle of Higher Education,* February 1, 2002.

20. Jackson, Pamela Braboy, and Monenique Finney. "Negative Life Events and Psychological Distress Among Young Adults." *Social Psychology Quarterly 2002,* Vol. 65, No. 2, p. 186.

21. Hertel, James. "College Students Generational Status: Similarities, Differences, and Factors in College Adjustment." *The Psychological Record,* Vol. 52, No. 1, Winter 2002, p. 3.

22. Park, Crystal, et al. "The Daily Stress and Coping Process and Alcohol Use Among College Students." *Journal of Studies on Alcohol,* Vol. 65, No. 1, January 2004, p. 126.

23. "In Case You Haven't Heard. . . ." *Mental Health Weekly,* Vol. 15, No. 3, January 17, 2004, p. 8.

24. Harrell, Shelly. "A Multidimensional Conceptualization of Racism-Related Stress: Implications for the Well-Being of People of Color." *American Journal of Orthopsychiatry,* Vol. 70, No. 1, January 2000.

25. Launier, Raymond. "Stress Balance and Emotional Life Complexes in Students in a Historically African American College."

Journal of Psychology, Vol. 131, No. 2, March 1997.

26. Rosenthal, Beth Spenciner, and Arleen Cedeno Schreiner. "Prevalence of Psychological Symptoms Among Undergraduate Students in an Ethnically Diverse Urban Public College." *Journal of American College Health,* Vol. 49, No. 1, July 2000.

27. Ibid.

28. Bowen-Reid, Terra, and Jules Harrell. "Racist Experiences and Health Outcomes: An Examination of Spirituality As a Buffer." *Journal of Black Psychology,* Vol. 28, No. 1, February 2002, p. 18.

29. Sax, Linda, et al. *The American Freshman.*

30. Hall, Cathy, et al. "Motivational and Attitudinal Factors in College Students With and Without Learning Disabilities." *Learning Disability Quarterly,* Vol. 25, No. 1, Spring 2002, p. 79.

31. Spalding, T. W., et al. "Aerobic Exercise Training and Cardiovascular Reactivity to Psychological Stress in Sedentary Young Normotensive Men and Women." *Psychophysiology,* Vol. 41, No. 4, July 2004, p. 552.

32. Shapiro, Deane, and Roger Walsh. *Beyond Health and Normalcy.* New York: Van Nostrand Reinhold, 1983.

33. Satcher, David. "Executive Summary: A Report of the Surgeon General on Mental Health." *Public Health Reports,* Vol. 115, No. 1, January 2000.

34. Russinova, Zlaytka, et al. "Use of Alternative Health Care Practices by Persons with Serious Mental Illness: Perceived Benefits." *American Journal of Public Health,* Vol. 92, March 2003, p. 1600.

35. Fiala, William, et al. "The Religious Support Scale." *American Journal of Community Psychology,* Vol. 30, No. 6, December 2002, p. 761.

36. Crocker, Jennifer, and Lora Park. "The Costly Pursuit of Self-Esteem." *Psychological Bulletin,* Vol. 130, No. 3, May 2004, p. 392.

37. Crocker, Jennifer, and Noah Nuer. "Do People Need Self-Esteem?" *Psychological Bulletin,* Vol. 130, No. 3, May 2004, p. 469.

38. Crocker and Park, "The Costly Pursuit of Self-Esteem."

39. Lawson, Willow. "The Glee Club." *Psychology Today,* January–February 2004, p. 34.

40. Seligman, Martin. *Authentic Happiness.* New York: Free Press, 2002.

41. Wart, Paula. "Why Be Happy?" *Health Plus,* Vanderbilt University, January 3, 2005.

42. Seligman, *Authentic Happiness.*

43. Lucas, R. F., et al. "Reexamining Adaptation and the Set Point Model of Happiness: Reactions to Changes in Marital Status." *Journal of Personality and Social Psychology,* Vol. 84, No. 3, March 2003, p. 527.

44. Seligman, *Authentic Happiness.*

45. Wart, Paula. "Be Optimistic: Improve Your Health." *Health Plus,* Vanderbilt University, January 3, 2005.

46. Levy, B. C. E., et al. "Longitudinal Benefit of Positive Self-Perceptions of Aging on Functional Health." *Journals of Gerontology. Series B Psychological Sciences and Social Sciences,* Vol. 57, No. 5, September 2002, pp. 409–417.

47. Wart, Paula. "Is Laughter Good for You?" *Health Plus,* Vanderbilt University, January 3, 2005.

48. Larsen, Randy. Personal interview.

49. Hales, Dianne. "Can Prayer Really Heal?" *Parade,* March 23, 2003, p. 4.

50. Storch, Eric, et al., "Religiosity and Depression in Intercollegiate Athletes." *College Student Journal,* Vol. 36, No. 4, December 2002, p. 526.

51. Koenig, Harold. Personal interview.

52. Palmer R. F., et al. "A Randomized Trial of the Effects of Remote Intercessory Prayer: Interactions with Personal Beliefs on Problem-Specific Outcomes and Functional Status." *Journal of Alternative and Complementary Medicine,* Vol. 10, No. 3, July 2004, p. 438.

53. McCaffrey A. M., et al. "Prayer for Health Concerns: Results of a National Survey on Prevalence and Patterns of Use." *Archives of Internal Medicine,* Vol. 164, No. 8, April 26, 2004, pp. 858–862.

54. Johnson M. R. "Faith, Prayer, and Religious Observance." *Clinical Cornerstone,* Vol. 6, No. 1, 2004, p. 17.

55. McCullough, Michael. personal interview.

56. "Survey Reveals Record Numbers of Students Involved in Service." *Black Issues in Higher Education,* Vol. 20, No. 10, July 3, 2003, p. 12.

57. Hermann, Karen, and Nancy Betz. "Path Models of the Relationships of Instrumentality and Expressiveness to Social Self-Efficacy, Shyness, and Depressive Symptoms." *Sex Roles: A Journal of Research,* Vol. 51, No. 1–2, July 2004, 55(12).

58. Kamdar, B. B., et al. "The Impact of Extended Sleep on Daytime Alertness, Vigilance and Mood." *Sleep Medicine,* Vol. 5, No. 5, September 2004, p. 441.

59. Vorona, R. D. et al. "Overweight and Obese Patients in a Primary Care Population Report Less Sleep than Patients with a Normal Body Mass Index." *Archives of Internal Medicine,* Vol. 165, No. 1, January 10, 2005, p. 25.

60. "Wake Up Call for Better Sleep." *Harvard Health Letter,* August 2004.

61. Ibid.

62. Kelly, William. "Sleep-Length and Life Satisfaction in a College Student Sample." *College Student Journal,* Vol. 38, No. 3, September 2004, p. 428(3) S.

63. Howell A. J., et al. "Sleep Quality, Sleep Propensity and Academic Performance." *Perception and Motor Skills,* Vol. 99, No. 2, October 2004, p. 525.

64. "Mounting Evidence Indicates Heart Disease Link." *Medical Letter on the CDC & FDA,* July 21, 2002, p. 14.

65. Vythilingam, Meena, et al. "Psychotic Depression and Mortality." *American Journal of Psychiatry,* Vol. 160, No. 3, March 2003, p. 425.

66. Strike, P. C., and A. Steptoe. "Depression, Stress, and the Heart." *Heart,* Vol. 88, No. 5, November 2002, p. 441.

67. Mussolino M. E., et al. "Depression and Bone Mineral Density in Young Adults: Results from NHANES III." *Psychosomatic Medicine,* Vol. 66, No. 4, July–August 2004, 533–537.

68. Tucker, Miriam. "History of Depression Predicts Physical Problems in Women: Current Depression Not Required." *Family Practice News,* Vol. 34, No. 12, June 15, 2004, p. 46(1).

69. Jonas, B. S., and A. C. Looker. "More College Students Seeking MH Services." *Mental Health Weekly,* Vol. 14, No. 13, March 29, 2004, p. 7(1).

70. Goode, Eric. "More in College Seek Help for Psychological Problems." *New York Times,* February 3, 2003, p. A11.

71. Benton, Sherry, et al. "Changes in Counseling Center Client Problems Across 13 Years." *Professional Psychology: Research and Practice,* Vol. 34, No. 1, January 2003, p. 66.

72. "Depression Is Up Among College Students." *The Brown University Child and Adolescent Behavior Letter,* Vol. 21, No. 1, January 2005, p. 2.

73. Bray, Steven, and Heidi Born. "Transition to University and Vigorous Physical Activity: Implications for Health and Psychological Well-Being." *Journal of American College Health,* Vol. 52, No. 4, January–February 2004, p. 181.

74. Spence, S. H., et al. "Mother's Depression in Early Childhood Increases the Risk of Adolescent Anxiety and Depression." *Evidence-Based Mental Health,* Vol. 6, No. 1, February 2003, p. 15.

75. Lenz, Brenda. "Tobacco, Depression, and Lifestyle Choices in the Pivotal Early College Years." *Journal of American College Health,* Vol. 52, No. 5, March–April 2004, p. 213.

76. McChargue, Dennis, et al. "Attachment and Depression Differentially Influence Nicotine Dependence among Male and Female Undergraduates: A Preliminary Study." *Journal of American College Health,* Vol. 53, No. 1, July–August 2004, p. 5.

77. Frankenberger, Kristi, et al. "Effects of Information on College Students' Perceptions of Antidepressant Medication." *Journal of American College Health,* Vol. 53, No. 1, July–August 2004, p. 35.

Chapter 8

1. Panel on Micronutrients, Subcommittees on Upper Reference Levels of Nutrients and Interpretation and Uses of Dietary Reference Intakes, and the Standing Committee on the Scientific Evaluation of Dietary Reference Intakes. *Dietary Reference Intakes for Energy, Carbohydrates, Fiber, Fat, Protein and Amino Acids.* Washington, DC: National Academy of Sciences Press, 2002.

2. Grandjean, Ann, et al. "The Effect on Hydration of Two Diets, One with and One without Plain Water." *Journal of the American College of Nutrition,* Vol. 22, April 2003, p. 165.

3. Gross, Lee, et al. "Increased Consumption of Refined Carbohydrates and the Epidemic of Type 2 Diabetes in the United States: An Ecologic Assessment." *American Journal of Clinical Nutrition,* Vol. 79, 2004, pp. 774–779.

4. *Dietary Guidelines for Americans 2005,* U.S. Department of Health and Human Services (USDHHS), U.S. Department of Agriculture (USDA), www.healthierus .gov/dietaryguidelines.

5. Harder, B. "Wholesome Grains: Insulin Effects May Explain Healthful Diet." *Science News,* Vol. 161, No. 20, May 18, 2002, p. 308.

6. Gannon, Mary. "Diet vs. Diet. To 'Low-Carb' or Not to 'Low-Carb.'" *Diabetes Forecast,* Vol. 56, No. 12, December 2003, p. 74.

7. Buchholz, Andrea, and Dale Schoeller. "Is a Calorie a Calorie?" *American Journal of Clinical Nutrition,* Vol. 79, No. 5, May 2004, p. 899S.

8. Stern, L., et al. "The Effects of Low-Carbohydrate Versus Conventional Weight Loss Diets in Severely Obese Adults: One-Year Follow-up of a Randomized Trial." *Annals of Internal Medicine,* Vol. 140, No. 10, May 18, 2004, pp. 778–785.

9. University of Sydney, Australia, Glycemic Index Testing Service, Human Nutrition Unit, www.glycemicindex.com.

10. Mozaffarian, Dariush, et al. "Cereal, Fruit, and Vegetable Fiber Intake and the Risk of Cardiovascular Disease in Elderly Individuals." *Journal of the American Medical Association,* Vol. 289, No. 13, April 2, 2003, p. 1659.

11. Liu, Simin. "Whole-Grain Foods, Dietary Fiber, and Type 2 Diabetes: Searching for a Kernel of Truth." *American Journal of Clinical Nutrition,* Vol. 77, 2003, pp. 527–529.

12. Panel on Micronutrients, Subcommittees on Upper Reference Levels of Nutrients and Interpretation and Uses of Dietary Reference Intakes, and the Standing Committee on the Scientific Evaluation of Dietary Reference Intakes. *Dietary Reference Intakes for Energy, Carbohydrates, Fiber, Fat, Protein and Amino Acids.*

13. "Position of the American Dietetic Association: Health Implications of Dietary Fiber." *Journal of the American Dietetic Association,* Vol. 102, No. 7, July 2002, p. 993.

14. German, J. B., and C. J. Dillard. "Saturated Fats: What Dietary Intake?" *American Journal of Clinical Nutrition,* Vol. 80, No. 3, September 2004, p. 550.

15. Erkkila, Arja, et al. "Fish Intake is Associated with a Reduced Progression of Coronary Artery Atherosclerosis in Postmenopausal Women with Coronary Artery Disease." *Journal of Clinical Nutrition,* Vol. 80, No. 3, September 2004, p. 626.

16. McKenna, Dolores, et al. "Intake of Omega-3 Polyunsaturated Fatty Acids Among College-Age Women." *Topics in Clinical Nutrition,* Vol. 19, No. 12, April–June 2004, p. 107(10).

17. *Dietary Guidelines for Americans 2005,* USDHHS, USDA. *Report of the Dietary Guidelines Advisory Committee on the Dietary Guidelines for Americans, 2005.*

18. Stear, Samantha, et al. "Effect of a Calcium and Exercise Intervention on the Bone Mineral Status of 16–18 Year-Old Adolescent Girls." *American Journal of Clinical Nutrition,* Vol. 77, No. 4, April 2003, p. 985.

19. Zemel, Michael. "Role of Calcium and Dairy Products in Energy Partitioning and Weight Management." *American Journal of Clinical Nutrition,* Vol. 79, No. 5, May 2004, p. 907S.

20. "African-American Health and Dairy Foods." *Journal of the American Dietetic Association,* Vol. 104, No. 3, March 2004, p. 500a.

21. *Dietary Guidelines for Americans 2005,* USDHHS, USDA.

22. Keinan-Bok, Lital, et al. "Dietary Phytoestrogens and Breast Cancer Risk." *American Journal of Clinical Nutrition,* Vol. 79, 2004, p. 282.

23. Radimer, K., et al. "Dietary Supplement Use by US Adults: Data from the National Health and Nutrition Examination Survey, 1999–2000." *American Journal of Epidemiology,* Vol. 160, No. 4, August 15, 2004, p. 339.

24. Brooks, George, et al. "Chronicle of the Institute of Medicine Physical Activity Recommendation: How a Physical Activity Recommendation Came to Be Among Dietary Recommendations." *American Journal of Clinical Nutrition,* Vol. 79, No. 5, May 2004, p. 921S.

25. Djoussé, Luc, et al. "Fruit and Vegetable Consumption and LDL Cholesterol: The National Heart, Lung, and Blood Institute Family Heart Study." *American Journal of Clinical Nutrition,* Vol. 79, No. 2, February 2004, p. 213.

26. Slattery, Martha, et al. "Plant Foods, Fiber, and Rectal Cancer." *American Journal of Clinical Nutrition,* Vol. 79, No. 2, February 2004, p. 274.

27. Moorman, P. G., and P. D. Terry. "Consumption of Dairy Products and the Risk of Breast Cancer: A Review of the Literature." *American Journal of Clinical Nutrition,* Vol. 80, 2004, p. 5.

28. Schulze, M. B., et al. "Sugar-Sweetened Beverages, Weight Gain, and Incidence of Type 2 Diabetes in Young and Middle-Aged Women." *Journal of the American Medical Association,* Vol. 292, No. 8, August 25, 2004, p. 927.

29. "Freshman College Student Dining Habits." *Food Service Director,* Vol. 15, No. 3, March 15, 2002, p. 1.

30. "Nutrition Knowledge of Collegiate Athletes." *Nutrition Research Newsletter,* Vol. 21, No. 4, April 2002, p. 3.

31. Gray, L. E., et al. "Assessment of Dietary Fiber Intake Among University Students." *Journal of the American Dietetic Association,* Vol. 104, No. 8, August 2004, p. A26.

32. *Dietary Guidelines for Americans 2005,* USDHHS, USDA.

33. Ibid.

34. Schlosser, Eric, *Fast Food Nation.* New York: Simon & Schuster, 2001.

35. Tanja, V. E. Kral, et al. "Combined Effects of Energy Density and Portion Size on Energy Intake in Women." *American Journal of Clinical Nutrition,* October 2004, Vol. 79, No. 6, p. 962.

36. Partnership for Food Safety, www .fightbac.org.

Chapter 9

1. Fontaine, K. R., et al. "Years of Life Lost Due to Obesity." *Journal of the American Medical Association,* Vol. 289, No. 2, April 9, 2003, p. 183.

2. Landers, Susan, "Policy-makers Take Aim at Obesity Rates." *American Medical News,* www.amednews.com, July 19, 2004.

3. Goel, Mita Sanghavi, et al. "Obesity Among U.S. Immigrant Subgroups by Duration of Residence." *Journal of the American Medical Association,* Vol. 292, No. 23, December 13, 2004, p. 2860.

4. "Global Strategy on Diet, Physical Activity and Health." World Health Organization, www.who.int/dietphysicalactivity/ publications/facts/obesity/en/.

5. Wald, Nicholas, and Walter Willett. "Reversing the Obesity Epidemic." *Lancet,* Vol. 364, July 10, 2004, p. 1040.

6. American Obesity Association, www .obesity.org.

7. Goel et al. "Obesity Among U.S. Immigrant Subgroups by Duration of Residence."

8. *Preventing Childhood Obesity: Health in the Balance (2005).* Washington, DC: Institute of Medicine, 2005.

9. National Center for Health Statistics, www.hhs.gov.

10. Ludwig, David, and S. Gortmaker. "Programming Obesity in Childhood." *Lancet,* Vol. 364, No. 9430, July 17, 2004, p. 226.

11. "State Efforts to Control Obesity." University of Baltimore, www.ubalt.edu/ experts/obesity/index.html.

12. Prince, J. R. "Why All the Fuss About Portion Size? Designing the New American Plate." *Nutrition Today,* Vol. 39, No. 2, March 2004, p. 59.

13. Pereira, M. A., et al. "Fast-food Habits, Weight Gain, and Insulin Resistance (the CARDIA study): 15-year Prospective Analysis." *Lancet,* Vol. 365, No. 9453, January 1, 2005, pp. 36–42.

14. Bray, Steven, and Heidi Born. "Transition to University and Vigorous Physical Activity: Implications for Health and Psychological Well-Being." *Journal of American College Health,* Vol. 52, No. 4, January–February 2004, p. 181.

15. Hu, Frank, et al. "Television Watching and Other Sedentary Behaviors in Relation to Risk of Obesity and Type 2 Diabetes Mellitus in Women." *Journal of American Medical Association,* Vol. 289, No. 14, April 9, 2003, p. 1785.

16. Pereira, Mark. Presentation, American Heart Association, Miami Beach, FL, February 2003.

17. Frank, L. D., et al. "Obesity Relationships with Community Design, Physical Activity, and Time Spent in Cars." *American Journal of Preventive Medicine,* Vol. 27, No. 2, August 2004, p. 87.

18. Health and Human Services Press Office. "Citing Dangerous Increase in Deaths, HHS Launches New Strategies Against Overweight Epidemic."

19. Whitaker, R. C. "Predicting Preschooler Obesity at Birth: The Role of Maternal Obesity in Early Pregnancy." *Pediatrics,* Vol. 114, No. 1, July 2004, p. 29.

20. Ludwig, David, and S. Gortmaker. "Programming Obesity in Childhood."

21. Elliott, M. A., et al. "Pediatric Obesity Prevention and Management." *Minerva Pediatrics,* Vol. 56, No. 3, June 2004, p. 265.

22. Delrue, M., and J. Michaud. "Fat Chance: Genetic Syndromes with Obesity." *Clinical Genetics,* Vol. 66, No. 2, August 2004, p. 83.

23. Huang, Terry, et al. "Overweight and Components of the Metabolic Syndrome in College Students." *Diabetes Care,* Vol. 27, No. 12, December 2004, p. 3000.

24. Graham, Melody, and Amy Jones. "Freshman 15: Valid Theory or Harmful Myth?" *Journal of American College Health,* Vol. 50, No. 4, January 2002, p. 171.

25. Lakdawalla, Darius, et al. "Are the Young Becoming More Disabled?" *Health Affairs,* Vol. 23, No. 1, January–February 2004, p. 168.

26. Moreira-Andres, M. N., et al. "Comparison of Anthropometric Parameters as Predictors of Serum Lipids in Premenopausal Women." *Journal of Endrocrinology Investigation,* Vol. 27, No. 4, April 2004, p. 340.

27. Deen, Darwin. "Metabolic Syndrome: Time for Action." *American Family Physician,* Vol. 69, No. 2, June 15, 2004, p. 2875.

28. U.S. Preventive Services Task Force (USP-STF), www.ahrq.gov/clinic/uspstfix.htm.

29. "More Evidence on the Cost of Obesity." *Occupational Health Management,* Vol. 15, No. 2, February 2004, p. 19.

30. Health and Human Services Press Office. "HHS Announces Revised Medicare Obesity Coverage Policy: Policy Opens Door to Coverage Based on Evidence," July 15, 2004.

31. "Researchers Question Relevance of Weight Gain on Race." *Obesity, Fitness & Wellness Week,* July 17, 2004, p. 7.

32. Taylor, Eric, et al. "Obesity, Weight Gain, and the Risk of Kidney Stones." *Journal of the American Medical Association,* Vol. 293, No. 4, January 26, 2005, p. 459.

33. Klein, Samuel, et al. "Weight Management Through Lifestyle Modification for the Prevention and Management of Type 2 Diabetes: Rationale and Strategies." *Diabetes Care,* Vol. 27, No. 8, 2004, pp. 2067–2073.

34. Calle, Eugenia, et al. "Overweight, Obesity, and Mortality from Cancer in a Prospectively Studied Cohort of U.S. Adults." *New England Journal of Medicine,* Vol. 348, No. 17, April 24, 2003, p. 1625.

35. Ibid.

36. Lahmann, P. H., et al. "Breast Cancer Risk in Overweight Postmenopausal Women." *Cancer Epidemiol. Biomarkers Prev.,* Vol. 15, No. 8, August 2004, p. 1414.

37. Vorona, Robert, et al. "Overweight and Obese Patients in a Primary Care Population Report Less Sleep than Patients with a Normal Body Mass Index." *Archives of Internal Medicine,* Vol. 165, No. 1, January 10, 2005, p. 25.

38. Flegal, Katherine, et al. "Excess Deaths Associated with Underweight, Overweight, and Obesity." *Journal of the American Medical Association,* Vol. 293, No. 15, April 20, 2005, p. 1861.

39. Gregg, Edward, et al. "Secular Trends in Cardiovascualr Disease Risk Factors According to Body Mass Index in U.S. Adults." *Journal of the American Medical Association,* Vol. 293, No. 15, April 20, 2005, p. 1868.

40. Mark, David. "Deaths Attributable to Obesity." *Journal of the American Medical Association,* Vol. 293, No. 15, April 20, 2005, p. 1918.

41. Johnston E., et al. "The Relation of Body Mass Index to Depressive Symptoms." *Canadian Journal of Public Health,* Vol. 95, No. 3, May–June 2004, p. 179.

42. Teixeira, P. J., et al. "Pretreatment Predictors of Attrition and Successful Weight Management in Women." *International Journal of Obesity Related Metabolic Disorders,* July 20, 2004.

43. Taylor, W. C. "Readiness to Change Physical Activity and Dietary Practices and Willingness to Consult Healthcare Providers." *Health Research Policy Systems,* Vol. 2, No. 1, June 2004, p. 2.

44. Hensrud, D. D. "Tackling Obesity in a 15-minute Office Visit: Physicians Can Start Patients on an Effective Weight-Loss Program, Despite Time Constraints." *Postgraduate Medicine,* Vol. 115, No. 1, January 2004, p. 59.

45. Huang, J., et al. "Physicians' Weight Loss Counseling in Two Public Hospital Primary Care Clinics." *Academic Medicine,* Vol. 79, No. 2, February 2004, pp. 156–161.

46. *Dietary Guidelines for Americans 2005,* U.S. Department of Health and Human Services, U.S. Department of Agriculture 2005, www.healthierus.gov/dietaryguidelines.

47. American Obesity Association. www.obesity.org.

48. Klein, "Weight Management Through Lifestyle Modification for the Prevention and Management of Type 2 Diabetes: Rationale and Strategies."

49. Tsai, Adam, and Thomas Wadden. "Systematic Review: An Evaluation of Major Commercial Weight Loss Programs in the United States." *Annals of Internal Medicine,* Vol. 142, No. 1, January 4, 2005, p. 56.

50. McTigue, Kathleen, et al. "Screening and Interventions for Obesity in Adults: Summary of the Evidence for the U.S. Preventive Services Task Force." *Annals,* Vol. 139, 2003, p. 930.

51. Dansinger, Michael, et al. "Comparison of the Atkins, Ornish, Weight Watchers, and Zone Diets for Weight Loss and Heart Disease Risk Reduction: A Randomized Trial." *Journal of the American Medical Association,* Vol. 293, No. 1, January 5, 2005, p. 43.

52. Tsai and Wadden, "Systematic Review."

53. Eckel, Robert. "The Dietary Approach to Obesity." *Journal of the American Medical Association,* Vol. 293, No. 1, January 5, 2005, p. 96.

54. Yancy, W. S., et al. "A Low-Carbohydrate, Ketogenic Diet Versus a Low-Fat Diet to Treat Obesity and Hyperlipidemia: A Randomized, Controlled Trial." *Annals of Internal Medicine,* Vol. 140, No. 10, May 18, 2004, p. 769.

55. Stern, Linda, et al. "The Effects of Low-Carbohydrate versus Conventional Weight Loss Diets in Severely Obese Adults: One-Year Follow-up of a Randomized Trial." *Annals of Internal Medicine,* Vol. 140, No. 10, May, 18, 2004, p. 778.

56. "The Skinny on Popular Diets." *Harvard Heart Letter,* February 2003, p. 1.

57. Willett, Walt. "Reduced-Carbohydrate Diets: No Roll in Weight Management?" *Annals of Internal Medicine,* Vol. 140, No. 10, May 18, 2004, p. 836.

58. Levine, James, et al. "Interindividual Variation in Posture Allocation: Possible Role in Human Obesity." *Science,* Vol. 307, No. 5709, January 28, 2005, p. 584.

59. Ibid.

60. McLaren, L., and L. Gauvin. "The Cumulative Impact of Being Overweight on Women's Body Esteem: A Preliminary Study." *Eating and Weight Disorders,* Vol. 7, No. 4, December 2002, p. 324.

61. Helmering, Doris, and Dianne Hales. *Think Thin, Be Thin.* New York: Broadway Books, 2005.

62. White, M. A., et al. "Mediators of Weight Loss in a Family-Based Intervention Presented over the Internet." *Obesity Research,* Vol. 12, No. 7, July 2004, p. 1050.

63. Womble, L. G., et al. "A Randomized Controlled Trial of a Commercial Internet Weight Loss Program." *Obesity Research,* Vol. 12, 2004, p. 1011.

64. National Weight Control Registry, www.lifespan.org/services/bmed/wt_loss/nwcr/.

65. White, M. A., et al. "Gender, Race, and Obesity-Related Quality of Life at Extreme Levels of Obesity." *Obesity Research,* Vol. 12, No. 6, June 2004, p. 949.

66. American Obesity Association, www.obesity.org.

67. Buchwald, Henry, et al. "Bariatric Surgery." *Journal of the American Medical Association,* Vol. 292, No. 14, October 13, 2004, p. 1724.

68. Gutzwiller, Joeanne, et al. "Eating Dysfunctions in College Women: The Roles of Depression and Attachment to Fathers." *Journal of American College Health,* Vol. 52, No. 1, July–August 2003, p. 27.

69. O'Dea, Jennifer, and Suzanne Abraham. "Eating and Exercise Disorders in Young College Men." *Journal of American College Health,* Vol. 50, No. 4, May 2002, p. 273.

70. Hales, Robert, and Stuart Yudofsky (eds.). *Textbook of Clinical Psychiatry,* 4th ed. Washington, DC: American Psychiatric Publ., 2003, p. 975.

71. Cummings, Sue, et al. "Position of the American Dietetic Association: Weight Management." *Journal of the American Dietetic Association,* Vol. 102, No. 8, August 2002, pp. 11, 1145.

Chapter 10

1. "The Bigger Worry: Heart Disease or Cancer?" *Harvard Health Letter,* February 2005.

2. Daviglus, Martha, et al. "Favorable Cardiovascular Risk Profile in Young Women and Long-term Risk of Cardiovascular and All-Cause Mortality." *Journal of the American Medical Association,* Vol. 292, No. 13, October 6, 2004, p. 1588.

3. "Young Adults Who Maintain Their Weight, Even if Overweight, Have Lower Risk Factor Levels for Heart Disease in Early Middle Age." *NIH News,* November 8, 2004.

4. Collins, Kristina, et al. "Heart Disease Awareness Among College Students." *Journal of Community Health,* Vol. 29, No. 5, October 2004, p. 405.

5. Green, John, et al. "Heart Disease Risk Perception in College Men and Women." *Journal of American College Health,* Vol. 51, No. 5, March 2003, p. 207.

6. Spencer, Leslie. "Results of a Heart Disease Risk-Factor Screening Among Traditional College Students." *Journal of American College Health,* Vol. 50, No. 6, May 2002, p. 291.

7. Gordon, Neil, et al. "Effectiveness of Therapeutic Lifestyle Changes in Patients with Hypertension, Hyperlipidemia, and/or Hyperglycemia." *American Journal of Cardiology,* Vol. 94, No. 12, December 15, 2004, p. 1558.

8. *Dietary Guidelines for Americans 2005.* U.S. Department of Health and Human Services, U.S. Department of Agriculture, www.healthierus.gov/dietaryguidelines

9. Myers, Jonathan. "Exercise and Cardiovascular Health." *Circulation,* Vol. 107, January 7–14, 2003, p. 2.

10. Marcovitch, Harvey. "Light Exercise Doesn't Protect Against Heart Disease." *British Medical Journal,* Vol. 327, No. 7407, July 19, 2003, p. 125.

11. Jensen, M. K., et al. "Intakes of Whole Grains, Bran, and Germ and the Risk of Coronary Heart Disease in Men." *American Journal of Clinical Nutrition,* Vol. 80, No. 6, December 2004, p. 1492.

12. Dallongeville, Jean, et al. "Fish Consumption Is Associated With Lower Heart Rates." *Circulation,* Vol. 108, 2003, pp. 820–825.

13. U.S. Preventive Services Task Force. *Routine Vitamin Supplementation to Prevent Cancer and Cardiovascular Disease.* Rockville, MD: Agency for Healthcare Research and Quality, 2003.

14. "Declining Prevalence of No Known Major Risk Factors for Heart Disease and Stroke Among Adults." *Journal of the American Medical Association,* Vol. 291, No. 17, May 5, 2004, p. 2069.

15. "Heart Disease and Stroke Statistics—2004." American Heart Association, 2004.

16. Wessel, Timothy, et al. "Relationship of Physical Fitness vs. Body Mass Index with Coronary Artery Disease and Cardiovascular Events in Women." *Journal of the American Medical Association,* Vol. 292, No. 10, September 8, 2004, p. 1179.

17. Blair, Steven, and Tim Church. "The Fitness, Obesity, and Health Equation." *Journal of the American Medical Association,* Vol. 292, No. 10, September 8, 2004, p. 1232.

18. Bauer, Jeff. "Intensity of Exercise Is What Counts When It Comes to Reducing Heart Disease Risk." *RN,* Vol. 66, No. 1, January 2003, p. 97.

19. Mitka, Mike. "Secondhand Smoke an Acute Heart Risk?" *Journal of the American Medical Association,* Vol. 291, No. 22, June 9, 2004, p. 3690.

20. Critchley, Julia, and Simon Capewell. "Mortality Risk Reduction Associated with Smoking Cessation in Patients with Coronary Artery Disease." *Journal of the American Medical Association,* Vol. 290, No. 1, July 2, 2003, p. 86.

21. Deen, Darwin. "Metabolic Syndrome: What Is It and What Can I Do About It?" *American Family Physician,* Vol. 69, No. 12, June 2004, p. 2887.

22. "Young Adults Who Maintain Their Weight." *NIH News.*

23. Huang, Terry, et al. "Overweight and Components of the Metabolic Syndrome in College Students." *Diabetes Care,* Vol. 27, No. 12, December 2004, p. 3000.

24. MayoClinic.com staff, "Metabolic Syndrome," www.mayoclinic.com.

25. Mitka, Mike. "Depression-Heart Disease Link Probed." *Journal of the American Medical Association,* Vol. 293, No. 3, January 19, 2005, p. 283.

26. Fitzgerald, Garret, et al. "Vioxx." *Circulation,* January 17, 2005.

27. Hampton, Tracy. "Experts Point to Lessons Learned from Controversy over Rofecoxib Safety." *Journal of the American Medical Association,* Vol. 293, No. 3, January 19, 2005, p. 413.

28. Jha, Ashish, et al. "Differences in Medical Care and Disease Outcomes Among Black and White Women with Heart Disease." *Circulation,* Vol. 108, No. 9, September 2003, p. 1089.

29. Forman, John, et al. "Folate Intake and the Risk of Incident Hypertension Among US Women." *Journal of the American Medical Association,* Vol. 293, No. 3, January 19, 2005, p. 320.

30. Muntner, Paul, et al., "Trends in Blood Pressure among Children and Adolescents." *Journal of the American Medical Association,* Vol. 291, No. 17, May 5, 2004, p. 2107.

31. Robertson, Rose Marie. Personal interview.

32. Chobanian, A. V., et al. "Seventh Report of the Joint National Committee on Prevention, Detection, Evaluation, and Treatment of High Blood Pressure." *Hypertension,* Vol. 42, No. 6, December 2003, p. 1206.

33. Forman, et al. "Folate Intake and the Risk of Incident Hypertension among US Women."

34. Grundy, Scott, et al. "Implications of Recent Clinical Trials for the National Cholesterol Education Program Adult Treatment Panel III Guidelines." *Circulation,* Vol. 110, 2004, p. 227; see also www.circulationaha.org.

35. Ridker, Paul, et al. "C-Reactive Protein Levels and Outcomes After Statin Therapy." *New England Journal of Medicine,* Vol. 352, No. 1, January 6, 2005, pp. 29–38.

36. Nissen, Steven, et al. "Statin Therapy, LDL Cholesterol, C-Reactive Protein, and Coronary Artery Disease." *New England Journal of Medicine,* Vol. 352, No. 1, January 6, 2005, pp. 29–38.

37. Ridker, et al. "C-Reactive Protein Levels and Outcomes After Statin Therapy."

38. Ringold, Sarah. "Cardiopulmonary Resuscitation." *Journal of the American Medical Association,* Vol. 293, No. 3, January 19, 2005, 388.

39. Women's Health Initiative Steering Committee. "Effects of Conjugated Equine Estrogen in Postmenopausal Women with Hysterectomy." *Journal of the American Medical Association,* Vol. 291, No. 14, April 14, 2004, p. 1701.

40. White, Halina, et al. "Northern Manhattan Study Interim Report." International Stroke Conference, January 2005.

Chapter 11

1. *Cancer Facts & Figures 2005.* Atlanta, GA: American Cancer Society, 2005, www.cancer.org.

2. Mitka, Mike. "New Cancer Figures Released." *Journal of the American Medical Association,* Vol. 291, No. 5, February 4, 2004, p. 552.

3. Kaklamani, Virginia. "TGFBR1*6A and Cancer Risk." *Journal of Clinical Oncology,* Vol. 21, No. 17, September 1, 2003, p. 3236.

4. "Cancer in Racial and Ethnic Minorities." *Cancer Facts & Figures 2005.* Atlanta, GA: American Cancer Society, 2005.

5. Calle, Eugenia, et al. "Overweight, Obesity, and Mortality from Cancer in a Prospectively Studied Cohort of U.S. Adults." *New England Journal of Medicine,* Vol. 348, No. 17, April 24, 2003, p. 1625.

6. "Cancers Linked to Infectious Diseases." *Cancer Facts & Figures 2005.* Atlanta, GA: American Cancer Society, 2005.

7. Willett, Walter. "Diet and Cancer." *Journal of American Medical Association,* Vol. 293, No. 2, January 12, 2005, p. 233.

8. van Gils, C. H., et al. "Consumption of Vegetables and Fruits and Risk of Breast Cancer." *Journal of American Medical Association,* Vol. 293, No. 2, January 12, 2005, p. 183.

9. Chao, A., et al. "Meat Consumption and Risk of Colorectal Cancer." *Journal of American Medical Association,* Vol. 293, No. 2, January 12, 2005, p. 172.

10. Poocharoen, Varee, and Clay Cockerell. "The War Against Skin Cancer." *Archives of Dermatology,* Vol. 141, April 2004, http://archderm.ama-assn.org.

11. Lamanna, Lenore. "College Students' Knowledge and Attitudes About Cancer and Perceived Risks of Developing Skin Cancer." *Dermatology Nursing,* Vol. 17, No. 2, April 2004, p. 161.

12. Mahler, Heike, et al. "Effects of UV Photographs, Photoaging Information, and Use of Sunless Tanning Lotion on Sun Protection." *Archives of Dermatology,* Vol. 141, March 2005, p. 373, http://archderm.ama-assn.org.

13. Ford, Leslie. Personal interview.

14. "Drinking Increases Risk." *Women's Health Weekly,* February 6, 2003, p. 2.

15. Li, Christopher, et al. "Relationship Between Long Durations and Different Regimens of Hormone Therapy and Risk of Breast Cancer." *Journal of the American Medical Association,* Vol. 289, No. 24, June 25, 2003, p. 3254.

16. Smith, R. A. "Screening Mammography." *Ca—A Cancer Journal for Clinicians,* Vol. 53, No. 3, 2003, p. 141.

17. "American Cancer Society Issues Updated Breast Cancer Screening Guidelines." News Release, May 15, 2003.

18. U.S. Multisociety Task Force on Colorectal Cancer. "Screening Guidelines for Colorectal Cancer." *Gastroenterology,* Vol. 124, February 2003, p. 544.

19. Nelson, William. "Prostate Cancer." *New England Journal of Medicine,* Vol. 349, No. 4, July 24, 2003, p. 366.

20. Strayer, Scott. "Vasectomy Not a Risk Factor for Prostate Cancer." *Journal of Family Practice,* Vol. 51, No. 9, September 2002, p. 791.

21. Johansson, Jan-Erik, et al. "Natural History of Early, Localized Prostate Cancer." *Journal of the American Medical Association,* Vol. 291, No. 22, June 9, 2004, p. 2713.

22. *Cancer Facts & Figures 2005.*

23. Cohen, S., et al. "Emotional Style and Susceptibility to the Common Cold." *Psychosomatic Medicine,* Vol. 65, No. 4, July–August, 2003, p. 652.

24. Barrett, B. P., et al. "Treatment of the Common Cold with Unrefined Echinacea. A Randomized, Double-Blind, Placebo-Controlled Trial." *American Family Physician,* Vol. 67, No. 7, April 1, 2003, p. 1589.

25. Kamath, Arati, et al. "Antigens in Tea-Beverage Prime Human V2V2 T Cells *In Vitro* and *In Vivo* for Memory and Non-memory Antibacterial Cytokine Responses." Proceedings of the National Academy of the Sciences, Vol. 100, No. 10, May 13, 2003, p. 6009.

26. Thompson, William, et al. "Influenza-Associated Hospitalizations in the United States." *Journal of the American*

Medical Association, Vol. 292, No. 11, September 15, 2004, p. 1333.

27. "CDC Recommendations to Prevent Influenza." *Journal of the American Medical Association,* Vol. 291, No. 1, January 7, 2004, p. 34.

28. Tsuang, Wayne, et al. "Influenza-like Symptoms in the College Dormitory Environment." *Journal of Environmental Health,* Vol. 66, No. 8, April 2004, p. 39.

29. "Meningococcal Disease: It's Not Just a College Problem." *Contemporary Pediatrics,* Vol. 22, No. 1, January 2005, p. 51.

30. Bruce, Michael, et al. "Risk Factors for Meningococcal Disease in College Students." *Journal of the American Medical Association,* Vol. 286, No. 6, August 8, 2001, p. 286.

31. "Meningococcal Disease: It's Not Just a College Problem."

32. Turner, James. "New Meningococcal Vaccine Recommendations under Consideration." *Journal of American College Health,* Vol. 53, No. 2, September–October 2004, p. 89.

33. Kuenzi, Lana. "Meningococcal Education: More Than Just a Vaccine." *Journal of American College Health,* Vol. 53, No. 2, September–October 2004, p. 93.

34. "Hepatitis C Fact Sheet." CDC, www.cdc.gov/hepatitis.

35. Torpy, Janet. "Body Piercing." *Journal of the American Medical Association,* Vol. 291, No. 8, February 24, 2004, p. 1024.

36. Spiegel, Allen. Personal interview.

37. Sherwin, Robert, Personal interview.

38. Parmet, Sharon. "Weight Gain and Diabetes." *Journal of the American Medical Association,* Vol. 292, No. 8, August 23, 2004, p. 998.

Chapter 12

1. Arnold, Matthew. "83 Million Consumers Go Online First for Health Info." *Medical Marketing & Media,* Vol. 39, No. 2, February 2004, p. 22.

2. Bard, Mark. Personal interview.

3. Escoffery, Cam, et al. "Internet Use for Health Information among College Students." *Journal of American College Health,* Vol. 53, No. 4, January–February 2004, p, 183.

4. Baker, Laurence, et al. "Use of the Internet and E-mail for Health Care Information." *Journal of the American Medical Association,* Vol. 289, No. 18, May 14, 2003, p. 2400.

5. Hales, Dianne. "The Best Medical Help Online." *Parade,* September 19, 2004, p. 9.

6. Hales, Dianne. "Take Your Meds—The Right Way." *Parade,* February 13, 2005.

7. *NCCAM,* http://nccam.nih.gov.

8. Barnes, P., E. Powell-Griner, K. McFann, and R. Nahin. "Complementary and Alternative Medicine Use Among Adults: United States, 2002." *CDC Advance Data Report #343,* May 27, 2004.

9. Zepf, Bill. "Evidence Basis for Four Commonly Used Herbs." *American Family Physician,* Vol. 67, No. 7, April 1, 2003, p. 1607.

10. Gold, Paul, et al. "The Lowdown on Ginkgo Biloba: This Popular Herbal Supplement May Slightly Improve Your Memory, But You Can Get the Same Effect by Eating a Candy Bar." *Scientific American,* Vol. 288, No. 4, April 2003, p. 86.

11. Rados, Carol. "Ephedra Ban: No Shortage of Reasons." *FDA Consumer Magazine,* March–April 2004.

12. Federal Drug Administration, www.cfsan.fda.gov/%7Edms/ds-warn.html.

13. Cherkin, D. C., et al. "A Review of the Evidence for the Effectiveness, Safety, and Cost of Acupuncture, Massage Therapy, and Spinal Manipulation for Back Pain." *Annals of Internal Medicine,* Vol. 138, No. 11, June 3, 2003, p. 898.

14. "Life Expectancy Improves But Infant Mortality Rate Up in 2002." *Public Health Reports,* Vol. 119, September–October 2004, p. 513.

15. Roizen, Michael. Personal interview.

16. "Healthy Behaviors Are the Foundation of Combating the Aging Process." *Obesity, Fitness & Wellness Week,* September 11, 2004, p. 238.

17. Birge, Stanley. "The WHI and the Brain: What Have We Learned?" *Sexuality, Reproduction & Menopause,* Vol. 2, No. 2, June 2004, p. 71.

18. Nestor, P. J., et al. "Advances in the Early Detection of Alzheimer's Disease." *Nature Medicine,* Supplement, July 10, 2004, p. S34–41.

19. "Osteoporosis Overview." The NIH Osteoporosis and Related Bone Diseases ~ National Resource Center, www.osteo.org.

20. Slovik, David (ed.). *Osteoporosis: A Guide to Prevention and Treatment.* Cambridge, MA: Harvard Medical School, 2005.

21. "Increasing Evidence That Osteoporosis Begins in the Womb." *Medical Letter on the CDC and FDA,* June 29, 2003, p. 32.

Chapter 13

1. Tuomilehto, Jaakko, et al. "Coffee Consumption and Risk of Type 2 Diabetes Mellitus among Middle-aged Finnish Men and Women." *Journal of the American Medical Association,* Vol. 291, No. 10, March 10, 2004, p. 1213.

2. Scott, William H., Jr., et al. "Effects of Caffeine on Performance of Low Intensity Tasks." *Perceptual and Motor Skills,* Vol. 94, No. 2, April 2002, p. 521.

3. "Fetal Alcohol Syndrome Is Still a Threat." *Harvard Mental Health Letter,* September 2004.

4. "Alcohol Consumption and Waist Circumference." *Nutrition Research Newsletter,* Vol. 22, No. 5, May 2003, p. 5.

5. Moore, Alison, et al. "Longitudinal Patterns and Predictors of Alcohol Consumption in the United States." *American Journal of Public Health.* Vol. 95, No. 3, March 2005, p. 458.

6. McCarthy, Carolyn. "Continuity of Binge and Harmful Drinking from Late Adolescence to Early Adulthood." *Pediatrics,* Vol. 114, No. 3, September 2004, p. 714.

7. "Binge Drinking a National problem." *Medical Letter on the CDC & FDA,* May 9, 2004, p. 11.

8. Frieden, Joyce. "Binge Drinking May Be Increasing." *Clinical Psychiatry News,* Vol. 32, No. 5, May 2004, p. 110.

9. Sullivan, Michelle. "Maternal Binge Drinking Tied to Childhood Problems: Risk of Behavior Problems Is 2.5 Times Higher for Bingers' Babies Than for Those Exposed to Less." *Clinical Psychiatry News,* Vol. 32, No. 4, April 2004, p. 74.

10. Foote, Jeffrey, et al. "A National Survey of Alcohol Screening and Referral in College Health Centers." *Journal of American College Health,* Vol. 52, No. 4, January–February 2004, p. 149.

11. Wilson, Gregory, et al. "Athletic Status and Drinking Behavior in College Students: The Influence of Gender and Coping Styles." *Journal of American College Health,* Vol. 52, No. 6, May–June 2004, p. 269.

12. Siebert, Darcy Clay, et al. "Differences in African American and White College Students' Drinking Behaviors: Consequences, Harm Reduction Strategies, and Health Information Sources." *Journal of American College Health,* Vol. 52, No. 3, November–December 2003, p. 123.

13. McKinnon, Sarah, et al. "Increased Risk of Alcohol Abuse Among College Students Living on the U.S.-Mexico Border: Implications for Prevention." *Journal of American College Health,* Vol. 51, No. 4, January 2003, p. 149.

14. Weitzman, Elissa. "Poor Mental Health, Depression, and Associations With Alcohol Consumption, Harm, and Abuse in a National Sample of Young Adults in College." *The Journal of Nervous and Mental Disease,* Vol. 192, No. 4, April 2004, p. 269.

15. Park, Crystal, et al. "The Daily Stress and Coping Process and Alcohol Use Among College Students." *Journal of Studies on Alcohol,* Vol. 65, No. 1, January 2004, p. 126.

16. Vickers, Kristin, et al. "Binge Drinking in Female College Students: The Association of Physical Activity, Weight Concern, and Depressive Symptoms." *Journal of American College Health,* Vol. 53, No. 3, November–December 2004, p. 133.

17. Delva, Jorge, et al. "A Study of the Relationship Between Protective Behaviors

and Drinking Consequences Among Undergraduate College Students." *Journal of American College Health,* Vol. 53, No. 1, July–August 2004, p. 19.

18. Ibid.

19. Mohler-Kuo, M., et al. "Correlates of Rape While Intoxicated in a National Sample of College Women." *Journal of Studies on Alcohol,* Vol. 65, No. 1, February 2004, p. 37.

20. Turner, James, and Jianfen Shu. "Serious Health Consequences Associated with Alcohol Use Among College Students: Demographic and Clinical Characteristics of Patients Seen in an Emergency Department." *Journal of Studies on Alcohol,* Vol. 65, No. 2, March 2004, p. 179(5).

21. Steinman, Kenneth. "College Students' Early Cessation from Episodic Heavy Drinking: Prevalence and Correlates." *Journal of American College Health,* Vol. 51, No. 5, March 2003, p. 197.

22. Mitchell, Rebecca, et al. "Alcohol Policies on College Campuses." *Journal of American College Health,* Vol. 53, No. 4, January–February 2005, p. 149.

23. Foote, et al. "A National Survey of Alcohol Screening and Referral in College Health Centers."

24. Weitzman, Elissa, et al. "Reducing Drinking and Related Harms in College: Evaluation of the 'A Matter of Degree' Program." *American Journal of Preventive Medicine,* Vol. 27, No. 3, October 2004, p. 187.

25. Wechsler, Henry, et al. "Drinking and Driving Among College Students: The Influence of Alcohol-Control Policies." *Journal of American College Health,* Vol. 53, No. 4, January–February 2005, p. 192.

26. Timmerman, M. A., et al. "Do the Designated Drivers of College Students Stay Sober?" *Journal of Safety Research,* Vol. 34, No. 2, 2003, p. 127.

27. Ringold, Sarah. "Alcohol Abuse and Alcoholism." *Journal of the American Medical Association,* Vol. 293, No. 13, April 6, 2005, p. 1694.

28. Johnston, L. D., P. M. O'Malley, J. G. Bachman, and J. E. Schulenberg. "*Cigarette Smoking Among American Teens Continues to Decline, But More Slowly Than in the Past.*" University of Michigan News and Information Services: Ann Arbor, MI, December 21, 2004, www .monitoringthefuture.org.

29. Ramsay, Jim, and Anne Hoffmann. "Smoking Cessation and Relapse Prevention Among Undergraduate Students: A Pilot Demonstration Project." *Journal of American College Health,* Vol. 53, No. 1, July–August 2004, p. 11(8).

30. Patterson, Freda. "Cigarette Smoking Practices Among American College Students: Review and Future Directions." *Journal of American College Health,*

Vol. 52, No. 5, March–April 2004, p. 203(8).

31. Ibid.

32. Ibid.

33. Lenz, Brenda. "Tobacco, Depression, and Lifestyle Choices in the Pivotal Early College Years." *Journal of American College Health,* Vol. 52, No. 5, March–April 2004, p. 213.

34. Ibid.

35. Rigotti, N., et al. "U.S. College Students' Exposure to Tobacco Promotions: Prevalence and Association with Tobacco Use." *American Journal of Public Health,* Vol. 95, No. 138, January 2004.

36. Wechsler, Henry, et al., "College Smoking Policies and Smoking Cessation Programs: Results of a Survey of College Health Center Directors." *Journal of American College Health,* Vol. 49, No. 5, March 2001, p. 205.

37. Bacon, C. G., et al. "Sexual Function in Men Older than 50 years of Age: Results from the Health Professionals Follow-up Study." *Annals of Internal Medicine,* Vol. 139, No. 3, August 5, 2003, p. l22.

38. Centers for Disease Control and Prevention, www.cdc.gov.

39. Ramsey and Hoffmann. "Smoking Cessation and Relapse Prevention Among Undergraduate Students."

40. Ibid.

41. Fiske, Susan. "Sad Facts." *Psychology Today,* March–April 2003, p. 41.

42. United Nations Office on Drugs and Crime. *2004 World Drug Report.* Vienna, Austria: Vienna International Centre, 2004.

43. Johnston, L. D., P. M. O'Malley, J. G. Bachman, and J. E. Schulenberg. *Monitoring the Future National Results on Adolescent Drug Use: Overview of Key Findings, 2004.* Bethesda MD: National Institute on Drug Abuse, 2005.

44. Mohler-Kuo, Mekchun, et al. "Trends in Marijuana and Other Illicit Drug Use among College Students: Results from 4 Harvard School of Public Health College Alcohol Study Surveys: 1993–2001." *Journal of American College Health,* Vol. 52, No. 1, July–August 2003, p. 17.

45. Boyd, C. J., et al. "Ecstasy Use Among College Undergraduates: Gender, Race, and Sexual Identity." *Substance Abuse Treatment,* Vol. 24, No. 3, April 2003, p. 209.

46. McCabe, S. E., et al. "Sexual Identity and Substance Use Among Undergraduate Students." *Substance Abuse,* Vol. 24, No. 2, June 2003, p. 77.

47. Eisenberg, M., and H. Wechsler. "Substance Use Behaviors Among College Students with Same-Sex and Opposite-Sex Experience: Results from a National Study." *Addictive Behaviors,* Vol. 28, No. 6, 2003, p. 899.

48. Engwall, Douglas, et al. "Gambling and Other Risk Behaviors on University Cam-

puses." *Journal of American College Health,* Vol. 52, No. 6, May–June 2004, p. 245.

49. Compton, Wilson, et al. "Prevalence of Marijuana Use Disorders in the United States." *Journal of the American Medical Association,* Vol. 291, No. 10, May 5, 2004, p. 1213.

50. "Reefer Rx: Marijuana as Medicine." *Harvard Health Letter,* September 2004.

51. Yacoubian, George, et al. "Correlates of Ecstasy Use Among Students Surveyed Through the 1997 College Alcohol Study." *Journal of Drug Education,* Vol. 33, No. 1, January 2003, p. 61.

52. Walters, Scott, et al. "The Agony of Ecstasy: Responding to Growing MDMA Use Among College Students." *Journal of American College Health,* Vol. 51, No. 3, November 2002, p. 139.

53. DEA Congressional Testimony by John B. Brown.

54. "Heroin." National Institute on Drug Abuse, www.nida.nih.gov.

55. Wu, L. T., et al. "Inhalant Abuse and Dependence Among Adolescents in the United States." *Journal of the American Academy of Child and Adolescent Psychiatry,* Vol. 43, No. 10, October 2004, p. 1206.

56. Johnston, Lloyd, et al. *Monitoring the Future: National Results on Adolescent Drug Use.* Bethesda, MD: National Institute on Drug Abuse, 2004.

57. Hall, Kristina, et al. "Illicit Use of Prescribed Stimulant Medication Among College Students." *Journal of American College Health,* Vol. 53, No. 4, January–February 2005, p. 167(8).

58. National Institute on Drug Abuse, www .nida.nih.gov.

Chapter 14

1. Centers for Disease Control and Prevention, www.cdc.gov.

2. Eisenman, Russell, and M. L. Dantzker. "Permissiveness and Male vs. Female Privileges in Hispanic College Students: Factor Analysis of a Sex Attitudes Scale." *Journal of Evolutionary Psychology,* Vol. 25, No. 1–2, March 2004, p. 2.

3. Goodson, P., et al. "Defining Abstinence: Views of Directors, Instructors, and Participants in Abstinence-Only-Until-Marriage Programs in Texas." *Journal of School Health,* Vol. 73, No. 3, March 2003, p. 91.

4. National Center for Health Statistics, www.cdc.gov/nchs.

5. "Smarter Sex Survey," www.SmarterSex .org.

6. Netting, N. S., and Matthew Burnett. "Twenty Years of Student Sexual Behavior: Subcultural Adaptations to a Changing Health Environment." *Adolescence,* Vol. 39, No. 153, Spring 2004, p. 19.

7. Johnson, Thomas, and Courtney Stahl. "Sexual Experience Associated with

Participation in Drinking Games." *Journal of General Psychology,* Vol. 131, No. 3, July 2004, p. 304.

8. Apostolopoulos, Y., et al. "HIV-Risk Behaviours of American Spring Break Vacationers: A Case of Situational Disinhibition?" *International Journal of STDs and AIDS,* Vol. 13, No. 11, November 2002, p. 733.

9. Blonna, Richard, and Jean Levitan. *Healthy Sexuality.* Belmont, CA: Wadsworth, 2005.

10. "It's Smart to Carry Condoms but . . . ." *Chain Drug Review,* Vol. 26, No. 13, August 16, 2004, p. 49.

11. Eisenberg, M. E. "The Association of Campus Resources for Gay, Lesbian, and Bisexual Students with College Students' Condom Use." *Journal of American College Health,* Vol. 51, No. 3, November 2002, p. 109.

12. Duncan, C., et al. "Barriers to Safer Sex Practices Among African American College Students." *Journal of National Medical Association,* Vol. 94, No. 11, November 2002, p. 944.

13. Gurman, Tilly, and Dina Borzekowski. "Condom Use Among Latino College Students." *Journal of American College Health,* Vol. 52, No. 4, January–February 2004, p. 169.

14. Tulloch, Heather, et al. "Partner Communication Skills and Condom Use Among College Couples." *Journal of American College Health,* Vol. 52, No. 6, May–June 2004, p. 263.

15. "The Truth About STDs." *SIECUS Fact Sheet,* March 2003.

16. National Center for Health Statistics, www.cdc.gov/nchs.

17. Weinstock, H., et al. "Sexually Transmitted Disease Among American Youth: Incidence and Prevalence Estimates, 2000." *Perspectives on Sexual and Reproductive Health,* Vol. 36, 2004, p. 6.

18. "Check Your Sexually Transmitted Disease Screening: More Young Adults Are at Risk for Chlamydia: One in 25 Young Americans are Infected with Chlamydia, Research Shows." *Contraceptive Technology Update,* Vol. 25, No. 8, August 2004, p. SI.

19. Ibid.

20. Miller, William, et al. "Prevalence of Chlamydial and Gonococcal Infections among Young Adults in the United States." *Journal of the American Medical Association,* Vol. 291, No. 18, May 12, 2004, p. 2229.

21. Golden, Matthew, et al. "Effect of Expedited Treatment of Sex Partners on Recurrent or Persistent Gonorrhea or Chlamydial Infection," *New England Journal of Medicine,* Vol. 352, No. 7, February 17, 2005, p. 676.

22. Weinstock, H., et al., "Sexually Transmitted Disease Among American Youth."

23. "Fluoroquinolone-Resistant Gonorrhea Rates on the Rise in the U.S." *Clinical Infectious Diseases,* Vol. 38, No. 12, June 15, 2004, p. iii(1).

24. Weinstock, H., et al., "Sexually Transmitted Disease Among American Youth."

25. Rosenberg, J. "Age at First Sex and Human Papillomavirus Infection Linked Through Behavioral Factors and Partner's Traits." *Perspectives on Sexual and Reproductive Health,* Vol. 34, No. 3, May–June 2002, p. 171.

26. Weinstock, H., et al., "Sexually Transmitted Disease Among American Youth."

27. "The Global HIV/AIDS Epidemic." *HIV/AIDS Policy Fact Sheet,* Menlo Park, CA: Kaiser Family Foundation, December 2004.

28. Gross, Michael. "When Plagues Don't End." *American Journal of Public Health,* Vol. 93, No. 6, June 1, 2003, p. 861.

29. Beck, A., et al. "Psychosocial Predictors of HIV/STI Risk Behaviours in a Sample of Homosexual Men." *Sexually Transmitted Infections,* Vol. 79, No. 2, April 2003, p. 142(5), www.cdc.gov.

30. Voelker, Rebecca. "Women Shoulder Growing HIV/AIDS Burden." *Journal of the American Medical Association,* Vol. 293, No. 3, January 19, 2005, p. 281.

31. *Morbidity and Mortality Weekly Report,* Vol. 52, 2003, pp. 540–544.

32. Marelich, William, and Tonya Clark. "Human Immunodeficiency Virus (HIV) Testing and False Disclosures in Heterosexual College Students." *Journal of American College Health,* Vol. 53, No. 3, November–December 2004, p. 109.

33. "HIV Testing in the United States." *HIV/AIDS Policy Fact Sheet,* Menlo Park, CA: Kaiser Family Foundation, June 2003.

Chapter 15

1. National Safety Council, www.nsc.org.

2. Villaveces, A. "Association of Alcohol-Related Laws with Deaths Due to Motor Vehicle and Motorcycle Crashes in the United States, 1980–1997." *American Journal of Epidemiology,* Vol. 157, No. 2, January 15, 2003, p. 131.

3. National Highway Traffic Safety Administration, www.nhtsa.dot.gov.

4. "National Safety Council Announces Motor Vehicle Safety Initiative." *Safety Compliance Letter,* No. 2441, May 2004, p. 15.

5. "CAA Reminds All Canadians to Buckle Down to Road Safety. Use Child Car Seats and Vehicle Seat Belts." *Canadian Corporate News,* April 6, 2004, p. NA.

6. Braver, E. R. "Race, Hispanic Origin, and Socioeconomic Status in Relation to Motor Vehicle Occupant Death Rates and Risk Factors Among Adults." *Accident Analysis and Prevention,* Vol. 35, No. 3, May 2003, p. 295.

7. Paschall, M. J. "College Attendance and Risk-Related Driving Behavior in a National Sample of Young Adults." *Journal of Studies of Alcohol,* Vol. 64, No. 1, January 2003, p. 43.

8. "Young Americans Still Shunning Seat Belts." *Health and Medicine Week,* August 25, 2003, p. 638.

9. Cummings, Peter, and Frederick Rivara. "Car Occupant Death According to Restraint Use of Other Occupants." *Journal of the American Medical Association,* Vol. 291, No. 3, January 21, 2004, p. 343.

10. "Risk of Death in Car Crashes Reduced If All Occupants Wear Seat Belts." *Health & Medicine Week,* February 2, 2004, p. 408.

11. Ferguson, Susan. "The Blue Ribbon Panel on Depowered and Advanced Airbags—Status Report on Airbag Performance." *Annual Proceedings/Association for the Advancement of Automotive Medicine,* Vol. 47, September 2003, p. 79.

12. Nerenberg, Arnold. Personal interview.

13. Strayer, David, et al. "Cell Phone Use Can Lead to Inattention Blindness Behind the Wheel." *Injury Insight,* February–March 2003.

14. Coffman S. "Bicycle Injuries and Safety Helmets in Children. Review of Research." *Orthopedic Nursing,* Vol. 22, No. 1, January–February 2003, p. 9.

15. Fisher, Bonnie, et al. *The Sexual Victimization of College Women.* Washington, DC: U.S. Department of Justice, December 2000.

16. Isely, P. J. "Sexual Assault of Men: College Age Victims." *National Association of Student Personnel Administrators Journal,* Vol. 35, No. 4, pp. 305–317. (Reported at webits3.appstate.edu.)

17. McDonald, Theodore, and Linda Kline. "Perceptions of Appropriate Punishment for Committing Date Rape: Male College Students Recommend Lenient Punishments." *College Student Journal,* Vol. 38, No. 1, March 2004, p. 44.

18. Gregg, Jillian, et al. "Urbanization Effects on Tree Growth in the Vicinity of New York City." *Nature,* Vol. 10, No. 424, July 2003, p. 183.

19. "Renewables Are So Right." *Energy & Environmental Management,* September–October 2004, p. 15.

20. *Second National Report on Human Exposure to Environmental Chemicals.* Atlanta, GA: Centers for Disease Control and Prevention, 2003, www.cdc.gov/exposurereport.

21. "American Radon Scientists Call on EPA to Act on Radon Exposure." *Health and Medicine Week,* June 9, 2003, p. 36.

22. Brown, Ray. "Mold: The New Asbestos?" *Architecture,* Vol. 92, No. 7, July 2003, p. 32.

23. Money, Nicholas. *Carpet Monsters and Killer Spores: A Natural History of Toxic Mold.* London: Oxford University Press, 2004.

24. "U.N. Organization Warns That Pesticide Waste Is Time Bomb in Poor Countries." *Health & Medicine Week,* October 4, 2004, p. 486.

25. "Parental Exposure to Pesticides Is Not Likely Linked to Childhood Brain Cancer." *Health and Medicine Week,* August 18, 2003, p. 64.

26. "Major Developments to Improve Hearing Health Reported." *Health & Medicine Week,* January 19, 2004, p. 543.

27. Voelker, Rebecca. "Access to Clean Water and Sanitation Pose 21st Century Challenge for Millions." *Journal of the American Medical Association,* Vol. 292, No. 3, July 21, 2004, p. 318.

28. "Are Cell Phones Safe? Research Hasn't Proved Any Hazards, But There May Be Cause for Concern." *Consumer Reports,* Vol. 68, No. 2, February 2003, p. 24(1).

Glossary

abscess A localized accumulation of pus and disintegrating tissue.

abstinence Voluntary refrainment from sexual intercourse.

acquired immune deficiency syndrome (AIDS) The final stages of HIV infection, characterized by a variety of severe illnesses and decreased levels of certain immune cells.

actin Thin myofilaments.

active stretching A technique that involves stretching a muscle by contracting the opposing muscle.

acupuncture A Chinese medical practice of puncturing the body with needles inserted at specific points to relieve pain or cure disease.

acute injuries Physical injuries, such as sprains, bruises, and pulled muscles, which result from sudden traumas, such as falls or collisions.

adaptive response The body's attempt to reestablish homeostasis or stability.

addiction A behavioral pattern characterized by compulsion, loss of control, and continued repetition of a behavior or activity in spite of adverse consequences.

aerobic exercise Physical activity in which sufficient or excess oxygen is continually supplied to the body.

affirmation A single positive sentence used as a tool for behavior change.

aging The characteristic pattern of normal life changes that occur as humans grow older.

alcohol abuse Continued use of alcohol despite awareness of social, occupational, psychological, or physical problems related to its use, or use of alcohol in dangerous ways or situations, such as before driving.

alcohol dependence Development of a strong craving for alcohol due to the pleasurable feelings or relief of stress or anxiety produced by drinking.

alcoholism A chronic, progressive, potentially fatal disease characterized by impaired control of drinking, a preoccupation with alcohol, continued use of alcohol despite adverse consequences, and distorted thinking, most notably denial.

altruism Acts of helping or giving to others without thought of self-benefit.

alveoli Tiny air sacs in the lungs where gas exchange takes place.

Alzheimer's disease A progressive deterioration of intellectual powers due to physiological changes within the brain; symptoms include diminishing ability to concentrate and reason, disorientation, depression, apathy, and paranoia.

amino acids Organic compounds containing nitrogen, carbon, hydrogen, and oxygen; the essential building blocks of proteins.

amphetamine Any of a class of stimulants that trigger the release of epinephrine, which stimulates the central nervous system; users experience a state of hyper-alertness and energy, followed by a crash as the drug wears off.

anaerobic exercise Physical activity in which the body develops an oxygen deficit.

angina pectoris A severe, suffocating chest pain caused by a brief lack of oxygen to the heart.

angioplasty Surgical repair of an obstructed artery by passing a balloon catheter through the blood vessel to the area of disease and then inflating the catheter to compress the plaque against the vessel wall.

anorexia nervosa A psychological disorder in which refusal to eat and/or an extreme loss of appetite leads to malnutrition, severe weight loss, and possibly death.

antibiotics Substances produced by microorganisms, or synthetic agents, that are toxic to other types of microorganisms; in dilute solutions, used to treat infectious diseases.

antioxidants Substances that prevent the damaging effects of oxidation in cells.

antiviral drug A substance that decreases the severity and duration of a viral infection if taken prior to or soon after onset of the infection.

anxiety A feeling of apprehension and dread, with or without a known cause; may range from mild to severe and may be accompanied by physical symptoms.

appetite A desire for food, stimulated by anticipated hunger, physiological changes within the brain and body, the availability of

food, and other environmental and psychological factors.

arteries The network of blood vessels that carry blood from the heart throughout the body.

arteriosclerosis Any of a number of chronic diseases characterized by degeneration of the arteries and hardening and thickening of arterial walls.

assertive Behaving in a confident manner to make your needs and desires clear to others in a nonhostile way.

atherosclerosis A form of arteriosclerosis in which fatty substances (plaque) are deposited on the inner walls of arteries.

atrium (plural **atria**) Either of the two upper chambers of the heart, which receive blood from the veins.

atrophy A decrease in the size of muscles because of inactivity.

autonomy The ability to draw on internal resources; independence from familial and societal influences.

Ayurveda A traditional Indian medical treatment involving meditation, exercise, herbal medications, and nutrition.

bacteria (singular, **bacterium**) One-celled microscopic organisms; the most plentiful pathogens.

ballistic stretching Rapid bouncing movements.

barbiturates Antianxiety drugs that depress the central nervous system, reduce activity and induce relaxation, drowsiness, or sleep; often prescribed to relieve tension and treat epileptic seizures or as a general anesthetic.

basal metabolic rate (BMR) The number of calories required to sustain the body at rest.

benzodiazepines Antianxiety drugs that depress the central nervous system, reduce activity, and induce relaxation, drowsiness, or sleep; often prescribed to relieve tension, muscular strain, sleep problems, anxiety, and panic attacks; also used as an anesthetic and in the treatment of alcohol withdrawal.

bidis Skinny, sweet-flavored cigarettes.

binge drinking For a man, having five or more alcoholic drinks at a single sitting; for a woman, having four drinks or more at a single sitting.

binge eating The rapid consumption of an abnormally large amount of food in a relatively short time.

biofeedback A technique of becoming aware, with the aid of external monitoring devices, of internal physiological activities in order to develop the capability of altering them.

blood-alcohol concentration (BAC) The amount of alcohol in the blood, expressed as a percentage.

body composition The relative amounts of fat and lean tissue (bone, muscle, organs, water) in the body.

body mass index (BMI) A mathematical formula that correlates with body fat; the ratio of weight to height squared.

botulism Possibly fatal food poisoning caused by a type of bacterium that grows and produces its toxin in the absence of air and is found in improperly canned food.

bulimia nervosa Episodic binge eating, often followed by forced vomiting or laxative abuse, and accompanied by a persistent preoccupation with body shape and weight.

calorie The amount of energy required to raise the temperature of 1 gram of water by 1 degree Celsius. In everyday usage related to the energy content of foods and the energy expended in activities, a calorie is actually the equivalent of a thousand such calories, or a kilocalorie.

capillary A minute blood vessel that connects an artery to a vein.

carbohydrates Organic compounds, such as starches, sugars, and glycogen, that are composed of carbon, hydrogen, and oxygen, and are sources of bodily energy.

carcinogen A substance that produces cancerous cells or enhances their development and growth.

cardiac muscle Heart muscle.

cardiopulmonary resuscitation (CPR) A method of artificial stimulation of the heart and lungs; a combination of mouth-to-mouth breathing and chest compression.

cardiorespiratory endurance Ability of the heart, lungs, and circulatory system to deliver oxygen to muscles working rhythmically over an extended period of time.

cardiorespiratory fitness The ability of the heart and blood vessels to circulate blood through the body efficiently.

cardiovascular system The heart and blood vessels; responsible for distributing nutrients and oxygen to the cells within the body and removing carbon dioxide and other waste materials from the body.

celibacy Abstention from sexual activity; can be partial or complete, permanent or temporary.

chanchroid A soft, painful sore or localized infection usually acquired through sexual contact.

chiropractic A method of treating disease, primarily through manipulating the bones and joints to restore normal nerve function.

chlamydia A sexually transmitted disease caused by the bacterium *Chlamydia trachomatis,* often asymptomatic in women but sometimes characterized by urinary pain; if undetected and untreated, may result in pelvic inflammatory disease (PID).

chlorinated hydrocarbons Highly toxic pesticides, such as DDT and chlordane, that are extremely resistant to breakdown; may cause cancer, birth defects, neurological disorders, and damage to wildlife and the environment.

cholesterol An organic substance found in animal fats; linked to cardiovascular disease, particularly atherosclerosis.

club drugs Illegally manufactured psychoactive drugs that have dangerous physical and psychological effects.

cocaine A white crystalline powder extracted from the leaves of the coca plant that stimulates the central nervous system and produces a brief period of euphoria followed by a depression.

collagen White fibers that provide support and structure in the connective tissue.

complementary and alternative medicine (CAM) A term used to apply to all healthcare approaches, practices, and treatments not widely taught in medical schools, not generally used in hospitals, and not usually reimbursed by medical insurance companies.

complementary proteins Incomplete proteins that, when combined, provide all the amino acids essential for protein synthesis.

complete proteins Proteins that contain all the amino acids needed by the body for growth and maintenance.

complex carbohydrates Starches, including cereals, fruits, and vegetables.

concentric contraction A type of isotonic contraction in which the muscle becomes shorter and applies force.

conditioning The gradual building up of the body to enhance one or more of the three main components of physical fitness: flexibility, cardiorespiratory or aerobic fitness, and muscular strength and endurance.

condom A latex sheath worn over the penis during sexual acts to prevent conception and/or the transmission of disease; some condoms contain a spermicidal lubricant.

cross-training Alternating two or more different types of fitness activities.

culture The set of shared attitudes, values, goals, and practices of a group that are internalized by an individual within the group.

daily values (DV) Reference values developed by the FDA specifically for use on food labels.

decibel (dB) A unit for measuring the intensity of sounds.

defense mechanism A psychological process that alleviates anxiety and eliminates mental conflict; includes denial, displacement, projection, rationalization, reaction formation, and repression.

delayed-onset muscle soreness (DOMS) The pain and soreness felt a day or two after a workout.

deleriants Chemicals, such as solvents, aerosols, glue, cleaning fluids, petroleum products, and some anesthetics, that produce vapors with psychoactive effects when inhaled.

dementia Deterioration of mental capability.

depression In general, feelings of unhappiness and despair; as a mental illness, also characterized by an inability to function normally.

diabetes mellitus A disease in which the inadequate production of insulin leads to failure of the body tissues to break down carbohydrates at a normal rate.

diastole The period between contractions in the cardiac cycle, during which the heart relaxes and dilates as it fills with blood.

diastolic blood pressure Lowest blood pressure between contractions of the heart.

dietary fiber The nondigestible form of carbohydrates found in plant foods, such as leaves, stems, skins, seeds, and hulls.

diminishing returns principle The principle that indicates that as you gain benefits as the result of physical activity, additional benefits will be more difficult to achieve.

distress A negative stress that may result in illness.

drug Any substance, other than food, that affects bodily functions and structures when taken into the body.

drug abuse The excessive use of a drug in a manner inconsistent with accepted medical practice.

drug misuse The use of a drug for a purpose (or person) other than that for which it was medically intended.

dual-energy X-ray absorptiometry (DXA) An assessment method using X rays to quantify the skeletal and soft tissue components of body mass; provides a direct measurement of body composition.

dynamic flexibility The ability to move a joint quickly and fluidly through its entire range of motion with little resistance.

dynamic training A training approach that focuses on muscle contractions that produce movement.

eating disorders Bizarre, often dangerous patterns of food consumption, including anorexia nervosa and bulimia nervosa.

eccentric contraction A type of isotonic contraction in which the muscle lengthens as it contracts.

ecosystem A community of organisms sharing a physical and chemical environment and interacting with each other.

ecstasy (MDMA) A synthetic compound, also known as methylenedioxymethamphetamine, that is similar in structure to methamphetamine and has both stimulant and hallucinogenic effects.

edema An excessive accumulation of fluid in connective tissue, causing swelling and pain.

elastin Yellow fibers that make the connective tissue elastic and flexible.

electromagnetic fields (EMFs) The invisible electric and magnetic fields generated by an electrically charged conductor.

emotional wellness The ability to express and acknowledge one's feelings and moods.

enabling factors The skills, resources, and physical and mental capabilities that shape our behavior.

endorphins Mood-elevating, pain-killing chemicals produced by the brain.

endothelium The specialized layer of tissue inside blood vessels.

environmental tobacco smoke Secondhand cigarette smoke; the third leading preventable cause of death.

essential nutrients Nutrients that the body cannot manufacture for itself and must obtain from food.

ethyl alcohol The intoxicating agent in alcoholic beverages; also called ethanol.

eustress Positive stress, which stimulates a person to function properly.

fast-twitch fibers Muscle fibers that contract rapidly and forcefully but fatigue quickly.

fellatio Sexual stimulation of a man's genitals by means of oral manipulation.

fetal alcohol effects (FAE) Milder forms of FAS, including low birthweight, irritability as newborns, and permanent mental impairment as a result of the mother's alcohol consumption during pregnancy.

fetal alcohol syndrome (FAS) A cluster of physical and mental defects in the newborn, including low birthweight, smaller-than-normal head circumference, intrauterine growth retardation, and permanent mental impairment caused by the mother's alcohol consumption during pregnancy.

FITT A formula that describes the frequency, intensity, type, and length of time for physical activity.

flexibility The range of motion allowed by one's joints; determined by the length of muscles, tendons, and ligaments attached to the joints.

folic acid A form of folate (water soluble B vitamin) used in vitamin supplements and fortified foods.

frostbite The freezing or partial freezing of skin and tissue just below the skin or even muscle and bone; more severe than frostnip.

frostnip Sudden blanching or lightening of the skin on hands, feet, and face, resulting from exposure to high wind speeds and low temperatures.

functional fiber Isolated, nondigestible carbohydrates with beneficial effects in humans.

fungi (singular, **fungus**) Organisms that reproduce by means of spores.

general adaptation syndrome (GAS) The sequenced physiological response to a stressful situation; consists of three stages: alarm, resistance, and exhaustion.

gingivitis Inflammation of the gums.

gonorrhea A sexually transmitted disease caused by the bacterium *Neisseria gonorrhoeae;* symptoms include discharge from the penis; women are generally asymptomatic.

guided imagery An approach to stress control, self-healing, or motivating life changes by means of visualizing oneself in a state of calmness, wellness, or change.

gum disease Inflammation of the gum and bones that hold teeth in place.

hallucinogen A drug that causes hallucinations.

hashish A concentrated form of a drug, derived from the cannabis plant, containing the psychoactive ingredient TCH, which causes a sense of euphoria when inhaled or eaten.

heart rate The number of heartbeats per minute.

heat cramps Painful muscle spasms caused by vigorous exercise accompanied by heavy sweating in the heat.

heat exhaustion Faintness, rapid heart beat, low blood pressure, an ashen appearance, cold and clammy skin, and nausea, resulting from prolonged sweating with inadequate fluid replacement.

heat stress Physical response to prolonged exposure to high temperature; occurs simultaneously with or after heat cramps.

heat stroke A medical emergency consisting of a fever of at least 105°F, hot dry skin, rapid heartbeat, rapid and shallow breathing, and elevated or lowered blood pressure caused by the breakdown of the body's cooling mechanism.

helminth A parasitic roundworm or flatworm.

hepatitis An inflammation and/or infection of the liver caused by a virus, often accompanied by jaundice.

herbal medicine An ancient form of medical treatment using substances derived from trees, flowers, ferns, seaweeds, and lichens.

herpes simplex A condition caused by one of the herpes viruses and characterized by lesions of the skin or mucous membranes; herpes virus type 2 is sexually transmitted and causes genital blisters or sores.

holistic An approach to medicine that takes into account body, mind, emotions, and spirit.

homeopathy A system of medical practice that treats a disease by administering dosages of substances that would in healthy persons produce symptoms similar to those of the disease.

homeostasis The body's natural state of balance or stability.

host A person or population that contracts one or more pathogenic agents in an environment.

human immunodeficiency virus (HIV) A type of virus that causes a spectrum of health problems, ranging from a symptomless infection to changes in the immune system, to the development of life-threatening diseases because of impaired immunity.

human papilloma virus (HPV) A pathogen that causes genital warts and increases the risk of cervical cancer.

hunger The physiological drive to consume food.

hydrostatic weighing Weighing a person in water to distinguish buoyant fat from denser muscle.

hypertension High blood pressure occurring when the blood exerts excessive pressure against the arterial walls.

hypertrophy An increase in the size of muscles brought on by working the muscles harder than normal.

hypothermia An abnormally low body temperature; if not treated appropriately, coma or death could result.

immune deficiency Partial or complete inability of the immune system to respond to pathogens.

immunity Protection from infectious diseases.

incomplete proteins Proteins that lack one or more of the amino acids essential for protein synthesis.

infiltration A gradual penetration or invasion.

inflammation A localized response by the body to tissue injury, characterized by swelling and the dilation of the blood vessels.

influenza Any of a type of fairly common, highly contagious viral diseases.

inhalants Substances that produce vapors having psychoactive effects when sniffed.

integrative medicine An approach that combines traditional medicine with alternative/complementary therapies.

intoxication Maladaptive behavioral, psychological, and physiologic changes that occur as a result of substance abuse.

irradiation Exposure to or treatment by some form of radiation.

isokinetic contraction A constant-speed contraction; exercise with specialized equipment that provides resistance equal to the force applied by the user throughout the entire range of motion.

isometric contraction A contraction in which muscles increase their tension without shortening in length, such as when pushing an immovable object.

isotonic contraction A construction involving movement where muscle tension remains the same, such as weight lifting or calisthenics.

joints The point or structure between two or more bones where movement occurs.

lactic acid A byproduct of the breakdown of glucose that causes muscle fatigue.

lacto-vegetarians People who eat dairy products as well as fruits and vegetables (but not meat, poultry, or fish).

lipoprotein A compound in blood that is made up of proteins and fat; a high-density lipoprotein (HDL) picks up excess cholesterol in the blood; a low-density lipoprotein (LDL) carries more cholesterol and deposits it on the walls of arteries.

listeria A bacterium commonly found in deli meats, hot dogs, and soft cheeses that can cause an infection called listeriosis.

locus of control An individual's belief about the source of power and influence over his or her life.

lumpectomy The surgical removal of a breast tumor and its surrounding tissue.

Lyme disease A disease caused by a bacterium carried by a tick; it may cause heart arrhythmias, neurological problems, and arthritis symptoms.

lymph nodes Small tissue masses in which some immune cells are stored.

macronutrients Nutrients required by the human body in the greatest amounts, including water, carbohydrates, proteins, and fats.

mainstream smoke The smoke inhaled directly by smoking a cigarette.

male pattern baldness The loss of hair at the vertex, or top, of the head.

mammography A diagnostic X-ray exam used to detect breast cancer.

marijuana The drug derived from the cannabis plant, containing the psychoactive ingredient THC, which causes a mild sense of euphoria when inhaled or eaten.

massage therapy A therapeutic method of using the hands to rub, stroke, or knead the body to produce positive effects on an individual's health and well-being.

mastectomy The surgical removal of an entire breast.

maximal oxygen uptake (VO₂ max) The greatest amount of oxygen a person can use in maximal exercise.

meditation A group of approaches that use quiet sitting, breathing techniques, and/or chanting to relax, improve concentration, and become attuned to one's inner self.

meningitis An extremely serious, potentially fatal illness that attacks the membranes around the brain and spinal cord; caused by the bacterium *Neisseria meningitis*.

mental wellness The ability to perceive reality as it is, to respond to its challenges, and to develop rational strategies for living.

metabolic syndrome A cluster of disorders of the body's metabolism that make diabetes, heart disease, or stroke more likely.

metastasize To spread to other parts of the body via the bloodstream or lymphatic system.

micronutrients Vitamins and minerals needed by the body in very small amounts.

mindfulness A method of stress reduction that involves experiencing the physical and mental sensations of the present moment.

minerals Naturally occurring inorganic substances, small amounts of some being essential in metabolism and nutrition.

mononucleosis An infectious viral disease characterized by an excess of white blood cells in the blood, fever, bodily discomfort, a sore throat, and kidney and liver complications.

mood A sustained emotional state that colors one's view of the world for hours or days.

muscle fibers The individual cells in a muscle.

muscular endurance The ability to perform muscular effort repeatedly over time.

muscular strength The maximum amount of force a muscle can produce in a single effort.

mutagen An agent that causes alterations in the genetic material of living cells.

mutation A change in the genetic material of a cell or cells that is brought about by radiation, chemicals, or natural causes.

myocardial infarction (MI) A condition characterized by the dying of tissue areas in the myocardium, caused by interruption of the blood supply to those areas; the medical name for a heart attack.

myocardium The heart muscle.

myofibrils Long threadlike structures found within muscle fiber.

myosin Thick myofilaments that, together with actin, allow for muscle contraction.

naturopathy An alternative system of treatment of disease that emphasizes the use of natural remedies such as sun, water, heat, and air. Therapies may include dietary changes, steam baths, and exercise.

neoplasm Any tumor, whether benign or malignant.

nonexercise activity thermogenesis (NEAT) Nonvolitional movement that can be an effective way of burning calories.

nongonococcal urethritis (NGU) Inflammation of the urethra caused by organisms other than the gonococcus bacterium.

nonopioids Chemically synthesized drugs that have sleep-inducing and pain-relieving properties similar to those of opium and its derivatives.

nonvolitional sex Sexual behavior that violates a person's right to choose when and with whom to have sex and what sexual behaviors to engage in.

norms The unwritten rules regarding behavior and conduct expected or accepted by a group.

nutrition The science devoted to the study of dietary needs for food and the effects of food on organisms.

obesity The excessive accumulation of fat in the body; a condition of having a BMI of 30 or above.

opioids Drugs that have sleep-inducing and pain-relieving properties, including opium and its derivatives and nonopioid, synthetic drugs.

optimism The tendency to seek out, remember, and expect pleasurable experiences.

organic Term designating food produced with, or production based on the use of, fertilizer originating from plants or animals, without the use of pesticides or chemically formulated fertilizers.

organic phosphates Toxic pesticides that may cause cancer, birth defects, neurological disorders, and damage to wildlife and the environment.

osteoporosis A condition common in older people in which the bones become increasingly soft and porous, making them susceptible to injury.

over-the-counter (OTC) drugs Medications that can be obtained legally without a prescription from a medical professional.

overload principle Placing a greater stress or demand on the body than it is normally accustomed to handling.

overloading Method of physical training involving increasing the number of repetitions or the amount of resistance gradually to work the muscle to temporary fatigue.

overtraining Working muscles too intensely or too frequently, resulting in persistent muscle soreness, injuries, unintended weight loss, nervousness, and an inability to relax.

overuse injuries Physical injuries to joints or muscles, such as strains, fractures, and tendinitis, which result from overdoing a repetitive activity.

overweight A condition of having a BMI between 25.0 and 29.9.

ovo-lacto-vegetarians People who eat eggs, dairy products, and fruits and vegetables (but not meat, poultry, or fish).

oxygen uptake (VO₂) The amount of oxygen the body uses per minute (measured in liters per minute).

passive stretching A stretching technique in which an external force or resistance (your body, a partner, gravity, or a weight) helps the joints move through their range of motion.

pathogen A microorganism that produces disease.

PCP (phencyclidine) A synthetic psychoactive substance that produces effects similar to other psychoactive drugs when swallowed, smoked, sniffed, or injected but may also trigger unpredictable behavioral changes.

pelvic inflammatory disease (PID) An inflammation of the internal female genital tract, characterized by abdominal pain, fever, and tenderness of the cervix.

periodontitis Severe gum disease in which the tooth root becomes infected.

physical dependence The physiological attachment to, and need for, a drug.

physical fitness The ability to respond to routine physical demands with enough reserve energy to cope with a sudden challenge.

phytochemicals Chemicals such as indoles, coumarins, and capsaicin, which exist naturally in plants and have disease-fighting properties.

plaque The sludgelike substance that builds up on the inner walls of arteries; the sticky film of bacteria that forms on teeth.

pollutant A substance or agent in the environment, usually the by-product of human industry or activity, that is injurious to human, animal, or plant life.

pollution The presence of pollutants in the environment.

predisposing factors The beliefs, values, attitudes, knowledge, and perceptions that influence our behavior.

prehypertension A condition of slightly elevated blood pressure, which is likely to worsen in time.

progressive overloading Gradually increasing physical challenges once the body adapts to the stress placed upon it to produce maximum benefits.

progressive relaxation A method of reducing muscle tension by contracting then relaxing, certain areas of the body.

proof The alcoholic strength of a distilled spirit, expressed as twice the percentage of alcohol present.

proprioceptive neuromuscular facilitation (PNF) A technique that involves fatiguing a muscle or muscle group through contracting and then stretching the muscle.

protein A substance that is basically a compound of amino acids; one of the essential nutrients.

protozoa Microscopic animals made up of one cell or a group of similar cells.

psychoactive Mood-altering.

psychological dependence The emotional or mental attachment to the use of a drug.

psychotropic Mind-affecting.

range of motion The fullest extent of possible movement in a particular joint.

rape Sexual penetration of a female or a male by means of intimidation, force, or fraud.

Rating of Perceived Exertion (RPE) A self-assessment scale that rates symptoms of breathlessness and fatigue.

reflexology A treatment based on the theory that massaging certain points on the foot or hand relieves stress or pain in corresponding parts of the body.

reinforcement Reward or punishment for a behavior that will increase or decrease one's likelihood of repeating the behavior.

reinforcing factors Rewards, encouragement, and recognition that influence our behavior in the short run.

relative risk The risk of developing cancer in persons with a certain exposure or trait compared to the risk in persons who do not have the same exposure or trait.

rep (or **repetition**) In weight training, a single performance of a movement or exercise.

1 repetition maximum (1RM) The maximum amount of weight a person can lift one time.

resistance The amount of weight that is lifted.

respiratory system The system of organs, consisting in particular of the lungs and air passages, that supply oxygen to the blood and expel waste gases.

resting heart rate The number of heartbeats per minute during inactivity.

sarcomere The basic contractile unit of muscle tissue.

satiety A feeling of fullness after eating.

saturated fat A chemical term indicating that a fat molecule contains as many hydrogen atoms as its carbon skeleton can hold. These fats are normally solid at room temperature.

self-actualization A state of wellness and fulfillment that can be achieved once certain human needs are satisfied; living to one's full potential.

self-efficacy Belief in one's ability to accomplish a goal or change a behavior.

self-esteem Confidence and satisfaction in oneself.

self-talk Repetition of positive messages about one's self-worth to learn more optimistic patterns of thought, feeling, and behavior.

sets In weight training, the number of repetitions of the same movement or exercise.

sex Maleness or femaleness, resulting from genetic, structural, and functional factors.

sexual coercion Sexual activity forced upon a person by the exertion of psychological pressure by another person.

sexually transmitted infections (STIs) Any of a number of diseases that are acquired through sexual contact.

sidestream smoke The smoke emitted by a burning cigarette and breathed by everyone in a closed room, including the smoker; contains more tar and nicotine than mainstream smoke.

simple carbohydrates Sugars; like all carbohydrates, they provide the body with glucose.

skeletal muscles Muscles attached to the bones or skeleton.

skinfold measurements A popular method of estimating body composition; taken by pinching the skin and then using calipers to measure the thickness of the two layers of skin and the underlying subcutaneous fat.

sliding filament theory A theory of muscle contraction describing how the sliding of thin filaments of actin along thick filaments of myosin generates the force causing contraction.

slow-twitch fibers Muscle fibers that contract slowly and are resistant to fatigue.

smog A grayish or brownish fog caused by the presence of smoke and/or chemical pollutants in the air.

smooth muscle Muscle that primarily lines hollow internal structures such as the stomach and arteries.

social isolation A feeling of unconnectedness with others caused by and reinforced by infrequency of social contacts.

social phobia A severe form of social anxiety marked by extreme fears and avoidance of social situations.

specificity principle Each part of the body adapts to a particular type and amount of stress placed upon it.

spiritual wellness The ability to identify one's basic purpose in life and to achieve one's full potential; the sense of connectedness to a greater power.

static flexibility The ability to assume and maintain an extended position at one end point in a joint's range of motion.

static stretching A gradual stretch held for a short time of 10 to 30 seconds.

static training A training approach that focuses on isometric contractions that produce little or no movement.

stimulant An agent, such as a drug, that temporarily relieves drowsiness, helps in the performance of repetitive tasks, and improves capacity for work.

stress The nonspecific response of the body to any demands made upon it; may be characterized by muscle tension and acute anxiety or may be a positive force for action.

stressor Specific or nonspecific agents or situations that cause the stress response in a body.

stroke A cerebrovascular event in which the blood supply to a portion of the brain is blocked.

stroke volume The amount of blood pumped by the heart in one contraction.

syphilis A sexually transmitted disease caused by the bacterium *Treponema pallidum* and characterized by early sores, a latent period, and a final period of life-threatening symptoms including brain damage and heart failure.

systemic disease A pathologic condition that spreads throughout the body.

systole The contraction phase of the cardiac cycle.

systolic blood pressure Highest blood pressure when the heart contracts.

target heart rate Sixty to eighty-five percent of the maximum heart rate; the heart rate at which one derives maximum cardiovascular benefit from aerobic exercise.

tendons The connective tissues that attach muscle to bone.

teratogen Any agent that causes spontaneous abortion, defects, or malformations in a fetus.

trans-fat Fats formed when liquid vegetable oils are processed to make table spreads or cooking fats and also found in dairy and beef products; considered to be especially dangerous dietary fats.

transient ischemic attack (TIA) A cerebrovascular event in which the blood supply to a portion of the brain is blocked temporarily; repeated attacks are predictors of more severe strokes.

transtheoretical model of change A model of behavioral change that focuses on the individual's decision making; it states that an individual progresses through a sequence of six stages as he or she makes a change in behavior.

triglyceride A blood fat that flows through the blood after meals and is linked to increased risk of coronary artery disease.

unsaturated fat A chemical term indicating that a fat molecule contains fewer hydrogen atoms than its carbon skeleton can hold. These fats are normally liquid at room temperature.

values The criteria by which one makes choices about one's thoughts and actions and goals and ideals.

vector A biological or physical vehicle that carries the agent of infection to the host.

vegans People who eat only plant foods.

veins Vessels that return blood to the heart.

ventricle Either of the two lower chambers of the heart, which pump blood out of the heart and into the arteries.

virus A submicroscopic infectious agent; the most primitive form of life.

visualization An approach to stress control, self-healing, or motivating life changes by means of guided, or directed, imagery.

vital signs Measurements of physiological functioning, specifically, temperature, blood pressure, pulse rate, and respiration rate.

vitamins Organic substances that are needed in very small amounts by the body and carry out a variety of functions in metabolism and nutrition.

waist-hip ratio The proportion of one's waist circumference to one's hip circumference.

wellness A state of complete well-being, including physical, psychological, spiritual, social, intellectual, and environmental components.

withdrawal Development of symptoms that cause significant psychological and physical distress when an individual reduces or stops drug use.

Photo Credits

Index